Human Memory

Human Memory, 4th edition, provides a comprehensive overview of research and theory on human memory. Written in an engaging style, the book is divided into three sections, providing an accessible introduction to the application and assessment of memory theory. Beginning with the history of memory, the first section explores basic methodology and neuroscience. The second section examines the key topics of memory such as the sensory registers, mechanisms of forgetting and short-term, nondeclarative, episodic, and semantic memory. The third section focuses on specialist topics such as amnesia, memory for space and time, autobiographical memory, memory and reality, memory and the law, metamemory and formal models of memory. Instructors could pick and chose which of these chapters best fit the goals of their course.

New to this edition:

- More prominent discussion of neuroscience findings.
- Coverage of a wider range of neuroscientific techniques.
- Greater emphasis on memory changes over time.
- New explanation of how to calculate a wider range of signal detection measures.
- Additional content on a wide range of topics including the mirror effect, sleep-related memory processes, vicarious autobiographical memories, inter-generational memory transmission, the impact of lying on memory, eyewitness collaboration, and aging and spatial memory.
- Expanded coverage of areas including theories of hypermnesia, chunking, serial order memory, prospective memory, threshold models, and eyewitness line-up identification.
- Updated companion resources, including PowerPoint slides and exam questions.

The book highlights the application of memory theory and findings to everyday experience, presents in-depth explorations of studies, and provides opportunities for students to explore the assessment of memory in more laboratory-based settings. Packed full of student-friendly pedagogy including study questions, Stop and Review and Try It Out sections, Study In Depth text boxes, and more, *Human Memory*, 4th edition, is an essential companion for all students of human memory.

Gabriel A. Radvansky received his BA from Cleveland State University under the supervision of Mark Ashcraft and Ben Wallace, and his MA and PhD from Michigan State University in 1992 under the supervision of Rose T. Zacks. He has been a faculty member in the Department of Psychology at the University of Notre Dame since 1993. He is an expert in human memory with over 100 publications. He has served as associated editor for the journals *Memory & Cognition*, the *Quarterly Journal of Experimental Psychology*, and *Collabra*.

"*Human Memory* has an unconventional and appealing organization. It covers critical topics that are omitted from most textbooks and weaves historical and modern research together into a format that will serve well for both beginning and advanced study of the topic. Most importantly, it covers both the theoretical and the applied side of human memory research, making it a valuable resource for understanding how and where the formal study of human memory fits into the social sciences more broadly."

– Aaron S. Benjamin, University of Illinois at Urbana-Champaign, U.S.A.

"This is an impressive text: Comprehensive, well-written and sure to be a winner. Radvansky provides a great blend of classic and contemporary research and the pedagogical features built into the book will be helpful for students."

– Henry L. Roediger III, Washington University in St. Louis, U.S.A.

Human Memory

Fourth Edition

Gabriel A. Radvansky

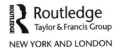
Routledge
Taylor & Francis Group

NEW YORK AND LONDON

Fourth edition published 2021
by Routledge
52 Vanderbilt Avenue, New York, NY 10017

and by Routledge
2 Park Square, Milton Park, Abingdon, Oxon, OX14 4RN

Routledge is an imprint of the Taylor & Francis Group, an informa business

First edition published by Willan 2008
Second edition published by Routledge 2009

Library of Congress Cataloging-in-Publication Data
A catalog record for this book has been requested

ISBN: 978-0-367-25291-5 (hbk)
ISBN: 978-0-367-25292-2 (pbk)
ISBN: 978-0-429-28703-9 (ebk)

Typeset in Stone Serif
by Apex CoVantage, LLC

Access the the companion website: www.routledge.com/cw/radvansky

For Amy

CONTENTS

FIGURES

TABLES

PREFACE

This book is a student's guide to human memory, its properties, theories about how memory works, and how an understanding of memory can give us a better idea of who we are and why we do what we do. Although I have tried to provide a reasonably comprehensive survey of many issues of the modern study of human memory, my main concern is the audience. Most college classes on human memory consist largely of psychology majors who are planning to go on to some field of psychology other than memory research, such as clinical or social psychology. Many others plan to go on to nonpsychology fields, such as medical or law school. Other students are not psychology majors, but they are taking the class because they think human memory would be something interesting to learn about (and they are right). Only a small minority of students plan to do research on memory. Thus, I have tried to write this book with the goals, interests, and backgrounds of the majority of the students in mind, while still providing enough information and detail to satisfy the "memory" student. I have taken several steps along these lines.

First, in addition to foundational topics that are necessary for a basic understanding of how memory works, I have tried to focus on topics that will be helpful and useful whatever the student's goal. I have tried to avoid going into detail about the minutiae of various topics and have instead focused on the big picture. However, there may be cases where I do present several different experimental outcomes or theoretical positions. I have done this to provide the student with a sense of the difficulty and complexity of studying human memory, and the degree of careful and rigorous thinking and action that are needed to get at the truth of the human condition.

I mention several times that a study was conducted using students from this college or that university so readers can associate with the information presented in this book. The participants in these studies are the same sort of people sitting in your classroom. I have tried to avoid language that would alienate a student, which can put up a barrier between the student and the material.

I have also tried to present the materials about memory from several different perspectives. Some of these come from experimental research on memory itself, such as perspectives from behavioral data, neurological data, and computational modeling. In addition, I present details about how various topics relate to work outside the realm of memory research, such as work in social, clinical, or developmental psychology, or even in fields as far-flung as law enforcement.

A quick survey of this book will reveal that it has a lot of chapters. Perhaps too many for a single class term. That is O.K. That was the intent. The field of memory is broad, and different classes place different emphases on different topics.

I would expect that most classes would assign and use Chapters 1–9 of this book. This is the background and core knowledge that one needs to understand human memory. Then, I would expect that the instructor would select out those choices from Chapters 10–18 that best suit their class and its goals. Of course, if you want to assign all 18 chapters, go for it!

I have also sprinkled throughout the book several boxes to highlight different things. These boxes serve to accomplish three goals. First, some of these are Try It Out boxes which provide descriptions of how to do studies that can illustrate salient findings in memory research. These are helpful for any students who might have a lab section associated with their course. Even if not, they give the student a better idea of how to set up and test memory, and the scientific enterprise more generally. Second, some of these are Study In Depth boxes which proved detailed accounts of actual studies in memory research, how they were set up, who was involved, the methods that were used, and the results that were found. These provide an opportunity for students to better grasp the scientific method as it is applied to the study of memory. This includes the identification of a problem, the derivation of the materials and the experimental design, the manipulation of various independent variables, the use of an appropriate dependent variable, the data collected, and how it was interpreted. Finally, some of these are Improve Your Memory boxes which illustrate, in a more direct way, how the basic findings and principles of research psychology can be extended to real life. Research studies in human memory can often seem artificial and so strongly laboratory-bound that it is hard for people who are not experts in the area to see what the value of this work may be to the bigger picture, and their own lives. I hope that these boxes go some way to achieving this aim.

Finally, I would like to thank the various people who have helped me along with the development of this book. These include Amy Radvansky for reading through every single chapter to make sure that what I wrote actually makes sense, all of my graduate students over the years, and all of my students in my learning and memory classes at Our Lady's university, and, finally, all of the assistance from people at Taylor & Francis/Routledge who worked so hard to make this book a reality. So, thanks!

PART 1

Background

CHAPTER 1

Overview and History of Memory Research

Memory is one of the most central aspects of human thought. Any question about human nature requires an understanding of memory. Memory makes us who we are, and it is one of the most intimate parts of ourselves. This may be why when we get close to someone there is a sharing of memories. Some people feel that the study of human memory is the closest one can get to a systematic study of the human soul. The aim of this book is to provide you with a survey and guide to what is known about human memory. As with most courses, there are a number of facts and ideas to learn. However, as any good instructor will tell you, the slow accumulation of facts is not the main point of course work. The primary aim is to provide you with a deeper understanding and appreciation of some aspect of the world—and, hopefully, yourself.

A SMATTERING OF DEFINITIONS

Before diving into the subject matter, we need to define how the terms *memory* and *learning* are used. Although it would seem to be straight-forward, precise, satisfactory definitions can be somewhat elusive. The primary subject of this book is, of course, memory. So what is memory? Well, the problem, and the beauty, of this term is that it has many meanings.

Memory

The word **memory** has three primary definitions (Spear & Riccio, 1994). First, memory is the location where information is kept, as in a storehouse, or memory store. Second, memory can refer to the thing that holds the contents of experience, as in a memory trace or **engram**. In this sense, each memory is a different mental representation. Finally, memory is the mental processes used to acquire (learn), store, or retrieve (remember) information. Memory processes are acts of using information to make that information available later or to bring that information back into the current stream of processing, the flow of one's thoughts.

Learning

The term **learning** refers to any change in the potential of people to alter their behavior because of the experience of regularities in the environment. Obviously, learning and memory are closely related. For something to be remembered, it must first be learned. Because of historical circumstances, these terms have become somewhat disconnected in the language of psychology. "Learning" has come to refer more to the acquisition of associations in the context of studies of conditioning often done using nonhuman animals, such as a rat learning a maze. In this book I use learning in the way it is conventionally used by people in the world, although I may occasionally use it in the more restricted sense.

METAPHORS FOR MEMORY

The human mind is the part of ourselves of which we have the most intimate awareness. Our experiences are our thoughts. That said, most of the mind's workings are not open to direct inspection. You cannot see "thinking." Moreover, every experience that the mind has changes it in some way. By reading this sentence, you are changed. These issues lead to several problems in trying to understand memory. One must be clever and develop ways to study memory (see Chapter 3). More relevant here is that there is no simple and direct way to talk about memory. Because of this, people often talk about it in indirect ways, using **metaphors for memory**. Roediger (1980) compiled a list of metaphors of memory that have been used over the centuries (see Table 1.1). Some of these express the idea that memory is a recorder of experience, such as a wax tablet, a record player, a writing pad, a tape recorder, or a video camera. Others imply that different types of memories, knowledge, and times in our lives are stored in different places. These include such

TABLE 1.1 *Various Metaphors for Memory*

Metaphor	Examples
Recorder of experience	Wax tablet, record player, writing pad, tape recorder, video camera
Storage locations	House, library, dictionary
Interconnections	Switchboard, network
Jumbled storage	Bird in an aviary, pocketbook, junk drawer, garbage can
Temporal availability	Conveyor belt
Content addressability	Lock and key, tuning fork
Forgetting of details	Leaky bucket, cow's stomach, acid bath
Reconstruction	Building an entire dinosaur skeleton from fossils
Active processing	Workbench, computer program

Source: adapted from Roediger (1980)

metaphors as memory being like a house, a library, or a dictionary. In contrast, another concept is that memories can also be intertwined and interconnected, like a switchboard or network.

Memory is not passive. Some metaphors capture its dynamic characteristics. For example, the process of retrieving one memory from the chaotic jumble that we have accumulated has led to the idea that searching for memories is like trying to catch birds in an aviary or looking for something in a junk drawer, or even a garbage can. This also goes along with the idea that memories are harder to get at over time, as if they were being led away on a conveyor belt. Often a search is required to find memories that meet a current need, like a lock and key, or a tuning fork resonating with a note. Memory retrieval is further complicated by the fact that much of what is stored is forgotten, leaving only a portion of the original, like water in a leaky bucket, or the degrading effects of a cows stomach or an acid bath. This loss of knowledge requires people to re-create the missing pieces of a memory, using a constructive process, perhaps like reconstructing a dinosaur from the fragments of bones left behind. Finally, there is the active manipulation of information, as if memory were a workbench or a computer program.

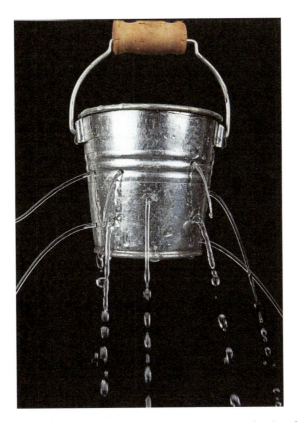

PHOTO 1.1 *According to one metaphor, memory is like a leaky bucket, being able to hold things for a period of time, but constantly losing information*

Source: ConstantinosZ/Shutterstock.com

The large number of metaphors should give you the idea that memory is a complex thing. Because of its ephemeral nature, we use our knowledge of more concrete and better understood concepts to help us make sense of it. The most dominant metaphor for memory is the literacy metaphor (Danziger, 2008). The advent of written language led people to view memories as things that are written down and put somewhere. This leads to the near universal conception of memory involving encoding, storage, and retrieval, much like writing books and storing them on a shelf. This metaphor treats memories as discrete units, like books or pages, which may or may not correspond to how the brain parses up our experiences. The dominant modern variant of this is the computer metaphor which drove the cognitive revolution of the mid-twentieth century.

Before moving on, let us look at one more metaphor that is very *inaccurate*: the idea that memory is a muscle. That is, the more you use your memory, the better it will be. In other words, simply memorizing things makes memory better. There is no evidence to support this idea. Instead, it is not how much you use your memory but how much information you have in it that is important. Memory is not like a muscle, but more like a key collection. The more keys that you have, the more locks that you can open.

Stop and Review

The terms *memory* and *learning* are used in specific ways in psychology. In general, *memory* refers to the storage and retrieval of information, and research is more likely to involve humans. *Learning* has a greater association with studies of conditioning that are more likely to involve nonhuman animals. Memory is not open to direct inspection, so we need metaphors to try to apprehend it. Each metaphor carries a degree of imprecision, but also captures some important characteristics. Various metaphors capture the idea that memory is a recorder of experience, is organized and interconnected, is jumbled and requires a search (better if you have the appropriate keys to unlock them), and actively operates on information. The most dominant metaphors are the computer and literacy metaphors which treat memories like files on a computer, or books stored on shelves.

HISTORY OF MEMORY RESEARCH

Questions about the nature of memory extend back millennia. However, the systematic, quantified, and rigorous assessment of the nature and limits of human memory did not begin until the end of the nineteenth century. In this section, we review some of the major players in the history of memory research, starting from the ancients.

Ancient and Pre-Modern Thinkers

Our understanding of memory has developed over time and has been influenced by people ranging from the great philosophers of ancient Greece to those from modern times. Keep in mind that it took a long time for people to realize that the brain was the seat of the mind, let alone memory. Previously, people thought that the mind resided in the heart (e.g., Aristotle), the ventricles (e.g., Leonardo Da Vinci), and the pineal gland (e.g., Rene Descartes) (Queenan et al., 2017). One of the first philosophers to record his thoughts on memory was Plato (ca. 428–347 B.C.). Plato was the seminal rationalist philosopher who emphasized thought as a means of understanding the world, and he deemphasized empirical observation, because it could be distorted by perception. He was a dualist who believed the mind was a different and separate entity from the body. His understanding of the mind and memory depended on understanding that the nature of innate, inborn knowledge was the foundation of human thought. Memory was the bridge between the perceptual world and the rational world of idealized abstractions (Viney & King, 1998).

Plato also provided the metaphor of memory as a wax tablet, holding the impressions of experience. This metaphor also conveys the idea that memory quality varies depending on the quality of the wax (the state of the person) and the pattern that is impressed (how well the information is encoded). The better the impression, the easier it is to retrieve it later or to compare it with other impressions. Furthermore, the wax can be altered or erased so an impression is lost, thus conveying the concept of forgetting.

Plato's most prominent pupil was Aristotle (384–322 B.C.). Like any good student, Aristotle's ideas were at odds with his mentor. Specifically, whereas Plato was a rationalist, Aristotle was an empiricist, who believed reality itself was the basis of inquiry, not an abstract, perfect realm. One of Aristotle's most important contributions was the idea that memories are composed of associations among various stimuli or experiences. As you will see, there are many theories of memory that are associationistic, such as accounts of priming, interference, or even the creation of some false memories. There is a pervasive idea that understanding how various elements are mentally linked to one another can capture the structure and processes of memory. These linking relationships often follow Aristotle's three laws of association: *similarity*, *contrast*, and *contiguity*. That is, memory associations provide links to ideas that are similar in nature, are the opposite on some critical dimension, or occurred near one another in time.

The desire to understand memory did not stop with these philosophers. This inquiry has been continuously pursued. For example, St. Augustine (354–430) spends a great deal of time in Book X of his *Confessions* on the topic of memory, covering the subject in a way that is familiar today. Some thinkers developed conceptions of memory that were often not pursued. For example, Robert Hooke (1635–1703) developed a surprisingly insightful theory of memory. However, his work was generally overshadowed by Sir Isaac Newton (1643–1727), which further hurried his ideas into obscurity (Hintzman, 2003).

Darwin and Evolution

One person who had a great impact on scientific thinking in general, including human memory, was **Charles Darwin** (1809–1882). Darwin, of course, is best known for his theory of natural selection, but his ideas influenced psychology as well (see the entire February–March 2009 issue of *American Psychologist*). The central idea is that within a species, changes occur as a result of variations that are either passed down to or removed from subsequent generations through the process of *natural selection*. Through this process species develop features or abilities that allow them to become better adapted to their environments. The same could be said of memory. Many theorists are either implicitly or explicitly guided by the idea that memory has evolved to capture many major characteristics of the environment and to perform specific tasks (Glenberg, 1997; Klein et al., 2002; Shepard, 1984). Different types of memories capture meaningfully different types of information. Also, because many species are evolving along similar trajectories, nonhuman animals can sometimes be used to study issues of memory that require more control than is either practically or ethically possible with humans.

This evolutionary aspect of memory has an influence on how people think about the mind, behavior, and genetic influences. In some sense all human behavior has a genetic component (Turkheimer, 1998). The very existence of our brains in the interiors of our skulls requires that we have human brain-building DNA, and all of our thoughts and memories depend on our biologically constructed brain. Any psychological state corresponds to a neural state. Thus, our thoughts and memories have an important genetic component. However, our DNA does not cause our brains to have the *exact* configuration that we have at the moment. This is due to our long history of experiences. Similarly, although our thoughts depend on neural hardware and processes, it does not mean that the most direct way to understand memory is by a detailed understanding of the underlying neurophysiology. That said, the more you understand the underlying neurological components and processes, the better you will understand the higher-order operations. For this reason, I include several descriptions of this influence to broaden your understanding.

Philosophy of Mind

Another important group of thinkers that has influenced ideas about memory are the British empiricists, including George Berkeley (1685–1753), John Locke (1632–1704), John Stuart Mill (1806–1873), and David Hume (1711–1776). Perhaps the most significant of their ideas involve association, a concept originally conceived by Aristotle, but worked up into grand form by the empiricists. Associationism maintains that memories are largely composed of interconnections among various simple concepts or ideas. The influence of this view is seen clearly in Chapter 18 when we discuss formal models of memory. This role of associations in memory can be easily illustrated. Things in the world are rarely treated by people as isolated entities or properties. Instead, we are often reminded of other, related experiences that included them. For example, when I eat a certain brand of cookies, I am reminded of my childhood because those were the kind of cookies my mother bought.

The empiricists' idea that memory is composed of associations has had a major influence on theories of human memory. However, the philosophical antagonists of the empiricists, the rationalists, including Rene Descartes (1596–1650) and

Immanuel Kant (1724–1804), have also had an influence. While the empiricists characterized memory as a passive collection of associations built up from the environment, the rationalists took the view that the mind is actively involved in the building of ideas. This can be seen in various theories of memory that involve the active construction and reconstruction of memories, such as those found in schema theories (see Chapter 9).

Early Memory Researchers in Psychology

Psychology as an independent discipline arose in the latter half of the nineteenth century. Since then many people have influenced memory research. While a few influential contributors are covered here, it should be kept in mind that the study of memory did not always move at a steady pace. Sometimes people develop ideas that have the potential to move the field forward but, for whatever reason, were not noticed at the time. These theories fall by the wayside, never to be heard from again. However, a few may capture the attention of future generations, who discover the earlier, neglected work. For example, in memory research, Richard Semon (1859–1918) had a theory of memory in the first decade of the twentieth century that incorporated many ideas about the process of retrieval. However, his contemporaries largely ignored these ideas, and his insights were not appreciated until 70 years later (Schacter et al., 1978). Now let us look at some people whose work had a more immediate impact.

One of the first students of memory in a scientific form was **Hermann Ebbinghaus** (1850–1909). He is best known for his 1885 publication *Memory: A Contribution to Experimental Psychology*. This work conveys detailed studies of memory, using himself as both experimenter and subject. This was a time of psychological research when the study of one's self was more acceptable. Currently, it is viewed as more objective if an experimenter tests another person who knows little to nothing about the experimental hypothesis. There are still some people who test their own memories, but these efforts are rare.

Ebbinghaus tried to study memory in what he considered as pure a form as possible, in the absence of an influence of prior knowledge. To do this, he devised test materials called **nonsense syllables**, which are consonant–vowel–consonant trigrams that have no clear meaning in the language. Examples of nonsense syllables for English are PAB, SER, and NID. Ebbinghaus created and used about 2,300 of these. These nonsense syllables have been used by researchers to study memory for decades, and they spent a great deal of effort studying them, even to the point where nonsense syllables were rated for meaningfulness (Glaze, 1928). For example, "BAL" is rated high in meaningfulness (because of "ball"), whereas "XAD" is rated very low.

Ebbinghaus memorized lists of nonsense syllables of various lengths, under various learning conditions, and for various retention intervals before he tested himself. (In some studies he did use some real words on the premise that it would have little effect.) For memory retrieval he would give himself the first nonsense syllable, and he would then try to recall the rest in the list. Using this approach, he was able to discover a wide range of basic principles of human memory that have withstood the test of time. It should be noted that although Ebbinghaus discovered these principles using nonsense syllables, these same patterns are observed with other types of information.

The **learning curve** is the idea that there is a period of time for information to be memorized. It can be affected by a few things, such as the amount of information to be learned. The learning curve is a negatively accelerated function in which most of the action occurs early on, with smaller and smaller benefits later on. So, the largest amount of information is learned in the first segment. In the second, although more is learned, the gain is not as great as during the first. A similar description applies to the third segment, and so on. Furthermore, Ebbinghaus showed that how he went about learning, in terms of the distribution of practice, influenced how well information was learned. Specifically, memory is better when practice is spread out over time, rather than lumped together—a distinction between what is known as **distributed practice** and **massed practice**.

The **forgetting curve** is the opposite of the learning curve. The forgetting curve, like the learning curve, is a negatively accelerating function. As we will see in Chapter 3, most of what is forgotten is lost during the initial period. As time goes on, forgetting continues but at a slower pace. The more time that passes, the slower the rate of forgetting.

Forgetting is the most problematic aspect of memory, and the forgetting curve suggests that we are doomed, sooner or later, to lose all our memories. However, this is not strictly the case. There is some knowledge that you have had for years and are unlikely to ever forget. This may happen by a process called **overlearning**, in which people continue to study information after perfect recall has been achieved, insulating them against forgetting. If there is substantial overlearning, forgetting may be delayed for quite some time, perhaps indefinitely.

When information has been forgotten to the point that nothing can be recalled with accuracy or reliability, it might seem that we must start at square one and repeat all of the previous effort. However, this is not the case. Ebbinghaus found that after seemingly complete forgetting, subsequent attempts to relearn the information required less effort than the first time. The difference between the amount of effort required on subsequent and initial learning attempts is called **savings**. The existence of savings is very important. It demonstrates that knowledge which appears to be lost may be residing somewhere in memory. It is no longer consciously accessible, but it can still exert an unconscious influence on behavior—in this case, serving as a platform on which to build a new set of consciously available memories.

Another major figure in the study of human memory is **Sir Fredrick Bartlett** (1886–1969). Bartlett was, in some ways, the opposite of Ebbinghaus. Whereas Ebbinghaus was interested in memory independent of prior knowledge, Bartlett was directly interested in how prior knowledge influenced memory. He found that prior knowledge profoundly influences memory. He suggested that memories are often fragmentary and incomplete. When people are remembering, they are reconstructing the information from the bits that they have along with prior knowledge about similar circumstances. This reconstruction is guided by "schemas" (an idea also used by the Gestalt psychologists). Schemas are general world knowledge structures

TRY IT OUT

One of the fundamental characteristics of memory that can be demonstrated is the forgetting curve. The aim of this Try It Out section is to assess the forgetting curve. For this task, first create some lists of 20 or so words to use as your materials. When you generate these lists, try to keep the words similar in some way, such as all being from the same class of words (e.g., nouns or verbs), being similar in length (e.g., 5–6 letters long with 2 syllables), and so on. If you want, you can try other kinds of items, such as pictures, sentences, odors, or any other kind of materials that may interest you.

When you present the materials to people, keep the presentation time constant for each item, such as 3–5 seconds. What is important here is the amount of time that has passed from when people first learn a list and when they later have their memory tested. A simple, straight-forward way to do this is to test people immediately, after 1 hour, after 1 day, and after 1 week, although you can use other retention intervals. The critical thing is to have different periods of time between when you test people.

Try to have at least 12 participants for each delay. These can either be different people for each retention interval, or the same people who are tested on different word lists at the different time delays. If you go with the second option, it is best if people memorize a different list of words for each retention delay, and even better if you separate out the lists and memory test delays. That is, do not give people all the word lists at once and then test them at different delays. This may confuse them. Instead, you might first give people the first list and then test them immediately. Then, you would give people the second list to learn and then wait an hour to test them. Then, give people the third list of words, and so on.

For the memory test, there are three ways that you can measure memory (see Chapter 3). They are recall, recognition, and savings. If all goes well, what you should find is that memory for the word lists will decline in a way that shows the greatest rate of forgetting soon after the list is encountered and a slower rate of forgetting at longer periods of time.

To assess memory using **recall**, have people report all of the items that they can remember by either writing them down on a piece of paper, typing them into a computer, saying them aloud, or whatever works best for you. To score this, count up the number of items from a given list that were correctly reported. Plot the number correct as a function of the amount of time that had elapsed.

To assess memory using **recognition**, give people a series of items and have them indicate "yes" or "no" whether each one was learned earlier. Ideally, half of the items will be ones that they studied earlier, and the other half, called lures, would be similar items that were not studied. This can be done by having people mark "yes" or "no" next to a series of items on a piece of paper, having them respond to flashcards, or showing people a series of PowerPoint slides, and so on. To score this, count up the number of studied items that were correctly identified, and subtract any incorrect items that a person erroneously said "yes" to (to correct for guessing). Finally, plot the corrected recognition scores as a function of the amount of time that had elapsed.

To assess memory using **savings**, instead of having people study each item for a set period of time, have people repeatedly go over the list until they can recall the entire set from memory. Then, after memorization, wait a given retention period, and have people relearn the list until it can be perfectly recalled again. To score this, calculate the difference in the memorization times used initially and after the retention interval. This difference is the savings score. Finally, plot the savings scores as a function of the amount of time that had elapsed.

about commonly experienced aspects of life (see Chapter 9). To illustrate the effects of schemas, Bartlett had people read a story and then later try to recall it anywhere from immediately after they read it to several months or years later. What he found was that as memories for the story became more fragmented, its content was altered to make it more consistent with a stereotypical story.

Another prominent early psychologists was **William James** (1842–1910).[1] Much of his influence comes through his book, *The Principles of Psychology* (1890/1950). James was a primary figure of the functionalist movement in early psychology. In terms of memory, James provided descriptions of memory that are similar to theories in use today. For example, his distinction between primary and secondary memory parallels the distinction between short-term and long-term memory. Similarly, he was one of the first academics to describe memory retrieval problems, such as the tip-of-the-tongue phenomenon (see Chapter 15) in which we are not able to remember something, such as someone's name, but there is this strong feeling that retrieval is imminent.

Gestalt Movement

The **Gestalt movement**, mostly advanced by German researchers such as Wolfgang Kohler (1887–1967), Max Wertheimer (1880–1943), and Kurt Koffka (1886–1941), suggested that strictly reductionistic approaches to mental life were incomplete. Instead, we need the idea that complex mental representations and processes have a quality that is different from the component parts that make them up. This is not to say that the Gestalt psychologists rejected reductionism. They most certainly did not. Instead, they argued that an understanding of more complex phenomena was important in its own right because it could be qualitatively different. For example, a melody is something that is qualitatively different from the individual notes that make it up, although it is certainly very dependent on them.

---

1 James is so highly regarded that it is not unusual to find a quote by James leading off a research or review article, particularly by Americans.

One of the ideas of the Gestalt movement that influences thinking about memory is that the whole is *different from* the sum of its parts. This can be seen in the idea that memories are built up of a configuration of simpler elements to take on a new quality. Gestalt psychologists also noted that the observed behavior of people depends on both the context in which they find themselves, as well as the frame of reference. This is reflected in the context effects that are observed in memory and perspective effects, such as the hindsight bias. Moreover, because our context and goals can change, the way we use and organize our memories change according to these demands as well (Danziger, 2008).

A final concept to come out of the Gestalt movement is the idea that mental representations are isomorphic. That is, their mental structure and operation are analogous to the structure and function of information in the world. This idea is clearly seen when spatial memory is discussed (see Chapter 11). The idea is that the structure of a memory trace reflects the structure of the event as it would be experienced, although the memory is not as complete. It should be noted that this isomorphism was a functional one. The memory trace functioned "as if" it had the same structure as external events, not that it actually did.

Behaviorism

As we will see in Chapter 6, there are many aspects of memory that operate on a basic and unconscious level. Some of these involve the encoding, storage, and retrieval of relatively simple contingencies that fall under the heading of "conditioning." This was the domain of the behaviorists. **Behaviorism** was a school of thought that sought to bring greater credibility to psychological science. It was a line of thinking that had a strong grip on psychology for much of the early to mid-twentieth century. Part of this effort was to avoid mentalistic constructs because they could not be objectively observed. Although the workings of the mind could not be observed, behavior could be. So, much of the experimental work done during the behaviorist era did not directly address issues of memory. However, there were some important insights and discoveries that are relevant here.

Two salient forms of conditioning are classical and operant conditioning. Classical conditioning is a form of memory that allows one to prepare for contingencies present in the environment, whereas operant conditioning allows one to remember the consequences of one's own actions. Both of these came into the vocabulary of psychology early on in the twentieth century. Classical conditioning was first described by the Russian physiologist Ivan Pavlov (1849–1936), who won the Nobel Prize for his work on digestion. Operant conditioning was first described by an until then little-known American named Edward Thorndike (1874–1949), who discovered these principles starting with his work as a graduate student.

The discovery and study of forms of conditioning are important because for decades they shaped much of the research in learning and memory. There was great interest in studying the principles that guided these forms of learning and the implications they had on behavior. One of the salient qualities of classical and operant conditioning is that one can take these principles pretty far without having

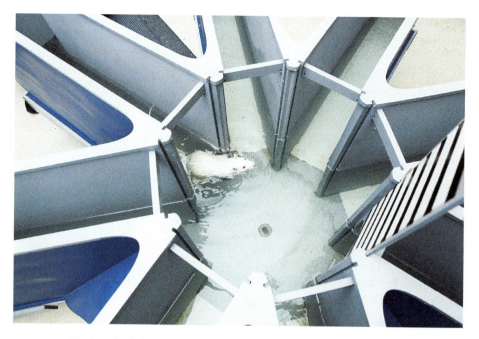

PHOTO 1.2 *During the behaviorist era, there was a heavy emphasis on observables, such as the behavior of a rat running a maze, and a de-emphasis on unobservables, such as the memory and thinking that goes on in the mind*

Source: IrinaK/Shutterstock.com

to posit much about what is going on mentally. One can just observe the stimulus conditions and the responses produced by an organism.

Despite the anti-mentalistic view of the behaviorist era, there were some behaviorists who had important insights into memory. For example, Edward Tolman (1886–1959) did a number of studies with rats running through mazes. According to strict behaviorist analyses of maze running, what the rat learns is to make specific turns at specific junctures. Each turn that the rat makes in the maze would be reinforced or not. If this is true, then any change in the maze should cause the rat to need to learn the route all over again. However, Tolman observed that rats adapted to changes very quickly. He suggested that his rats had a mental representation in memory that he called the "mental map." The rats consulted this mental map to adapt to changes in the maze. Thus, working within the behaviorist context, people such as Tolman were able to bring a discussion of memory and mental activity back into mainstream psychology.

Tolman was a molar behaviorist, although the term he preferred was "purposive behaviorism." That is, he was interested in larger behaviors as opposed to the more microscopic behaviors that interested many of his colleagues. An example of a molar behavior might be something like getting to the end box of a maze or going to a movie, whereas a microscopic behavior might be an action like "turn left." This interest in molar behavior can be seen in an approach to memory that takes into account the goals and context of a person in the memory situation.

Verbal Learning

The **verbal learning** tradition existed in the context of a behaviorist psychology and stemmed from Ebbinghaus's work with nonsense syllables. The term "verbal learning" itself reflects the behaviorism of many of its practitioners, although what was being studied was a form of memory. Because of this context, these studies often had clearly defined stimulus and response components. Memorization was referred to as "attachment of responses to stimuli," and forgetting was "loss of response availability." (For a summary of verbal learning and its relationship to memory, see Tulving & Madigan, 1970.[2]) The verbal learning tradition was a way to study memory during the anti-mentalistic era of behaviorism.

A dominant method in the verbal learning tradition is **paired associate** learning, a paradigm developed by Mary Calkins (1894). In this approach, people memorize pairs of items, often words, letters, or nonsense syllables. An example of a pair would be "BIRD–FANCY." During testing, people would be presented with the first item of the pair and would be told to produce the second (e.g., "BIRD–?"). The first item served as the stimulus and the second as the response.

There were many variations on this theme. The simple A–B paradigm would present people with a list of paired associates and have them recall the B items in the presence of the A cues. Other paradigms are more complicated, where people must learn a second list of items. If this second list is unrelated to the first, this is an A–B C–D paradigm (easy). An example of this would be learning the pair "BIRD–FANCY" in the first list and "TABLE–ARROW" in the second. If the second list retains the initial cues with the first list, it is an A–B A–D paradigm (hard). An example of this would be learning the pair "BIRD–FANCY" in the first list and "BIRD–ARROW" in the second. Alternatively, have the second list be combinations of the A items with synonyms of the B items, called an A–B A–B′ paradigm (very hard). An example of this would be learning the pair "BIRD–FANCY" in the first list, and "BIRD–DRESSY" in the second. Finally, if there are recombinations of the A and B items from the first list, this is an A–B A–Br paradigm (very, very hard). An example of this would be learning the pairs "BIRD–FANCY" and "TABLE–ARROW" in the first list and "BIRD–ARROW" and "TABLE–FANCY" in the second. Often researchers were assessing the effects of interference of prior learning on new learning. Issues of interference continue to be of interest, and some still use paired associate learning. We will see some of these ideas explored in the sections on interference in Chapter 8.

Early Efforts in Neuroscience

Memories are stored in the brain, and the brain is a complex and busy place. So, where exactly is each memory stored? Is it possible to find individual memories in the brain? This is the basic question asked by neuropsychologists such as **Carl Lashley** (1890–1958). Lashley (1950) did a series of studies in search of the "engram"—the neural representation of a memory. Lashley first trained rats to run through a maze and then surgically removed part of the rats' brains. After the rats recovered from the

---

2 This chapter by Tulving and Madigan is one of the most wonderfully snarky papers I've ever read. I wish I could write papers like this.

surgery, they were placed back into the maze. If memories for the maze were localized in one part of the brain, then destroying that part would destroy the memory and the rats would then run the maze just as if they were entering it for the first time. The major outcome was that no matter what part of the brain was removed, these rats were able to perform better than control rats that were put in the maze for the first time. The critical factor was how much tissue had been removed, not where (see Figure 1.1).[3] Lashley concluded that engrams were not localized in one part of the brain but are distributed throughout the cortex. While more recent work has shown that some forms of memory may be localized in different parts of the brain, the general conclusion that many different and distributed parts of the brain are used during memory processing is well supported.

In addition to understanding what different parts of the brain do, it is important to understand how the brain works. That is, how do the interconnections among neurons influence memory? One of the pioneers along this line of research was **Donald Hebb** (1904–1985). Through his classic book *The Organization of Behavior* (1949), Hebb became one of the forerunners of computational neuroscience—the mathematical modeling of brain activity. According to Hebb, memories were encoded in the nervous system in a two-stage process. In the first stage, neural excitation would reverberate around in cell assemblies. A collection of cells that

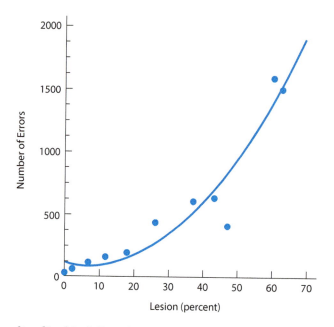

FIGURE 1.1 *Results of Lashley's Experiment with Brain Ablation*

Source: created from data reported in Lashley, K. S. (1950). In search of the engram. *Symposia of the Society for Experimental Biology: Physiological Mechanisms of Animal Behavior (Vol. 4).* New York: Academic Press

3 A similar study was done by J. P. Flourens, with pigeons, in the nineteenth century, as reported by Danziger, 2008.

corresponds to a new pattern or idea would be stimulated, and this stimulation would continue for some time. In the second stage, the interconnections among the neurons would physically change, with some connections growing stronger. The classic phrase here is "neurons that fire together, wire together." This is similar to the idea of long-term potentiation, discussed in Chapter 2. It takes some time for memories to move from stage 1 to stage 2. This is why if people suffer a trauma to the brain, such as a blow to the head, they may lose recent memories (see Chapter 10). In addition, Hebb's ideas of neural organization and change help lead to the development of computational models of the nervous system, such as the parallel distributed processing (PDP) models, discussed in Chapter 18.

The Cognitive Revolution

Over time, psychologists became frustrated with the constraints of behaviorism. There was a desire to study mental activity as mental activity, not as a black box between the input of the stimulus and the output of the behavior. The **cognitive revolution** of the 1950s and 1960s marked a return of mental states to legitimate study. The study of memory was palatable once again.

Many people contributed to the cognitive revolution. We focus here on one whose efforts serve as an example of the work and ideas that brought about this change. George Miller (1920–2012) provided a number of important findings for memory research, such as his work on the capacity of short-term memory in his paper "The Magical Number Seven: Plus or Minus Two" (Miller, 1956). This work took the idea of mental processing seriously and demonstrated how it was a limited system, much like a computer's processing is limited by the amount of memory it has. These studies were some of the first to show that memory could be studied with the methodological rigor that the behaviorists were so fond of.

Miller also showed that how people mentally organized information influences memory. The more highly organized a set of information was, the better the memory. In other words, how information is actively thought about can improve memory. In addition, the knowledge that people had stored in long-term memory can influence current memory performance in profound ways. Thus, work by Miller, and people like him, showed that to understand how memory works in the current situation, we must understand how it is structured over the long term.

Stop and Review

The study of memory stretches back to ancient times, with philosophers such as Plato and Aristotle. Other important thinkers to consider memory include St. Augustine, Robert Hooke, Charles Darwin, as well as the various philosophy of mind figures. The scientific study of human memory began with people such as Hermann Ebbinghaus, Sir Frederick Bartlett, and William James. Current thinking and research is also guided by work of the Gestalt psychologists and the behaviorists. The verbal learning tradition, which emerged out of the behaviorist era, and efforts in neuroscience evolved into our current cognitive science approach to memory.

THE MODAL MODEL OF MEMORY

The standard model of memory, or the **modal model** (Atkinson & Shiffrin, 1968), is a heuristic guide for understanding how memory works. It has successfully limped along for years as a framework for discussing issues about how information is stored over time. This model has four primary components: (1) sensory registers, (2) short-term store, (3) long-term store, and (4) control processes (for a historic overview, see Malmberg et al., 2019). An outline of the model is shown in Figure 1.2.

The first component, the **sensory registers**, is a collection of memory stores. Each corresponds to a different sensory modality. There is a sensory register for vision, one for audition, one for touch, and so on. The world is full of information that is in a constant state of flux. Our sensory registers allow us to hold on to this information for brief periods of time to determine if it is worthy of further attention. If we did not possess such memory stores, our minds would be constantly locked into only the very current state of affairs. We would not be able to detect patterns that involve very brief memories, such as determining that two frames of a film can be interpreted as continuous movement or that a sequence of sounds forms a word.

Once information has been attended to, it needs to be kept in the current stream of thought. Because what we are currently thinking about constantly changes, this information needs to be kept available for a short period of time. This **short-term memory** generally retains information for less than a minute if nothing is actively done with it. If consciousness is associated with any part of memory, it would be here. This is knowledge that is either currently in conscious awareness or just beyond it. Another characteristic of short-term memory is its capacity—the amount of information that can be held in an active state. This amount is humblingly small—somewhere on the order of seven items or less. The topic of the sensory registers and short-term memory are considered in detail in Chapter 4.

The third part of the modal model is the idea that there are **control processes** that manipulate information in short-term memory. This can include rehearsing information, transferring knowledge to and from long-term memory, or perhaps even reasoning. This component of memory makes it an active participant in reality

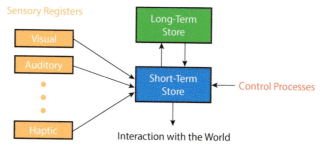

FIGURE 1.2 *The Modal Model of Memory*

Source: adapted from Atkinson, R. C., & Shiffrin, R. M. (1968). Human memory: A proposed system and its control processes. *The Psychology of Learning and Motivation*, 2, 8–195

rather than just a passive absorption and retrieval mechanism. The idea that control processes work with knowledge in the service of some goal has led to the idea that short-term memory should be considered more of a working memory system. Issues of working memory are considered in Chapter 5.

The fourth component of memory—the one that interests most people and that much of this text is devoted to—is long-term memory. **Long-term memory** encompasses a wide variety of long-term knowledge and different ways of using that knowledge. Issues of long-term memory are covered in Chapters 6 through 18.

Again, it should be noted that the modal model is a heuristic for thinking about memory, but it is not an accurate theory of memory. For example, incoming information does not need to pass through short-term memory to reach long-term memory. Instead, the information may activate knowledge in long-term memory, which is then actively manipulated as short-term memory (van der Meulen et al., 2009).

Stop and Review

The modal model of memory is a heuristic that is used as a guide to discuss memory. This model includes the sensory registers, a short-term memory system that holds small amounts of information for short periods of time (usually under a minute), control processes for manipulating information, and a long-term memory system.

Improve Your Memory

At this point, we have not said much about how memory works. This section outlines some basic principles that you can follow to improve your learning and memory in this and any other class. Many of these points touch on issues that are discussed at different points in the book. For now, a few "best practices" are listed so that you can do better in your classes, perhaps with less time and effort (because you will not waste your time doing things that do not work). You should:

- Read the assignment **before** you come to class. You only have one opportunity to hear a lecture. Reading the material ahead of time gives you a better foundation to identify what is more or less important in a lecture, and what it means. The more you can remember from a lecture, the less time and effort is needed later.
- **Preview** the text prior to reading. Often sections of a chapter have headings, and there are key terms set off in bold. If you know what ground will be covered prior to reading, you can build a scaffolding in your mind ahead of time. Then, as you read, you can fill in this mental framework, allowing you to better retain what you are reading.
- Come up with **questions** to have in mind as you read. Seeking answers to these questions helps you process and remember the material. If you write

these questions down ahead of time, this small amount of extra effort at the beginning can save you more effort later.

- Make sure that you **read** the text carefully, trying to link up the material with what you already know, and making sure you understand new words and jargon. If you give yourself enough time to learn as you read, you will remember it better and save yourself time later.

- After reading, try to **recite** answers for the questions that you came up with ahead of time. If you wrote them down before reading, this will be easier. If you can answer those questions, then you can be more confident that you have learned the material. However, if you struggle, then this highlights which material was not well learned. Another good strategy is to **produce** something by writing down a summary of the material you read. This sounds like a lot of work. However, doing this will help organize the material in your mind and save you study time later. Even the act of saying something aloud can boost memory.

- Much of what you learn can be forgotten. To help maintain this knowledge, you need to **review** the material again to boost knowledge that may be weak or forgotten.

- When you study, try to do so in a **quiet** setting. This will minimize competition for your thoughts and allow you to better learn the material. Also, try to study in **different places** and at **different times** of the day if you can. This can help the knowledge from being tied to a specific setting. You want the things that you are learning to be available under any setting, such as when you are taking an exam.

- Humans are visual animals. So, if you are having a hard time learning something, try to form a **mental image** in your head. This may make it easier to remember, especially if you can imagine several things interacting.

- Try to spread your study time out in a **distributed** manner. Cramming is not effective for long-term learning. If you study your class materials every day, you will learn them better, and will need to spend less time later trying to relearn things that you have forgotten.

- Much of your studying is done alone. However, if you find other people to study with, this can aid learning and memory. First, after class, **compare** notes with someone else. This helps you identify material that you may have missed. Also, quiz each other over the material. Ideally, this would be done about once a week. The act of **generating** questions to ask people improves your memory, and the act of **testing** yourself also improves memory. You can also test yourself using things like flashcards. Quizzing allows you to identify those aspects of the material that you do not know well.

- Finally, there are many neurological processes that help memory that occur when you **sleep**. If you get enough sleep at night, you will have better memory for the class material. Relatedly, if you can take a nap during the day, this can be helpful too.

MULTIPLE MEMORY SYSTEMS

As is illustrated by the modal model, memory is not unitary. It has several subcomponents that have evolved as a result of selection pressures to handle different jobs (Klein et al., 2002; Sherry & Schacter, 1987). There are a number of classifications schemes for long-term memory. One is Tulving's (1985) **Triarchic Theory of Memory**, shown in Figure 1.3. This view divides long-term memory into three classes: nondeclarative, semantic, and episodic. These divisions reflect the different tasks required of memory, as well as different levels of conscious awareness.

Procedural memory is an evolutionarily old system. Even primitive organisms have some kind of procedural memory. Some refer to this as the nondeclarative memory and have grouped semantic and episodic memory together as declarative memory. This **declarative–nondeclarative distinction** is reflected in the organization shown in Figure 1.4. Declarative memory refers to memories that are easy for people to articulate and talk about. In contrast, nondeclarative memory refers to memories that are difficult to articulate but still influence our lives. As can be seen in Figure 1.4, nondeclarative memories can be divided into different types, and in Chapter 6 we discuss many of these. One type of nondeclarative memory is the procedural memory of Tulving's classification. This is memory for how to do things, such as ride a bicycle or speak your native language. Other types of memories are also included in this category, including unconscious, implicit memory processing. This memory system is described as *anoetic* (a: "no"; -noetic: "thinking") in Tulving's system because it does not require conscious awareness.

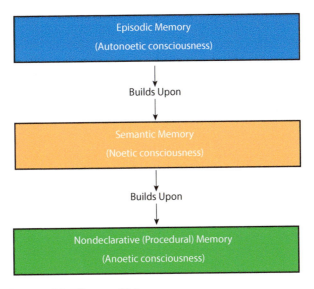

FIGURE 1.3 *Tulving's Triarchic Theory of Memory*

Source: adapted from Tulving, E. (1985). How many memory systems are there? *American Psychologist*, 40, 385–398

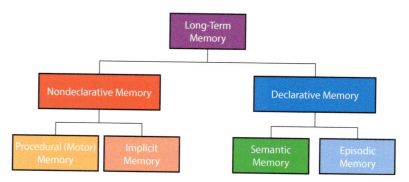

FIGURE 1.4 *The Division of Long-Term Memory Systems*

Source: adapted from Squire, L. R. (1988). Mechanisms of memory. *Science*, 232, 1612–1619

As shown in Figure 1.4, declarative memory can be divided into two categories as defined by the **episodic–semantic distinction** (Tulving, 1972). Semantic memories are generalized and encyclopedic and are not tied to a specific time or place. This is stable knowledge that you share with your community. For example, knowing what a bird is, what a stop sign means, and what you do in a restaurant are all semantic memories. Semantic memories are highly interrelated and are forgotten rather slowly once established. In Tulving's Triarchic Theory, semantic memory is *noetic* ("thinking") because it requires conscious awareness. You have to be consciously aware to know that an object is a bird or a tree, and that it is similar to other members of that category.

Episodic memories refer to specific episodes or events in our lives. They are tied to the time and place in which the information was learned. For example, where did you go on your first date? Who told you that funny joke? Did you just see the word "apple" in a list of words? Also, unlike semantic memories, episodic memories are more compartmentalized and forgotten rapidly. Episodic memory uses *autonoetic* (auto: "self"; -noetic: "thinking") knowledge in Tulving's Triarchic Theory because it requires knowledge of the self. For example, to know whether you have recently seen an action film, you need to have some memory of yourself as a separate identity to which past events can be referenced. In fact, neurological measures, such ERP recordings (see Chapter 2), show different types of brain activity for memories that refer to the self in some way compared to semantic memories (Magno & Allen, 2007). More generally, semantic and episodic memories overlap in terms of many neural structures, although there are some differences (for a detailed discussion, see Renoult et al., 2019).

In addition to the different types of memory systems, we can also point out differences in how people use their memories. One is the **explicit–implicit distinction** (Schacter, 1987). The idea here is how information is retrieved from memory, not the information content. Explicit memory refers to when people actively and consciously try to remember something. When you try to recall someone's name or when you recognize a suspect in a police lineup, this is explicit memory. Implicit memory refers to when people are unaware that memory is being used. For example, to be able to read, you need to remember what the various squiggles on a page correspond to. You do not really feel like you are pulling information out of memory to do this, and yet you are. Even though most of this book is dedicated to issues of explicit memory, much of our lives, both thinking and action, are governed by implicit memory. The fact that familiar things are recognized more quickly, are preferred in choices, and guide our thinking are all examples of the influence of implicit memory.

Stop and Review

Memory is divided into multiple systems that do different things with different types of information. These divisions may capture levels of consciousness awareness, as with the Triarchic Theory, and include the declarative–nondeclarative distinction or the implicit–explicit processes distinction.

RECURRING ISSUES

Before we move on to the specific topics, there are some issues that bear highlighting. These issues reoccur throughout the book, so it is helpful to alert you to them.

Neurological Bases

Memory is a property of the nervous system. The better you understand the nervous system, the better you can understand memory. If nothing else, knowing that theoretical mental processes are associated with neural processes lends confidence to findings and ideas. As we advance into the future, cognitive neuroscience is becoming more and more important.

Retention Over Time

Memory is for retaining information over time. This is the most important point of Ebbinghaus's (1885) early work. Science should be predictive, and in order to predict how much will be remembered after a period of time, we need to know how it is changing over time. As such, when retention and forgetting curves are available, I try to present them.

Emotion

More memory researchers are incorporating emotion into their theories (see Kensinger, 2009). In general, memory is better for emotional materials. Emotion facilitates memory consolidation as well as (a) increases attention to emotional aspects of events, (b) makes event memories more distinct, and (c) results in more information organization (Talmi, 2013). Certain topics, such as flashbulb memories, are critically dependent on emotion.

Multiple Memory Sources

Memory often uses multiple sources. This is reflected in what are known as **fuzzy trace theories** (e.g., Brainerd et al., 1999) in which there are two or more memory traces involved in any act of remembering. One is a memory that contains detailed information. The other captures more general information. Remembering reflects a combination of these. Detailed memory dominates when a person has a good memory of an event. In contrast, general memory trace dominates when memory for an event is poor or if knowledge is being used in a general way, such as trying to remember what a flywheel is.

Embodied Cognition

Embodied cognition[4] can mean many different things (Wilson, 2002), but the basic idea is that mental activity is grounded in the type of world our bodies inhabit and the ways we use our bodies; our sensory and motor processes (Ianì, 2019). Memory is affected by the situations people find themselves in, such as using context to help guide encoding and retrieval. Also, memory often operates in real time as events are unfolding. As anyone taking an exam knows, memories need to be adequately retrieved in a set time limit.

Scientific Rigor and Converging Evidence

Memory is a tricky thing to study. Each person's memories are different from everyone else's. There are also aspects of memory that are qualitatively different. To have the clearest picture of what our memories are like and who we are, we need to take as objective a view as possible. We need to avoid being led astray by our biases, momentary intentions, and other prejudices. Taking a rigorous, scientific approach can do this. Psychology, after all, is a science. To emphasize this, various approaches or methods of looking at the data from studies are presented throughout the text to illustrate how the data from memory studies can be analyzed and interpreted to gain better insight into the depths of our mental storehouses. Also, opinions and theories formed as a science are better supported when evidence comes from different methods of collecting and analyzing data. If these multiple sources of information are consistent with the same explanation, this gives us greater confidence that the theory is closer to the truth. This is known as **converging operations**. This is important as ideas about memory that emerge largely from relatively limited and simplistic methods and views can distort our thinking about and understanding of human memory (Hintzman, 2011).

---

4 Although the term "grounded cognition" (Barsalou, 2008) is more descriptive and inclusive, we use the phrase "embodied cognition" to be consistent with the majority of the literature.

Stop and Review

There are a number of recurring threads that reappear across the topics that are discussed about memory. These include an increased desire to understand the neurological underpinnings of memory, how memories change over time, the involvement of emotions in memory, the division of information across multiple memories, and the need to understand how memory operates in the real world. All of the topics in memory are approached from a scientific perspective that seeks to derive answers that help us have an accurate and durable understanding of ourselves.

PUTTING IT ALL TOGETHER

Understanding memory is one of the most introspective tasks you can undertake. By looking at how your memories are created, structured, stored, retained, forgotten, and retrieved, you can gain a better insight into who you are. The study of memory, however, is difficult. Even with explicit definitions of learning and memory, there are many things that go uncaptured. Memory is complex and not open to direct observation, so we need metaphors to capture its essential qualities. People have been trying since ancient times to uncover the mysteries of human memory. The scientific study of memory began in earnest with work by Ebbinghaus. Using himself and lists of nonsense syllables he discovered several basic principles of memory. Bartlett used the concept of a schema to capture general knowledge of the world. The Gestalt psychologists understood the impact of context or setting on what is remembered. Finally, the behaviorists provided an approach of experimental rigor that continues to be used. The verbal learning tradition, along with efforts in neuroscience, led to the emergence of the current cognitive tradition. Over the past several decades we have gained a clearer and more consistent picture of what memory is. There are different kinds of memory that cover different spans of time and are for processing different types of information. This book surveys human memory, often touching on neuropsychological issues, changes over time, the impact of emotions, and multi-trace influences, all within the context of using appropriate scientific rigor.

STUDY QUESTIONS

1. What do the terms *learning* and *memory* mean in the context of this chapter? How are they referring to similar things? How do they diverge?
2. Why do we need metaphors for memory? What are some metaphors? What do they tell us about the nature of memory?

3. What were some of the major figures and some of the major schools of thought that dominated thinking about human memory? What were the contributions of each?

4. What are some of the major components of the modal model of memory? How do these components interact?

5. What are some of the major divisions of human memory? What sort of processing is done by each of those divisions?

6. What are some of the emerging themes that will be recurring at various points in our discussion of memory?

KEY TERMS

- behaviorism
- cognitive revolution
- control processes
- converging operations
- declarative–nondeclarative distinction
- distributed practice
- embodied cognition
- engram
- episodic–semantic distinction
- explicit–implicit distinction
- forgetting curve
- fuzzy trace theories
- Gestalt movement
- learning
- learning curve
- long-term memory
- massed practice
- memory
- metaphors for memory
- modal model
- nonsense syllable
- overlearning
- paired associate
- recall
- recognition
- savings
- sensory registers
- short-term memory
- Triarchic Theory of Memory
- verbal learning

EXPLORE MORE

Here are some additional readings that you can explore to provide yourself better insight into the history and basics of human memory.

Barsalou, L. W. (2008). Grounded Cognition. *Annual Review of Psychology, 59,* 617–645.

Danziger, K. (2008). *Marking the Mind.* Cambridge, UK: Cambridge University Press.

Ebbinghaus, H. (1885/1964). *Memory: A Contribution to Experimental Psychology.* Translated by H. A. Ruger & C. E. Bussenius. New York: Dover.

Hebb, D. O. (1949). *The Organization of Behavior.* New York: Wiley.

Hintzman, D. L. (2011). Research strategy in the study of memory: Fads, fallacies, and the search for the "coordinates of truth." *Perspectives on Psychological Science, 6,* 253–271.

James, W. (1890 / 1950). *The Principles of Psychology.* New York: Dover.

Mandler, G. (2011). *A History of Modern Experimental Psychology: From James and Wundt to Cognitive Science.* Cambridge, MA: MIT Press.

REFERENCES

Atkinson, R. C., & Shiffrin, R. M. (1968). Human memory: A proposed system and its control processes. *The Psychology of Learning and Motivation, 2*, 89–195.

Barsalou, L. W. (2008). Grounded Cognition. *Annual Review of Psychology, 59*, 617–645.

Brainerd, C. J., Reyna, V. F., & Mojardin, A. H. (1999). Conjoint recognition. *Psychological Review, 106*, 160–179.

Calkins, M. W. (1894). Association. *Psychological Review, 1*, 476–483.

Danziger, K. (2008). *Marking the Mind*. Cambridge, UK: Cambridge University Press.

Ebbinghaus, H. (1885/1964). *Memory: A Contribution to Experimental Psychology*. Translated by H. A. Ruger & C. E. Bussenius. New York: Dover.

Glaze, J. A. (1928). The association value of nonsense syllables. *Journal of Genetic Psychology, 35*, 255–269.

Glenberg, A. M. (1997). What is memory for? *Behavioral and Brain Sciences, 20*, 1–55.

Hebb, D. O. (1949). *The Organization of Behavior*. New York: Wiley.

Hintzman, D. L. (2003). Robert Hooke's mode of memory. *Psychonomic Bulletin & Review, 10*, 3–14.

Hintzman, D. L. (2011). Research strategy in the study of memory: Fads, fallacies, and the search for the "coordinates of truth". *Perspectives on Psychological Science, 6*, 253–271.

Ianì, F. (2019). Embodied memories: Reviewing the role of the body in memory processes. *Psychonomic Bulletin & Review, 26*(6), 1747–1766.

James, W. (1890 / 1950). *The Principles of Psychology*. New York: Dover.

Kensinger, E. A. (2009). *Emotional Memory Across the Adult Lifespan*. New York: Psychology Press.

Klein, S. B., Cosmides, L., Tooby, J., & Chance, S. (2002). Decisions and the evolution of memory: Multiple systems, multiple functions. *Psychological Review, 109*, 306–329.

Lashley, K. S. (1950). In search of the engram. *Symposia of the Society for Experimental Biology: Physiological Mechanisms of Animal Behavior*, Vol. 4. New York: Academic Press.

Magno, E., & Allan, K. (2007). Self-reference during explicit memory retrieval: An event-related potential analysis. *Psychological Science, 18*, 672–677.

Malmberg, K. J., Raaijmakers, J. G. W., & Shiffrin, R. M. (2019). 50 years of research sparked by Atkinson and Shiffrin (1968). *Memory & Cognition, 47*(4), 561–574.

Miller, G. A. (1956). The magical number seven, plus or minus two: Some limits on our capacity for processing information. *Psychological Review, 63*, 81–97.

Queenan, B. N., Ryan, T. J., Gazzaniga, M. S., & Gallistel, C. R. (2017). On the research of time past: The hunt for the substrate of memory. *Annals of the New York Academy of Sciences, 1396*(1), 108–125.

Renoult, L., Irish, M., Moscovitch, M., & Rugg, M. D. (2019). From knowing to remembering: The semantic–episodic distinction. *Trends in Cognitive Sciences, 23*(12), 1041–1057.

Roediger, H. L. (1980). Memory metaphors in cognitive psychology. *Memory & Cognition, 8*, 231–246.

Schacter, D. L. (1987). Implicit memory: History and current status. *Journal of Experimental Psychology: Learning, Memory, and Cognition, 13*, 501–518.

Schacter, D. L., Eich, J. E., & Tulving, E. (1978). Richard Semon's theory of memory. *Journal of Verbal Learning and Verbal Behavior, 17*, 721–743.

Shepard, R. N. (1984). Ecological constraints on internal representation: Resonant kinematics of perceiving, imagining, thinking, and dreaming. *Psychological Review, 9*, 417–447.

Sherry, D. F., & Schacter, D. L. (1987). The evolution of multiple memory systems. *Psychological Review, 94*, 439–454.

Spear, N. E., & Riccio, D. C. (1994). *Memory: Phenomena and Principles*. New York: Allyn & Bacon.

Squire, L. R. (1988). Mechanisms of memory. *Science, 232*, 1612–1619.

Talmi, D. (2013). Enhanced emotional memory: Cognitive and neural mechanisms. *Current Directions in Psychological Science, 22*, 430–436.

Tulving, E. (1972). Episodic and semantic memory. In E. Tulving & W. Donaldson (Eds.), *Organization of Memory* (pp. 381–403). New York: Academic Press.

Tulving, E. (1985). How many memory systems are there? *American Psychologist, 40,* 385–398.

Tulving, E., & Madigan, S. A. (1970). Memory and verbal learning. *Annual Review of Psychology, 21,* 437–484.

Turkheimer, E. (1998). Heritability and biological explanation. *Psychological Review, 105,* 782–791.

van der Meulen, M., Logie, R. H., & Della Sala, S. (2009). Selective interference with image retention and generation: Evidence for the workspace model. *Quarterly Journal of Experimental Psychology, 62,* 1568–1580.

Viney, W., & King, D. B. (1998). *A History of Psychology: Ideas and Context.* Boston, MA: Allyn & Bacon.

Wilson, M. (2002). Six views of embodied cognition. *Psychonomic Bulletin & Review, 9,* 625–636.

CHAPTER 2

Neuroscience of Memory

How are memories encoded? Where are they stored? How are they retrieved? Using the computer analogy, thoughts and memories are the software and data, and the nervous system is the hardware. We can understand many aspects of the software without knowing much about the hardware. How many computer users do not really understand how the hardware of their various devices works, but can still operate the software that they run? That said, to gain a truer insight into the software, how it represents and processes information, why some processes are faster and others are slower, one needs an understanding of the hardware. The same is true for memories and the nervous system.

Memory is an **emergent property** of the nervous system. That is, it is not a property of the individual neurons themselves, but it emerges when they work together. To illustrate the idea of what an emergent property is, think of six square boards. None of the boards alone have the property of containment. However, when they are arranged to make a box, then it is possible to place something inside it. The property of containment emerges out of the arrangement of the elements that lack that property individually (see Minsky, 1986).

Without a basic understanding of the nervous system, your knowledge of memory is limited. The aim here is to provide information about the major components of the nervous system and how they are involved in memory. We first consider neural structure, how neural communication occurs, and how this changes as a result of experience (memory). After that, we skip to higher levels of processing and discuss some of the major components of the brain, such as the cortex. Finally, we examine ways to study the underlying neurobiology and how findings in memory research are related to neurological structures and processes.

NEURONS

To adequately understand how underlying neurophysiology relates to psychological experience and the operation of memory, you need a working understanding of the nervous system. We start with the basic components of individual neurons, followed by a consideration of neural communication.

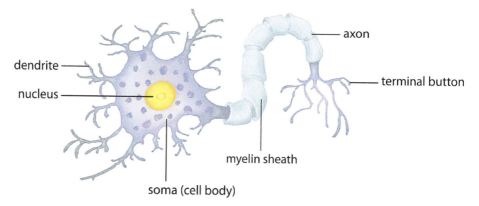

FIGURE 2.1 *A Neuron*

Neural Structure

The most basic parts of the nervous system are neurons. A **neuron** is a specialized cell for the transmission and retention of information. The structure of a neuron is shown in Figure 2.1. Some of a neuron's components are shared with other cells. For example, a neuron has a cell body, or **soma**, that contains all of the general cell processing components, such as mitochondria, ribosomes, RNA, and so on.

Other cell structures are important for the specialized jobs of neurons. Extending out of each neuron are dendrites. **Dendrites** are used for receiving signals either from sensory cells or from other neurons. Dendrites collect information for the neuron. Neurons also have another structure protruding from them called an axon. **Axons** transmit information out of the neuron either to other neurons or to muscles and glands. Thus, axons are responsible for sending information out of the neuron.

At the end of each axon are nodules called **terminal buttons** that contain the neurotransmitters. **Neurotransmitters** are the chemicals that are used to send signals to other neurons. Because axons can sometimes be quite lengthy, to avoid the loss or confusion of signals, some neurons have axons that are encased in a fatty substance known as a **myelin sheath** that acts as an insulator. If a neuron has a myelin sheath, the myelin is not created by the neuron, but by glial cells associated with it.[1] The myelin sheath is not continuous but has gaps along its length called the **nodes of Ranvier**. These gaps facilitate the transmission of information within a neuron by allowing the neural signal to jump from one point to the next (one gap to the next) without having to continuously traverse the entire length of the axon. Thus, the distance that the neural signal travels is functionally shortened, allowing the signal to travel more quickly.

The Action Potential

We now look at the transmission of information. Neural communication can be broken down into two components, one electrical and the other chemical. The electrical component that occurs within a neuron is the **action potential**. When

---

1 Oligodendrocytes in the central nervous system and Schwann cells in the peripheral nervous system.

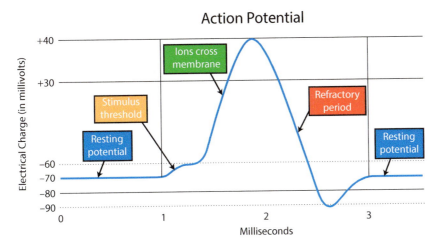

FIGURE 2.2 *The Action Potential over Time*

a neuron is sufficiently stimulated, an action potential occurs, and the neuron is said to "fire" (see Figure 2.2). When a neuron is not being stimulated, it has a resting electrical charge of −70 mV (millivolts). This is because there are a number of negatively charged ions in the interior of the neuron. When a neuron is stimulated, there is a depolarization of its electrical potential. If this depolarization shifts the neuron's electrical charge in a positive direction, the electrical charge may reach −50 mV. At this point there is a dramatic change in the charge of the neuron, shifting to +40 mV. This is the action potential. After a neuron fires, there is a recovery period where it prepares itself to fire again and resets itself at the resting potential of −70 mV. This electrical charge is the basis of some neuroimaging and neurostimulation techniques described later. It should be noted that the action potential operates on the all-or-none principle. That is, there is either an action potential, which is always the same, or there is not.

The action potential does not exist in the entire neuron at once. Rather, there is a wave of activity flowing down the axon. When a neuron fires, sodium ions in the extracellular fluid flow into the neuron because depolarization causes sodium "gates" on the cell membrane to open. The sodium ions are positively charged, and this produces the positively charged action potential. The wave flowing down the axon is the wave of sodium gates opening and allowing these ions to enter the cell, much a like a row of dominos falling. Each domino causes the next to falter. Immediately behind this wave of positive charge, there is a second wave of potassium ions being sent out of the cell. This is part of recovering the cell's resting potential level of electrical charge.

Neurotransmitters and the Synapse

The chemical component of neural communication occurs at the **synapse** between two neurons. Although a single neuron may communicate with large numbers of other neurons, especially in the cortex, there is no direct physical connection between them. There is a small gap. This gap is about 100 to 200 angstroms wide (1 angstrom = 1/10,000th of a millimeter). Neurons communicate across the synapse using chemicals called neurotransmitters. Neurotransmitters reside in the terminal buttons of one neuron, inside synaptic vesicles, and are forced out into the synapse when there is an action potential. These are often absorbed by the subsequent neuron, altering its electrical potential.

While many neurotransmitters are involved in memory in some way, either directly or indirectly, some are more important than others. One is **acetylcholine** (**ACh**). When acetylcholine effects are enhanced, memory can improve, and it declines when acetylcholine effects are suppressed (Mishkin & Appenzeller, 1987). Acetylcholine may enhance the strength of synaptic potentials during long-term potentiation (see later). **Glutamate** (**Glu**) is an excitatory neurotransmitter involved in altering synapses and creating new memories. In comparison, gamma-amino butyric acid (**GABA**) is an inhibitory neurotransmitter, also critically involved in new memory formation. GABA is strongly related to glutamate in that GABA is formed by modifying the glutamate molecule. **Norepinephrine** is involved in the consolidation of memories, and **Dopamine** is important to memory processing. One problem in Parkinson's disease is the low level of dopamine.

There are two general classes of neurotransmitters. *Excitatory* neurotransmitters encourage the subsequent neuron to fire, causing the ion gates on the neuron's cell membrane to open and let in the sodium ions. In contrast, *inhibitory* neurotransmitters encourage the subsequent neuron to *not* fire, encouraging the ion gates to stay closed. If the goal of neural communication is to transmit information, why would one neuron inhibit the firing of a subsequent neuron? The reason is that one way that information is coded in the nervous system is as a pattern of activity across a wide assembly of neurons. To create this pattern, some neurons need to be firing and others not. As an analogy, computers code information as a pattern of 1s (on) and 0s (off). This is roughly the same idea, although in a different form, and with much greater complexity. Waves of neural firing that are dominated by excitation and little inhibition can occur and are called seizures.

Another important point about neurotransmitters is that they do not operate alone. Other chemicals can affect them. For example, neuromodulators can accentuate or diminish the influences of neurotransmitters. This adds a level of variability to neural processing. Also, while some neurons interact with the body directly, such as through muscles, other neurons may make contact with the glands that can release hormones into the body. Thus, the nervous system can influence parts of the body outside of itself.

Neural Change in Learning

Although communication between neurons occurs at the synapse, how are these connections altered during learning? One way is through the process of **long-term potentiation**, or **LTP** (Bliss & Collingridge, 1993; Bliss & Lomo, 1973), which was first observed in rabbits (see Patihis, 2018 for a historical overview, and Nicoll, 2017 for a review). LTP is often investigated using cells from the hippocampus (see later). LTP strengthens the connections between neurons by altering the ease with which postsynaptic neurons fire. The majority of the change occurs at the dendrites. Along the cell membrane, there is an increase in the number of receptor cites for the neurotransmitters, as well as the growth of dendritic spines, although there may be some changes in the presynaptic neuron's axon as well (Emptage et al., 2003). As a result, more neurotransmitters can bind to the postsynaptic cell. Note that there is an analogous process called **long-term depression** or **LTD** that weakens connections between neurons, which is also important for learning (e.g., Duffy, Labrie, & Roder, 2008).

LTP can last for days or weeks, but it eventually dissipates. This dissipation may come from interference from new memories. In a study by Abraham et al. (2002), LTP was induced in rats. They were then placed in environments that were either enriched or impoverished. It was found that LTP faded for the enriched environment rats, but was still present in impoverished environment rats a year later. Thus, LTP is the type of neural change that occurs in memory formation early on, but another process is needed for information to be stored more permanently in other parts of the brain.

Stop and Review

The fundamental building blocks of the nervous system are neurons. Memory is an emergent property of collections of neurons working together. Understanding how neurons work and communicate provides a better understanding of memory. Neurons have important features, such as dendrites and axons that are involved in neural communication. The electrical component of neural communication is captured in the action potential and a chemical component by the neurotransmitters. Neurons form memories by altering their connections to one another.

CORTICAL LOBES

Up to this point, we have been talking about low-level processes. Now we are going to jump up to much larger levels of neural organization. There are many structures that make up the brain. Those that are more directly involved in memory can be classified into two broad categories: (1) the lobes of the cortex and (2) subcortical structures, which are parts of the brain that lie beneath the cerebral cortex.

The phylogenetically newest, and most prominent, part of the brain is the cerebral cortex. This is the wrinkly part that sits on top and is what most people think of when they picture a brain. The wrinkled appearance is because there is so much surface area crammed into such a small volume. The brains of other animals, such as reptiles and amphibians, may be smooth in their entirety. In contrast, our brains are more powerful, because we have many more neurons. However, this increase in brain size brings with it an increase in head size. If the head becomes too large, then other problems arise, such as difficulty giving birth and supporting and controlling such a large structure on the neck.

To keep the head reasonably small, while increasing the number of neurons, the cortex has become folded and wrinkled. If you removed a cortex and lay it flat, you would see that it is very large. The average adult cortex covers about 1,800 square cm (about 2 square feet) and is 2 to 3 mm thick. The wrinkling preserves the size of the surface area while reducing the volume occupied. An analogy is trying to get a sheet of paper into a cup. The paper will not go in lying flat. However, if you wrinkle it up and stuff it in, you have taken a large surface area and enclosed it in a small volume.

The cortex is divided into several major regions. First, there are the two hemispheres, a left and a right hemisphere. Some memory functions are more dependent on one hemisphere than the other. This dominance of one hemisphere over the other is **laterality**. For now, note that the left hemisphere is generally better at analytic processing, such as language and math, and the right hemisphere is better at holistic processing, such as spatial or music processing.

TRY IT OUT

One issue that is raised in this chapter is the idea of hemispheric lateralization for different mental processes. This lateralization includes memory. In addition to processing different kinds of information, keep in mind that the hemispheres are primarily responsible for controlling the opposite sides of the body. This is called a *contralateral connection*. One manifestation of this is handedness. Most of us are right-handed, but some of us are left-handed. Our handedness can influence how we process information from memory, including whether we like something or not, and how we respond to and process information (Casasanto & Jasmin, 2010).

For this task, first create a list of 20 or so product types, such as detergent, cars, breakfast cereals, and so on. What you should do for each person is have them describe one version of the product that they like and another for one they do not like. Be sure to tell people that they can gesture with their hands if they like. What you need to do is keep track of which hand they gesture with when they describe products they like and dislike. You should have four categories of responses: (1) left hand mostly, (2) right hand mostly, (3) both equally, and (4) neither. While they are talking, keep track of which hand is used to gesture as they describe the products. After you have collected your data, ask each person whether they are right-handed or left-handed.

After you have finished, average the number of times each person used one of the four gesturing categories when describing products that they felt positively and negatively about. Be sure to classify the responses as being dominant or non-dominant hand so that you can collapse the data across both right- and left-handers. When you look at your data, what you may find is that which hand people used to make gestures varies with whether they liked a product. It has been found that people are more likely to gesture with their dominant hand (right for right-handers, left for left-handers) when making positive statements about things they like and are more likely to use the other hand for negative statements about things they dislike.

Each hemisphere is divided into four subsections called lobes (see Figure 2.3). Each lobe is associated with different functions. At the back of the brain is the **occipital lobe**, which is primarily involved in visual processing. In front of the occipital lobe, on the top of the brain and just behind the central fissure, is the **parietal lobe**. This is responsible for sensory processing from throughout the body, as well as spatial processing (e.g., knowing where something is). In front of the occipital lobe and below the parietal lobe, under the lateral fissure, is the **temporal lobe**. This is responsible for auditory processing and retaining knowledge about the identity of things in the world. Finally, at the front of the brain, in front of the central fissure and above the lateral fissure, is the **frontal lobe**. This is the evolutionarily most recently developed part of the cortex and is involved in the control of action, emotion, and thought. The frontal lobes help a person select those memories that are most relevant on a given occasion. They also coordinate various types of information into a coherent memory trace.

To help you localize different parts of the cortex, throughout the text there will be both verbal descriptions of the location as well as a number that refers to the

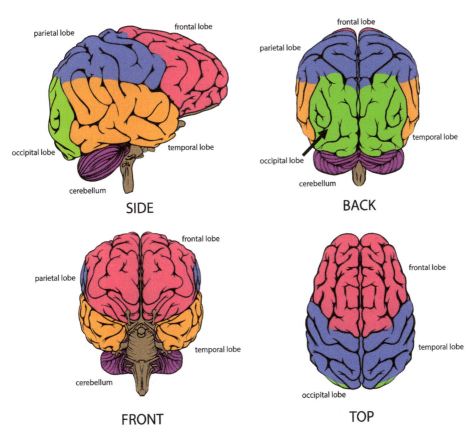

FIGURE 2.3 *The Organization of the Cortical Lobes*

Source: Christos Georghiou/Shutterstock.com

Brodmann Area (e.g., BA 20). This is a reference to a part of the cortex that has been identified on a Brodmann atlas. Copies of the Brodmann atlas are provided in the end pages of this book for your easy reference.

Occipital Lobes

The occipital lobes are involved more in perception than memory. However, there are some aspects that can be interpreted as memory. The occipital lobes detect features in the environment (Hubel & Wiesel, 1965), but the sensitivity to these features is based on experiences with the world. For example, if kittens are reared in an environment in which they only see horizontal lines, when they are adults, they will walk into a table leg because they cannot see vertical lines. They lack the feature detectors for vertical objects (Blakemore & Cooper, 1970). This suggests that our perceptual experiences are based on mental representations for visual world components. These components are stored in the perceptual system over the long term. As such, they can be considered a form of very long-term memory representations for the bits and pieces that make up the world.

Parietal Lobes

The parietal lobes are less often thought of as being involved in memory than the temporal and frontal lobes, but they are used in a wide range of circumstances. For example, working memory processes for visual memory or the spatial manipulation of information (see Chapter 8) involve the parietal lobes (Mishkin & Appenzeller, 1987). This would include doing a task that involves mental imagery, such as scanning a mental image. Animals that have had their parietal lobes surgically removed have trouble remembering spatial relations.

Temporal Lobes

The lobes most closely associated with memory are the temporal lobes. This is not surprising as they surround the hippocampus, which, as you will soon see, is one of the more important structures for memory. The part of the temporal lobe that is often studied regarding memory is directly adjacent to or surrounding the hippocampus. The area adjacent to the hippocampus is often referred to as the medial temporal lobe. The temporal lobes are where many of our long-term memories for different types of information may be stored. Damage to this part of the brain often results in some memory loss. This part may be involved in remembering events from one's own life, something called autobiographical memory (see Chapter 12). It may also be the source of remembering ideas related to concepts you are pondering at the time. For example, having the idea "wood" become more accessible after hearing the word "lumber." This is a memory process called priming (see Chapter 3).

Frontal Lobes

The frontal lobes are also important to memory. They are involved in the coordination of information, so they are critical for working memory (see Chapter 5). In general, the most caudal (backward) regions of the frontal lobe are for motor and premotor control, the mid portion for contextual control (such as knowing if something is relevant), and the most rostral (frontward) regions are for schematic control (such as knowing the sequence of actions needed to prepare breakfast) (Badre & Nee, 2018). Sometimes we have situations where information becomes separated, such as when we recall something but cannot remember where we know it from. For example, did you hear about that secret from your friend Jordan or from Riley? Alternatively, we may remember that someone told us *something*, but we cannot remember what it was. Knowledge of the information content, as well as knowing where it came from, must be put together using a process of source monitoring (see Chapter 13). The frontal lobes are also involved in remembering what we need to do in the future, something called prospective memory (see Chapter 7). A failure to remember to tell your roommate that his mother called may be due to a problem with the memory processes controlled by the frontal lobe.

The Default Mode Network

The various hemispheres and lobes of the cortex are involved in different mental processes in and of themselves, but they also work together in various ways. One example of different brain regions working together is the **default mode network**, or **DMN** (Buckner et al., 2008). The DMN is a collection of brain structures whose activity is highly correlated. The DMN is more active when people do not have attention strongly engaged in some activity. That is, the activation of the DMN is negatively correlated with activity in various attention networks in the brain (Andrews-Hanna, 2012). In some sense, this network in the brain is more active by default when people are colloquially thinking about "nothing in particular," such as when they are daydreaming, mind-wandering, autobiographical remembering, or perhaps engaging in episodic future thinking about their own lives or people they know. This network is also active when people are watching a television show or a film (Hasson et al., 2008; Lerner et al., 2011) and so may be involved in basic comprehension.

The DMN is made up of a number of structures, including parts of the parietal lobe, such as the posterior cingulate cortex (BAs 23 & 31), the angular gyrus (BA 39), and the precuneus (BA 7), parts of the frontal lobe, such as the dorsomedial and medial prefrontal cortices (BA 11), and parts of the temporal lobe, including its lateral portions and the anterior pole, as well as parts of the hippocampal complex such as the hippocampus, parahippocampus, and retrosplenial cortices (see the next section) (Andrews-Hanna et al., 2014). Keep in mind that the DMN is just one example of a collection of structures working together. There are others.

Stop and Review

The brain is made up of specialized substructures. The most prominent of these are the two hemispheres. Each hemisphere is divided into four lobes. The temporal lobe plays a prominent role in memory, along with the frontal and parietal lobes, whereas the occipital lobe is the least involved. Different parts of the cortex are involved in specialized processes. They coordinate with one another to accomplish various tasks, as with the default mode network.

SUBCORTICAL STRUCTURES

In addition to the cortical lobes, there are several subcortical structures that are centrally involved in memory. The most important of these is the hippocampus. There is also some coverage of the amygdala, basal ganglia, and diencephalon.

Hippocampus

The subcortical structure that gets the most attention in memory research is the **hippocampus** (see Figure 2.4). This is a seahorse-shaped structure (hence the name). The hippocampus, as well as the related surrounding complex of areas, is important

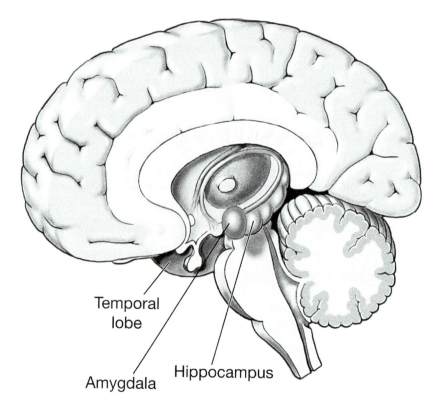

Temporal
lobe

Amygdala Hippocampus

FIGURE 2.4 *The Hippocampus and the Amygdala*

for conscious memories of events (Mishkin & Appenzeller, 1987). Much of the research on long-term potentiation has been done by studying neurons from the hippocampus. While it is strongly associated with LTP, and thus may be able to retain information for up to several weeks, it does not appear to be where very long-term declarative memories are stored. Instead, it may be involved in helping to encode these memories into other parts of the cortex, where they are held for longer periods of time (see the later section on consolidation). The hippocampus may serve as a waystation for knowledge on the journey to permanent encoding (if it makes it that far).

The hippocampus, like many brain structures, is divided into several subregions, as shown in Figure 2.5, and is surrounded by important cortical areas that are collectively known as the hippocampal complex. In terms of the hippocampus itself, it is composed of the *dentate gyrus*, regions *CA1, CA2, CA3,* and *CA4* (with areas CA1 and CA3 being more important for memory processing) and the *subiculum*.

Outside the hippocampus proper, there are several associated areas of concern, as shown in Figure 2.6. First, for processing spatial information there is the *parahippocampal cortex* which is posterior (behind) and inferior (below) to the hippocampus. Next, for processing object information, there is the *perirhinal cortex* which is inferior to the hippocampus and anterior to (in front of) the parahippocampal cortex (BA 35). Finally, there is the *entorhinal cortex* (BAs 28 & 34), which is anterior to and inferior to the hippocampus. The entorhinal cortex takes information from the parahippocampal and perirhinal cortices and passes it along to the hippocampus itself.

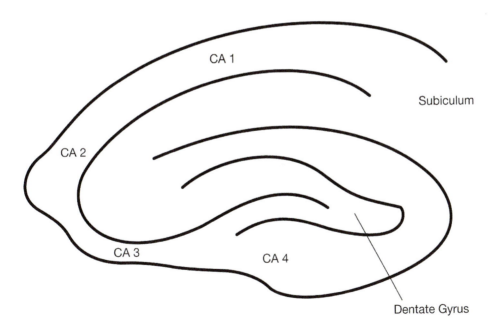

FIGURE 2.5 *The Structure of the Hippocampus*

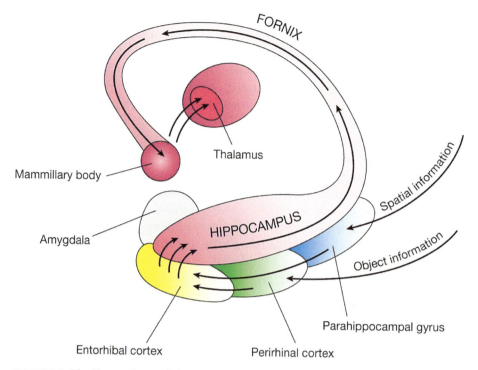

FIGURE 2.6 *The Connections of the Hippocampus to the Cortex*

In addition to processing what and where objects are, their importance or emotional value is signaled by the orbital frontal cortex of the frontal lobe (BA 11) and the amygdala (see below). These signals are processed through the perirhinal and entorhinal cortices. Thus, across the hippocampus-related brain regions, an array of connections allows the hippocampus to integrate and bind information about the spatial–temporal context, objects, and their value.

The dentate gyrus and area CA3 receive inputs from the medial entorhinal cortex. Moreover, the dentate gyrus also sends signals to area CA3. In comparison, area CA1 receives inputs from the lateral entorhinal cortex and passes this information on to the subiculum. Area CA1 also receives inputs from area CA3. The subiculum sends its processes on to the entorhinal cortex. Some hippocampal fibers also travel to the *fornix*, the *mammillary bodies* and the *thalamus*.

A great deal of research on the hippocampus is focused on its role in the formation and storage of new memories. Damage to the hippocampus can lead to severe declarative memory deficits (Mahut et al., 1982), such as anterograde amnesia (see Chapter 10). That said, it also involved in the retrieval and the replaying or re-experiencing of prior events (Karlsson & Frank, 2009) and the imagining of future event possibilities (Hassabis et al., 2007).

In addition to long-term memory, the hippocampal complex is involved in processing spatial information. For example, place cells (which are active when an organism is in a particular location) are found in the hippocampus (O'Keefe,

& Dostrovsky, 1971), grid cells are found in the entorhinal cortex (Hafting et al., 2005), and boundary cells are found in the subiculum and entorhinal cortex (Solstad et al., 2008). Thus, hippocampal areas are important for encoding and processing context. There is also evidence for hippocampal time cells that track when events occur (Howard & Eichenbaum, 2013). Thus, the hippocampus is important for processing the spatial–temporal framework within which episodic memory events occur.

Overall, the hippocampus is specialized for processing and binding conjunctions of stimuli that appear together in the environment. It is well designed for the rapid encoding and binding of episode-specific conjunctions—that is, whatever is co-occurring at the moment. This includes the spatial and temporal contexts, as well as the objects within the current event. The hippocampus does this by processes of pattern separation (segmenting experience) and completing missing elements from general world knowledge (Behrendt, 2013). That is, the hippocampus binds together information from a variety of sources to create integrated memories of individual scenes or events (Maguire & Mullally, 2013). There is evidence that when an event is complete, there is an increase in hippocampal activity at event boundaries as it closes up one event and opens up a new one (Ben-Yakov et al., 2013).

Other Subcortical Structures

Another important subcortical structure is the amygdala (see Figure 2.4). The **amygdala** is an almond-shaped structure (hence the name) located at the lower, anterior part of the hippocampus. It is involved in processing emotional aspects of memories (Davis, 1997; Mishkin & Appenzeller, 1987). For example, if there is an emotional reaction to an event, that reaction would be encoded into the memory trace via the amygdala.

The **basal ganglia** are a collection of subcortical structures (including the caudate nucleus, the putamen, the globus pallidus, and the subthalamic nucleus) located above and around the thalamus (see Figure 2.7). These structures are important for motor memory—that is, the control of the voluntary muscle groups. The basal ganglia are implicated in memory for habits and motor skills, such as riding a bicycle. A related set of findings is observed with the **cerebellum**. This is a phylogenetically old structure located at the back of the brain (see Figure 2.3). Like the cortex, it has a convoluted surface, so it looks like a little brain underneath the larger one (and hence its name). The cerebellum is associated with fine motor control and coordination. Thus, it is used in memory for procedural skills that involve the complex coordination and control of the muscles, such as walking. This is a more primitive form of memory, but very important, nonetheless.

The **diencephalon**, including the **thalamus** and **hypothalamus**, serves as a routing station for signals from different parts of the brain. It is also involved in memory for conscious, factual knowledge. The diencephalon is important in processing the temporal sequence of events. More indirectly, the diencephalon is involved in controlling the neurotransmitters that are present in the nervous system at any given time, and so it has an influence on memory.

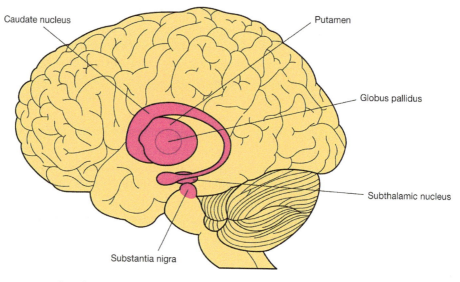

Caudate nucleus

Putamen

Globus pallidus

Subthalamic nucleus

Substantia nigra

FIGURE 2.7 *Basal Ganglia Structures*

Stop and Review

The most important subcortical structure for memory is the hippocampus and its related brain structures. Anterior hippocampal connections are involved more in the processing of objects and identities, whereas the posterior hippocampal connections are involved more in the processing of spatial–temporal contexts. There are also inputs relating to the emotional and evaluative components of processing. Other important subcortical structures for memory include the amygdala, which is involved in processing emotion, the cerebellum and basal ganglia, which are involved in motor memories, and the diencephalon, which is involved in the routing and coordinating of information.

NEUROLOGICAL MEASURES AND STIMULATION

One of the most exciting areas of research is the development of methods and tools to allow us to look at how the brain works to encode, store, and retrieve memories. Some of these methods are described here. In this section we look at measures of brain structure, functions based on cortical electrical activity and blood flow, as well as ways in which we may actively stimulate the brain.

Structural Measures

Although it is important to know the functions that operate in the brain, it also helps to know its structure, especially of a specific person or group of people. Sometimes clues to patterns in the way people think can be gained by understanding how their brains might be physically different from the norm. One thing to keep in mind about the brain is that its physical structure is not uniform; it differs from person to person, in much the same way that each person's face is unique. The best way to view the physical structure of a brain is to remove it from the skull (after death, of course). However, this approach has its limits. Another way is to open up the skull of a living person and examine the brain, which can happen during surgery.

Short of death and brain surgery, there are other ways to examine living brain structure. One way is to take a series of x-rays, each of them taking a different "slice" of the head, and then examine the brain structures revealed. This is known as a **computer-assisted tomography** scan, or **CT** scan (also known as a CAT scan). An example of a CT scan of the right and left hemispheres of the brain is shown in Figure 2.8. CT scans show the structure of a brain and can reveal things such as the location of a tumor, damage from a stroke, or the general condition of a brain.

A popular neuroimaging technique is **magnetic resonance imaging**, or **MRI** (sometimes called nuclear magnetic resonance imaging). MRI works with the resonant frequencies of different molecules in the brain. First, a person is placed in a strong, controlled magnetic field. This is the magnetic part of MRI. This magnetic field affects the spin of all of the atoms of a certain type in the body, such as all of the hydrogen atoms, causing the protons in those atoms to line up along a

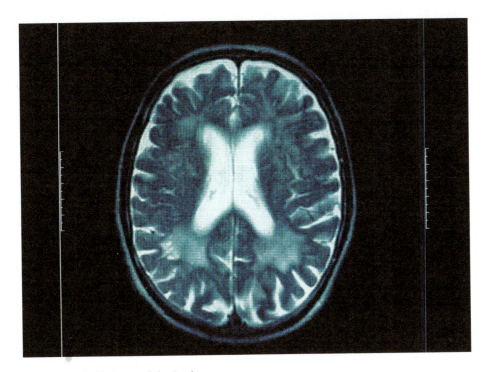

FIGURE 2.8 *A CT Scan of the Brain*

Source: SvedOliver/Shutterstock.com

specific axis, with about half oriented in each direction along that axis. After this, a radio frequency pulse is passed through the body. This pulse causes unmatched protons to spin in a different direction at a specific frequency. Concurrently, a set of gradient magnets are cycled on and off, which alter the primary magnetic field, allowing images or slices of the brain to be acquired. When this pulsing stops, the hydrogen atoms go back to their normal state and release the energy absorbed from the pulses. This is the resonance in MRI. This energy is detected by the coils in the machine and sent to a computer for analysis. The computer then interprets the data and creates the MRI image.

An MRI brain scan is shown in Figure 2.9. Typically, the density of water molecules, which contain hydrogen, is used to determine structure. The density of hydrogen atoms varies as a function of whether a particular region contains unmyelinated neurons, myelinated axons, cerebral spinal fluid, and so on. An advantage of MRI is that it is not necessary to inject a chemical into the body, as with PET scans (see later), or use harmful radiation, as with CT scans. Perhaps the biggest advantage of MRI scans is their clarity. These images are of a higher quality than those from a CT scan.

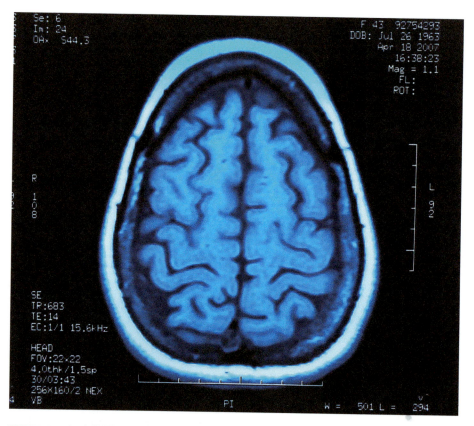

FIGURE 2.9 *An MRI Scan of the Brain*

Source: Allison Herreid/ Shutterstock.com

Electrical Measures

This section examines measures of electrical activity generated by action potentials in the brain. Be sure to read the Study In Depth box to learn about an early attempt by Wilder Penfield in the 1950s to use electrical stimulation to recover otherwise lost memories.

Wilder Penfield (1891–1976) was a Canadian neurosurgeon held in high regard for his mapping of the sensory and motor homunculi in the cortex. He did this by probing people's brains with a mild electrical charge during surgery. These people had some intractable condition, so parts of the cortex were removed in an attempt at relief (with a reasonable level of success). While the patient was awake, a section of the skull was removed. This was done so that the patient could report what effects the stimulations had. This allowed Penfield to identify those parts of the brain that were critically important. Although many functions rely on similar areas of different people's brains, there is some variability. While probing, Penfield would sometimes get interesting reports when a portion of the temporal lobe was probed. These reports were as if people were re-experiencing memories of their lives. Here is one example.

> The patient then said something about "street corner." The surgeon asked him, "Where?" and he replied "South Bend, Indiana, corner of Jacob and Washington." When asked to explain, he said he seemed to be looking at himself—at a younger age.
> (Penfield, 1955, p. 52)

Penfield reported that he had several responses of this nature from different patients. He interpreted these reports as memories. What was striking to Penfield was that they were not the events that people typically recall from their lives but were rather boring and mundane memories. The vividness of these reports and their everyday quality led Penfield to suggest that the brain records the stream of consciousness throughout a lifetime. Long-term memory acts like a videorecorder. The electrical probe that he had applied allowed people to remember and replay otherwise forgotten aspects of their lives.

Although this is striking, there are some caveats (Loftus & Loftus, 1980). First, it is unclear to what extent the reports were actually memories or were experiences generated at the time. These "memories" may be created in much the same way that dreams are. Because the brain does not like randomness, it imposes structure on the information it is getting. To do this, it uses readily available information that is reasonably close to the stimulation. This is information in long-term memory. Penfield's patients were getting random stimulation, and their brains were trying to make sense of this random input with whatever knowledge was available in memory. If so, then these reports were mental constructs created at the time from random inputs from the probe along with information that was stored in memory.

Another problem is that there were very few of these reports. Of the 1,132 of Penfield's patients, only 40 (3.5%) had what he interpreted as memories, and most of these were not full-blown reports. Twenty-four had auditory experiences (e.g., hearing voices or music), 19 had visual experiences (seeing familiar people or objects), and only 12 gave what appeared to be complete memory reports. Thus, there is very little evidence to work with.

Some of these reports could not possibly have been re-experiences of past events. For example, in the report just given, the patient states that he can see himself standing on a street corner. If memories of experiences were faithfully recorded, this could not happen. You cannot look at yourself from a distance without a mirror or a TV camera, for example.

The most direct use of electrical component of neural processing is **single-cell recording**. In this method, an electrode is used to probe an individual living cell somewhere in the nervous system. The researcher is then able to determine when the cell fires. Each time the electrical charge flows down the axon it is recorded (this also picks up activity of other neurons in the proximity of the probe). The experimenter then has the subject engage in the task of interest, watching to see how the firing pattern of that individual cell changes.

Obviously, this is a very micro level of analysis. Information is only gathered about the operation of one cell in a brain made up of billions of neurons. Nevertheless, this technique can provide information about how different cells in the brain are processing different types of information. Also, this technique is very invasive, so it is typically limited to animal research.

That said, there are studies emerging that use information from single-cell recording in humans who have had these electrodes embedded in the medial temporal lobe or hippocampus for clinical reasons (e.g., Suthana & Fried, 2012). This approach is **intracranial electroencephalography**, or **iEEG** (Fox et al., 2018). This provides a more direct assessment of neural functioning. Each electrode can record the activity of cell assemblies of 200,000–500,000 neurons.

While single-cell recording provides information about what is going on in one cell, other measures provide information about large groups of cells and are noninvasive, and so can be used with ordinary people, doing more complex tasks, such as remembering a poem. For this procedure electrodes are attached to the scalp to record the electrical activity in the underlying part of the brain. These recordings are called **electroencephalography**, or **EEG** waves. Often there are several electrodes at regularly spaced and predetermined locations over the skull to help localize the recorded activity.

EEG waves can be used to measure **event-related potentials**, or **ERPs**. An ERP is a regular change in the pattern of electrical energy measured as a function of the particular task or event that the person is thinking about (Coles et al., 1990). Researchers have people engage in various tasks at predetermined points in time. These are the "events" of event-related potentials. Then the researchers look at the EEG waves that were recorded at that time relative to when the events occurred. These electrical "potentials" in the EEG waves are what are "related" to the earlier "events"—hence the name event-related potentials, or ERPs.

If you have ever seen an EEG wave, it looks like a random bunch of squiggles. And for each trial of an ERP study, this is largely what it is. Keep in mind that the brain is actively doing many things other than the task at hand, so there is a lot of electrical activity from these processes. To get a clearer idea of what is going on, researchers need to average the potentials across many trials. This averaging process washes out much of the noise, leaving a clearer signal. As more trials are averaged together, the ERP wave becomes more pronounced. This ERP signature is often a relatively large wave of positive or negative electrical charge in a region of the brain occurring at a point in time after the target event. The ERP can then be related to theories of memory. The ERP wave suggests that mental work is taking place. A difference between two waves corresponding to two different conditions in the study corresponds to different types of mental processes.

An advantage of ERPs is temporal resolution—that is, knowing when things happen. Recordings can be made at 1 ms time slices. Thus, it is clear when certain processes are kicking in or when different regions of the brain are involved. People often talk about ERPs in terms of interesting components in the waveform and the nature of these components. For example, we might talk about a P300 wave, which refers to an electrically positive wave occurring about 300 ms after the beginning of an event. An N400 wave refers to a negative wave occurring about 400 ms after the beginning of an event (Bentin, 1989).

There are some disadvantages to ERPs. One is that the spatial resolution—*where* things happen in the brain—is poor. We can get a general idea about what part of the brain is involved, but determining a precise location is difficult. This is complicated by the fact that there is a lot of "stuff" between the electrodes and the brain—skin, blood vessels, meninges, and bone. In some ways, using EEG recordings to figure out what is going on in the brain is like trying to figure out what is going on in a factory by listening through the wall.

While ERPs provide information about a level of positive or negative electrical charge at a point in time, there is other information that can be extracted from EEG signals. The nervous system has a tendency to have various oscillators throughout it. That is, groups of cells tend to fire together. Although these are primarily neurons, it is possible that glial cells (astrocytes) may also be involved (Fellin, et al., 2009). This oscillation is called synchronization, and when this increases after an event it is called **event-related synchronization**, or **ERS**. When people are at rest, synchronization is stable. However, when people engaged in a mental activity, there may be a desynchronization. This is called **event-related desynchronization**, or **ERD**. These oscillations occur at different frequency bands, depending on how fast the oscillations are. One way of dividing up the frequency bands is to have different regions separated by about 2 Hz each, using a person's base frequency as a reference point, defining the Delta band as –8 to –6 Hz, the Theta band as –6 to –4 Hz, the Lower 1 Alpha band as –4 to –2 Hz, the Lower 2 Alpha band as –2 to 0 Hz, and the Upper Alpha band as 0 to +2 Hz (Dopplemayr et al., 1998). Changes in any of these bands can vary as a function of the memory task.

Such patterns are related to memory performance. For example, during effective memory processing, there is decreased alpha synchronization and increased theta synchronization (Klimesch, 1999). Essentially, the resting alpha synchronization is disrupted by activity of a particular type. The theta synchronization is associated with increased activity in the hippocampus and surrounding structures. Moreover, changes in alpha and theta band power have been related to activation and inhibitory processes in memory (Herweg et al., 2020; Klimesch, 2012). Finally, the distinction between episodic and semantic memory is supported by ERD work showing greater upper alpha de-synchronization for semantic memory and increased theta band synchronization for episodic encoding (Klimesch, 1999).

Another neuroimaging method is **magnetoencephalography** or **MEG** which uses magnetic fields to measure cortical electrical activity. Many parts of the brain are always active, doing lots of different things at any one time. To get an idea of what part of the brain is involved in a process measured in a MEG scan, the **subtractive method** is used. With the subtractive method, scans are taken both when people are doing the mental activity of interest as well as a control condition in which they are not thinking about anything in particular. The brain activity of the control condition is subtracted from the activity recorded during the process of interest. The difference in activity tells the researchers which parts of the brain are more or less active for that type of processing. This subtractive method is also used with other types of neuroimaging, such as PET and fMRI scans (see the following section).

Overall, researchers can use MEG to pinpoint which parts of the brain may be active for various memory tasks. MEG scans have better spatial resolution than EEG and have a good temporal resolution of about 10 ms. While not as good as ERP, it is still respectable. As one example of using MEG, Kim et al. (2008) tested recognition memory for words. The MEG scans revealed that medial temporal lobes are more involved when there is a delay prior to recognition compared to when it is more immediate.

Blood Flow Measures

Not all neuropsychological methods use electrical impulses. Some involve measures of cerebral blood flow. Collections of neurons that are working harder need more nutrients to be replenished and keep going. As a result, blood flow to those areas increases to compensate for this. The discovery of a relationship between blood flow and neural activity was somewhat serendipitous (Posner & Raichle, 1994). In the early twentieth century, Walter K. had an abnormality in the blood vessels in his brain. There was a large clump of vessels over his occipital lobes. Walter complained of a constant humming in his ears, which was the blood rushing through these vessels. He noticed the humming decreased when his eyes were closed and increased when his eyes were open. The increased activity in the occipital lobes was associated with increased blood flow. Here, we look at two measures that use blood flow to assess brain activity.

For *positron emission tomography*, or **PET**, people are injected with a radioactive isotope of oxygen (oxygen-15 or ^{15}O). This isotope decays (to ^{16}O), which is reasonably stable. The level of radioactivity is low and short-lived (it has a half-life of just over two minutes), so there is little harm to the body. Once the isotope

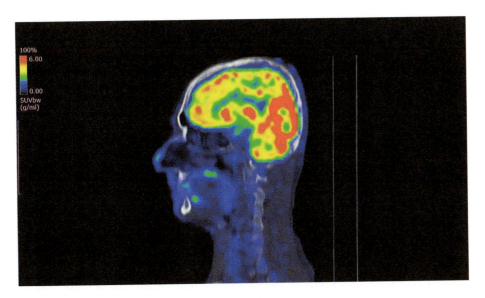

FIGURE 2.10 *A PET Scan Image*
Source: springsky/Shutterstock.com

is in the bloodstream, people are placed in a scanner that measures the levels of the isotope in the brain. Recording levels in control conditions are compared with experimental conditions where people are engaging in the type of thought that is of interest for the study. Depending on the task, different parts of the brain are more or less active. A sample PET scan image is shown in Figure 2.10. These different levels of activity can be used to help determine which parts of the brain are being used.

Compared to ERPs, the spatial resolution in PET scans is better. However, with PET it takes a long time for a good image to be generated, typically no faster than 20 seconds. How many different thoughts you could have if you were lying on your back in a scanner for 20 seconds? Thus, while the spatial resolution is better, the temporal resolution is relatively poor. So, we can determine *where* something is occurring in the brain but not *when*.

The MRI technology discussed earlier can be adapted to look at function as well as structure. This is called **functional MRI** or **fMRI**. fMRI uses the detection of oxygen atoms as a measure of mental activity. The density of oxygen molecules is associated with the operation of neural assemblies and the flow of blood to fortify those cells. After all, the delivery of oxygen is one of the primary purposes of the bloodstream. An fMRI scan has an advantage over PET because no injection is required, and the images can be taken in a shorter period of time, on the order of a few seconds. Still, fMRI scans cannot match the temporal accuracy of EEG measurements.

At this point, several neuroimaging methods have been mentioned. Each of these is used to take a picture of either the structure of the brain or the neurological operations that occur. There can be no question that such methods provide unique, intriguing, and valuable insights. So, why not use such methods exclusively? Well, it should be kept in mind that these methods provide only information about neurological structure and activity. They do not tell us much about how information is represented or processed by the brain—that is the content of thoughts and memories—they only tell us the output of the imaging device (de-Wit et al., 2016). To know *what* a person is remembering, we still need behavioral methods.

Neural Stimulation

In addition to recording brain activity as either electrical impulses or blood flow, another approach is to actively stimulate the brain. This can be done is through **transcranial *m*agnetic stimulation (TMS)**. TMS uses electromagnetic induction to create a magnetic field to alter the electrical charges of the neurons in a targeted part of the brain, thereby exciting those neurons. This either further enhances the processing of those cells or takes out that region as a kind of temporary lesion in otherwise normal brains. An advantage of TMS is that it allows a researcher to explore how different parts of the brain are used in different tasks by selectively affecting neurons in various areas. As one example of the use of TMS to study memory, Kirschen et al., (2006) used TMS to disrupt the phonological similarity effect in working memory (see Chapter 5).

Another method is **transcranial *d*irect *c*urrent *s*timulation (tDCS)** in which an electric current is applied to the scalp (Reinhart et al., 2017). This direct current (DC) is applied for several minutes, often using a 9-volt battery. This mild electric current passes through the head from the anode to the cathode of the device, stimulating the underlying neurons. While tDCS uses direct current, there is also **transcranial *a*lternative *c*urrent *s*timulation (tACS)**, and **transcranial *r*andom *n*oise stimulation (tRNS)**.

Altered Brains

Another source of insight into neurological underpinnings of memory comes from **case studies** of people who have suffered some damage or lesion to the brain. This might be from an external event, such as a car accident or a gunshot; an internal event, such as a stroke or a virus; or, in rare cases, from surgery. By examining the memories that are affected following damage to a specific part of the brain, some inferences can be made about what role that structure plays. For example, if the damage leads a person to be able to remember very little in the short term, it suggests that short-term memory uses this structure. Because of their very nature, a single case may be studied in depth to help understand what happened, what went wrong, and what techniques can be used to improve the situation.

Although brain lesions provide valuable insights, they are imperfect. First, seldom is there a pure lesion, with one structure being affected and the other structures remaining unharmed. Lesions are often messy and affect several structures. This is true for both accidents and diseases affecting humans, as well as animal studies in which lesions are intentionally made surgically. Another problem with lesion studies is that there are never two cases of people with identical lesions. Thus, it cannot be determined whether the consequences of the damage are unique to that person or are a generalizable consequence. Finally, lesions are haphazard both in terms of where and when they occur. They do not afford the sort of control one would have in a systematic study. Thus, while important and valuable information can be gained from case studies, there are clear limitations to the conclusions that can be drawn.

Studies of **special populations** of people who have a neurological condition also provide useful data. For example, when we discuss amnesia (see Chapter 10), you will see studies using chronic alcoholics who have acquired Korsakoff's syndrome. Also, there are systematic neurological changes that occur because of the natural aging process. Thus, age-related changes in memory can be viewed as neurological assessment of memory (see Chapter 17). Finally, some diseases, such as Alzheimer's, have systematic effects on the central nervous system. In these special populations, there is some regularity in the change that occurs, so we can observe a systematic change in neurological function that results in altered thoughts and behaviors. Of course, there may be some preexisting conditions that can complicate an assessment—for example, epilepsy can alter the brain's organization and structure.

Special populations are advantageous sources of information because they provide many people with a prespecified condition that has standard neurological changes associated with it. This allows for the removal of idiosyncratic changes that occur and present in case studies. Because these groups are large, it also allows for a better understanding of the condition and, hopefully, will lead to better treatments.

Stop and Review

Several methods have been developed to assess brain structure and function. Some of these, such as CT and MRI scans, provide information about structural characteristics of a living brain. Others allow researchers to look at brain function. Some of these are based on the electrical activity such as single-cell recordings, MEG scans, and EEG recordings, as well as measures that are derived from EEG recordings, such as ERP measures and assessments of event related (de)synchronization. In addition, changes in blood flow can be measured to assess neural activity, as with PET and fMRI scans. It is also possible to stimulate the electrical activity of the nervous system using TMS and tDCS. Finally, it is also possible to assess cases of brain damage, as well as groups of people who have well-known changes in brain function, such as older adults. It is always possible to explore memory using multiple measures. For example, Anderson et al. (2018) used by EEG and MEG to explore stages of memory processing.

THE PERMANENCE OF MEMORY

When you are thinking about something, different parts of your brain are active, depending on the contents of that thought. These reflect the active firing of the neural assemblies that correspond to the material at hand. The information that is currently being thought is in short-term/working memory in the language of the modal model of memory. However, for information to be useful beyond the current moment, it needs to be stored in a state that does not require active neural firing.

The process of making memories more stable is **consolidation**. New knowledge and experiences physically alter the structure of the brain over long periods of time. This is true, in some form, of every experience we have. Our brains and our memories are in a constant state of flux as we encounter new events, thoughts, and experiences.

A great deal of the evidence for consolidation comes from work on brain damaged people, particularly those with retrograde amnesia (see Chapter 10). Essentially, people are more likely to lose recent memories, while older memories remain intact (Nadel & Moscovitch, 1997). This is Ribot's gradient (Ribot, 1882). The idea is that newer memories have not yet been sufficiently consolidated, and so they are easier to disrupt in the face of head trauma. In comparison, older memories are more consolidated, and so are harder to disrupt.

While memory consolidation is going on all of the time (Carr et al., 2011; Tambini & Davachi, 2019), these processes become more intense when people sleep (Rasch & Born, 2008; Stickgold, 2005). Moreover, if you dream about what you learned prior to sleep, you are more likely to remember it later (Wamsley et al., 2010). One reason we sleep is to provide our brain with an opportunity to engage in activities that are not possible or are less effective when we are awake. This improved memory with sleep is due to a decline in the loss or forgetting of memories rather than a boost of previously weaker memories (Fenn & Hambrick, 2013). These sleep benefits occur not only for nightly sleep, but any sleep that you get from taking a nap, although the benefit is greater for nocturnal sleep (Lo et al., 2014).

Finally, in addition to sleep, some memory consolidation can also be boosted through physical exercise (McNerney & Radvansky, 2015; Voss et al., 2013). The benefits of increased brain activity from physical activity can increase memory consolidation (Robertson & Takacs, 2017. This benefit not only comes from traditional exercise, but also from activities such as dancing and playing music instruments (Tomporowski & Pesce, 2019). There are benefits of both long-term exercise regimens, as well as short-term benefits from recent exercise (Moreau & Chou, 2019).

Improve Your Memory

This chapter covers issues about the underlying neuroscience of human memory. While it is easy to see how these issues are important for understanding how memory works, it may be harder to see how these topics can be used to improve your own memory. One issue covered here is the idea that memory consolidation is aided by sleep and exercise. This is a point that you can clearly apply to your own life. First off, you should try to get enough sleep each night, and to exercise regularly. You will learn more quickly and hold on to information longer if you do. Additionally, information that is learned closer to when you fall asleep or exercise is more likely to benefit from consolidation. Thus, it is to your advantage to study material for your classes prior to going to sleep or around the time that you exercise. Moreover, if you are fortunate enough to be able to nap during the day after your classes, you should do so.

The next section of the chapter discusses two kinds of consolidation, synaptic and systems consolidation (Alvarez & Squire, 1994), as well as the process of reconsolidation. It should be noted that our discussion is focused on declarative memory consolidation. There are consolidation processes for non-declarative memories, but these involve different neural systems, such the basal ganglia and cerebellum (Shadmehr & Holcomb, 1997).

Synaptic Consolidation

Synaptic consolidation is the creation of relatively enduring memories that have just been actively thought about. For declarative memories, some synaptic consolidation occurs in the hippocampus through LTP. This is a relatively rapid process that involves information that is currently active in the firing neural assemblies of short-term/working memory. If people are given an opportunity to briefly rest (say 2.5 seconds) after viewing information, this gives synaptic consolidation an opportunity to occur without further incoming and interfering items (Bayliss et al., 2015). Moreover, from what we know about LTP, we can estimate that synaptically consolidated memories may be retained for a few days or weeks. However, this type of consolidation is transient and is not the final permanent storage of memories. That is, while this is considered long-term memory for the modal model of memory, it is not permanent memory storage.

Systems Consolidation

After synaptic consolidation, there is a wider consolidation that occurs in larger brain systems (Abraham, 2006). Less is known about **systems consolidation**, other than it involves long-term memories becoming more independent of the hippocampus. One study that looked at this was done by Takashima et al. (2006). They used fMRI recordings for remembering pictures of natural landscapes 1, 2, 30, and 90 days after learning. They found that neural activity in the hippocampus decreased over time. In contrast, activity in the cortex, particularly in areas of the frontal lobe, increased with greater retention intervals. Thus, as memories become consolidated in the cortex, the hippocampus is less involved in storage, and the cortex is more involved. That said, the hippocampus is still involved in memory retrieval (Barry & Maguire, 2019). It has also been reported that there may be an influence of some glial cells (astrocytes) on long-lasting memory (beyond 48 hours) (Pinto-Duarte et al., 2017).

The Process of Consolidation

Memory consolidation is a multiple stage process (McGaugh, 2000; Meeter & Murre, 2004) illustrated in the top of Figure 2.11. After information has been encoded, it is held in an active state where it can be manipulated. However, when new information is processed, this older information quickly becomes lost. This is illustrated by the blue curve in the graph at the bottom of Figure 2.11. This corresponds to short-term/working memory in the modal model.

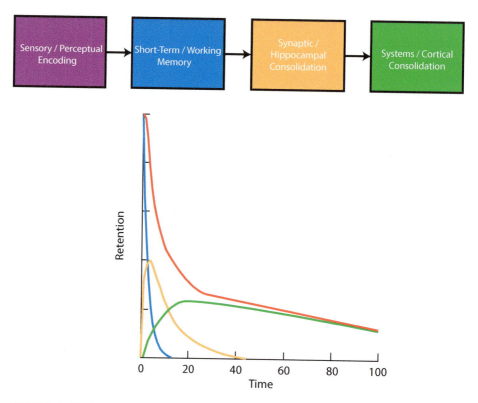

FIGURE 2.11 *Trajectory of Availability Because of Various Consolidation Processes*

Information that is active in short-term/working memory can undergo synaptic consolidation associated with the hippocampus. Information is initially consolidated relatively rapidly, within a few seconds or minutes. It then remains available for several days or weeks. This is illustrated by the gold curve in Figure 2.11. This stage corresponds to long-term memory in the modal model.

The final stage is systems consolidation that occurs in the cortex for information held in the hippocampus, although there may be some fast mapping of memories directly into the cortex (Hebscher et al., 2019). Information takes longer to be consolidated in this system, anywhere from several minutes, day, weeks, months, or years. No one really knows at this point. These memories are retained for long periods of time, up to a lifetime, although there is likely to be some loss over time. This is illustrated by the green curve in Figure 2.11. This stage also corresponds to long-term memory in the modal model.

What should be noted further about Figure 2.11 is the line in red. This is the availability of a given memory trace. It is the sum of the three other components. This is a negatively accelerating function, as is observed with Ebbinghaus's forgetting/retention curve. This is the case even though the three functions that give rise to it each have different shapes. Thus, the forgetting curve that is derived from memory data may reflect the operation of multiple, different underlying processes that each have their own characteristics.

Reconsolidation

As memories become more consolidated, they become less prone to forgetting. And, for the most part, this is what seems to happen. However, this does not mean that consolidated memories cannot be changed. A process of **reconsolidation** can occur when a memory has been consolidated and is later remembered. This causes it to be reactivated and this reactivated memory is then reconsolidated. What is interesting is that during reactivation, a memory enters a fluid, malleable state where it can be changed! This is another example of the principle that remembering can cause forgetting. That said, the older and more strongly consolidated a memory is, the less malleable it is following retrieval, and the harder it is to change. While consolidation and reconsolidation use similar neurological processes, there are some ways that they differ. That said, there is also some suggestion that reconsolidation is just a portion of the entire process of consolidation (Alberini, 2005).

There are two ways for memories to be altered during the reconsolidation. The first is for information to be lost from the original memory. If a consolidated memory is retrieved and then disrupted, the consolidated memory is lost. In a study by Nader et al. (2000), rats were trained to fear an aversive stimulus (a tone paired with a foot shock). After their fear memories had consolidated, the rats were reminded of the original fear-inducing events. During this time, the rats were given an infusion of a protein synthesis inhibitor, causing the consolidated memories to be disrupted. This disruption did not occur if the inhibitor was given when the rats had not been reminded of the unpleasant events.

Similarly, in a study with humans, Schwabe and Wolf (2009) had people recall autobiographical events from their lives. Then, immediately after, they had people memorize a story or not. This immediate memorization disrupted the memories for events from their own lives. People who memorized the story later remembered fewer autobiographical events, although this was limited to neutral events, not emotionally positive or negative events. Also, Zhu et al. (2016) found that reactivating declarative memories of previously learned paired associates rendered them more prone to interference from newly learned items.

Another way for reconsolidation to have an influence is for new information to be added to a trace. Here, a previously consolidated memory is retrieved, and then new information is presented at the same time. This new material is then incorporated into the memory. For example, Forcato et al. (2007) gave people lists of words to remember. Then, after that memory had consolidated over 24 hours, people were reminded of the first list and were also given a second list. They found that the new words were incorporated and reconsolidated with the original list. In other words, when people remember an event from their past and encounter new information at that time, this new information may be reconsolidated with the original memory, changing it.

A potential practical use of reconsolidation may be to help people who have troubling memories from their past, as with PTSD. By altering or removing them, these people would be less tortured by these memories. This idea is still in its infancy and its effectiveness is uncertain. While there is some evidence that it may

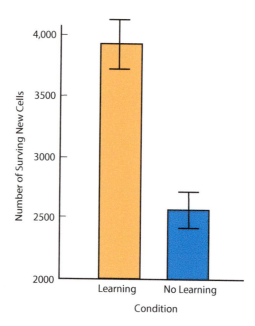

FIGURE 2.12 *Number of Surviving New Cells from Neurogenesis after Either a Period of No Learning or the Learning of New Information*

Source: adapted from Shors, T. J. (2014). The adult brain makes new neurons, and effortful learning keeps them alive. *Current Directions in Psychological Science, 23,* 311–318

be possible (Weems et al., 2014), there have also been failures to find an effect (Wood et al., 2015).

Neurogenesis

Another process that may aid in the formation of permanent memories is **neurogenesis**. While you already have most of the neurons that you will have to work with, your brain is still creating new ones all the time (Gage, 2002). Thousands of new neurons are created in the hippocampus each day (Shors, 2014). However, the fate of many of these new neurons is to die off. That said, there is some evidence that if an organism engages in new learning during the day, more of these newly created neurons stick around, perhaps because they are part of networks of knowledge created during learning. This can be seen in Figure 2.12. Thus, it seems likely that the more you learn, the more of these new neurons you will retain. This gain in neural mass can then aid your ability to learn even more information later. So, study hard.

Stop and Review

Memories become permanent over time through the process of consolidation. Early on, there is a phase of synaptic consolidation in the hippocampus. Then, there is a slower phase of systems consolidation involving more broad-based cortical processes.

Consolidated memories can be changed by reactivating and reconsolidating them. This involves either removing information from a memory or adding new information. Finally, memory permanence can be aided through neurogenesis.

PUTTING IT ALL TOGETHER

Memory depends on the operation of the nervous system, and its structure can be assessed using CT and MRI scans. Remembering involves multiple sites with changes in the nervous system during memory encoding, storage, and retrieval. Memory encoding involves changes in the dendrites of your neurons. This can be seen in changes in the firing rate of individual neurons using single cell recordings. Of course, neurons work together in cell assemblies, cortical nuclei, substructures, and networks, as with the default mode network.

Memory storage involves the process of consolidation. This includes synaptic consolidation in the hippocampus and systems consolidation across the cortex. Consolidated memories can be changed through disruptions, such as external electrical activity, as with ECT, or through normal processes, such as reconsolidation and neurogenesis.

Memory retrieval is observed by assessing changes in electrical activity and blood flow. Your brain's electrical activity can be assessed using EEG and MEG scans. EEG recordings can be used to assess ERP waves and changes in the neural (de)synchronization. We can measure changes in blood flow using PET and fMRI scans. Such measures reveal the brain areas that are important for memory processing, such as the temporal lobe, the hippocampus, the amygdala, the basal ganglia, and the diencephalon.

STUDY QUESTIONS

1. What are the basic components of a neuron?
2. How does the nervous system communicate information? What is the electrical component? What is the chemical component?
3. How do neurons change to store information in memory?
4. What are the lobes of the cortex and how are they involved in memory? What do characteristics, such as the default mode network, mean for how the cortical lobes work?
5. What is the hippocampus, and how is it critically involved in memory? What are other subcortical structures that have an influence on memory?
6. What are some of the various neuroimaging methods available? Which are good for assessing structure? Which are good for recording electrical activity? Which are good for recording blood flow?
7. What are some of the various neurostimulation methods available? How can they affect cortical activity?
8. In what ways can changes in brain structure be used to assess memory?

9. How do memories become more permanently stored in the brain?
10. What is the difference between the various types of consolidation, and what is the difference between consolidation and reconsolidation?
11. How does neurogenesis contribute to the formation of memories over long periods of time?

KEY TERMS

- Acetylcholine (Ach)
- action potential
- amygdala
- axons
- basal ganglia
- Brodmann Areas (BA)
- case studies
- cerebellum
- computer-assisted tomography (CT)
- consolidation, default mode network (DMN)
- dendrites
- diencephalon
- dopamine
- electroencephalography (EEG)
- emergent property
- event-related desynchronization (ERD)
- event-related potentials (ERP)
- event-related synchronization (ERS)
- frontal lobe
- functional magnetic resonance imaging (fMRI)
- GABA
- glutamate (Glu)
- hippocampus
- hypothalamus
- *intracranial electroencephalography* (iEEG)
- laterality
- long-term depression (LTD)
- long-term potentiation (LTP)
- magnetic resonance imaging (MRI)
- magnetoencephalography (MEG)
- myelin sheath
- neurogenesis
- neuron
- neurotransmitters
- nodes of Ranvier
- norepinephrine
- occipital lobeparietal lobe
- positron emission tomography (PET)
- reconsolidation
- single-cell recording
- soma
- special populations
- subtractive method
- synapse
- synaptic consolidation
- systems consolidation
- temporal lobe
- terminal buttons
- thalamus
- transcranial alternating current stimulation (tACS)
- transcranial direct current stimulation (tDCS)
- transcranial magnetic stimulation (TMS)
- transcranial random noise stimulation (tRNS)

EXPLORE MORE

Here are some additional readings that you can explore to provide you better insight into the neuroscience of memory.

Barry, D. N., & Maguire, E. A. (2019). Remote memory and the hippocampus: A constructive critique. *Trends in Cognitive Sciences, 23*(2), 128–142.

Bliss, T. V. P., & Collingridge, G. L. (1993). A synaptic model of memory: Long-term potentiation in the hippocampus. *Nature, 232*, 31–39.

Buckner, R. L., Andrews-Hanna, J. R., & Schacter, D. L. (2008). The brain's default network: Anatomy, function, and relevance to disease. *Annals of the New York Academy of Sciences, 1124*(1), 1–38.

McGaugh, J. L. (2000). Memory—a century of consolidation. *Science, 287*(5451), 248–251.

Meeter, M., & Murre, J. M. (2004). Consolidation of long-term memory: Evidence and alternatives. *Psychological Bulletin, 130*(6), 843–857.

Patihis, L. (2018). The historical significance of the discovery of long-term potentiation: An overview and evaluation for nonexperts. *American Journal of Psychology, 131*(3), 369–380.

Posner, M. I., & Raichle, M. E. (1994). *Images of Mind*. New York: Scientific American Library/Scientific American Books.

Ramachandran, V. S. (2012). *The Tell-Tale Brain: A Neuroscientist's Quest for What Makes Us Human*. New York: W. W. Norton.

REFERENCES

Abraham, W. C. (2006). Memory maintenance: The changing nature of neural mechanisms. *Psychological Science, 15*, 5–8.

Abraham, W. C., Logan, B., Greenwood, J. M., & Dragunow, M. (2002). Induction and experience-dependent consolidation of stable long-term potentiation lasting months in the hippocampus. *Journal of Neuroscience, 22*(21), 9626–9634.

Alberini, C. M. (2005). Mechanisms of memory stabilization: Are consolidation and reconsolidation similar or distinct processes? *Trends in Neurosciences, 28*(1), 51–56.

Alvarez, P., & Squire, L. R. (1994). Memory consolidation and the medial temporal lobe: A simple network model. *Proceedings of the National Academy of Sciences, 91*(15), 7041–7045.

Anderson, J. R., Borst, J. P., Fincham, J. M., Ghuman, A. S., Tenison, C., & Zhang, Q. (2018). The common time course of memory processes revealed. *Psychological Science, 29*(9), 1463–1474.

Andrews-Hanna, J. R. (2012). The brain's default network and its adaptive role in internal mentation. *The Neuroscientist, 18*(3), 251–270.

Andrews-Hanna, J. R., Smallwood, J., & Spreng, R. N. (2014). The default network and self-generated thought: Component processes, dynamic control, and clinical relevance. *Annals of the New York Academy of Sciences, 1316*(1), 29–52.

Badre, D., & Nee, D. E. (2018). Frontal cortex and the hierarchical control of behavior. *Trends in Cognitive Sciences, 22*(2), 170–188.

Barry, D. N., & Maguire, E. A. (2019). Remote memory and the hippocampus: A constructive critique. *Trends in Cognitive Sciences, 23*(2), 128–142.

Bayliss, D. M., Bogdanovs, J., & Jarrold, C. (2015). Consolidating working memory: Distinguishing the effects of consolidation, rehearsal and attentional refreshing in a working memory span task. *Journal of Memory and Language, 81*, 34–50.

Behrendt, R-P. (2013). Conscious experience and episodic memory: Hippocampus at the crossroads. *Frontiers in Psychology, 4*, 304.

Bentin, S. (1989). Electrophysiological studies of visual word perception, lexical organization, and semantic processing: A tutorial review. *Language and Speech, 32*, 205–220.

Ben-Yakov, A., Eshel, N., & Dudai, Y. (2013). Hippocampal immediate poststimulus activity in the encoding of consecutive naturalistic episodes. *Journal of Experimental Psychology: General, 142*, 1255–1263.

Blakemore, C., & Cooper, G. F. (1970). Development of the brain depends on the visual environment. *Nature, 228,* 477–478.

Bliss, T. V. P., & Collingridge, G. L. (1993). A synaptic model of memory: Long-term potentiation in the hippocampus. *Nature, 232,* 31–39.

Bliss, T. V. P., & Lomo, T. (1973). Long-lasting potentiation of synaptic transmission in the dentate area of the anaesthetized rabbit following stimulations of the perforant path. *Journal of Physiology, 232,* 331–356.

Buckner, R. L., Andrews-Hanna, J. R., & Schacter, D. L. (2008). The brain's default network: Anatomy, function, and relevance to disease. *Annals of the New York Academy of Sciences, 1124*(1), 1–38.

Carr, M. F., Jadhav, S. P., & Frank, L. M. (2011). Hippocampal replay in the awake state: A potential substrate for memory consolidation and retrieval. *Nature Neuroscience, 14*(2), 147–153.

Casasanto, D., & Jasmin, K. (2010). Good and bad in the hands of politicians: Spontaneous gestures during positive and negative speech. *PLoS One, 5*(7), e11805.

Coles, M. G. H., Gratton, G., & Fabiani, M. (1990). Event-related brain potentials. In J. T. Cacioppo & L. G. Tassinary (Eds.), *Principles of Psychophysiology: Physical, Social, and Inferential Elements* (pp. 413–455). Cambridge, UK: Cambridge University Press.

Davis, M. (1997) Neurobiology of fear responses: The role of the amygdala. *Journal of Neuropsychiatry, 9,* 382–402.

de-Wit, L., Alexander, D., Ekroll, V., & Wagemans, J. (2016). Is neuroimaging measuring information in the brain? *Psychonomic Bulletin & Review, 23*(5), 1415–1428.

Doppelmayr, M. M., Klimesch, W., Pachinger, T., & Ripper, B. (1998). The functional significance of absolute power with respect to event-related desynchronization. *Brain Topography, 11,* 133–140.

Duffy, S., Labrie, V., & Roder, J. C. (2008). D-serine augments NMDA-NR2B receptor-dependent hippocampal long-term depression and spatial reversal learning. *Neuropsychopharmacology, 33,* 1004–1018.

Emptage, N. J., Reid, C. A., Fine, A., & Bliss, T. V. P. (2003). Optical quantal analysis reveals a presynaptic component of LTP at hippocampal Schaffer-associational synapses. *Neuron, 38,* 797–804.

Fellin, T., Halassa, M. M., Terunuma, M., Succol, F., Takano, H., Frank, M. G., Moss S. J., & Haydon, P. G. (2009). Endogenous nonneuronal modulators of synaptic transmission control cortical slow oscillations in vivo. *Proceedings of the National Academy of Sciences, 106*(35), 15037–15042.

Fenn, K. M., & Hambrick, D. Z. (2013). What drives sleep-dependent memory consolidation: Greater gain or less loss? *Psychonomic Bulletin & Review, 20*(3), 501–506.

Forcato, C., Burgos, V. L., Argibay, P. F., Molina, V. A., Pedreira, M. E., & Maldonado, H. (2007). Reconsolidation of declarative memory in humans. *Learning & Memory, 14*(4), 295–303.

Fox, K. C. R., Foster, B. L., Kucyi, A., Daitch, A. L., & Parvizi, J. (2018). Intracranial electrophysiology of the human default network. *Trends in Cognitive Sciences, 22*(4), 307–324.

Gage, F. H. (2002). Neurogenesis in the adult brain. *The Journal of Neuroscience, 22*(3), 612–613.

Hafting, T., Fyhn, M., Molden, S., Moser, M. B., & Moser, E. I. (2005). Microstructure of a spatial map in the entorhinal cortex. *Nature, 436*(7052), 801–806.

Hassabis, D., Kumaran, D., Vann, S. D., & Maguire, E. A. (2007). Patients with hippocampal amnesia cannot imagine new experiences. *Proceedings of the National Academy of Sciences of the United States of America, 104,* 1726–1731.

Hasson, U., Furman, O., Clark, D., Dudai, Y., & Davachi, L. (2008). Enhanced intersubject correlations during movie viewing correlate with successful episodic encoding. *Neuron, 57*(3), 452–462.

Hebscher, M., Wing, E., Ryan, J., & Gilboa, A. (2019). Rapid cortical plasticity supports long-term memory formation. *Trends in Cognitive Sciences, 23*(12), 989–1002.

Herweg, N. A., Solomon, E. A., & Kahana, M. J. (2020). Theta oscillations in human memory. *Trends in Cognitive Sciences, 24*(3), 208–227.

Howard, M. W., & Eichenbaum, H. (2013). The hippocampus, time, and memory across scales. *Journal of Experimental Psychology: General, 142,* 1211–1230.

Hubel, D. H., & Wiesel, T. N. (1965). Receptive fields and functional architecture in two nonstriate visual areas (18 and 19) of the cat. *Journal of neurophysiology, 28*(2), 229–289.

Karlsson, M. P., & Frank, L. M. (2009). Awake replay of remote experiences in the hippocampus. *Nature Neuroscience, 12*(7), 913–918.

Kim, M. S., Kim, J. C., & Chung, C. K. (2008). Neural correlates of immediate and delayed word recognition memory: An MEG study. *Brain Research, 1240*, 132–142.

Kirschen, M. P., Davis-Ratner, M. S., Jerde, T. E., Schraedley-Desmond, P., & Desmond, J. E. (2006). Enhancement of phonological memory following Transcranial Magnetic Stimulation (TMS). *Behavioural Neurology, 17*, 187–194.

Klimesch, W. (1999). EEG alpha and theta oscillations reflect cognitive and memory performance: A review and analysis. *Brain Research Reviews, 29*, 169–195.

Klimesch, W. (2012). Alpha-band oscillations, attention, and controlled access to stored information. *Trends in Cognitive Sciences, 16*(12), 606–617.

Lerner, Y., Honey, C. J., Silbert, L. J., & Hasson, U. (2011). Topographic mapping of a hierarchy of temporal receptive windows using a narrated story. *The Journal of Neuroscience, 31*(8), 2906–2915.

Lo, J. C., Dijk, D. J., & Groeger, J. A. (2014). Comparing the effects of nocturnal sleep and daytime napping on declarative memory consolidation. *PLOS:One, 9*(9), e108100.

Loftus, E. F., & Loftus, G. R. (1980). On the permanence of stored information in the human brain. *American Psychologist, 35*, 409–420.

Maguire, E. A., & Mullally, S. L. (2013). The hippocampus: A manifesto for change. *Journal of Experimental Psychology: General, 142*, 1180–1189.

Mahut, H., Zola-Morgan, S., & Moss, M. (1982). Hippocampal resections impair associative learning and recognition memory in the monkey. *The Journal of Neuroscience, 2*, 1214–1229.

McGaugh, J. L. (2000). Memory—a century of consolidation. *Science, 287*(5451), 248–251.

McNerney, M. W., & Radvansky, G. A. (2015). Mind racing: The influence of exercise on long-term memory consolidation. *Memory, 23*, 1140–1151.

Meeter, M., & Murre, J. M. (2004). Consolidation of long-term memory: Evidence and alternatives. *Psychological Bulletin, 130*(6), 843–857.

Minsky, M. L. (1986). *The Society of Mind*. New York: Simon & Schuster.

Mishkin, M., & Appenzeller, T. (1987). The anatomy of memory. *Scientific American, 256*, 80–89.

Moreau, D., & Chou, E. (2019). The acute effect of high-intensity exercise on executive function: A meta-analysis. *Perspectives on Psychological Science, 14*(5), 734–764.

Nadel, L., & Moscovitch, M. (1997). Memory consolidation, retrograde amnesia and the hippocampal complex. *Current Opinion in Neurobiology, 7*(2), 217–227.

Nader, K., Schafe, G. E., & LeDoux, J. E. (2000). Reply—Reconsolidation: The labile nature of consolidation theory. *Nature Reviews Neuroscience, 1*(3), 216–219.

Nicoll, R. A. (2017). A brief history of long-term potentiation. *Neuron, 93*(2), 281–290.

O'Keefe, J., & Dostrovsky, J. (1971). The hippocampus as a spatial map: Preliminary evidence from unit activity in freely-moving rat. *Brain Research, 34*, 171–175.

Patihis, L. (2018). The historical significance of the discovery of long-term potentiation: An overview and evaluation for nonexperts. *American Journal of Psychology, 131*(3), 369–380.

Penfield, W. (1955). The permanent record of the stream of consciousness. *Acta Psychologica, 11*, 47–69.

Pinto-Duarte, A., Roberts, A. J., Ouyang, K., & Sejnowski, T. J. (2019). Impairments in remote memory caused by the lack of Type 2 IP3 receptors. *Glia, 67*(10), 1976–1989.

Posner, M. I., & Raichle, M. E. (1994). *Images of Mind*. Scientific American Library/Scientific American Books.

Rasch, B., & Born, J. (2008). Reactivation and consolidation of memory during sleep. *Current Directions in Psychological Science, 17*(3), 188–192.

Reinhart, R. M. G., Cosman, J. D., Fukuda, K., & Woodman, G. F. (2017). Using transcranial direct-current stimulation (tDCS) to understand cognitive processing. *Attention, Perception, & Psychophysics, 79*(1), 3–23.

Ribot, T. A. (1882). *Diseases of Memory: An Essay in the Positive Psychology*. London: Kegan Paul & Trench.

Robertson, E. M., & Takacs, A. (2017). Exercising control over memory consolidation. *Trends in Cognitive Sciences, 21*(5), 310–312.

Schwabe, L., & Wolf, O. T. (2009). New episodic learning interferes with the reconsolidation of autobiographical memories. *PLoS One, 4*(10), e7519.

Shadmehr, R., & Holcomb, H. H. (1997). Neural correlates of motor memory consolidation. *Science, 277*(5327), 821–825.

Shors, T. J. (2014). The adult brain makes new neurons, and effortful learning keeps them alive. *Current Directions in Psychological Science, 23*, 311–318.

Solstad, T., Boccara, C. N., Kropff, E., Moser, M. B., & Moser, E. I. (2008). Representation of geometric borders in the entorhinal cortex. *Science, 322*(5909), 1865–1868.

Stickgold, R. (2005). Sleep-dependent memory consolidation. *Nature, 437*(7063), 1272–1278.

Suthana, N., & Fried, I. (2012). Percepts to recollections: Insights from single neuron recordings in the human brain. *Trends in Cognitive Sciences, 16*(8), 427–436.

Takashima, A., Nieuwenhuis, I. L. C., Jensen, O., Talamini, L. M., Rijpkema, M., & Fernández, G. (2009). Shift from hippocampal to neocortical centered retrieval network with consolidation. *The Journal of Neuroscience, 29*(32), 10087–10093.

Tambini, A., & Davachi, L. (2019). Awake reactivation of prior experiences consolidates memories and biases cognition. *Trends in Cognitive Sciences, 23*(10), 876–890.

Tomporowski, P. D., & Pesce, C. (2019). Exercise, sports, and performance arts benefit cognition via a common process. *Psychological Bulletin, 145*(9), 929–951.

Voss, M. W., Vivar, C., Kramer, A. F., & van Praag, H. (2013). Bridging animal and human models of exercise-induced brain plasticity. *Trends in Cognitive Sciences, 17*(10), 525–544.

Wamsley, E. J., Tucker, M., Payne, J. D., Benavides, J. A., & Stickgold, R. (2010). Dreaming of a learning task is associated with enhanced sleep-dependent memory consolidation. *Current Biology, 20*(9), 850–855.

Weems, C. F., Russell, J. D., Banks, D. M., Graham, R. A., Neill, E. L., & Scott, B. G. (2014). Memories of traumatic events in childhood fade after experiencing similar less stressful events: Results from two natural experiments. *Journal of Experimental Psychology: General, 143*(5), 2046–2055.

Wood, N. E., Rosasco, M. L., Suris, A. M., Spring, J. D., Marin, M. F., Lasko, N. B., Goetz, J. M., Fischer, A. M., Orr, S. P., & Pitman, R. K. (2015). Pharmacological blockade of memory reconsolidation in posttraumatic stress disorder: Three negative psychophysiological studies. *Psychiatry Research, 225*(1), 31–39.

Zhu, Z., Wang, Y., Cao, Z., Chen, B., Cai, H., Wu, Y., & Rao, Y. (2016). Cue-independent memory impairment by reactivation-coupled interference in human declarative memory. *Cognition, 155*, 125–134.

CHAPTER 3

Methods and Principles

Memory is an intimate part of who we are. However, we have little conscious awareness of it. Intuitively, memory seems very ethereal. As noted in Chapter 1, for most of history, memory was thought to be beyond objective study. It was not until the late nineteenth century that it was systematically studied. Because it is impossible to get a direct look at memory, we need reliable methods to measure and test it. We need *empirical evidence* of memory representations and processes. These methods often involve an experimenter manipulating what is to be remembered, recording an act of remembering, and then making inferences about memory based on what is observed. This may sound artificial, but it is not unlike how other sciences proceed or how we conduct our day-to-day lives. For example, astronomers looking at computer readings can draw conclusions about planets circling distant stars without ever laying eyes on them.

In this chapter we first address what an experiment is and how it compares to other types of data collection. Then we examine various methods of memory research. We first look at the learning situation, followed by tasks that can be used to test memory. Finally, we consider issues of conscious introspection. Along with these methods we look at some basic, well-established principles of memory whose discovery can be attributed, at least in part, to these methods. For those interested students, ways of calculating some memory measures, perhaps for a laboratory section or a research project, are provided in the Appendix.

COMPONENTS OF MEMORY RESEARCH

We approach memory from a scientific perspective to gain an objective understanding and minimize subjective biases. The ideas about memory covered here reflect the work of scientists. To help you understand how these people do their job, we first discuss just what an experiment is and the different types of variables a researcher measures and controls.

What Is an Experiment?

Most of our scientific knowledge about memory comes from experiments. So, just what *is* an experiment? An **experiment** is a controlled situation in which a researcher manipulates variables of interest, measuring the effect of this manipulation, while controlling for irrelevant variables. Furthermore, participants are randomly assigned to conditions to reduce any unwanted systematicity. Let's unpack what the components of an experiment are and what they mean.

In an experiment, there are two variables of primary interest: the independent variable and the dependent variable. The **independent variable** is the variable that is being manipulated by the researcher. Independent variables in a memory experiment might be how much information people have to remember, how long they have to remember it, and so on. For example, suppose you are doing an experiment in which you want to know whether students learn better by studying consistently throughout a week or by cramming right before they are tested. In this experiment the independent variable is the type of studying. You would randomly assign people to two conditions. Condition A would be studying consistently, and Condition B would be cramming. Because these variables are being manipulated gives the researcher a great deal of control. In our example, you can be confident that the memory differences you observed are due to how people studied because you manipulated this independent variable.

The other variable of primary interest is the **dependent variable**, the one being measured. Dependent variables in a memory experiment might be how much is remembered, how accurate the memories are, how fast they are remembered, and so

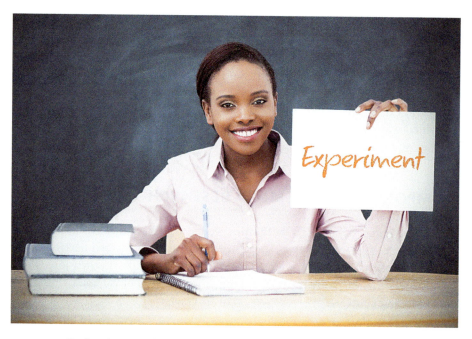

PHOTO 3.1 *Performing experiments is critical to an objective and accurate understanding of human memory*

Source: wavebreakmedia/Shutterstock.com

on. Continuing our example, to assess whether studying consistently or cramming results in better memory, you might use the number of correct answers on a multiple-choice test as your dependent variable. You could then see whether people score higher in Condition A or Condition B.[1] Different dependent variables have different advantages and disadvantages. Which one is selected in an experiment is a function of what theory or ideas are being tested.

Irrelevant aspects of the situation are **control variables**. A control variable is any aspect of the experiment that could potentially have an impact on the observed results but is not a factor of interest. Control variables can include things such as the room lighting, the instructions, the apparatus used, and so on. For example, suppose for a learning study if people in Condition A are always tested in room 261, and people in Condition B are always tested in room 265, and room is not a variable of interest in the study. Here there is an unwanted systematicity, and the results would be problematic because conditions are confounded with testing room. You did not adequately account for a control variable. This could have been controlled for by having half of the people in each group tested in each of the rooms. A good experimenter makes sure that control variables are not confounded with the independent variables to ensure that the results are interpretable.

Other Types of Studies

An experiment is not the only way to gather data about memory. Other methods are suitable when experimental control is difficult or impossible. One alternative is a **correlation** study, where the performance of a dependent measure is assessed as a function of some preexisting factors. For example, you can look at memory as a function of age. Age cannot be experimentally controlled, but it is information that can be used to make inferences about memory.

Alternatively, a researcher may do a **quasi-experiment** in which preexisting conditions are combined with the controlled assignment of independent variables—for example, suppose there are age groups, college students and older adults. Half of the people in each age group are put in a condition in which they study consistently throughout the week, and the rest learn by cramming. Here, people's ages are a preexisting condition, but the assignment of study group is manipulated as it would be in an experiment.

Finally, in some situations, it is not possible to assess large numbers of people. Instead, a researcher can do a **case study**. When we look at the effects of brain damage, we may test memory in specific people because they are the only ones with a specific type of deficit.

Theories and Hypotheses

To study memory, a researcher should have a theory of how it works or at least some part of it. A **theory** is a principled explanation for how some process in the world is structured or operates. For example, a theory of gravity is an explanation for how gravity works. A theory of evolution is an explanation of how evolution unfolds. A

---

1 What you would find is that people who study consistently score higher than people who cram.

theory of memory is an explanation of how memory works. Scientifically, saying that something is theoretical does not necessarily mean that the phenomenon is hypothetical. No rational person would question the existence of human memory. Instead, saying that something is a theory of a phenomenon means that it is an explanation of it. Of course, a theory can be wrong or have elements that are incorrect, but this does not deny that there is a phenomenon in the world to be explained.

In memory research, theories can be broad and encompass large aspects of memory, or they can be narrow and focus on explanations of a specific phenomenon. What kind of theory is used is a function of the researchers' goals and the need to keep things tractable. Memory and cognition are incredibly complex. It is nearly impossible to track every aspect of memory when doing any given experiment. Part of this comes from the fact that for a given task, not every memory representation and process that people have is going to come into play. For example, if you are trying to remember if a word was on a list that you studied, your memory for how to play the piano is unlikely to be of much importance. Thus, sometimes memory researchers are better off using mini theories that focus on particular aspects of a process that are of interest.

Using a theory, one can derive a hypothesis about the outcome of a study. A **hypothesis** is an educated guess or prediction about how variations of an independent variable are related to the outcome of the dependent variables. Typically, this is cast in theoretical language about how memory is operating in the context of the experiment. It is often advantageous not to test a single hypothesis, but to put two or more hypotheses in competition, each derived from different theories. In doing so, we can distinguish between those theories and decide which account is closer to the truth. In this way, we can accept some theories, reject others, or, in some cases, modify existing theories to better capture the patterns observed in the data.

Stop and Review

There are a variety of ways to study memory. The most common way is do an experiment in which you have control over the variables of interest and can better assess what is affecting the outcome. The independent variables are what are manipulated, the dependent variables are what are measured, and the control variables are factors that could affect the outcome, so are either held constant or randomly varied. In addition to experiments, you can do correlational, quasi-experimental, and case studies. These allow for tests of memory under circumstances where some factors cannot be explicitly manipulated. Finally, scientific studies require theories to provide explanations. From these theories you can derive hypotheses. Studies provide the data to support or refute theories or encourage theory modification.

ASPECTS OF LEARNING

To properly assess memory, some information must first be learned. How this happens is important. Was the material something that was consciously learned, or was it something that was just picked up along the way? What kind of information was it, visual or verbal?

Intentional versus Incidental Learning

Methods. An important factor is whether people explicitly *try* to learn. Explicit memorization is called **intentional learning**. The alternative is that people just happen to learn something during the course of other activities. This is called **incidental learning**. Intentional learning is when you study for this or any other class. Incidental learning is knowledge that you have picked up without having to try, such as knowing how many movies you have seen in the past month.

An experimenter can explicitly alert people that they are going to test people for their memory of the material. These intentional learning instructions are direct, and they lead people to treat information more elaboratively. This can involve building upon the information in some way, such as making inferences or creating mental images. Elaborative processing profoundly affects memory. Alternatively, if an experimenter gives incidental memory instructions, they have people attend to and think about the information but not expend any extra effort memorizing it. In such cases, a cover task is given to orient people to the material. These cover tasks vary, and can include things such as pleasantness ratings, sensibility ratings, or sorting items into categories. Thus, these cover tasks direct attention to the material, allowing for the possibility for it to be stored in memory even though people do not actively memorize it.

Principles. Memory is often better with intentional than incidental learning (Block, 2009). This section outlines principles of memory that demonstrate the importance of the type of learning: levels of processing, mental imagery, the generation effect, and the automaticity of encoding.

An influence of effort exerted during memorization is illustrated by the **levels of processing** framework (Craik & Lockhart, 1972). This refers to the degree to which people elaborate on information during study. When people try to learn, they may simply repeat the information over and over. This is called **rote rehearsal**. In general, recall memory does not improve much with rote rehearsal, and recognition is only slightly improved (Glenberg et al., 1977). The results of a study by Nickerson and Adams (1979) are an example of the poor effectiveness of rote rehearsal. In this study, students at Brown University were shown drawings of pennies like those in Figure 3.1. They were asked to indicate whether each was correct. These students had seen thousands of pennies during their lives. See if you can identify which penny is the correct one. Students in this study were able to identify the correct drawing only 50% of the time. The penny that had the highest rate of acceptance (67%) was an incorrect version.[2] Thus, repeated exposure alone does not improve memory.

In contrast, the more people actively think about the meaning of information, the more likely they are to use knowledge that they already have, making inferences and elaborating on the to-be-learned information. This connecting and generation of knowledge to build on what is given is called **elaborative rehearsal**.

Information that receives little elaboration is processed less. For example, suppose a task is to think about a set of words and only say whether each is printed in upper- or lower-case letters. This is shallow processing because it requires little attention

---

2 See Blake et al. (2015) for a replication of this finding with the Apple Computer logo, and Vendetti et al. (2013) for memory of frequently used elevator buttons.

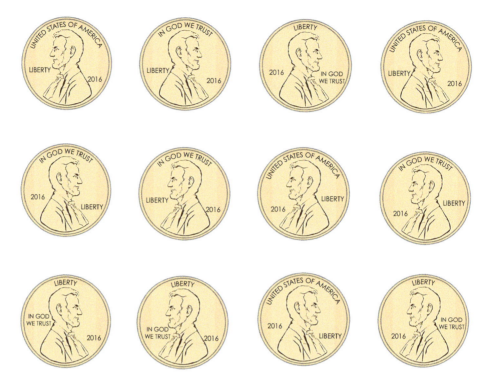

FIGURE 3.1 *Which Penny Is the Correct One?*

Source: adapted from Nickerson, R. S., & Adams, M. J. (1979). Long-term memory for a common object. *Cognitive Psychology, 11*, 287–307

to meaning and prior knowledge. However, if the task is to determine whether the word makes sense in a sentence, this is deeper processing. In some sense, shallow processing evokes more incidental learning, whereas elaborative processing is more like intentional learning, although there may not be an overt effort to memorize. The levels of processing effect occur for both incidental and intentional encoding (Hyde & Jenkins, 1973), although it is more likely to be seen with intentional learning.

One way to elaborate on information, and engage in deeper processing, is to use **mental imagery** to create a mental picture of what is being learned. As an example, to remember that you need to get some green peppers and a loaf of bread at the grocery store, you might form a mental image of a green pepper sandwich. Mental images improve memory (Schnorr & Atkinson, 1969), as shown in Figure 3.2, in this case for students at Stanford University. Memories are better when you form mental images than when you simply rehearse the information. You need to make an effort to form mental images. They do not appear spontaneously.

The benefit to memory of mental images led to the development of **Dual Code theory** (Paivio, 1969). According to this view, people store information in memory in at least two forms: a verbal/linguistic code of what they are reading or hearing and a mental image code that they create from their imaginations. These two codes can be associated if they refer to the same thing. One is a verbal code for the words that were read, and the other is an image code of the mental picture

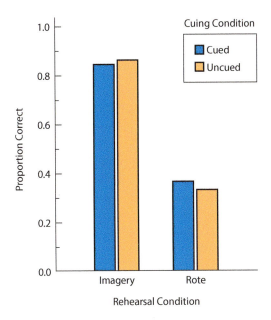

FIGURE 3.2 *Impact of Mental Imagery on Later Memory*

Source: created from data reported in Schnorr, J. A., & Atkinson, R. C. (1969). Repetition versus imagery instructions in the short- and long-term retention of paired-associates. *Psychonomic Science, 15*, 183–184.

that was created. Memory improves because there are multiple retrieval pathways to the same information and more memory traces containing the desired information. This makes successful remembering more likely.

For the levels of processing framework, the more information is elaborated upon, the better it is remembered. This is also shown by the **generation effect**: information that a person generates is remembered better than material that is simply read or heard (Slamecka & Graf, 1978; see Bertsch et al., 2007, for a meta-analysis). For example, suppose people are presented with a series of word stems, such as TAB_____, with the task of completing the word. This is a generation task because people generate the rest of the information. Alternatively, if they simply read a series of complete words, nothing is being created. As a more everyday example of the generation effect, think of your conversations from the past week. What do you remember best from them? Typically, it will be the things that you said. This is because you generated those statements.

A generation effect is also observed when people solve a puzzle or a problem. This is called the **"aha" effect** (Auble, et al., 1979). For example, you may have trouble initially understanding a sentence such as "The man's back ached because the ends were too large." At some point, there is an awareness that this sentence is about using barbells and you have an "aha" experience. Because people generated their own solutions, memory is better.

In addition to generating words and ideas, memory is better when we actually perform a task rather than watch someone else do it or read about it. This is the **enactment effect** (Engelkamp & Zimmer, 1989). Like the generation and "aha" effects, this involves elaborative rehearsal (Senkfor et al., 2008). Any type of performed action seems to produce a benefit and take advantage of embodied aspects of cognition. Moreover, we are mentally organizing and structuring information when we perform the action (Koriat & Pearlman-Avnion, 2003). However, this memory benefit only occurs when people enact only some of the items, not all of them (Dodd & Shumborski, 2009), suggesting that there is some distinctiveness to enactment. If people enact all of the items, then none of them are distinctive from the rest.

A cousin of the enactment effect is the **production effect** (MacLeod, et al., 2010; see Fawcett, 2013 for a meta-analysis), in which people are asked either to say aloud what they are trying to learn or to read it silently. Generally, we remember more if we read things aloud (we "produce" them) than if we do not. The production effect is not limited to saying things aloud. It can also occur if people mouth the material, whisper it, write it, or even type it (Forrin et al., 2012). However, the results are best when things are said aloud. The production effect is due to several factors, including the elaboration and distinctiveness that comes with producing something (Forrin & MacLeod, 2018).

A production effect is also observed when we make even simple drawings of things (Fernandes et al., 1989; Wammes et al., 2016). The superior memory from drawings is shown in Figure 3.3. By drawing we are both elaborating on the information and capitalizing on the benefits of visual memory.

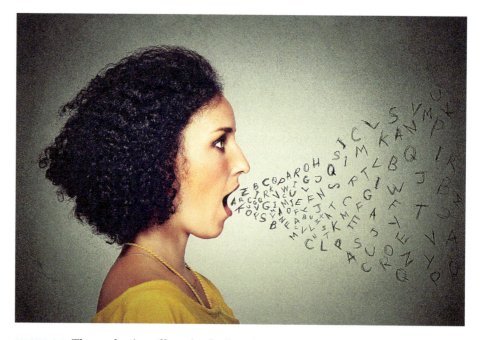

PHOTO 3.2 *The production effect, the finding that saying things aloud, or even writing them down, can improve memory, shows the importance of going beyond simple reading*

Source: pathdoc/Shutterstock.com

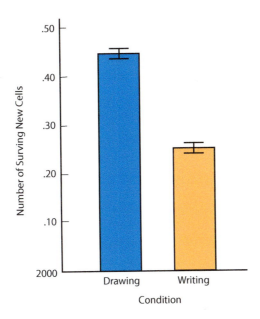

FIGURE 3.3 *Influence of Drawing Versus Writing on Later Memory*

Source: created from data reported in Wammes, J. D., Meade, M. E., & Fernandes, M. A. (2016). The drawing effect: Evidence for reliable and robust memory benefits in free recall. *Quarterly Journal of Experimental Psychology, 69*, 1752–1776.

Overall, doing something with the information aids memory. So long as you engage with the information, you will remember it better. Even the simple act of making a choice (e.g., which of the following is a sport: *tennis* or *toast*?) can boost memory (Coverdale & Nairne, 2019; Perlmuter et al., 1971).

It should be noted that, under some conditions, the type of learning does not matter much. Memory is similar with incidental and intentional encoding, depending on how people thought about the information at the time (Postman & Adams, 1956) and intentional/incidental effects may not be present with certain memory tests, such as recognition (Eagle & Leiter, 1964). In some cases, there is an **automaticity of encoding** (Hasher & Zacks, 1979; 1984) in which information is remembered with little effort. With automatic encoding, further efforts at learning do not provide much additional benefit. Information that is more automatically encoded includes event frequency, time, and location. For example, think of how many times in the past month you have eaten out. The answer comes to mind easily, and it is unlikely that you deliberately learned this as it was occurring. If you think about the knowledge that you have, some of it was very easy to learn, whereas some of it was learned only with a great deal of effort.

Finally, there are cases where incidental encoding leads to better memory than intentional encoding. In a study by Helbing et al. (2020), students at Goethe University Frankfurt navigated virtual environments (e.g., kitchen, bathroom, office etc.) with the goal of either *memorizing* certain objects in the space (intentional) or simply *searching* and finding those objects (incidental). Memory was better when people searched for objects compared to when they tried to memorize them. Thus, cognition is tuned to encoding into memory those items that are consistent with our goals as part of our everyday interactions.

Improve Your Memory

This chapter provides a wealth of information about how to improve your memory using basic principles that we covered here. For example, using the depth of processing framework as a guide, you have learned that the more you exert some effort to deeply process information, the more you will remember later. This can be done by elaborating on the material that you are trying to learn, forming mental images of items covered, acting things out if you can, or at least saying things aloud or writing them down, and so on. A good step that you can take to achieve this is to write a summary of the class material after you have completed your readings or listened to a lecture. This provides more organization of the information, causing you to mentally elaborate on it, leading to better memory, and reducing the amount of study time you will need later. The more often you do this with the material, the more overlearning there will be, the stronger your memories will be, and the better you will do in your courses. This sounds like a lot of extra work. However, most of the extra work is done up front. By taking these steps, you may exert less work on the whole, possibly leading you to spend less time studying overall because you are being more efficient and effective with the time that you do have.

Stop and Review

When exploring memory, one thing that you need to consider is whether the material was learned intentionally or incidentally. The levels of processing framework is oriented around the idea that how much attention and processing a set of information receives during learning affects later memory. The more deeply that information is processed, the better it will be remembered later. Various ways to deeply process materials include forming mental images as well as generating and producing information. Finally, some types of information are more automatically encoded into memory. In these cases, intentional encoding does not improve memory much beyond what is learned more spontaneously and incidentally.

Material Characteristics

During learning, it is possible to manipulate not only what people are doing but also the nature of the materials. As has already been mentioned, some types of knowledge are easy to learn and remember. In contrast, others require more effort, and are more likely to be forgotten.

Methods. It is important to take into consideration what research participants think about the experiment. An adequate **task analysis** is needed. If not, it is possible that the researcher and the participant may interpret the task in different ways. What an experimenter thinks the participant is memorizing is the **nominal stimulus**. The stimulus the participant identifies and thinks about is the **functional stimulus**. Usually, these are the same thing, but in some cases, they are very different. For example, a researcher might give people a list of nonsense syllables, one of them "DAX." In the experimenter's mind, this is a meaningless series of letters. However, if the participant is an avid *Star Trek* fan, he or she would recognize this as the name of a character in the series.

Principles. Memory can vary depending on the nature of the materials being memorized. This section outlines principles that have been derived from studies with different materials, including the principle of savings, the influence of using pictures and concrete materials compared to verbal and abstract materials, and the roles of emotion and frequency on memory.

Materials affect memory in a few ways. One of these, discovered by Ebbinghaus (1885), is the principle of **savings**. After information has been learned and forgotten, people require less effort to learn it a second time. For example, if it took you ten repetitions to learn something the first time and only three repetitions the second time, this would be a saving of seven. The principle of savings is important for two reasons. First, this nicely illustrates the fact that although we may not be consciously aware of knowledge from our past, it may still affect our ability to learn and remember. Second, it shows that information we are already familiar with, even if we are not conscious of it, is easier to remember than something we encounter for the first time. In general, the more information taps into our prior knowledge, the easier it is to remember. Thus, the meaning of a stimulus varies from person to person depending on the individual's experiences with it.

In general, human are visual animals. As such, it is not surprising that pictures are remembered extremely well (Brady et al., 2008; Shepard, 1967; Standing, 1973), even when they are learned incidentally (Goetschalckx et al., 2019). A similar finding is observed with videos (Ferguson et al., 2017). This is the **picture superiority effect**. It occurs because we are better attuned to processing perceptual than linguistic information. Also, a picture is more likely to be unique and contain a higher degree of detail. Consider a study by Fioravanti & Di Cesare (1992) in which people were either tested for memory for short narratives or pictures of animals and objects. The result, shown in Figure 3.4, was that memory was better for pictures than stories, and this benefit was still present two days later.

However, even pictures can vary in how easily they are remembered depending on how meaningful they are (Goetschalckx et al., 2018). For example, people find it easier to remember pictures of faces than pictures of snowflakes or inkblots (Goldstein & Chance, 1970). Moreover, the picture superiority effect is magnified with dynamic images (e.g., video) over static images (Matthews et al. 2007).[3] That said, pictures memory is detailed initially, but becomes more gist-like over time (Gloede & Gregg, 2019), with people remembering only general things (e.g., it was a chair sitting in a stream).

---

3 See Crutcher and Beer (2011) for an auditory analog to the picture superiority effect, and Hutmacher and Kuhbandner (2018) and Pensky et al. (2008) for a haptic (touch) analog.

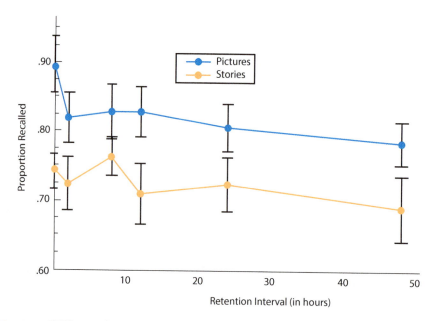

FIGURE 3.4 *Difference between Memory for Pictures and for Stories, as Well as How This Changes over Time*

Source: created from data reported in Fioravanti, M., & Di Cesare, F. (1992). Forgetting curves in long-term memory: Evidence for a multistage model of retention. *Brain and Cognition, 18*(2), 116–124.

Pictures and words are treated differently by memory, even at a neurological level. The right hippocampus is more active for processing pictures, whereas the left is more active for words (Papanicolaou, et al., 2002). Furthermore, using fMRI, Vaidya et al. (2002) found that during the encoding of pictures there is bilateral activation of the fusiform area (BA 37), the lingual–medial occipital lobe (BA 18, 19), and the inferior temporal gyrus (BA 20). Moreover, a subset of these areas, namely the fusiform area and the inferior temporal gyrus is also activated during retrieval for items studied as pictures, even if the memory probes are words. Thus, the picture superiority effect reflects the use of a broader range of brain regions.

Related to the picture superiority effects, and also emphasizing the role of perceptual information, it has also been found that concrete materials—words like "car," "house," or "book"—are remembered better than abstract materials— words like "truth," "betrayal," or "redemption." This is the **concreteness effect**. Concreteness aids memory because it involves more perceptual qualities: concrete information is more likely to have an additional image code. This distinction between concrete and abstract information is supported neurologically. Concrete words are associated with greater basal extrastriate cortex activation (BA 19), suggesting more perceptual processing (although there is some involvement of abstract information as well; Martin-Loeches et al., 2001). Finally, there is greater activation of the right hemisphere for concrete words, whereas abstract words tend to involve more left hemisphere processing (Kounios & Holcomb, 1994).

Memory can also be influenced by **emotions**. Emotional memories are often better remembered than neutral memories (Kensinger, 2009). That said, the benefit of emotion on memory is often not observed immediately but appears after a delay (e.g., Anderson et al., 2006; Kleinsmith & Kaplan, 1963), such as an hour, a day, or a week.

Emotional memories are more vivid and contain more detail (Kensinger & Corkin, 2003). Emotional information, over the long term, seems to be preferred for consolidation during sleep (Payne & Kensinger, 2010). Less emotionally intense emotions tend to involve an influence of the frontal lobes (LaBar & Cabeza, 2006), whereas more intense emotions, involve an influence of the amygdala. This then carries over and affects memory functioning in the hippocampus and medial temporal lobes, perhaps because the amygdala helps direct attention to more emotionally relevant aspects of the world, although this may come at a cost to less emotional details (Mather, 2007). More emotionally intense events may affect memory because of their more primitive, visceral, and survival-based qualities. In contrast, emotional, but less intense, events may influence memory based on their seeming importance.

In addition to emotional intensity, memory may be affected by emotional valence. That is, whether something is emotionally positive (e.g., "courage") or negative (e.g., "ordeal"). According to the **Pollyanna principle**, there is a tendency to better remember positive than negative information. For example, positive words are learned faster than negative words (Anisfeld & Lambert, 1966; Stagner, 1933). However, there are circumstances where negative information is remembered better (Ortony et al., 1983), such as with flashbulb memories for surprising, and often negative, events (see Chapter 12). Negative words are learned faster than emotionally neutral words (like "wood") (Carter, 1936; Carter et al., 1934). Finally, relative to neutral information, negative memories are more likely to benefit from consolidation during sleep (Payne et al., 2008).

Returning to the idea of concrete and abstract information, while it is clear that concrete information is embodied via sensory experience (e.g., what a "barn" looks like), abstract concepts may be embodied because they may elicit emotions (e.g., "trust" may elicit a positive emotion) (e.g., Casasanto, 2009). Abstract and emotional materials show similar patterns of memory over time. For example, a study by Butter (1970) assessed memory for paired associates in which the cue words were concrete versus abstract, or emotional versus neutral. The results, shown in Figure 3.5, were that while memory for concrete and neutral cues show a decline, abstract and emotional cues actually improved.

Another quality that can affect memory is event **frequency**, that is, how often a given item is encountered. The word frequency is operationalized in terms of how often a word occurs in the language. Frequency is a bit odd in some respects. Memory is better for frequent information for recall tests (Taft, 1979), but it is better for infrequent information for recognition tests. Common things are easier to recall because there are more ways to get at them. However, with recognition, less frequent items have fewer competitor memories, so they are recognized more easily (see the following sections on recall and recognition).

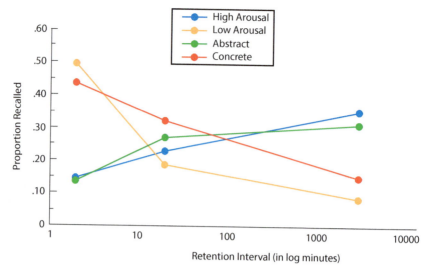

FIGURE 3.5 *Changes in Memory over Time as a Function of Whether Materials Were Emotionally Arousing or Not, and Whether They Were Concrete or Abstract*

Source: created from data reported in Butter, M. J. (1970). Differential recall of paired associates as a function of arousal and concreteness-imagery levels. *Journal of Experimental Psychology, 84*(2), 252–256.

Stop and Review

Learning is influenced by the nature of the memorized materials. The principle of savings illustrates that even material that was previously learned, but which people claim has been forgotten, may still have representations in memory. Also, some materials are easier to learn than others, such as pictures and concrete concepts. This may reflect embodied aspects of memory. Moreover, information that is emotionally charged is easier to remember than neutral content, although this typically emerges over time. Over time there is also a bias to remember positive memories more than negative memories. Finally, how frequent or commonly materials are encountered can influence memory, with more frequent things being easier to recall, but less frequent things being easier to recognize.

ASSESSING THE CONTENTS OF MEMORY

Questions about memory often center on issues of what is in memory, what can be remembered later, and how easily it is remembered. There are a number of ways of getting at the contents of memory, and each has its advantages and disadvantages.

Recall

Methods. A straightforward way to test memory is a **recall** test. For recall, people generate and report whatever knowledge that they can access from memory. There are many types of recall tests, and three are considered here, namely, free recall, forced recall, and cued recall.

The most basic type of recall test is **free recall**, in which people report as much information as they can. This is similar to answering an essay question on an exam. Because there is very little additional information provided, free recall is a good way to find out what people know well. Presumably, what is known well is what is reported. Information that is known, but not very well, is less likely to be reported because people are less likely to successfully retrieve it, or they may not have confidence in the memory, and so hold back their responses.

Free recall data is not only appropriate for knowing what people accurately remember, but it can also be used to study errors of omission (what people do not remember) and errors of commission (information that is reported, but was not, in fact, part of the event). Errors of commission are called **intrusions**, and they can be important when studying things such as false memories (see Chapter 13). Moreover, studying **recall order**, that is the order in which people report things on a free recall test, can give some insight into how memories are structured. For example, when recalling sports teams, people may recall teams in the same division or conference together, suggesting that this knowledge is stored together in memory. Also, stronger memories are more likely to be reported early in free recall, whereas weaker memories are likely to be reported later.

One problem with free recall is that there might be information that people remember, perhaps faintly, but they are unwilling to report it because they lack confidence in those memories and withhold them in case they might be wrong. One way to encourage people to report weaker memories is to give a **forced recall** test. Unlike a free recall, where people can report as much or as little as desired, in a forced recall test people are supposed to report a certain amount of information. For example, if people were presented with a list of 20 words to learn, they could be asked to report 20 items on a forced recall test. Typically, the amount of information reported on a forced recall test is more than what would have been reported under free recall.

Using this approach, weaker knowledge in memory can be evaluated as being present in some way. Typically, weaker knowledge is provided toward the end of forced recall. Forced recall is also more likely to elicit intrusions. These errors can be informative about the processes people use to recover memories by illustrating how those processes can break down. In other words, the mistakes that people make are not random, but follow certain principles. Studying these errors can provide insight into how memory works.

Memories are often associated with a context or setting. To study how this influences memory retrieval, a **cued recall** test can be used. During memorization, people learn a set of information. The experimenter designates some of this information as target information to be recalled. Associated with this is other information that serves as retrieval cues. Thus, the experimenter can control the context that will be relevant later. The paired associate learning tasks discussed in Chapter 1 are a good example of this sort of cue and target knowledge learning.

During retrieval, the experimenter provides a set of cues, and the task is to report what goes with them. For example, if people learned the word pair "goose–marble," the experimenter would give the word "goose" and the participants would need to recall the word "marble." Thus, the experimenter controls the context and can observe how it influences memory. Retrieval in cued recall tests is more constrained than under free recall. During cued recall, people respond to either as many cues as they can or to all of the cues, much like a forced recall test. Again, both accuracy and errors can be used to help understand the contents of memory.

During recall, people need to mentally organize information to be able to retrieve it later. This includes both recalling information that has not yet been reported as well as avoiding reporting something that has already been recalled. To monitor memory retrieval, people develop a strategy known as a **retrieval plan**. This is a set of self-generated retrieval cues used to guide people through the material. If this retrieval plan is thwarted or disrupted by external influences, then performance declines.

TRY IT OUT

This chapter has several ideas for research projects on memory. For many of these, you can simply create a list of 20 or so words and use these as your materials. When you generate these lists, try to keep the words similar in some way, such as all being from the same class of words (e.g., nouns or verbs), being similar in length (e.g., 5–6 letters long with two syllables), and so on. When you present the information to people, try to keep the presentation time constant in the different conditions. Typically, for word lists, people might see each word for about one to three seconds each (you could write each word on an index card or something). To encourage some forgetting, have people do a distractor task, such as solve three-digit math problems (294 + 603 = ?) for two minutes. Ideally you should have at least 12 participants for each of these tasks, with at least 12 people in each group if you decide to vary things in your experiment between groups. Now, with these basic ground rules, here are some things that you could do.

Test the difference between incidental and intentional learning. Have one group of people (incidental) rate each word for pleasantness and another group (intentional) study each word knowing that they will get a memory test later. After the distractor period, have people write down as many words as they can. People in the incidental learning condition should remember fewer words than those in the intentional learning condition.

Test the effectiveness of imagery by giving a list of words to two groups of people. Have one group (control) simply try to learn the words as effectively as possible. Have the other group (experimental) try to form mental images of each study word. After the distractor period, have people write down as many words as they can remember. People in the experimental (imagery) condition should remember more than people in the control condition.

To show the effectiveness of concreteness, have two groups of people. For one group, keeping everything else the same, give them a list of nouns for concrete objects (e.g., "truck"), and for the other group, give them nouns for abstract concepts (e.g., "trust"). After the distractor period, have people write down as many words as they can remember. People in the concrete condition should remember more words than those in the abstract condition.

Recognition

During recall, people need to generate the information, at least in part. However, in some cases, people need only to identify something already in the environment as being familiar or old, and thus recognized, or as being unfamiliar or new, and thus unrecognized. **Recognition** is a process in which the contents of the environment are compared with the contents of memory. If there is a match, then recognition occurs; otherwise it does not.

Methods. The simplest form of recognition testing is old–new recognition. For this method people are given an item and are asked to indicate whether it is old or new. Memory is assessed based on the pattern of responses. This method simplifies the retrieval situation, making it easier to track and analyze. A great deal of information can be derived from such simple tasks. For example, EEG recordings show that when items are recognized, there is an initial increase in synchronization of theta activity around the parietal lobe, followed by decreased synchronization in the upper and lower alpha bands around the temporal lobe (Burgess & Gruzelier, 2000).

For old–new responses, some accurately reflect memory, but others involve a degree of uncertainty, and are guesses. Suppose a memory test has 50 old items (to which people should respond "yes") and 50 new items (to which people should respond "no"). Now suppose that one person, Amy, identified the 50 old items by correctly responding "yes" to them on a recognition memory test. If she also had no incorrect answers of responding "yes" to the new items, then it would seem that her memory was very accurate. However, now suppose that another person, Scott, also identified the 50 old items by responding "yes" to them. If he also incorrectly responded "yes" to the 50 new items on the recognition memory tests, then it is clear that his memory is actually pretty poor and that he was guessing for the entire test. What is needed is a way to correct for guessing on a recognition test, to provide a more accurate estimate of memory.

Before discussing ways to correct for guessing, we first identify the four kinds of responses people can make on a recognition test (see Figure 3.6). The first kind of response is *correctly* responding "yes" to a memory item that is old (learned before). This is called a **hit**. The second kind of response is *incorrectly* responding "yes" to a memory item that is new (not learned before). This is called a **false alarm**. The third kind of response is *incorrectly* responding "no" to a memory item that is old. This is called a **miss**. Finally, the last kind of response is *correctly* responding "no" to a memory item that is old. This kind is called a **correct rejection**.

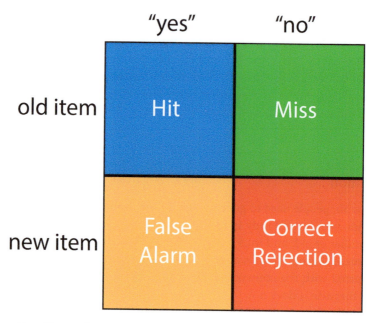

	"yes"	"no"
old item	Hit	Miss
new item	False Alarm	Correct Rejection

FIGURE 3.6 *Four Types of Possible Recognition Responses*

When correcting for guessing, you do not need to use the rate of responding for all four of these. If you take a minute and think about it, half of these are redundant with the other half. For example, if you know that a recognition memory test has 100 old items on it, and a person has 83 hits, then you also know that they had 17 misses. Thus, the hit and the miss rates are redundant. Similarly, if you know that there were 100 new items, and a person had 12 false alarms, you know that they had 88 correct rejections. Thus, the information in the false alarm and correct rejection rates are redundant. As such, we only need two of these measures. By convention, researchers use the hit and false alarm rates to correct for guessing.

A simple way to correct for guessing is to calculate a measure, called *Pr*, in which we simply subtract the number of false alarms from the number of hits. Guessing on a recognition test can be affected by two pieces of information. One is the degree to which old items can be distinguished from new ones in memory. This is called **discrimination**. Sometimes discrimination is relatively easy, such as identifying whether a person is a famous actor versus someone you have never heard of before. Other times it may be more difficult, such as identifying whether a person is a classmate of yours from ten years ago or their twin sister.

The second piece of information is the degree to which people are willing to accept what is remembered as new or old. This is called **bias**. Sometimes people adopt a strict criterion and have a "conservative" bias. In this situation, people accept only cases in which they are very sure that the information is old to avoid false alarms. A situation in which people might be motivated to adopt a conservative bias would be eyewitness identification. The eyewitness wants to be sure that the person identified is the perpetrator. Picking out the wrong person could lead to an innocent person being punished and leaving the guilty party at large, free to commit more crimes. In other cases, people may adopt a loose criterion and thus have a "liberal" bias. In this situation, people are more willing to accept a memory that has a more remote possibility of being old to avoid making any miss responses. A situation in which people might be motivated to adopt a liberal bias would be in looking for a lost set of keys. The searcher wants to be sure that all plausible locations are checked, and the consequences of a false alarm are fairly insignificant.

A method for estimating discrimination and bias is **signal detection theory** (Banks, 1970; Lockhart & Murdock, 1970). This approach has been adopted from psychophysicists studying sensation and perception, who, in turn, borrowed it from communications theory. By using this approach, one can derive a measure of discrimination, often called d', and of bias, often called β (see Snodgrass & Corwin, 1988, and the Appendix).

The basic idea behind signal detection theory is to assess the ability to detect the signal (an accurate memory) from the noise (inaccurate memories). The thinking is illustrated in Figure 3.7. This approach assumes that there are two distributions: one for the old items and one for the new items, along some dimension, such as familiarity. The further apart these two distributions are, the easier it is to discriminate between them. Conversely, the more these two distributions overlap, the harder it is to discriminate between them. Keeping the distance between the two distributions constant, we can see how bias affects memory performance. The criterion people use to separate out what is identified as old and new is measured by β. If β is set very far to the right, people have adopted a conservative criterion, and very few memories will be accepted as old. However, if β is set far to the left, people have adopted a liberal criterion, and very few memories will be accepted as new.

Another form of recognition is when people are given several items and are asked to indicate which one is old. This is **forced choice recognition**. Typically, there are two, three, or four alternatives. Forced choice recognition allows a researcher to manipulate the incorrect items in terms of the degree to which they resemble the correct one. Such manipulations can provide insight into what kinds of knowledge

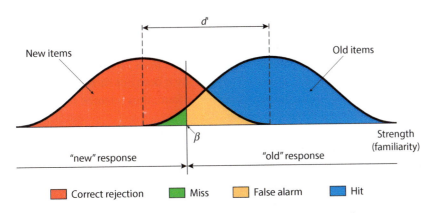

FIGURE 3.7 *Illustration of the Underlying Logic for Signal Detection Theory*

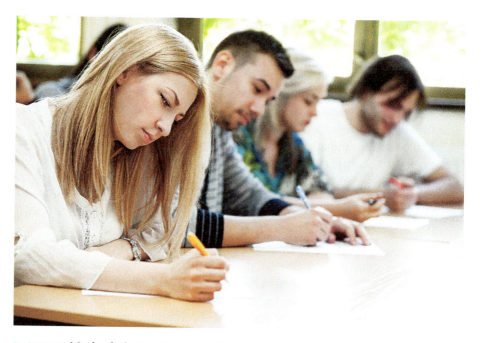

PHOTO 3.3 *Much of what we know about memory comes from having people take recall and recognition tests for the critical material at hand*

Source: Lucky Business/Shutterstock.com

people are using at retrieval. The wrong items that are more often selected as "old" would more closely match the information in memory. In addition, when forced choice recognition is used, particularly when there are three or more choices, the rate of chance performance is lower than the 50 percent for old–new recognition.

Principles. The use of recall and recognition tests has revealed several things about human memory. This includes both insight into how well information is learned as well as how it is structured in memory. This section outlines some principles of memory that have been derived from using recall and recognition tests. These included the forgetting curve, overlearning, reminiscence, and hypermnesia.

The clearest finding to come out of research using recall tests is that the more time that has passed, the less likely people will remember. Alternatively, people forget more as time passes. The pattern of data that has been observed is the **forgetting curve**, shown in Figure 3.8, although technically it does not show forgetting, per se. Instead what it is showing is the amount of information retained over time. Thus, it can also be called a **retention curve**.

A forgetting curve is a negatively accelerating function. That is, most of the forgetting occurs right after the information was learned. Research has shown that the forgetting curve follows a power function (Wixted & Ebbesen, 1991). However, it is unclear whether this is because of some fundamental neurological process or because of some artifact of averaging across many trials (Anderson & Tweney, 1997). For example, rather than a power function, the decay of individual traces may be

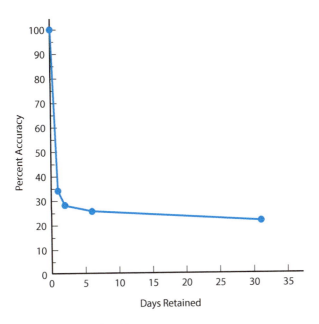

FIGURE 3.8 *Ebbinghaus's Forgetting Curve*

Source: created from data reported in Ebbinghaus, H. (1885/1964). *Memory: A Contribution to Experimental Psychology*. Translated by H. A. Ruger & C. E. Bussenius. New York: Dover

more exponential. Careful work suggests that individual memory traces are forgotten at an exponential rate, but the averaging across them is best fit by a power function (Murre & Chessa, 2011).

As time passes, although the cumulative amount of forgetting loss grows larger, the rate of forgetting slows down accordingly. In other words, the rate of forgetting captured in the power function grows smaller and smaller. This change in the forgetting function is captured by **Jost's Law** (1897; as cited in Wixted, 2004), shown in Figure 3.9. Jost's Law is that, for memories of a similar strength, the older memories decay slower than the newer memories. Another way of stating this is that the rate of forgetting is not constant but slows down as the memories become older (and not yet forgotten). Note that in the figure, both groups of memories are remembered at the same rate at time 5, but, then, older memories are forgotten more slowly.

While there is a truth in the forgetting curve, it is not always the case that forgetting inevitably occurs. Another principle that Ebbinghaus discovered using recall was overlearning. **Overlearning** occurs when people continue to study information after it is already possible to recall it without errors. This continued practice causes the forgetting curve to lessen and possibly disappear altogether. In such cases, the information becomes chronically available and is resistant to forgetting. Thus, many of the fundamentals you remember from your schooling, such as the "A, B, C" song, have been greatly overlearned, and you are unlikely to forget that knowledge. This is one reason why education emphasizes repetition and practice.

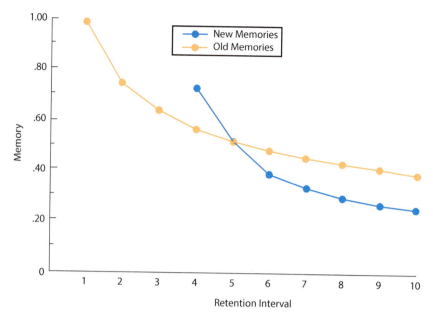

FIGURE 3.9 *Illustration of Jost's Law in which an older memory is forgotten at a slower rate than a newer memory*

Source: adapted from Wixted, J. T. (2004). On Common Ground: Jost's (1897) law of forgetting and Ribot's (1881) law of retrograde amnesia. *Psychological Review, 111*(4), 864

Not only do we forget things, but we can also remember things that were once forgotten. The remembering of previously forgotten information is **reminiscence** (Ballard, 1913). Generally, reminiscence is more often observed with a recall task, particularly free recall. Although reminiscence can occur, so does forgetting. Thus, if the occasions that people try to remember are spread out, even though reminiscence may occur (memory gains), people continue to forget (memory losses) and may be remembering less overall.

That said, there are cases where rate of memory gains may be greater than the rate of losses. Under these circumstances the people are cumulatively remembering more and more each time (Erdelyi & Becker, 1974). This increased memory over multiple attempts is called **hypermnesia** (the opposite of amnesia). Hypermnesia is not typically observed. It is more likely to be seen with pictures (Payne, 1987). It is also more evident with recall than with recognition (Otani & Hodge, 1991), and the magnitude of the hypermnesia effect does not appear to change over time (e.g., weeks later) (Wallner & Bäuml, 2018).

There are several theories of hypermnesia (see Wallner & Bäuml, 2018). For the *cumulative retrieval hypothesis*, the two retrieval tests are considered one attempt with a disruption in the middle (Roediger et al., 1982). However, this requires that the tests be close in time. For the *cue set change hypothesis*, over time the set of internally generated cues for people's retrieval plans change, and includes using the previously retrieved memories as cues to retrieve even more. Because different cues are used, different memories are retrieved (Roediger & Thorpe, 1978). For the *retrieval strategy hypothesis*, people improve their strategies (Erdelyi & Becker, 1974). However, this only works with free recall. Finally, the *retrieval practice hypothesis* (Wallner & Bäuml, 2018) the initial retrieval of some memories strengthens them. Then reminiscence capitalizes on those boosted memories, resulting in hypermnesia.

The existence of reminiscence and hypermnesia has practical significance. When it seems that you have completely forgotten something, putting it out of your mind for a period of time may help you remember it later. Of course, as with any type of memory, the more elaborately you think about the information during learning, the more successful later attempts to remember will be, even for appearance of the effects of reminiscence and hypermnesia.

One final principle is observed with recognition involving the hit and false alarm rates is the **mirror effect**. This is a finding that conditions that decreased in hit rates are accompanied by increased false alarm rates, and vice versa (Glanzer & Adams, 1985). This occurs because, as time passes, along with the forgetting of previously studied information (lower hit rate), people become more liberal in responding and accept memories that they previously would have rejected (higher false alarm rate).

Stop and Review

Two common ways to test memory are recall and recognition. Recall involves producing information. A free recall test is one in which people report as much as they can remember. The data from free recall tests tell us things about memory based not only on what was recalled, but also based on any intrusions that may occur, and the order in which items are reported. To encourage people to report memories that they are not confident in, a forced recall task might be used. Finally, cued recall can be used to elicit memories in response to cues. This is a way of manipulating context and its influence on memory. Often people need a retrieval plan to organize their recall efforts. There is also recognition. The basic type of recognition test is old–new recognition in which people indicate whether things were encountered before. When using recognition data, we need some way to correct for guessing, such as doing a signal detection analysis. Forced choice recognition can also be used. It has the advantage of allowing you to manipulate the nature of the distractors to reveal some aspects of memory. Recall and recognition tests have helped illustrate the principles of the forgetting curve, overlearning, reminiscence, and hypermnesia.

ASSESSING MEMORY STRUCTURE AND PROCESS

This section covers ways of assessing memory structure and the processes that are used in retrieval. The structure of memories refers to both the organization of multiple pieces of information within a single memory as well as across multiple memories. The processes of memory are the mental activities that people engage in when trying to retrieve knowledge. Basically, *how* do we remember?

Mental Chronometry

A frequently used source of information is the speed of responding. How fast your mind does something is *mental chronometry*. In many cases this **response time** is recorded on the order of milliseconds or seconds.[4] The idea is that faster response times reflect simpler memory processes and/or more familiar memories, whereas slower response times reflect more complex memory processes and/or more unfamiliar memories.

Methods. Response time is measured from the onset of some stimulus. For example, when asked to identify whether a series of faces has been seen before, time is recorded from the moment a picture was shown to the time people respond. The time for any given memory is not very informative by itself. That time must be placed in the context of others to know whether it is fast or slow. While there are many variations on this idea, the use of response times can be classified into two broad categories: subtractive and additive factors logic.

The first approach to mental chronometry is Donders' **subtractive factors logic**. This is outlined in Figure 3.10. The idea is to have at least two conditions that are identical except for the inclusion of one processing step. For example, both conditions include the same encoding (factor A) and response (factor B) processes. However, the condition of interest involves an extra step (factor X). After collecting the times, the time for the simpler process (A + B) is subtracted from the time for the more complex one (A + X + B). What is left over should be the time for the critical process. For example, in a simple condition one could have people indicate whether a picture of a face is old or new. In a more complex condition people would indicate whether a picture of a face is old or new and whether the individual is living or dead. Based on subtractive factors logic, the difference between these two conditions reflects the time it takes to remember a person's current health status.

While subtractive factors logic is appealing, it has several problems. For one, it is unclear whether the process of interest is added in a way that does not disrupt or

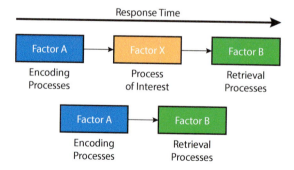

FIGURE 3.10 *Donders' Subtractive Factors Logic for Response Times*

---

4 Some researchers use the term **reaction time** rather than **response time**. Following Luce (1986), the term response time is preferred. As Luce states, "response time is a generic term and reaction time refers only to experiments in which response time is made a major focus of attention for the subject. The experimenter may request the subject to respond as fast as possible, or to maintain the response times in a certain temporal interval, and so on" (p. 2). Thus "reaction time" is for when people respond as quickly as possible when a stimulus appears, and "response time" more generally, as is the case for all the studies reported here.

change other processes and that the process of interest occurs at a time when these other processes are not taking place. Another approach is **additive factors logic**, developed by Sternberg (and Chapter 4). This approach is outlined in Figure 3.11. Rather than having two conditions that differ by the presence or absence of a mental stage, in additive factors logic the critical stage of interest (factor X) is always present. What varies is its degree of involvement—that is, how much of that process is added relative to a comparison condition. For example, it may be a stage that people need to go through many times or that involves various numbers of memory traces. By looking at the differences between conditions, one can get an estimate of the influence of each increment of complexity. This approach is more likely to preserve a greater array of mental processes across conditions, making the comparison more reliable and meaningful.

Most studies use *mean* response times for different conditions to assess memory, and this works well in many contexts. That said, response times typically do not produce normal bell-curve distributions. Instead, they are positively skewed, with long tails to the right for very long response times. There are approaches that take advantage of this. Response time distributions are a mixture of two underlying distributions (Balota & Yap, 2011). For reference, see Figure 3.12. One of the distributions is the normal bell curve, also known as a Gaussian distribution. The other is an exponential distribution that starts out high for fast response times and tapers off for longer response times. The observed response time distribution is an Ex-Gaussian distribution that reflects these two components. Importantly, the Gaussian and exponential distributions may reflect

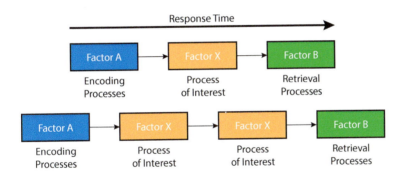

FIGURE 3.11 *Sternberg's Additive Factors Logic for Response Times*

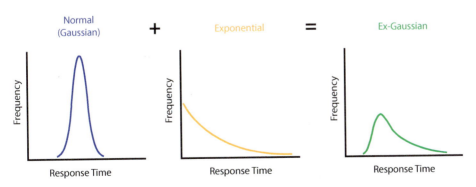

FIGURE 3.12 *Normal (Gaussian) and Exponential Distributions, Which Can Combine to Form an Ex-Gaussian Distribution. This Is the Form of Distribution Typically Observed in Response Time Studies*

different underlying memory processes. Statistical procedures can provide estimates of these two distributions, providing greater insight into how memory works. For example, the Gaussian distribution may reflect the speed of initiating a memory process, whereas the exponential component reflects individual differences in working memory capacity. A drawback of this approach is that it requires a large number of observations to derive stable estimates of the two underlying distributions.

Most research involves a manual response, such as pressing a button on a computer keyboard, screen, or mouse. Another source of response time data comes from the eyes, as with **eye-tracking**. What eye-trackers do is tell a researcher what people are looking at and for how long. The time spent looking at something, called a *fixation*, can indicate whether something is stored in memory. For example, if you have already encountered something you are likely to spend less time looking at it than if you are seeing it for the first time.

Another eye-based methodology is **pupillometry** which involves recording the size of people's pupils and assessing how the size changes in different conditions. Pupils are larger when there is greater mental effort, such as when people need to remember more (Goldinger & Papesh, 2012) and for things that are better remembered later (Kafkas & Montaldi, 2011). For example, pupil sizes are larger when people hear melodies that they heard before (Weiss et al., 2016).

Principles. Response time data has yielded a wealth of information about memory. One prominent principle is priming. **Priming** is a speed up in response time to items that immediately follow related items. For example, when making lexical decision judgments (that is, deciding whether a string of letters is a word or not), people are faster to say that the string "doctor" is a word if it immediately follows "nurse" than if it follows "bread" (Meyer & Schvaneveldt, 1971). The idea is that "nurse" activates or primes knowledge of nurses in long-term memory. The concept "doctor" is very related to "nurse," and so has been primed. Thus, information about doctors is retrieved faster than it would have been had the person just been thinking about something unrelated (like bread).

STUDY IN DEPTH

An influential study of memory is Meyer and Schvaneveldt's (1971) study of semantic priming. The aim of this study was to assess whether the meaningfulness of the information in memory can influence the ease of retrieval of other information. To assess this, they used a paradigm that is a classic memory research, and which continues to be used to this day. This is the *lexical decision task*. For a lexical decision task, participants are presented with a series of letter strings. The task is simply to say whether the letter strings correspond to a word or not. So, for example, "doctor" is a word, but "ductyr" is not. Because people are often near perfect at this task, in terms of their accuracy, what is of importance here is the speed at which they respond. As such, response time, recorded in terms of milliseconds, is the critical dependent measure.

What Meyer and Schvaneveldt did was to test 12 high school students. They presented each student with a series of 240 letter string pairs, with each string being 3–7 letters long. These 240 pairs were broken up in the following way: (a) 48 **nonword pairs**, such as "ductyr–prenct," (b) 96 **word-nonword pairs**, such as "krepst–office," (c) 48 pairs of unrelated words, such as "horse–butter", and, most importantly, (d) 48 pairs of associated words, such as "nurse–doctor."

After a brief practice period, the letter string pairs were presented, one pair at a time, on a screen. The letter strings were presented one on top of the other. People were told to respond by pressing one of two buttons, using one finger from each hand, as quickly and as accurately as possible. The right hand was used for "yes' if both of the letter strings were words, and the left hand for "no" if either or both were nonwords. Each pair was preceded by a ready signal so that people could prepare. After each trial, there was feedback indicating whether the response was correct or not. Each session lasted about 45 minutes.

After the data were collected the response time data were analyzed considering only times for correct responses. For the (a) nonwords pairs ($M = 884$ ms) and (b) word–nonword pairs ($M = 996$ ms), people were slightly slower, which is typical for negative "no" responses. This likely indicates extra processing taken to make sure that the letter strings were not words stored somewhere in memory. More importantly, people were slower to respond "yes" when the letter strings were (c) unrelated words ($M = 940$ ms) than if they were (d) associated word pairs ($M = 855$ ms). Thus, this shows that when people retrieve information from memory, it is easier if the two memories are related than if they are not. One memory primes or facilitates the availability of those memories that are related to it. For example, in this case, the retrieval of the memory that "nurse" is a word spread to related memories about what a nurse is. As a result, the processing and retrieval of "doctor" was made easier and faster because the idea of *doctor* is highly related to the idea of *nurse*. That is, *nurse* primes *doctor*. Thus, we not only activate the memory we need at the moment, but we also activate other strongly related knowledge that may be useful, even if those memories are not completely retrieved.

Cluster Analysis

Some research methods are aimed at assessing how information is organized in memory. Knowing this can provide insight into how things such as remindings occur and why our thoughts drift in some ways, but not in others. There are several ways to approach this issue. Data from priming studies is one way. Regardless of the method, what is going on is an attempt to look at clusters of memories. There is a special domain of statistics known as cluster analysis where the goal is to detect groups or clusters of information in a set of data.

Methods. There are number of clustering methods that can be used. An example of the output from a hypothetical cluster analysis of memory is shown in Figure 3.13. Here we focus on two relatively simple measures to give you a feel for how this approach works.

A time-based method for assessing memory organization with recall is if you track the amount of time between each recalled item. What you will find is that there is not a uniform pattern. Instead, people report a burst of a few items, then a pause, then a burst of a few more, pause, and so on (Patterson et al., 1971). By using these

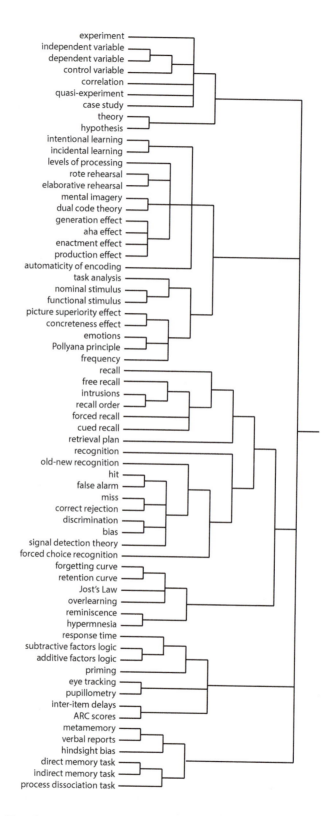

FIGURE 3.13 *Hypothetical output from a cluster analysis. Note that similar concepts are clustered closer together, and more distant concepts are clustered further apart*

inter-item delays, we can make inferences about memory structure. Memories that are structured together are likely to be recalled together during a burst. However, information that is stored apart is more likely to be separated by a pause.

We can also obtain memory clusters by looking at the content of recall, specifically the order in which information was reported. Pieces of information that are stored together in memory are likely to be recalled together. In many cases you can make a reasonable guess about how a set of information could be organized. For example, a set of words can be organized into categories. It then becomes possible to test whether people use that organization. This can be done by calculating **Adjusted Ratio of Clustering** (or **ARC**) scores (Roenker et al., 1971). ARC scores index the degree to which recall conforms to predetermined categories, taking into account how much organization would be expected by chance. The formula for calculating ARC scores is given in the Appendix. There are many measures of knowledge organization. For example, the **ARC′** score measures the degree to which a recall conforms to a sequential order (Pellegrino, 1971). The method for calculating ARC′ scores is also provided in the Appendix.

Apart from using more objective means of organizing information, such as categories, it is also possible that people organize information in idiosyncratic and subjective ways. There are ways to get at subjective organization. One approach is a measure that produces an ordered cluster tree (Reitman & Rueter, 1980). Basically, people recall a complete set of information several times. What measures such as this do is look for consistencies in these repeated recalls, both in terms of the clusters that might be present as well as any stable sequential orders that might be produced.

Principles. Clustering methods show that memories are highly structured. The more structure people impose on information, the better memory will be (Mandler, 1967). When people are given a set of information, they often adopt a hierarchical structure, which is seen in how they remember the information. For example, in a study by Bousfield (1953), students at the University of Connecticut were given a list of 60 words to memorize. These words were from four categories (animals, people's names, vegetables, and professions), but they were presented in a random order. When people later recalled the words there was a strong tendency to recall them in clusters based on the four categories. Moreover, as time passed and people had more experience with the information, their memories become more organized (e.g., Bousfield & Bousfield, 1966). In fact, experts in a domain have highly organized knowledge bases.

Finally, even when given a random set of information, people impose a subjective organization upon it (Tulving, 1962). This subjective organization takes into account the idiosyncratic interpretations people place on a set of materials to create a structure that helps them remember. While space may abhor a vacuum, the human brain abhors randomness. It is always searching for regularities and structure.

Stop and Review

There are a number of ways to assess memory structure and function. Mental chronometry (response times) is a popular way to study memory. Priming is a classic example of the use of mental chronometry. While the subtractive factors logic can be used, some form of additive factors logic is more common. With enough observations, more complex analyses can be done on the normal and exponential components of response time distributions. Memory structure and organization can also be assessed using eye movements and pupillometry to index changes in mental effort. Cluster analyses more directly convey how some types of knowledge are organized. These analyses can be done using the gaps in time that occur during recall, by evaluating which items tend to be recalled together, or by simply asking people to put items together in some way.

CONSCIOUS EXPERIENCE OF MEMORY

Metamemory Measures

Another important characteristic to consider is the phenomenological experience of memory. What does it feel like to remember? How do you know if you know something or not? The awareness of your own memory and memory processes is **metamemory** and is highlighted in Chapter 15. A brief coverage of metamemory issues is presented here to illustrate how to study the experience and awareness of memory.

Methods. Metamemory studies ask people to report on their own memory processes. The method of introspection has a long and checkered past dating back to the early days of experimental psychology, and some people are still cautious about using **verbal reports** (Nisbett & Wilson, 1977) because many of our mental processes lie outside of conscious awareness. However, despite this, there are still cases where verbal reports can provide insights into cognition (Ericsson & Simon, 1980), especially if one is concerned with the conscious experience and its consequences.

There are a number of metamemory methods. A common one is *remember* vs. *know* judgments (Gardiner, 1988). With this method, people are asked to recall or recognize a set of information. For those things that are recalled or identified as old, people then rate whether the information is something they consciously remember learning or something they know they encountered before but have no conscious memory of learning. For example, if you can recollect where and when you learned of your acceptance into college, then you would say that you remember it. In contrast, if you have no conscious memory of this event, but you know it must have occurred, then you would say that you only know it.

Principles. Several insights have been gained by assessing what people attribute to their own memory processes. People can be led astray and become biased. This is illustrated by the hindsight bias (Fischhoff, 1975). The **hindsight bias** is a tendency to distort memories so they conform to one's current goals, circumstances, or knowledge. For example, people might be asked to make predictions about how likely an event is to occur, such as which team will win a football game and by how much. Then, at some time afterward, one group (the experimental group) is presented with information about the actual outcome. Another group (the control group) is not given this information. If everyone then is asked to report their original estimates, those in the experimental group are more likely to "misremember" their original estimates as being closer to the actual outcome. This is also one of the reasons why students may sometimes feel that they did not learn much during a class. They forget their prior ignorance and are not aware of just how much they have learned. We discuss this more in Chapter 15.

Implicit Memory

Again, implicit memory refers to memories and memory processes that are unconscious. It is rare that memory uses only implicit or explicit processes. Performance almost always reflects a mixture. There are methods that allow for the influence of each of these to be separated to some degree.

Methods. Measures that are aimed more at implicit memory use tasks in which people are not aware that memory is being tested or when there is little to no conscious control over the process. It is difficult, if not impossible, to have a memory task that purely taps either implicit or explicit memory. Thus, memory *tasks* are referred to as either **direct memory tasks**, which directly ask people for a memory report (such as recall and recognition), or **indirect memory tasks**, which assess memory by focusing on people's attention on another aspect of the task. In general, direct memory tasks involve more explicit memory, whereas indirect memory tasks involve more implicit memory. Indirect memory tasks often either tap into preexisting knowledge or present people with information and test memory some time afterward. In the latter case, the memory tests are given under the guise of being unrelated to what had been done previously so people are not motivated to consciously remember. Indirect memory measures include such things as word fragment completion, perceptual identification, and priming.

As an example of an indirect memory test, suppose that in the first part of a study, people rate a series of words for pleasantness. Then, afterward, the experimenter thanks them and says that because there is still some time left, they will do another, unrelated study. At this point the experimenter might give a series of word fragments with the task of having people complete them with the first word that comes to mind. The researcher can then assess how often people completed the word fragments with words that had been seen before as compared to a group of people who had not seen those words previously. The difference reflects the operation of implicit memories of the previously seen words from the first part of the study.

One method for separating out implicit and explicit memory processes is the **process dissociation procedure**. This procedure can help estimate the relative influence of implicit and explicit memory (Jacoby, 1991; Yonelinas & Jacoby, 2012). For example, suppose people have read a list words and then take a word fragment completion test. The process dissociation procedure works by using two conditions. In the *inclusion* condition, people complete a series of word fragments with whatever words they can think of, even if they were from the prior list. In the *exclusion* condition, people use any word they can think of so long as they are *not* words that were on the previous list. Using data from these two conditions, it is possible to get estimates of explicit and implicit memory. The procedures for calculating these components are given in the Appendix.

Stop and Review

It is important to know what it consciously feels like to remember and what we consciously know we remember. The awareness of your own memory is metamemory. Metamemory studies reveal how accurate or inaccurate our insights into our own memories are. An example of a metamemory measure is remember–know judgments. Metamemory studies have revealed phenomena such as the hindsight bias. That said, many memory processes occur outside of conscious awareness, involving implicit memory. To assess it, you need clever methods that minimize or separate out conscious influences on remembering. This involves using indirect tests of memory or by using a process dissociation procedure.

PUTTING IT ALL TOGETHER

This chapter covered several methods for assessing memory and some basic principles that they illustrate. Each method has its strengths and limitations. Memory is a slippery and ethereal thing that is difficult to grasp. The use of experiments, correlational studies, quasi-experiments, and case studies allows a more objective perspective. From the data gathered from these approaches we have derived principles, theories, hypotheses, and predictions about the limits and capabilities of human memory. The conscious introspection into memories is only appropriate for exploring metamemory issues.

Using the methods of scientific psychology, we have already revealed a range of principles. We know that the effort put into intentional learning leads to better memory. This is seen with the various forms of deep processing, such as using mental images, generating information, the "aha" effect, the enactment effect, and the production effect. That said, some types of materials are more automatically learned in an incidental manner. Even when some effort is required, some things are learned more easily than others, such as pictures, concrete ideas, and emotional experiences. Moreover, the ease of learning is greatly influenced by whether you have encountered something before, which allows us to observe some savings.

Memory can be assessed directly using recall and recognition, with their various accuracy, intrusion, and response time measures. Alternatively, indirectly using measures such as stem completion, eye tracking, and pupillometry can also be used. Each of these has advantages and limitations. There is always more information in memory than a given test will reveal. Although memory follows Ebbinghaus's forgetting curve, which can be attenuated through overlearning, some things that are forgotten that may later be remembered, as revealed by the principles of reminiscence and hypermnesia. Finally, memory is always seeking ways to structure and organize information to make it easier to remember. That organization comes from the materials themselves or may be subjectively imposed.

To gain a more accurate picture of memory, it is important to use multiple methods and **converging operations**. The more methods that point to the same answer, the more reliable that answer will be. However, if different methods lead to different answers, then something may be wrong. For example, if people are more accurate and slower in one condition of a study than another there is a **speed–accuracy tradeoff**. People are making fewer errors and slowing down because they are being more careful. The data may not reflect anything about memory per se. Overall, there is a concern in psychological research to be able to replicate findings. Some studies do not have enough power and may be too variable (that is, not enough data were gathered to be sure that the pattern of results are not due to random chance) to be replicable (e.g., Stanley et al., 2018).

STUDY QUESTIONS

1. What is an experiment? What are the primary components of an experiment? Why is experimentation a preferred way to study memory?
2. What are other ways to study memory besides experiments? What are their advantages and disadvantages?
3. What are theories and hypotheses and how do they relate to one another?
4. What are some ways to learn information so it will be better remembered later? Is this true of all kinds of information?
5. What kinds of information are easier to remember? What kinds are more difficult?
6. What is the difference between recall and recognition tests of memory?
7. What are the various sorts of recall tests, and what can they reveal about memory?
8. What are the various sorts of recognition tests, and what can they reveal about memory?
9. What are some of the ways to correct for guessing on memory tests?
10. What is the nature of the forgetting curve? How is it modified by aspects such as Jost's Law?
11. How can mental chronometry be used to assess characteristics of memory? What is an example of some phenomenon of memory that is clearly shown using mental chronometry?
12. How can we use changes in a people's eyes to assess memory?
13. How are cluster analyses used to study memory?
14. What is metamemory, and what does it tell us about how people use their memories?
15. What is implicit memory, and why is it important to memory functioning more generally?
16. What better ways to approach doing research? What kinds of evidence can reveal a problem with how a study was done?

KEY TERMS

- additive factors logic
- Adjusted Ratio of Clustering (ARC)
- "aha" effect
- associated words
- automaticity of encoding
- bias, case study
- concreteness effect
- control variable
- converging operations
- correct rejection
- correlation
- cued recall
- dependent variable
- direct memory task
- discrimination
- Dual Code theory
- elaborative rehearsal
- emotions
- enactment effect
- experiment
- eye-tracking
- false alarm
- forced choice recognition
- forced recall

- forgetting curve
- free recall
- frequency
- functional stimulus
- generation effect
- hindsight bias
- hit, hypermnesia
- hypothesis
- incidental learning
- independent variable
- indirect memory task
- intentional learning
- inter-item delays
- intrusions
- Jost's Law
- levels of processing
- mental imagery
- metamemory
- mirror effect
- miss
- nominal stimulus
- nonword pairs
- old–new recognition
- overlearning
- picture superiority effect

- Pollyanna principle
- priming
- process dissociation procedure
- production effect
- pupillometry
- quasi-experiment
- recall
- recall order
- recognition
- reminiscence
- response time
- retention curve
- retrieval plan
- rote rehearsal
- savings
- signal detection theory
- speed–accuracy tradeoff
- subtractive factors logic
- task analysis
- theory
- unrelated word
- verbal reports

EXPLORE MORE

Here are some additional readings that you can explore to provide yourself (with) better insight into basic principles of memory.

Averell, L., & Heathcote, A. (2011). The form of the forgetting curve and the fate of memories. *Journal of Mathematical Psychology, 55*(1), 25–35.

Craik, F. I. M., & Lockhart, R. S. (1972). Levels of processing: A framework for memory research. *Journal of Verbal Learning and Verbal Behavior, 12,* 671–684.

Ebbinghaus, H. (1885/1964). *Memory: A Contribution to Experimental Psychology.* Translated by H. A. Ruger & C. E. Bussenius. New York: Dover.

Macmillan, N. A., & Creelman, C. D. (2004). *Detection Theory: A User's Guide.* New York: Psychology Press.

Sadoski, M., & Paivio, A. (2012). *Imagery and Text: A Dual Coding Theory of Reading and Writing*. New York: Routledge.

Wheeler, M. A., & Roediger, H. L. (1992). Disparate effects of repeated testing: Reconciling Ballard's (1913) and Barlett's (1932) results. *Psychological Science*, 3, 240–245.

Wixted, J. T. (2004). On common ground: Jost's (1897) law of forgetting and Ribot's (1881) law of retrograde amnesia. *Psychological Review, 111*, 864–879.

REFERENCES

Anderson, R. B., & Tweney, R. D. (1997). Artifactual power curves in forgetting. *Memory & Cognition, 25*(5), 724–730.

Anderson, A. K., Yamaguchi, Y., Grabski, W., & Lacka, D. (2006). Emotional memories are not all created equal: Evidence for selective memory enhancement. *Learning & Memory, 13*(6), 711–718.

Anisfeld, M., & Lambert, W. E. (1966). When are pleasant words learned faster than unpleasant words? *Journal of Verbal Learning and Verbal Behavior, 5*, 132–141.

Auble, P. M., Franks, J. J., Soraci, S. A. (1979). Effort toward comprehension: Elaboration or "aha"? *Memory & Cognition, 7*, 426–434.

Ballard, P. B. (1913). Oblivescence and reminiscence. *British Journal of Psychology Monograph Supplements, 1*, 1–82.

Balota, D. A., & Yap, M. J. (2011). Moving beyond the mean in studies of mental chronometry: The power of response time distributional analyses. *Current Directions in Psychological Science, 20*(3), 160–166.

Banks, W. P. (1970). Signal detection theory and human memory. *Psychological Bulletin, 74*, 81–99.

Bertsch, S., Pesta, B. J., Wiscott, R., & McDaniel, M. A. (2007). The generation effect: A meta-analytic review. *Memory & Cognition, 35*, 201–210.

Blake, A. B., Nazarian, M., & Castel, A. D. (2015). The Apple of the mind's eye: Everyday attention, metamemory, and reconstructive memory for the Apple logo. *Quarterly Journal of Experimental Psychology, 68*(5), 858–865.

Block, R. A. (2009). Intent to remember briefly presented human faces and other pictorial stimuli enhances recognition memory. *Memory & Cognition, 37*, 667–678.

Bousfield, A. K., & Bousfield, W. A. (1966). Measurement of clustering and of sequential constancies in repeated free recall. *Psychological Reports, 19*, 935–942.

Bousfield, W. A., (1953). The occurrence of clustering in the recall of randomly arranged associates. *Journal of General Psychology, 49*, 229–240.

Brady, T. F., Konkle, T., Alvarez, G. A., & Oliva, A. (2008). Visual long-term memory has a massive storage capacity for object details. *Proceedings of the National Academy of Sciences, 105*(38), 14325–14329.

Burgess, A. P., & Gruzelier, J. H. (2000). Short duration power changes in the EEG during recognition memory for words and faces. *Psychophysiology, 37*, 596–606.

Butter, M. J. (1970). Differential recall of paired associates as a function of arousal and concreteness-imagery levels. *Journal of Experimental Psychology, 84*(2), 252.

Carter, H. D. (1936). Emotional correlates of errors in learning. *Journal of Educational Psychology, 27*, 55–67.

Carter, H. D., Jones, H. E., & Shock, N. W. (1934). An experimental study of affective factors in learning. *Journal of Educational Psychology, 25*, 203–215.

Casasanto, D. (2009). Embodiment of abstract concepts: good and bad in right-and left-handers. *Journal of Experimental Psychology: General, 138*(3), 351–367.

Coverdale, M. E., & Nairne, J. S. (2019). The mnemonic effect of choice. *Psychonomic Bulletin & Review, 26*(4), 1310–1316.

Craik, F. I. M., & Lockhart, R. S. (1972). Levels of processing: A framework for memory research. *Journal of Verbal Learning and Verbal Behavior, 12,* 671–684.

Crutcher, R. J., & Beer, J. M. (2011). An auditory analog of the picture superiority effect. *Memory & Cognition, 39*(1), 63–74.

Dodd, M. D., & Shumborski, S. (2009). Examining the influence of action on spatial working memory: The importance of selection. *Quarterly Journal of Experimental Psychology, 62,* 1236–1247.

Donders, F. C. (1868). Over de snelheid van psychische processen. Onderzoekingen gedaan in het Physiologisch Laboratorium der Utrechtsche Hoogeschool, 1868–1869. *Tweede reeks, II,* 92–120.

Eagle, M., & Leiter, E. (1964). Recall and recognition in intentional and incidental learning. *Journal of Experimental Psychology, 68,* 58–63.

Ebbinghaus, H. (1885/1964). *Memory: A Contribution to Experimental Psychology.* Translated by H. A. Ruger & C. E. Bussenius. New York: Dover.

Engelkamp, J., & Zimmer, H. D. (1997). Sensory factors in subject-performed tasks. *Acta Psychologica, 96,* 43–60.

Erdelyi, M. H., & Becker, J. (1974). Hypermnesia for pictures: Incremental memory for pictures but not words in multiple recall trials. *Cognitive Psychology, 6,* 159–171.

Ericsson, K. A., & Simon, H. A. (1980). Verbal reports as data. *Psychological Review, 87,* 215–251.

Fawcett, J. M. (2013). The production effect benefits performance in between-subject designs: A meta-analysis. *Acta Psychologica, 142*(1), 1–5.

Ferguson, R., Homa, D., & Ellis, D. (2017). Memory for temporally dynamic scenes. *Quarterly Journal of Experimental Psychology, 70*(7), 1197–1210.

Fernandes, M. A., Wammes, J. D., & Meade, M. E. (2018). The surprisingly powerful influence of drawing on memory. *Current Directions in Psychological Science, 27*(5), 302–308.

Fioravanti, M., & Di Cesare, F. (1992). Forgetting curves in long-term memory: Evidence for a multistage model of retention. *Brain and Cognition, 18*(2), 116–124.

Fischhoff, B. (1975). Hindsight is not equal to foresight: The effect of outcome knowledge on judgment under uncertainty. *Journal of Experimental Psychology: Human Perception and Performance, 1,* 288–299.

Forrin, N. D., & MacLeod, C. M. (2018). This time it's personal: The memory benefit of hearing oneself. *Memory, 26*(4), 574–579.

Forrin, N. D., MacLeod, C. M., & Ozubko, J. D. (2012). Widening the boundaries of the production effect. *Memory & Cognition, 40*(7), 1046–1055.

Gardiner, J. M. (1988). Functional aspects of recollective experience. *Memory & Cognition, 16,* 309–313.

Glanzer, M., & Adams, J. K. (1985). The mirror effect in recognition memory. *Memory & Cognition, 13*(1), 8–20.

Glenberg, A. M., Smith, S. M., & Green, C. (1977). Type I rehearsal: Maintenance and more. *Journal of Verbal Learning and Verbal Behavior, 16,* 339–352.

Gloede, M. E., & Gregg, M. K. (2019). The fidelity of visual and auditory memory. *Psychonomic Bulletin & Review, 26*(4), 1325–1332.

Goetschalckx, L., Moors, J., & Wagemans, J. (2019). Incidental image memorability. *Memory, 27*(9), 1273–1282.

Goetschalckx, L., Moors, P., & Wagemans, J. (2018). Image memorability across longer time intervals. *Memory, 26*(5), 581–588.

Goldinger, S. D., & Papesh, M. H. (2012). Pupil dilation reflects the creation and retrieval of memories. *Current Directions in Psychological Science, 21*(2), 90–95.

Goldstein, A. G., & Chance, J. E. (1970). Visual recognition memory for complex configurations. *Perception & Psychophysics, 9,* 237–241.

Hasher, L., & Zacks, R. T. (1979). Automatic and effortful processes in memory. *Journal of Experimental Psychology: General, 108,* 356–388.

Hasher, L., & Zacks, R. T. (1984). Automatic processing of fundamental information: The case of frequency of occurrence. *American Psychologist, 39,* 356–388.

Helbing, J., Draschkow, D., & Võ, M. L. H. (2020). Search superiority: Goal-directed attentional allocation creates more reliable incidental identity and location memory than explicit encoding in naturalistic virtual environments. *Cognition, 196,* 104–147.

Hutmacher, F., & Kuhbandner, C. (2018). Long-term memory for haptically explored objects: Fidelity, durability, incidental encoding, and cross-modal transfer. *Psychological Science, 29*(12), 2031–2038.

Hyde, T. S., & Jenkins, J. J. (1973). Recall for words as a function of semantic, graphic, and syntactic orienting tasks. *Journal of Verbal Learning and Verbal Behavior, 12,* 471–480.

Jacoby, L. L. (1991). A process dissociation framework: Separating automatic from intentional uses of memory. *Journal of Memory and Language, 30,* 513–541.

Jost, A. (1897). Die Assoziationsfestigkeit in ihrer Abhängigkeit von der Verteilung der Wiederholungen [The strength of associations in their dependence on the distribution of repetitions]. *Zeitschrift für Psychologie und Physiologie der Sinnesorgane, 16,* 436–472.

Kafkas, A., & Montaldi, D. (2011). Recognition memory strength is predicted by pupillary responses at encoding while fixation patterns distinguish recollection from familiarity. *Quarterly Journal of Experimental Psychology, 64*(10), 1971–1989.

Kensinger, E. A. (2009). *Emotional Memory Across the Adult Lifespan.* New York: Psychology Press.

Kensinger, E. A., & Corkin, S. (2003). Memory enhancement for emotional words: Are emotional words more vividly remembered than neutral words? *Memory & Cognition, 31,* 1169–1180.

Kleinsmith, L. J., & Kaplan, S. (1963). Paired-associate learning as a function of arousal and interpolated interval. *Journal of Experimental Psychology, 65,* 190–193.

Koriat, A., & Pearlman-Avnion, S. (2003). Memory organization of action events and its relationship to memory performance. *Journal of Experimental Psychology: General, 132,* 435–454.

Kounios, J., & Holcomb, P. J. (1994). Concreteness effects in semantic processing: ERP evidence supporting dual-code theory. *Journal of Experimental Psychology: Learning, Memory, and Cognition, 20,* 804–823.

LaBar, K. S., & Cabeza, R. (2006). Cognitive neuroscience of emotional memory. *Nature Reviews: Neuroscience, 7,* 54–64.

Lockhart, R. S., & Murdock, B. B. (1970). Memory and the theory of signal detection. *Psychological Bulletin, 74,* 100–109.

Luce, R. D. (1986). *Response Times: Their role in inferring elementary mental organization.* New York: Oxford University Press.

MacLeod, C. M., Gopie, N., Hourihan, K. L., Neary, K. R., & Ozubko, J. D. (2010). The production effect: Delineation of a phenomenon. *Journal of Experimental Psychology: Learning, Memory, and Cognition, 36*(3), 671–685.

Mandler, G. (1967). Organization and memory. In K. W. Spence and J. T. Spence (Eds.), *The Psychology of Learning and Motivation.* New York: Academic Press.

Martin-Loeches, M., Hinojosa, J. A., Fernandez-Frias, C., & Rubia, F. J. (2001). Functional differences in the semantic processing of concrete and abstract words. *Neuropsychologia, 39,* 1086–1096.

Mather, M. (2007). Emotional arousal and memory binding: An object-based framework. *Perspectives on Psychological Science, 2,* 33–52.

Matthews, W. J., Benjamin, C., & Osborne, C. (2007). Memory for moving and static images. *Psychonomic Bulletin & Review, 14,* 989–993.

Meyer, D. E., & Schvaneveldt, R. W. (1971). Facilitation in recognizing pairs of words: Evidence of a dependence between retrieval operations. *Journal of Experimental Psychology, 90,* 227–234.

Murre, J. M. J., & Chessa, A. G. (2011). Power laws from individual differences in learning and forgetting: Mathematical analyses. *Psychonomic Bulletin & Review, 18*(3), 592–597.

Nickerson, R. S., & Adams, M. J. (1979). Long-term memory for a common object. *Cognitive Psychology, 11,* 287–307.

Nisbett, R. E., & Wilson, T. D. (1977). Telling more than we can know: Verbal reports on mental processes. *Psychological Review, 84,* 231–259.

Ortony, A., Turner, T. J., & Antos, S. J. (1983). A puzzle about affect and recognition memory. *Journal of Experimental Psychology: Learning, Memory, and Cognition, 9,* 725–729.

Otani, H., & Hodge, M. H. (1991). Does hypermnesia occur in recognition and cued recall? *American Journal of Psychology, 104,* 101–116.

Paivio, A. (1969). Mental imagery in associative learning and memory. *Psychological Review, 76,* 241–263.

Papanicolaou, A. C., Simos, P. G., Castillo, E. M., Breier, J. I., Katz, J. S., & Wright, A. A. (2002). The hippocampus and memory of verbal and pictorial material. *Learning and Memory, 9,* 99–104.

Patterson, K. E., Meltzer, R. H., & Mandler, G. (1971). Inter-response times in categorized free recall. *Journal of Verbal Learning and Verbal Behavior, 10,* 417–426.

Payne, D. G. (1987). Hypermnesia and reminiscence in recall: A historical and empirical review. *Psychological Bulletin, 101,* 5–27.

Payne, J. D., & Kensinger, E. A. (2010). Sleep's role in the consolidation of emotional episodic memories. *Current Directions in Psychological Science, 19*(5), 290–295.

Payne, J. D., Stickgold, R., Swanberg, K., & Kensinger, E. A. (2008). Sleep preferentially enhances memory for emotional components of scenes. *Psychological Science, 19,* 781–788.

Pellegrino, J. W. (1971). A general measure of organization in free recall for variable unit size and internal sequential consistency. *Behavior Research Methods & Instruments, 3,* 241–246.

Pensky, A. E. C., Johnson, K. A., Haag, S., & Homa, D. (2008). Delayed memory for visual-haptic exploration of familiar objects. *Psychonomic Bulletin & Review, 15,* 574–580.

Perlmuter, L., Monty, R. A., & Kimble, G. A. (1971). Effect of choice on paired-associate learning. *Journal of Experimental Psychology, 91*(1), 47–53.

Postman, L., & Adams, P. A. (1956). Studies in incidental learning: IV. The interaction of orienting tasks and stimulus materials. *Journal of Experimental Psychology, 51,* 329–333.

Reitman, J. S., & Rueter, H. H. (1980). Organization revealed by recall orders and confirmed by pauses. *Cognitive Psychology, 12,* 554–581.

Roediger, H. L., Payne, D. G., Gillespie, G. L., & Lean, D. S. (1982). Hypermnesia as determined by level of recall. *Journal of Verbal Learning and Verbal Behavior, 21*(6), 635–655.

Roediger, H. L., & Thorpe, L. A. (1978). The role of recall time in producing hypermnesia. *Memory & Cognition, 6*(3), 296–305.

Roenker, D. L., Thompson, C. P., & Brown, S. C. (1971). Comparison of measures for the estimation of clustering in free recall. *Psychological Bulletin, 76,* 45–48.

Schnorr, J. A., & Atkinson, R. C. (1969). Repetition versus imagery instructions in the short- and long-term retention of paired-associates. *Psychonomic Science, 15,* 183–184.

Senkfor, A. J., Van Petten, C., & Kutas, M. (2008). Enactment versus conceptual encoding: Equivalent item memory but different source memory. *Cortex, 44,* 649–664.

Shepard, R. N. (1967). Recognition memory for words, sentences, and pictures. *Journal of Verbal Learning and Verbal Behavior, 6,* 156–163.

Slamecka, N. J., & Graf, P. (1978). The generation effect: Delineation of a phenomenon. *Journal of Experimental Psychology: Human Learning and Memory, 4,* 592–604.

Snodgrass, J. G., & Corwin, J. (1988). Pragmatics of measuring recognition memory: Applications to dementia and amnesia. *Journal of Experimental Psychology: General, 117,* 34–50.

Stagner, R. (1933). Factors influencing the memory value of words in a series. *Journal of Experimental Psychology, 16,* 129–137.

Standing, L. (1973). Learning 10,000 pictures. *Quarterly Journal of Experimental Psychology, 25,* 207–222.

Stanley, T. D., Carter, E. C., & Doucouliagos, H. (2018). What meta-analyses reveal about the replicability of psychological research. *Psychological Bulletin, 144* (12), 1325–1346.

Taft, M. (1979). Recognition of affixed words and the word frequency effect. *Memory & Cognition, 7,* 263–272.

Tulving, E. (1962). Subjective organization in free recall of "unrelated" words. *Psychological Review, 69,* 344–354.

Vaidya, C. J., Zhao, M., Desmond, J. E., & Gabrieli, J. D. (2002). Evidence for cortical encoding specificity in episodic memory: Memory-induced re-activation of picture processing areas. *Neuropsychologia, 40*(12), 2136–2143.

Vendetti, M., Castel, A. D., & Holyoak, K. J. (2013). The floor effect: Impoverished spatial memory for elevator buttons. *Attention, Perception, & Psychophysics, 75*(4), 636–643.

Wallner, L. A., & Bäuml, K. H. T. (2018). Hypermnesia and the Role of Delay between Study and Test. *Memory & Cognition, 46,* 878–894.

Wammes, J. D., Meade, M. E., & Fernandes, M. A. (2016). The drawing effect: Evidence for reliable and robust memory benefits in free recall. *Quarterly Journal of Experimental Psychology*, *69*, 1752–1776.

Weiss, M. W., Trehub, S. E., Schellenberg, E. G., & Habashi, P. (2016). Pupils dilate for vocal or familiar music. *Journal of Experimental Psychology: Human Perception and Performance*, *42*(8), 1061–1065.

Wixted, J. T. (2004). On common ground: Jost's (1897) law of forgetting and Ribot's (1881) law of retrograde amnesia. *Psychological Review*, *111*, 864–879.

Wixted, J. T., & Ebbesen, E. B. (1991). On the form of forgetting. *Psychological Science*, *2*(6), 409–415.

Yonelinas, A. P., & Jacoby, L. L. (2012). The process-dissociation approach two decades later: Convergence, boundary conditions, and new directions. *Memory & Cognition*, *40*(5), 663–680.

PART 2

Core Memory Topics

CHAPTER 4

Sensory and Short-Term Memory

When people think about memory, they typically think about retaining knowledge over long periods of time. When people speak of short-term memory, they often refer to remembering over a few hours or days. However, for cognitive scientists, memory in the short term means much briefer spans of time, often less than a minute. What is the point of studying such fleeting memories? Are not changes in the world from one moment to the next rather trivial? Well, no. Without these short-term memories, we would live in the permanent, absolute present—the eternal now. Language as we know it would not be possible. You would not be able to watch a film. Much of the world involves events that are spread out over time. Take the example of hearing a word. All words are made up of stream of sounds occurring at different points in time. To hear this stream as a whole word, you must integrate the sounds together. What allows you to do this is the memory of what occurred before, so the information you remember over time helps you link the sounds into the whole word.

Two types of brief memories are covered here. The first are very short memories, known as sensory registers. These modality-specific systems allow us to do important sensory identification and integration, such as the preceding example of word identification. The second is more formally known as short-term memory. This type of memory stores ideas that are within or close to conscious awareness.

SENSORY MEMORY

The briefest memory systems are the **sensory registers**. These are modality-specific, with each one retaining information specific to a sensory modality. For example, the visual sensory register retains visual information. The primary purpose of the sensory registers is low-level processing that involves the sensory information itself. Because different sensory systems process information with different properties, each register has different qualities and characteristics. Some consideration is given here to three sensory registers: (1) the visual sensory register, or iconic memory, (2) the auditory sensory register, or echoic memory, and (3) the haptic sensory register for touch information. There are others, but these three provide a broad understanding. The first two have been given a great deal of study. The third has received less attention, but it is included to show how a sensory register operates even in a modality for which humans are not particularly well suited.

ICONIC MEMORY

The first sensory memory considered is the visual sensory register or **iconic memory**. Humans are primarily visual animals and iconic memory is the most extensively studied sensory register. Information is represented in iconic memory to capture visual stimulation from our retinas, although there are important differences across species. The mental representation in iconic memory is an *icon* (hence the name *iconic* memory). To understand the role iconic memory plays, we need to understand how much information is held in iconic memory, how long an iconic representation is retained, and how it is used to build up mental representation of the visual world, even though at any moment we only see a small bit of it.

Span and Duration of Iconic Memory

The first two issues addressed about the visual sensory register memory are how much information can iconic memory hold, and how long can it hold it? In one study, Averbach (1963) presented two people (himself and another) sets of 1 to 13 dots for brief periods of time, anywhere from 40 to 600 milliseconds. The task was to say how many dots were in the display. The results are shown in Figure 4.1.

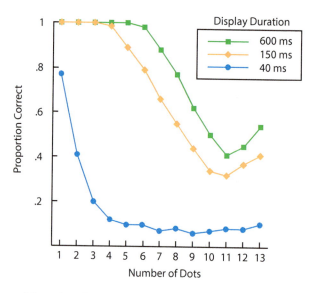

FIGURE 4.1 *Span of Apprehension Averaged across Participants*

Source: created from data reported in Averbach, E. (1963). The span of apprehension as a function of exposure duration. *Journal of Verbal Learning and Verbal Behavior, 2,* 60–64.

For the briefest display (40 ms), they were fairly accurate when there was one dot, but they were pretty lousy when there were more than one. For the longer two durations (150 and 600 ms), they were fairly accurate when there were up to four or five dots, with performance declining after that. Although there is a large time difference between the second and third conditions, the pattern of performance is roughly the same. The additional time did not provide much benefit.

Because this study looked at briefly presented displays, it assessed iconic memory. From these data it is tempting to conclude that the amount of information held in iconic memory is four or five items. Any more is beyond that capacity. Within that range people can make an accurate assessment of how many items are present. However, this is an incorrect conclusion. In a study by Sperling (1960; see also Sternberg, 2016), people saw brief displays, similar to Averbach (1963). They saw letters, instead of dots, and there were always 12 (in a 3 x 4 matrix). The task was to recall as many letters as possible. This display was presented for 50 milliseconds. In the control condition (also called the *whole report* condition) people reported as many of the letters as possible. In this case, people were able to name four or five. Again, by itself, this could be interpreted as showing that the number of items in iconic memory is four or five.

However, there was an experimental condition in Sperling's (1960) study (also called the *partial report* condition). Here, one of three tones sounded to indicate

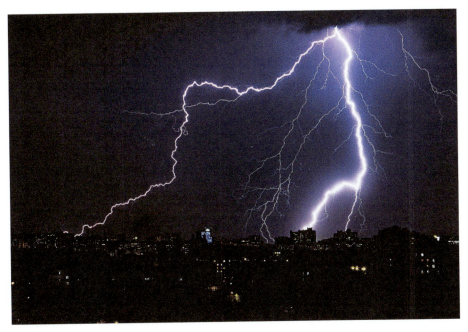

PHOTO 4.1 *Rapid visual stimuli, such as lightning strikes, appear to last longer than they are actually present in the world because of the persistence of the image in iconic memory*

Source: eugenegurkov/Shutterstock.com

which row of the display to report. A high tone indicated the top row, a medium tone for the middle row, and a low tone for the bottom row. Moreover, this tone occurred anywhere from just prior to the display being removed to one second after the display was removed. Sperling used the sum of the performance at each row to estimate how much information was initially available in iconic memory. If people could always report all four items in a cued row, this would indicate that all of the information was represented but that it decayed quickly. Alternatively, if they could report all four items from the top row but very few, if any, from the other rows, this would suggest that iconic memory can hold only very few items.

The results are shown in Figure 4.2. Performance was near ceiling (very close to perfect) when the tone cue was presented at the time the display was removed. However, as time increased before the tone, there was a decline in memory. Nearing the quarter-second mark (250 milliseconds), people approached performance in the whole-report condition. This indicates that a large amount of information is held in iconic memory—perhaps just about anything entering the visual system. However, iconic memory has a very brief duration. By about one-quarter of a second, nearly everything that was initially in iconic memory was lost. This is deterministic, not random, suggesting some influence of higher-order processes (Gold et al., 2005). Anything that is left was presumably transferred from iconic memory into short-term memory before it was lost. Note that, while typically the number of items transferred from iconic memory is 4–5, this can be increased if there is a semantic or functional (interactive) relationship between the items (O'Donnell et al., 2018).

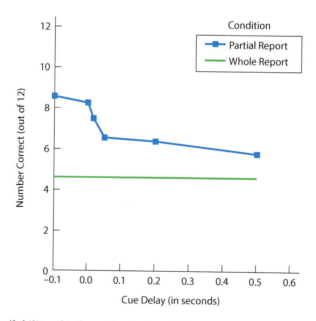

FIGURE 4.2 *Availability of Information in Iconic Memory*

Source: created from data reported in Sperling, G. (1960). The information available in brief visual presentations. *Psychological Monographs: General and Applied, 74 (11)*, 1–29.

Trans-Saccadic Memory

We do not view the world in one glance. Instead, we must move our eyes, head, and body to scan our surroundings. In doing so, we view different parts of the world and then integrate them to build a complete mental picture. A typical eye movement is a **saccade**. When our eyes land on some point in space, it is a **fixation**. Fixations typically last around 300 milliseconds and saccadic eye movements typically take about 30 ms to execute. Moreover, we mostly process information during the fixations. This is important because it places demands on iconic memory. We need to integrate information across saccades to build up a picture of the world. This involves (a) selecting where our eyes will move to, (b) holding onto information across the saccade, (c) checking that our eyes have fixated where we want them, and (d) comparing what we are seeing with the knowledge in iconic memory (Van der Stigchel & Hollingworth, 2018). Thus, there needs to be a **trans-saccadic memory** (e.g., Irwin, 1996) aspect of iconic memory to do this. There are a few ideas about how this is done.

One was that trans-saccadic memory uses retinal coordinates, the position of an image on the retinas of your eyes. This makes sense in that iconic memory is a visual memory, and the eyes provide the initial basis for this kind of information. However, this is incorrect. For example, suppose people are presented with two displays composed of portions of a 3 x 3 grid of eight dot locations. If the two grids were overlaid on top of one another, one could pick out the location of a missing ninth dot. This is easy to do when the two grids are presented in the same position and people do not have to move their eyes. The process of using this idea to test trans-saccadic memory is shown in the left column of Figure 4.3. The first display appears where people are currently looking. Then a cross appears in the periphery, indicating where people should look next. As people move their eyes to the new location, the first display is erased, and a second is presented where the eyes have

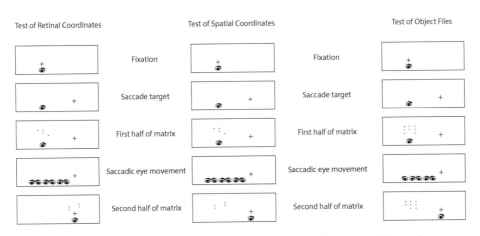

FIGURE 4.3 *Testing Retinally Based, Spatially Based, and Object-Based Ideas about Trans-Saccadic Memory*

Source: adapted from Irwin, D. E., Brown, J. S., & Sun, J. S. (1988). Visual masking and visual integration across saccadic eye movements. *Journal of Experimental Psychology: General, 117,* 276–287

moved to. This second display overlaps the first in retinal coordinates (that is, the same place on a person's eye). Under these conditions, people are *not* able to integrate these two displays to find the missing dot location. Thus, where images fall on the eyes does not appear to be important for trans-saccadic memory.

Alright, does trans-saccadic memory use spatial information—that is, where things are in space? This makes sense because people need to know how the world is structured beyond themselves. Thus, it could be that iconic memory uses information about where things are in space to build up an understanding of the world, similar to the way you could build up a larger picture by overlapping photographs taken from different positions. A similar procedure used to test the idea of retinally based integration can be used to test this idea. This is shown in the middle column of Figure 4.3, where the two dot patterns are in the same spatial location, even though the eyes are in motion. However, this does not work either. People cannot do well even though the two images are in the same spatial location (Irwin et al., 1983).

Instead, although trans-saccadic memory does use retinal and spatial information, with retinal being more accurate (Golomb & Kanwisher, 2012), it appears that it uses representations of objects, called **object files** (Kahneman et al., 1992). That is, individual objects or entities serve as the basis for how we assemble our understanding of the visual world. Trans-saccadic memory keeps track of basic characteristics of an object. Evidence for this comes from studies in which people can detect that something has been changed after an eye movement (Henderson & Anes, 1994). For example, in the right column of Figure 4.3, the task would require a response to indicate whether the dot pattern changed from one display to the next. This is a task that people can do quite readily. Moreover, change detection is more likely to occur when the entity is at the focus of attention rather than in the background. Thus, although we subjectively experience the world as stable and full of detail, this impression relies in part on our memories to fill in the gaps with what we have seen before or with what long-term memory assumes should be there.

Although trans-saccadic memory seems fairly simple, it can have important influences on more complex processing. That is, you cannot do some kinds of thinking while your eyes move. For example, if we need to mentally rotate an image, such as an inverted sign (see Chapter 5), this takes longer if we have to concurrently make an eye movement (Irwin & Brockmole, 2000). The execution of an eye movement and active operation of trans-saccadic memory puts other memory processes on hold while the eyes do their thing. This may be because the same part of memory is needed to do both, and these two very simple cognitive operations, moving the eyes and mentally turning something, use the same underlying machinery. It should also be noted that no mental processing is done when you blink or move your eyes (Irwin & Robinson, 2016).

Change Blindness

The lack of detail in iconic memory has interesting consequences. For example, there are often errors in feature films that go unnoticed by most of the audience, such as objects appearing and disappearing across cuts, clothes changing, and so on. These are called *continuity errors*. In a set of studies, people saw films in which objects changed across cuts. For example, dinner plates might change from red to white. However, people are very poor at detecting these changes and did so less than 2% of the time (Levin & Simons, 1997).

In one study, people watched films in which one actor was changed across film cuts (the two people were of the same gender and ethnicity). Only 33% of people noticed the change (Levin & Simons, 1997). In another example, an experimenter asked an individual (the subject) on the Cornell University campus for directions. While giving directions, two people passed between them carrying a door, thus blocking the person's view of the experimenter. At this time, a second experimenter switched places with the first. After the door had passed, many people continued giving directions even though they were now talking to a different person. Only about 50% of the people noticed the switch (Simons & Levin, 1998).

Visual memory reflects our expectations. For briefly presented scenes, people are more likely to detect a change in an object if it belongs in the scene (e.g., a blender in a kitchen) than if it does not (e.g., a live chicken in a kitchen) (Hollingworth & Henderson, 2003). This prior knowledge and expectation includes social constraints. In person-change experiments, college students were more likely to detect a person-switch when the experimenters were dressed like students than when they were dressed like construction workers. Students are in the same social group as the people being tested, but construction workers are not, so less attention is paid to them.

ECHOIC MEMORY

Echoic memory serves a similar purpose for audition as iconic memory does for vision. The mental representation in echoic memory is called the **echo**. Because the demands on this system are different from vision, echoic memory differs in important ways. Specifically, it must consider the fleeting and temporary nature of sound.

Span and Duration of Echoic Memory

As a parallel to iconic memory, let us look at the capacity and duration of echoic memory. In an analog to Sperling's (1960) study, Darwin et al. (1972) presented people wearing headphones with three lists of three digits. One list was presented only to the right ear, a second to only the left ear, and a third to both ears (so that it sounded like it was in the middle of the listener's head). Afterward, the task was to report as many digits as possible (whole report control condition) or to report only one list based on a visual cue that indicated left, right, or middle. The data are in Figure 4.4. As with Sperling's study of iconic memory, performance in the cued conditions indicated that more was available in echoic memory than was suggested by the whole report condition. Thus, echoic memory retains a large amount of information.

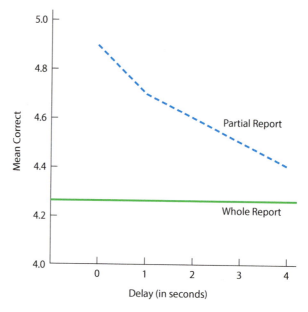

FIGURE 4.4 *Assessment of Echoic Memory*

Source: adapted from Darwin, C. J., Turvey, M. T., & Crowder, R. G. (1972). An auditory analogue of the Sperling partial report procedure: Evidence for brief auditory storage. *Cognitive Psychology, 3*, 255–267.

Now consider the duration of echoic memory. As shown in Figure 4.4, unlike iconic memory, echoic information is retained for a longer duration, about 4 seconds. This makes sense, given the nature of auditory information. For vision, stuff in the environment is typically present all at once. Moreover, the eyes are constantly shifting to new locations, so old information must be removed to make way for the new. If we need to reprocess something, we often need to look at the thing again. In contrast, auditory information is stretched out over time and can typically be heard only once. Consequently, echoic memory needs to keep larger chunks of information and retain it long enough so it can be properly analyzed to more accurately figure out what is being heard.

HAPTIC SENSORY MEMORY

Although iconic and echoic memories have received the most attention, each sensory modality has its own store, with characteristics unique to it. For example, memory for touch, **haptic sensory memory**, takes into account qualities such as pressure and temperature. Moreover, it needs to account for both the spatial extent of what is in contact with the body, as well as how it changes over time. Thus, this sensory register is more like iconic memory than echoic memory. Furthermore, different parts of the body are differentially sensitive to tactile information (e.g., the hands and face are more sensitive than the knees or back). Thus, the sensory register gives differential preference to touch information from different parts of the body.

Span and Duration of Haptic Sensory Memory

Let us look at the capacity and duration of haptic sensory memory. A study by Bliss et al. (1966), modeled on the Sperling (1960) study, had people receive small jets of air at different locations on the fingers of each hand. People gave whole reports of all the locations that were stimulated or gave partial reports after a light or a tone to indicate which parts of the fingers were relevant. In the whole report condition people could report three or four skin locations, but in the partial report condition, performance was better, with people having access to nearly all the locations. There was also a rapid decay of information such that by about 1.3 seconds, much of the information was lost.

Stop and Review

Some kind of memory is needed for even brief periods of time, and each sensory modality has a register dedicated to it. Iconic memory, the sensory register of vision, has a large capacity, but a short duration, as was made clear from the work by Sperling and his partial report method. The integration of trans-saccadic visual information over time is done in a systematic, object-based way. Finally, work on change blindness reveals that we are actively processing only small parts of the visual world. Echoic memory, the sensory register of hearing, also has a large capacity and a short duration, although it holds onto information longer than iconic memory does, most likely because useful auditory information is stretched out over time. Haptic sensory memory also has a large capacity, but a short duration, and its processes are oriented toward the features of touch, such as pressure and spatial extent.

SHORT-TERM MEMORY

Short-term memory is responsible for processing and retaining information beyond the sensory registers, but not for much longer than a minute or so (without active attention). Short-term memory is unique in that its contents include consciousness. Thus, when we think, we are using information in short-term memory. We examine the active manipulation of information in Chapter 5 when we consider working memory.

Although it has been studied for years, the precise nature of short-term memory is still unclear. Some researchers think of short-term memory as a qualitatively different part of human memory (e.g., Norris, 2017). In contrast, others view it as just a portion of long-term memory that is currently active (e.g., Cowan, 1988; Oberauer, 2002), with no clear distinction between short- and long-term memory, rather a continuum of activity in a single memory system. Regardless of which view is closer to the truth, there are aspects of memory that are salient during short time periods. It is these aspects that are of concern here.

SHORT-TERM MEMORY CAPACITY

A striking aspect of short-term memory is its limited capacity. Only a small number of things can be actively held at once. This is easily demonstrated. For a quick, at-home study, have a friend read you lists of random digits at the rate of about one per second. At the end of the list, recall the digits in the order that you heard them. Start with a short list, with only two or three digits, and then progress to longer lists. What you will find is that your short-term memory capacity is very small. Although this task starts out easy, it quickly becomes difficult. Most people are able to remember between five and nine digits in the correct order. In everyday experience you may run up against this limit if a person rattles off a telephone number too fast, or too quickly gives you a list of things to buy at the grocery store.

This small amount of information that can be held in short-term memory has been found for different types of information. A common idea is that our memory span is around seven items. The idea of short-term memory being an information processing bottleneck was first laid out in a classic paper entitled "The Magical Number Seven, Plus or Minus Two" (Miller, 1956[1]). Thus, memory span is often described as being 7 ± 2 chunks of information. The term *chunk* is important because what can serve as a unit of information is flexible.

TRY IT OUT

In this chapter there are a number of ideas for research on short-term memory. In this Try It Out section we look at how to assess its capacity. You should have at least 12 participants for this task, with at least 12 people in each group if you decide to vary things in your own study between groups. Here is what you could do to assess short-term memory capacity. Give a group of people progressively larger, randomly ordered, sets of items to remember. These can be digits, letters, or even simple words. Start with relatively small sets of items, such as 2, and work up to larger set sizes, with 5 lists for each set size. Present each list one item at a time, with a 1 second interval between items. At the end of the list, the participant should write the items down in the order that they were heard. If they cannot get any of the lists correct at a given level (none of the 5 item lists), then you can stop. Afterward score each person in terms of the highest level at which they could recall a list. If people get only one of the lists at the highest-level, score that level as a half. However, if they get two or more, give them full credit for that level. Most people should have a highest recall level between five and nine.

Although the 7 ± 2 figure is often cited as the capacity of short-term memory, some researchers have argued that capacity is actually only about 4 ± 1 items

---

1 See Cowan (2015) for a historical perspective on this paper and the handling of ideas that are out of step with current lines of scientific thinking.

(Cowan, 2000). People remember more because they are using other cognitive resources to extend the functional size of short-term memory. For example, we may chunk the information or use long-term memory to augment short-term memory (Chekaf et al., 2016).

Regardless of whether the capacity of short-term memory is seven or four units, this is still not a lot. Yet, we can think about larger amounts of knowledge than this limit implies. We have rather complex thoughts during the course of a day. How do we do it? There are ways to expand short-term memory capacity. The most widely discussed is the concept of chunking. **Chunking** occurs when we take smaller units of information and group them into a larger unit. This effectively frees up capacity in short-term memory (Thalmann et al., 2019). For example, the words "door" and "knob" can be chunked as "doorknob" This can be done in one of two ways: *redintegration* and *data compression* (Norris et al., 2020). For redintegration, knowledge in long-term memory is used to reconstruct elements in short-term memory. For data compression, the new information is recoded into a new form with fewer bits of information.

For example, if you were given a list of letters to remember, you may recall about seven of them. However, if those letters are grouped into words, then you can remember seven unrelated words, and the number of letters that you remember increases. A word serves as a chunk to organize the letters. Every time there is an opportunity for chunking, there is an opportunity to hold more information in short-term memory. Thus, when you are trying to learn something new, you are more likely to be able to retain it if you can place it into some organization or structure.

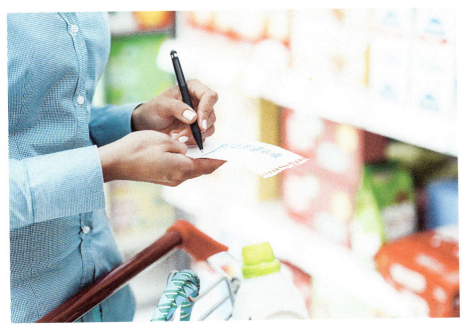

PHOTO 4.2 *If we can group lists of items, such as a list of items needed at the grocery store, into meaningful chunks, such at what to get in the produce section, bakery, canned goods, etc., then our memory for that information will be better*

Source: Stokkete/ Shutterstock.com

What guides chunking? Prior knowledge is a major influence. The more you know, the easier it is to form chunks by identifying patterns in information. The more knowledge you have, and the more efficient your application of it becomes, the greater your memory capacity will seem, even though it really stays about the same. Thus, memory can be improved by gaining expertise. As such, expose yourself to a wide range of different kinds of experiences to improve your memory. Another basis for organizing chunks are people. We more readily organize information around representations of people (Ishiguro & Saito, 2019), perhaps because we are such social animals.

Improve Your Memory

To have better memory in the long run, it is best if your memory operates effectively in the short run. An effective technique for improving memory is chunking, or grouping information together into larger meaningful units. That is, organize information by putting things together into groups. This can be based on some structure already present in the information (such as common categories, like produce, meat, and dairy) or by some structure that you make up for yourself. By doing this, you will remember more information overall. Moreover, this boost in remembering in the short-term can help you in the long term as well. This is why creating an outline of what you are trying to learn can help. Thus, to improve your memory, look for ways to structure or organize sets of material. The more that you group together information in any way that makes sense to you, the faster that you will learn it, and the more that you will remember.

Very Large Capacity

The influence of expertise on short-term memory capacity is clearly seen in a study by Ericsson et al. (1980). In this study at Carnegie-Mellon University, they had a person, S. F., go to the memory lab to assess his short-term memory span for digits. At the beginning of the study his digit span was about nine items. They continued to test him for over a year and a half. As shown in Figure 4.5, his digit span grew larger and larger over time. At the end of the study he could repeat back, in the correct order, over 80 digits that he had just heard read at the rate of 1 per second. Note that each list was different each time. How did he achieve this superhuman feat of reaching such a large digit span?

Well, S. F. was a runner. He grouped the digits into chunks based on race lengths and running times, as well as using other devices, such as famous dates. For example, the sequence 3492 was recoded as "3 minutes, 49 point 2 seconds, near world-record mile time," and 1944 as "near the end of World War II." The increase in S. F.'s memory span was a result of his using long-term knowledge to organize information in short-term memory. This made his short-term memory capacity seem larger. Note that his chunks were each often made up of three or four digits. The fact that S. F.'s short-term memory span, per se, did not actually grow larger is illustrated by the fact that after his digit span had grown to gargantuan proportions, when he was given a set of letters, his memory span dropped back down to six.

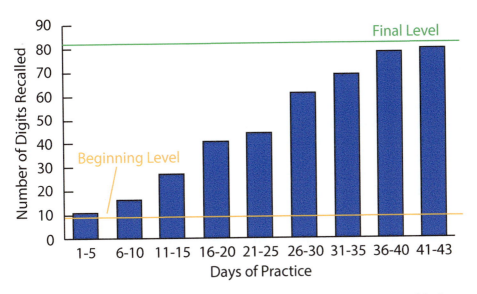

FIGURE 4.5 *Example of Expertise Influences on Short-Term Memory Span. In This Case, S. F.'s Digit Span Improved with Practice*

Source: adapted from Ericsson, K. A., Chase, W. G., & Faloon, S. (1980). Acquisition of a memory skill. *Science, 208*, 1181–1182

Another example of the influence of expertise is memory for chessboards. In one study people were first given a picture of a chessboard with pieces arranged on it. This board was then removed, and people reconstructed the positions of the pieces. Chess experts were much better at remembering where the pieces were on the board compared to people who are novice chess players. The chess experts were drawing on their knowledge of the game to help them chunk the pieces and remember their original locations. This is highlighted by conditions in which people were given chessboards that were not from the middle of a game, but had pieces randomly placed on the board. Under these circumstances, everyone's memory declined, and the chess masters did no better than the novices (Chase & Simon, 1973).

Another way that short-term memory capacity may be affected is if people have **synesthesia**. These people have involuntary sensory experiences in addition to normal ones (see Hochel & Milán, 2008 for a review). For example, people may experience colors when reading words. Two likely causes of synesthesia are a decreased ability to sufficiently suppress inappropriate feedback loops in perception (Grossenbacher & Lovelace, 2001) or an incomplete pruning of cortical connections during development (Maurer, 1997). Accounts of the effects of synesthesia on memory began with Luria's (1968) subject S. (see Chapter 15). He had a phenomenal verbatim memory, in part because he used his synesthetic experience as a memory aid. In general, synesthetes do better on short-term memory tests, such as memory for simple word lists (Radvansky et al., 2011; Yaro & Ward, 2007). They appear to use the additional sensory experiences to help them retain and remember items in short-term memory.

Synesthesia does not uniformly improve memory. For example, if synesthetes and controls are given items to learn that are (a) printed in black, (b) colors congruent with the synesthetic experience, or (c) colors incongruent with that experience, then synesthetes do better than the controls on memory for items presented in congruent colors but worse when the items are in incongruent colors (Radvansky et al., 2011; Smilek et al., 2002). This suggests that synesthesia can impair memory when the experience is inconsistent with the information in the world. Synesthetes also do not show a von Restorff effect (see Chapter 7) if the unique word in a list is identified by color (e.g., a red word among a list of black words) (Radvansky et al., 2011). Finally, they do not appear to be any better than normal at processing information beyond the individual word level, such as at the event model level (Radvansky et al., 2014). So, just because there are larger memory span scores does not necessarily lead to superior comprehension and understanding.

DURATION OF SHORT-TERM MEMORY AND FORGETTING

Not only does short-term memory have a small capacity, but it also retains information for short periods of time. Without active attention, information in short-term memory is largely forgotten within 30 seconds. The trick in showing this is that people must first think about something so that it enters short-term memory and then not think about it again until memory is tested.

There are several problems with this. First, it is next to impossible to *not* think about anything (Wegner, 1989). Our minds are always drifting around searching for something, anything, to think about. Second, whatever thoughts people have cannot be related to what we are trying to test. Otherwise, they are attending to it, and we cannot study how it is forgotten.

There have been several attempts to assess short-term memory forgetting. A major issue has been whether forgetting is due to decay or interference. For **decay**, the primary cause of forgetting is the passage of time or at least some process that is strongly correlated with time, like the decay of neural connections (Hardt et al., 2013). The more time that passes, the more a memory trace has decayed and forgetting has occurred. An early piece of evidence to support a decay interpretation was reported more or less simultaneously by Brown (1958) and by Peterson and Peterson (1959). As such, it is known as the Brown–Peterson paradigm (see Ricker et al., 2016 for a historical overview).

In the Petersons' study, students at Indiana University at Bloomington were given consonant trigrams (e.g., TPZ) to remember. To keep them from actively rehearsing these, after seeing the trigram they gave the students a three-digit number (e.g., 274), with the task of saying the number aloud and then counting backward by threes (e.g., 274, 271, 268, 265,) until they were told to stop, at which point they were to recall the trigram. The amount of time between the presentation of the trigram and the cue to recall the information was varied. The data are in Figure 4.6, which shows a nice forgetting curve. The more time that had elapsed, the less likely it was that the trigram was remembered. By 18 seconds, nearly all the information was lost. Because the to-be-remembered information was not involved in the current stream of thought, the only mechanism that seemed a likely reason for forgetting was decay.

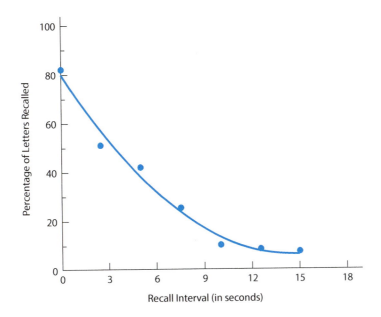

FIGURE 4.6 *Results from Peterson and Peterson's Short-Term Memory Experiment*

Source: Peterson, L. R., & Peterson, M. J. (1959). Short-term retention of individual verbal items. *Journal of Experimental Psychology, 58,* 193–198

While the decay theory has some intuitive appeal and is relatively simple (and science prefers simpler explanations), there are serious challenges to it. Most of these rest on the idea that forgetting is caused by interference. With **interference**, information in short-term memory interferes with or in some way blocks, displaces, or otherwise hinders the retrieval of other information. Because short-term memory has a limited capacity, if new information is put into it, it will compete with the information that is already there.

One study that supported the interference idea was by Keppel and Underwood (1962). They suggested that some of the forgetting in the Brown–Peterson paradigm was due to interference from items learned on previous trials. That is, prior letter trigrams remained in memory and competed with the new ones that were supposed to be remembered. What they did was to have only three trials in the entire experiment. With this approach, they found that there was virtually no forgetting on the first trial. Performance was essentially perfect. Forgetting only started to appear on the second and third trials. Thus, when there was no source of interference from prior trials, there was no short-term memory forgetting.

In a study by Waugh and Norman (1965) people got lists of 16 digits. At the end of each list was a probe digit, which was also marked with a tone. The task was to state what digit followed the earlier occurrence of the probe digit in the series that was just heard. In this way they could control how much interference people had experienced. The further back in the list the probe digit was, the more interference there was. To get at issues of decay, they presented the digits at either a slow (one per second) or fast rate (four per second). The results are shown in Figure 4.7. The more intervening items between the probe and its prior occurrence—that is, the

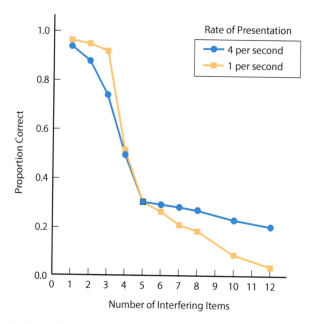

FIGURE 4.7 *Results from Waugh and Norman's Interference Experiment*

Source: created from data reported in Waugh, N. C., & Norman, D. A. (1965). Primary memory. *Psychological Review, 72,* 89–104

more interference there was—the greater the forgetting. The rate of forgetting was similar in both the slow and fast presentation conditions. Thus, short-term memory forgetting is more of a function of the amount of interference than the amount of time that has passed. Forgetting was observed in the Brown–Peterson task because counting backward produced interference and caused the forgetting of the trigrams.

In sum, interference is the primary cause of forgetting in short-term memory. That said, there may be at least some involvement of decay (Berman et al., 2009; Portrat et al., 2008; Ricker et al., 2020). Altmann and Schunn (2012) make a compelling argument that the classic Waugh and Norman (1965) data actually reflects a mixture of both decay and interference, with interference having a greater influence.

Forgetting via interference with new information entering short-term memory has implications for everyday life. For example, if you are trying to keep information in mind, such as a telephone number or a person's name and are disrupted by something else, it is likely that you will forget the information. When you are reading or listening to something, you may need to keep track of several ideas to understand what is being communicated. If you are not able to do so effectively, then your comprehension, and memory will suffer. In a study by Zeamer and Fox Tree (2013), students remembered less from a lecture if there were additional distracting sounds, such as audience laughter, murmuring, construction noises, and so on. Thus, to improve your memory, it is best to keep sources of interference to a minimum.

Overall, if there is interfering information in the environment, this displaces the information that you need in short-term memory. If you try to study with the television on, your ability to understand and remember what you are studying is compromised. If you try to reason through something, you often need to consider various possibilities and outcomes. This places a strain on short-term memory. We all have been in situations in which there was a lot going on around us while we made a decision, and because we were not able to think clearly due to an interference, we were left with a choice we later regretted.

Stop and Review

Short-term memory can hold only a small amount of information for a few seconds. We can increase our capacity by chunking information into larger units. When forgetting occurs, this is due to processes correlated with the passage of time, primarily the intrusion of new, interfering information that blocks, displaces, or otherwise hinders memory for the target information.

RETRIEVAL IN SHORT-TERM MEMORY

If we encode information into the limited capacity of short-term memory and avoid decay and interference sufficiently to retain it, it may be necessary to then use it. At that point it needs to be retrieved. For example, suppose you are on the phone with someone who tells you a list of names of people who will be attending a surprise party just as you are walking into the dining hall. There you see a friend, and now you need to remember if that person's name was in the set of names you just heard. The contents of short-term memory must be searched to select the one item (that person's name) that is needed. How do you do this? As you can read in the Study In-Depth Box, people seem to be using a serial self-terminating search in which they search through items one at a time in short-term memory and produce a response after going through all of the items.

A notable attempt to address the search of short-term memory was a series of studies by Sternberg (1966; 1969; 1975). In one of his studies (1966) he used an experimental paradigm in which eight students at the University of Pennsylvania were given lists of one to six digits (e.g., 5, 2, 4, 3, 8, 0) to hold in short-term memory. These digits were presented one at a time, for 1.2 seconds each. Note that these list sizes are well within the capacity of short-term memory. At the end of the list, after a 2-second delay, people were then given a memory probe (e.g., 4) with the task of pressing a button to indicate whether the probe was in the list. For a dependent measure Sternberg recorded how long it took to respond as a function of how many items were in the set, and whether the probe was in the set. There were 24 practice trials and 144 experimental trials, with half of each requiring a "yes" response and half "no."

Using this approach Sternberg tested three theories of short-term memory search. The first is a **parallel search** in which all the items in short-term memory are available more or less at once and accessed in parallel. This makes sense if one assumes that the

STUDY IN DEPTH

contents of short-term memory are either in or close to consciousness. If people search short-term memory in parallel, then the amount of information in the search set should not matter. All the information is available at once regardless of the size of the search set. As a result, response times should not vary with set size, and there should be no difference between the "yes" and "no" responses.

A second alternative is a **serial self-terminating search**. This involves going through items one at a time, that is, in serial. Once people get to the target item, the search stops or terminates. In this type of search there is an increase in response time with an increase in set size. By going through the items one by one, the larger the set, the longer it should take. There is also a difference in the slope of the response times for "yes" and "no" responses. For "no" responses, the function is relatively steep because people always need to go through the entire set to verify that the probe item is not there. However, for "yes" responses, there is an increasing response time slope, but it should be half that of "no" responses. This is because people are going through the items one at a time, and on average, they get about halfway through the set before getting to the target item.

The final alternative is a **serial exhaustive search**. This again involves people going through things one at a time, in serial. However, rather than stopping when they get to what they were looking for, people continue until they go through the entire set. This search process would also result in an increasing response time function with increasing set size. However, if people searched in a serial exhaustive fashion, there would be no difference in the response time slope for the "yes" and "no" responses. This is because in both cases they are going through the entire set of information.

The results of a study by Theios et al. (1973) that replicated Sternberg's results are shown in Figure 4.8. As you can see, the data support a serial exhaustive search. This

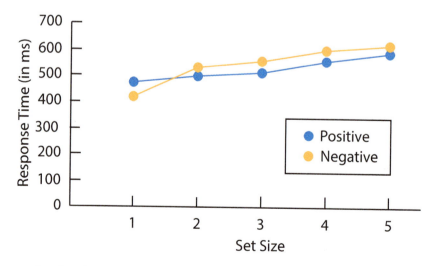

FIGURE 4.8 *Results of Sternberg's Search of Short-Term Memory Task*

Source: adapted from Theios, J., Smith, P. G., Haviland, S. E., Traupmann, J., & Moy, M. C. (1973). Memory scanning as a serial self-terminating process. *Journal of Experimental Psychology, 97*(3), 323–336

outcome is instructive in two ways. First, it shows how short-term memory is searched. The other lesson is about our ability to report on our own memories. When I list out the three possible outcomes in my classes and ask students to state which one they think is true, most people pick serial self-terminating search. It may, in some way, be consistent with subjective experience. The fact that so many people get this wrong is important because we are talking about a simple process that occurs repeatedly in our lives in a part of memory that is very close to conscious awareness. This is why memory researchers do so many studies trying to understand what may sometimes seem like a simple question. It is not unusual for the results of experiments to produce counterintuitive results. We do not have much conscious awareness of how our own memories operate. We need objective measures to test our theories.

Serial versus Parallel Issues

An important point about the search of short-term memory is that not everyone agrees that a serial process is involved. This pattern of data could result from parallel processing in which there are limited cognitive resources. When multiple elements are held in short-term memory, these resources are divided among them. This is like sending water down a pipe and then dividing the pipe into several smaller pipes, resulting in less water flowing down any one pipe. As a result, the more finely divided cognitive resources are, the less there is available to any one item, and thus, the longer it takes for retrieval to occur.

This issue of serial versus parallel processes has a long and tortuous history in memory research (Townsend, 1990). It is not unusual for one researcher to claim that a given memory process is either serial or parallel and then to have another come along and demonstrate that the opposite could be true. It is difficult to distinguish between the two.

For every complex memory process there are probably both parallel and serial components intermixed in a **cascading process**. The brain is composed of billions of neurons that are all regularly engaged in some sort of processing. Thus, because several neural assemblies are often simultaneously being used for memory, there is some element of parallel processing. For example, when people try to remember where they heard something, they need to know both what the information is and the source of the information. Memory processes can also involve stages in which latter steps simply cannot be done without the results of other, earlier steps.

Serial Position Curves

We now consider temporal influences on the retrieval of information from short-term memory. One of the most durable effects is the **serial position curve**, shown in Figure 4.9 (Rundus, 1971). It has been studied at least since the early work of Mary Whiton Calkins in the late nineteenth century (Madigan & O'Hara, 1992). A serial position curve is a U-shaped function, with memory being better for

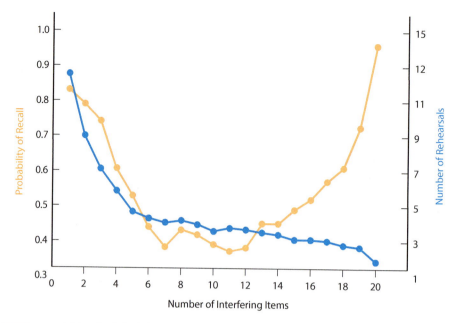

FIGURE 4.9 *A Standard Serial Position Curve in Short-Term Memory. Green Dots Show Short-Term Memory, and Red Dots Indicate the Mean Number of Rehearsals per Item*

Source: Rundus, D. (1971). Analysis of rehearsal processes in free recall. *Journal of Experimental Psychology, 89*, 63–77

information at the beginning and end of a set, whereas information in the middle is less well remembered (Murdock, 1962). A serial position curve is found for various information types and set sizes.

Better memory for information at the beginning of a set is the **primacy effect**. Traditionally, the primacy effect is attributed to long-term memory. The idea is that items at the beginning have more opportunity to be rehearsed and are more likely to have been consolidated into long-term memory. For example, for the first item, no other items have yet been given, so all of the rehearsal effort can be devoted to it. Thus, the first item has the highest probability of being transferred to long-term memory. For the second item, attention is now split between the first and second items, so it is less likely that the second item will make it to long-term memory. This logic can then be extended to the rest of the set. After a number of items, the amount of additional rehearsal benefit is negligible. The relationship between practice and later memory for items is also shown in Figure 4.9. Rundus (1971) tracked how much each item was rehearsed by having people say their rehearsals aloud during learning. As you can see, for the primacy effect, the more rehearsals of a given item, the more likely it was remembered later.

If people are given more time to rehearse information, then the primacy effect gets larger. The predicted pattern of results is shown in Figure 4.10, with single, double, and triple referring to the amount of time people have to study each item. This was confirmed in a study by Glanzer and Cunitz (1966) in which people

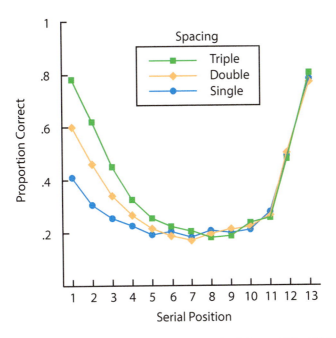

FIGURE 4.10 *Effects of Additional Rehearsal Time on the Primacy Effect Using Hypothetical Data*

were given information at different speeds. When the presentation rate was slow, memory was better and the primacy effect was larger, but the recency effect was unaffected. The idea that the primacy effect depends more on long-term memory is further supported by fMRI data showing that early items (primacy effect) involve more activation of brain areas associated with long-term verbal memory, such as the left hippocampus and parts of the left temporal lobe (BA 36), whereas late items (recency effect) show increased activation of parietal lobe areas, such as the right inferior portions (BAs 39 & 40) (Talmi et al., 2005).

Superior memory for items at the end of the set is the **recency effect**. The recency effect is attributed to short-term memory (Davelaar et al., 2005). These items have not been displaced by later interfering information and so are less likely to be forgotten. In Rundus's (1971) study, the later items are not rehearsed as much. They are remembered not because of how much they were rehearsed, but because they are likely to still be in short-term memory. As such, to maximize performance, it is best to try to recall the most recent things first, before you encounter potentially interfering information, and then move to whatever is stored in long-term memory. This is shown in Figure 4.11 in which there are various retention intervals that are filled with a distractor task to displace information from short-term memory. Glanzer and Cunitz's (1966) study confirmed this aspect of the serial position curve. In a second experiment, people waited a time during which they did a distractor task before they recalled the information. The longer the filled delay at the end of the list, the less pronounced the recency effect. However, the primacy portion of the curve, which is attributed to long-term memory, was unaffected.

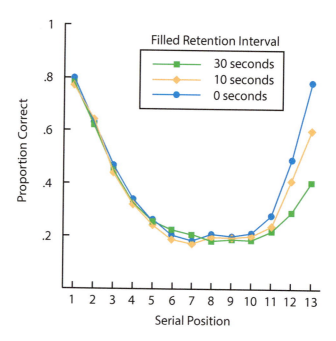

FIGURE 4.11 *Effects of Different Filled Retention Intervals (in Seconds) on the Recency Effect Using Hypothetical Data*

TRY IT OUT

The storage of information in short-term memory is affected by the order in which items were encountered. This is clear when one looks at serial position curves for information beyond the capacity of short-term memory. To demonstrate serial position curves (see Zechmeister & Nyberg, 1982), first assemble a list of 15–20 single syllable words. These are the words that you will read to your participants.

After this, gather 12 or more people to be your participants. Give each person a piece of paper on which to write their responses. Have them listen while you read aloud your list of 15–20 words. Read these words clearly at a rate of about 1 word per second. At the end of the list have your participants write down as many of these words as they can remember. For this task, the order in which they write them down is of less importance, but that is something that you can manipulate if you wanted to. You should give about five minutes to recall as much as they can remember.

After the participants are done recalling, collect their response sheets. Then you should tabulate which words were recalled as a function of the order in which they appeared on the list. What you should find is that people remember more from the beginning and end and fewer from the middle. You can do a number of variations of this by altering list lengths, giving a second group of people a 30-second distractor task of math problems (e.g., 935 + 135 =?) at the end (to eliminate the recency effect), or have people verbalize their rehearsals to see the relationship of these with the primacy effect.

Changing the Serial Position Curve

While the serial position curve is a robust finding, it is not always observed. There are things that can reduce the primacy or recency effect or eliminate them altogether. Most research on serial position curves uses verbal materials, such as lists of words. In comparison, in terms of memories for recently performed actions, although performed actions are remembered better than words (see Chapter 3), there is still some forgetting. Again, this is the enactment effect. This forgetting is influenced by serial position, but with performed actions there is no primacy effect (Seiler & Engelkamp, 2003). Doing something leads people to focus more on the individual actions. As such, there is less opportunity to rehearse those that were done previously, and so this information is less likely to be transferred to long-term memory. As a result, no primacy effect is seen for performed actions.

Also, when people are given a sequence of odors, they show a strong recency effect, but only a weak or absent primacy effect (Miles & Hodder, 2005). Conversely, for tactile stimulation, there is a clear primacy effect, but little or no recency effect (Johnson et al., 2016). Thus, for things that are hard to name, this can result in poorer processing of information in memory. That said, both primacy and recency effects have been noted for tastes (Daniel & Katz, 2018).

Another serial position phenomenon is the **suffix effect**. With the suffix effect, the recency effect is diminished when extra information is presented at the end of a list (Conrad, 1960; Crowder & Morton, 1969). For example, suppose you heard a list of words in a short-term memory study. Then, at the end of the list, the experimenter either said nothing or said the word "go" to indicate that you should recall the list. In this case, the word "go" is a suffix. Memory is worse in the "go" condition than in the silence condition. The word "go" interferes with information in short-term memory, causing forgetting. As a real-world illustration of the suffix effect, Schilling and Weaver (1983) had students call a telephone operator to request a phone number. After giving the number, when the operator concluded the call with the phrase "Have a nice day," memory for the phone number that was just heard was worse. The pleasantry at the end served as a suffix, causing more forgetting of the target information (the phone number).

The size of the suffix effect is related to the nature of the suffix itself. The more it is like the items on a list, the greater the interference and the greater the effect (Ayers et al., 1979). As shown in Figure 4.12, when the suffix was human speech, the recency effect was reduced, but not when it was an unrelated sound, like a buzzer. It is also important what people think the suffix is. When we hear a list of words and then hear a "baa" sound, if we are told that the sound was made by a person,

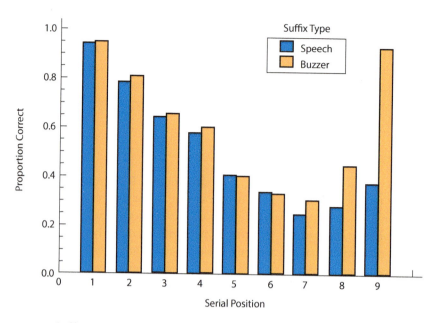

FIGURE 4.12 *Suffix Effects with Human Speech and Nonhuman Nonspeech Sound*

Source: adapted from Crowder, R. G. (1972). Visual and auditory memory. In J. F. Kavanagh, & I. G. Mattingly (Eds.), *Language by Ear and by Eye*. Cambridge, MA: MIT Press

there is a larger suffix effect than if we are told it was made by a sheep, even though the same sound is used (Neath et al., 1993).

In general, the suffix effect is influenced by the physical characteristics of a suffix, leading many researchers to consider it as part of echoic memory. This was hammered out in a marathon series of 15 experiments reported by Morton et al. (1971). They found that the suffix effect was unaffected by the meaning of the suffix, its frequency, or its emotionality. However, the effect was reduced if the suffix came from a different location in space, was in a different timbre (human voice versus noise), or was from a different person, particularly one of a different gender. Thus, the suffix effect is influenced by both perceptual qualities and conceptual understanding of what is being heard (Bloom, 2006). Finally, the suffix effect can also occur for visual information, lip reading, tactile stimuli, and odors (Campbell & Dodd, 1982; Mahrer & Miles, 1999; Parmentier et al., 2004). This presence of a suffix effect in all these sensory modalities suggests that it is a general property of short-term memory.

TRY IT OUT

The recency portion of the serial position curve reflects the idea that information that is still being held in short-term memory has not yet been displaced by new information. It should be possible to reduce or eliminate the recency effect by giving people other non-list items after the last list item to produce a suffix effect. Before you do the study, set up 11 lists of digits (from 1 to 9) in which there are 8 digits, in a random order, on each list. Make sure there are no repeats within a list and that there are no sequential runs in a list (e.g., 7, 8, 9).

After you have your lists, you will need two groups of at least 12 people in each. Read aloud the list of digits. The task is for people to recall the digits, in the order they hear them, after the end of a list. They can write their responses on a sheet of paper in which there is a box for each of the eight digits in a given list. Have people write a digit in each box at the position in which they remember it. They can put an "X" in a box if they cannot remember the digit at a given position. In the *control* group, people should start recalling when you finish reading a list of eight digits. In the *suffix* group, at the end of each list give the digit 0. Tell those people that when they hear the 0, this is their cue to start remembering.

After you have given all 11 lists, collect the response sheets and look at what people wrote down. Throw out the first list as practice. Then, count up the number of errors people made. What you should find is that memory for the lists will be worse in the suffix group than in the control group (see Zechmeister & Nyberg, 1982).

Stop and Review

Retrieval from short-term memory is affected by how much information is in memory, similar to what would be expected with a serial exhaustive search. That said, there are other possibilities, such as a parallel search with limited resources. Short-term memory retrieval is also affected by the order in which items were encountered. People often show serial position curves, with a primacy effect (better memory for things early on) and a recency effect (better memory for the most recent items). This latter finding can be disrupted with a suffix.

MEMORY FOR SERIAL ORDER

Short-term memory not only retains information content, but also the **serial order** in which items were encountered. If someone gives you a telephone number, remembering just the digits is not sufficient. You need to know the proper sequence as well. For the most part, people are fairly good at remembering serial orders (provided the amount of information is within normal short-term memory capacity). There is a strong forward-order bias in remembering. We can report things in the reverse order, but this is often harder (see Donolato et al., 2017, for a review). When people do forget, they do not do so randomly, but in systematic ways. For example, there is a serial position effect, with elements at the beginning and end of an order remembered in their correct location better than those in the middle. Also, for things that are remembered out of order, they are likely to be close to one another. For example, if you mess up the telephone number 123–4567, you are more likely to misremember it as 123–5467 than as 163–4527. Using an organization adopted by Henson (1998) we look at three classes of theories of memory for serial order in short-term memory.

Chaining Models

For **chaining models** (Ebbinghaus, 1885/1964; Lewandowsky & Murdock, 1989) it is assumed that in short-term memory there are a series of associative links. Order information is recovered by moving along the chain. A problem is that if people cannot remember an item, then the chain should be broken, and they should not be able to continue. However, some approximation of the lost item could be used to pick up items further along, perhaps using more remote associations with items not immediately following a given item. Typically, forgetting results in only a partial loss of information.

Along these lines, there is evidence that serial order short-term memory is supported by language (Acheson & McDonald, 2009). For example, people can use long-term memory for syntactic information, such as "itchy window" (e.g., Epstein, 1961; Marks & Miller, 1964). These syntactic benefits are present if the words are presented in a typical syntactic order (e.g., itchy window) than the reverse (e.g., window itchy) (Perham et al., 2009). People use this syntactic information to help reconstruct the serial order in memory (Jones & Farrell, 2018).

Ordinal Models

For **ordinal models**, serial order is captured by information about where a given item occurs along a dimension *relative* to the others. For example, in the **perturbation model** (Estes, 1972) information is organized as a hierarchy of chunks. Every item is regulated by a control unit that manages the chunk. These control units themselves may be grouped together by higher-order control units. One such a hierarchy is shown in Figure 4.13. The item-to-control unit associations convey order information. This accounts for the fact that misorderings are more likely to occur at a local level and within chunks than across them. For example, a phone number, like 123–4567, is divided into two chunks: 123 and 4567. It is more likely that we will misorder 4 and 5, because they are in the same chunk, than 3 and 4, because they are in different chunks.

Another ordinal model is the **inhibition model** (Burgess & Hitch, 1992) which suggests that inhibition, a mechanism of attention, is used to recover serial order. The idea is that as we go through a list, the retrieval process selects the most active or accessible item, which is usually the first in the series. As each is retrieved and reported, it is inhibited and activation is sent to the next item in the order, which is now the most active. Inhibition keeps prior items from being recalled again.

The inhibition of recently processed short-term memory information is seen in the phenomenon of **repetition blindness** (Kanwisher, 1987). This is observed when people read sentences using rapid serial visual presentation (or RSVP). Essentially, words are rapidly shown one at a time in the same location on a screen, but still

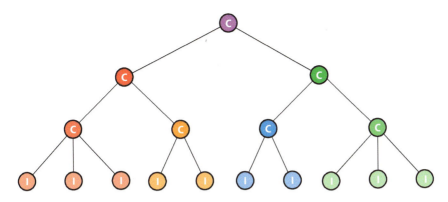

FIGURE 4.13 *A Hierarchy of Control Units as Theorized by the Perturbation Model*

Source: adapted from Estes, W. K. (1972). An associative basis for coding and organization in memory. In A. W. Melton & E. Martin (Eds.), *Coding Processes in Human Memory*, pp. 161–190. New York: Wiley

slow enough that they can be read. If the same word is repeated within a short time span, people claim to not have seen the second occurrence of it. For example, for the sentence "When she spilled the ink, there was ink all over" people are likely to not report the second "ink," even though this makes the sentence ungrammatical. This is because "ink" had been recently processed and inhibited in short-term memory. Thus, people have trouble processing it again, even though they are looking right at it.

Positional Models

For **positional models**, serial order is conveyed by associating each item with its position in a sequence. The simplest versions are **slot-based models** (Conrad, 1965) that assume that short-term memory is a series of ordered slots (or boxes) and that information is dropped into each one as it is encountered. To convey order, we simply read off what is in the slots. Here, item and order information are stored together because each item is put in a slot in a predetermined order. However, there is little evidence to support this. A more refined version of this is the *mental whiteboard hypothesis*, which assumes that we track serial position using embodied, spatial processes to keep track of where something is in a sequence (Abrahamse et al., 2017).

More sophisticated versions include **context-based models** (Burgess & Hitch, 1992) that exploit the fact that context is constantly in flux, even if at a subtle level. This includes both what is going on in the environment, as well as the internal context of our physiological, emotional, and cognitive states. This shifting context varies in regular ways, as with neural oscillators, which can then be used to identify positions in a series. As you will see in Chapter 7, context information is stored in memory. This can be used to determine serial order information by reconstructing order from the way that context is changing. Here, misorderings occur because the contexts were similar. Items that are close in time are likely to have similar contexts than items farther apart. This explains why local misorderings are more common than distant ones.

Finally, positional models take into account salient positions in a series, such as the first and last positions, which are distinctive (Henson, 1998). People can use these positions to help reproduce a serial order. Such theories can account for people sometimes making errors in which an item from a previous series is misremembered in the current one. Such an error is called a **protrusion**. When these occur, the incorrect item is remembered in the same position as it was in the prior series. This suggests that position, in some way, is stored with the items in short-term memory.

Neurological Support

The fact that there are different theories of serial order memory suggests that how we figure out how to put things in a proper sequence is a complex process that involves different types of information used in different ways. It has even been suggested that memory is not really designed to remember order information at all (Hintzman, 2016). Marshuetz (2005) showed that several brain regions are involved, each playing a different role. An explicit need to remember order information requires the hippocampus, perhaps because the order itself becomes a source of content to be learned. Also, serial order memory involves increased activity in the prefrontal and parietal regions. The dorsolateral prefrontal cortex (BAs 9 & 46) is involved in the allocation of the attention needed to encode and extract a sequence of items. Also, the part of the parietal cortex used to code numerical magnitude (e.g., knowing that 8 is larger than 4) is also involved.

There is also evidence that the premotor cortex (BA 6) is involved in chunking items into a sequence and the timing of that sequence. Moreover, the motor cortex (BA 4) is involved in more detailed aspects of serial order. This makes sense from an embodied cognition perspective. Serial order is critical for many motor behaviors that would be impossible without doing things in the proper order (e.g., walking, eating, or tying your shoelaces).

Stop and Review

Retrieval from short-term memory can involve retrieving a serial order. Serial order memory is a complex process that is influenced by the associations formed between items, how the elements are chunked, and knowledge of where in a series a given item was encountered. Chaining models emphasize the associative links. Ordinal models assume that serial order is captured in relative order information. Finally, positional models assume that spots in a series are directly represented in short-term memory. These different types of serial order information are associated with different neurological processes or regions.

PUTTING IT ALL TOGETHER

Dealing with information on a more immediate time scale involves sensory and short-term memories. The recurrent issues for these memory systems are how much information can a system hold, for how long, and how is it lost? In terms of capacity, for the sensory registers, regardless of whether you are talking about iconic memory, echoic memory, haptic memory, or whatever, the capacity is very large—essentially whatever can be processed by the sensory receptors. In comparison, the bottleneck of the system is short-term memory, which can hold a small number of items, either 7 or 4, depending on how you count. This limit can be increased by structuring or chunking the knowledge. If you have synesthesia, it can help with this process. In addition to knowledge about content (what is remembered), short-term memory also keeps track of the sequence in which things were encountered. This is done by linking items into a chain, chunking knowledge into a hierarchical structure (like your social security number), suppressing recently encountered items, or exploiting regular changes in context.

How long can these memory systems hold on to information? For the sensory registers, these are very brief periods of time, anywhere from a quarter of a second to four seconds, depending on the modality. Thus, not very long at all. This allows you to continually bring in and process new sensory data. Short as it is, it is long enough for us to build up a picture of the world, as suggested by work in trans-saccadic memory. For short-term memory, if you continue to attend to things, they can stay in short-term memory for a long time. However, when your attention moves away, the memory only hangs around for 30 seconds or so. Early items in a set may be transferred to long-term memory, but later items are less likely to have that happen.

Again, an important issue in memory is not remembering but forgetting. For the sensory registers, forgetting happens with the passage of time. The more time that has passed, the less there is. For short-term memory, while there may be some memory loss through a decay process, the bulk of the forgetting is due to interference from other items. The absence of immediate inference is what produces the recency effect, which itself can be disrupted by any subsequent inference that serves as a suffix. If it is remembered, this information is likely to be retrieved in a way consistent with either a serial exhaustive or parallel, limited capacity manner.

STUDY QUESTIONS

1. What is the point of having sensory registers as memory systems?
2. What are the basic principles of iconic memory, and why does it have these characteristics? Echoic memory? Haptic sensory memory?
3. What are some of the basic characteristics of trans-saccadic memory?
4. What does the existence of change blindness say about the nature of visual short-term memory?
5. What is the capacity and duration of short-term memory? How can this be extended?
6. How can the presence of synesthesia influence people's short-term memory for information?
7. How does forgetting typically occur in short-term memory?
8. How is information retrieved from short-term memory?
9. How easy or difficult is it to distinguish between serial and parallel processes in human memory?

10. What is the serial position curve, and what does it have to do with short-term memory?

11. How is short-term memory able to keep track of the order in which things occur? What are the three basic classes of theories of short-term serial order memory?

KEY TERMS

- cascading processes
- chaining models
- chunking
- context-based models
- decay
- echo
- echoic memory
- fixation
- haptic sensory memory
- icon
- iconic memory
- inhibition model

- interference
- object files
- ordinal models
- parallel search
- perturbation model
- positional models
- primacy effect
- protrusion
- recency effect
- repetition blindness
- saccade
- sensory registers

- serial exhaustive search
- serial order
- serial position curve
- serial self-terminating search
- short-term memory
- slot-based models
- suffix effect
- synesthesia
- trans-saccadic memory

EXPLORE MORE

Here are some additional readings that you can explore to get better insight into sensory and short-term memory.

Brown, G. D. A. (1997). Formal models of memory for serial order: A review. In M. A. Conway (Ed.), *Cognitive Models of Memory* (pp. 47–78). Cambridge, MA: MIT Press.

Cowan, N. (2000). The magical number 4 in short-term memory: A reconsideration of mental storage capacity. *Behavioral and Brain Sciences*, *24*, 87–185.

Goldinger, S. D., & Papesh, M. H. (2012). Pupil dilation reflects the creation and retrieval of memories. *Current Directions in Psychological Science*, *21*(2), 90–95.

Hardt, O., Nader, K., & Nadel, L. (2013). Decay happens: The role of active forgetting in memory. *Trends in Cognitive Sciences*, *17*(3), 111–120.

Miller, G. A. (1956). The magical number seven, plus or minus two: Some limits on our capacity for processing information. *Psychological Review*, *63*, 81–97.

Radvansky, G. A., Gibson, B. S., & McNerney, M. W. (2011). Synesthesia and memory: color congruency, von Restorff, and false memory effects. *Journal of Experimental Psychology: Learning, Memory, and Cognition*, *37*(1), 219.

REFERENCES

Abrahamse, E. L., van Dijck, J. P., & Fias, W. (2017). Grounding verbal working memory: The case of serial order. *Current Directions in Psychological Science, 26*(5), 429–433.

Acheson, D. J., & McDonald, M. C. (2009). Twisting tongues and memories: Explorations of the relationship between language production and verbal working memory. *Journal of Memory and Language, 60*, 329–350.

Altmann, E. M., & Schunn, C. D. (2012). Decay versus interference A new look at an old interaction. *Psychological Science, 23*(11), 1435–1437.

Averbach, E. (1963). The span of apprehension as a function of exposure duration. *Journal of Verbal Learning and Verbal Behavior, 2*(1), 60–64.

Ayers, T. J., Jonides, J., Reitman, J. S., Egan, J. C., & Howard, D. A. (1979). Differing suffix effects for the same physical suffix. *Journal of Experimental Psychology: Human Learning and Memory, 5*, 315–321.

Berman, M., Jonides, J., & Lewis, R. L. (2009). In search of decay in verbal short-term memory. *Journal of Experimental Psychology: Learning, memory, and Cognition, 35*, 317–333.

Bliss, J. C., Crane, H. D., Mansfield, P. K., & Townsend, J. T. (1966). Information available in brief tactile presentations. *Perception & Psychophysics, 1*, 273–283.

Bloom, L. C. (2006). Two-component theory of the suffix effect: Contrary evidence. *Memory & Cognition, 34*, 648–667.

Brown, J. (1958). Some tests of the decay theory of immediate memory. *Quarterly Journal of Experimental Psychology, 10*, 12–21.

Burgess, N., & Hitch, G. J. (1992). Toward a network model of the articulatory loop. *Journal of Memory and Language, 31*, 429–460.

Campbell, R., & Dodd, B. (1982). Some suffix effects on lipread lists. *Canadian Journal of Psychology, 36*, 508–514.

Chase, W. G., & Simon, H. A. (1973). Perception in chess. *Cognitive Psychology, 4*, 55–81.

Chekaf, M., Cowan, N., & Mathy, F. (2016). Chunk formation in immediate memory and how it relates to data compression. *Cognition, 155*, 96–107.

Conrad, R. (1960). Very brief delay of immediate recall. *Quarterly Journal of Experimental Psychology, 12*, 45–47.

Conrad, R. (1965). Order error in immediate recall of sequences. *Journal of Verbal Learning and Verbal Behavior, 4*, 161–169.

Cowan, N. (1988). Evolving conceptions of memory storage, selective attention, and their mutual constraints within the human information processing system. *Psychological Bulletin, 104*(2), 163–191.

Cowan, N. (2000). The magical number 4 in short-term memory: A reconsideration of mental storage capacity. *Behavioral and Brain Sciences, 24*, 87–185.

Cowan, N. (2015). George Miller's magical number of immediate memory in retrospect: Observations on the faltering progression of science. *Psychological Review, 122*, 536–541.

Crowder, R. G. (1972). Visual and auditory memory. In J. F. Kavanagh & I. G. Mattingly (Eds.), *Language by Ear and by Eye*. Cambridge, MA: MIT Press.

Crowder, R. G., & Morton, J. (1969). Precategorical acoustic storage (PAS). *Perception & Psychophysics, 5*, 365–373.

Daniel, T. A., & Katz, J. S. (2018). Primacy and recency effects for taste. *Journal of Experimental Psychology: Learning, Memory, and Cognition, 44*(3), 399–405.

Darwin, C. J., Turvey, M. T., & Crowder, R. G. (1972). An auditory analogue of the Sperling partial report procedure: Evidence for brief auditory storage. *Cognitive Psychology, 3*, 255–267.

Davelaar, E. J., Goshen-Gottstein, Y., Ashkenazi, A., Haarmann, H. J., & Usher, M. (2005). The demise of short-term memory revisited: Empirical and computational investigations of recency effects. *Psychological Review, 112*, 3–42.

Donolato, E., Giofrè, D., & Mammarella, I. C. (2017). Differences in verbal and visuospatial forward and backward order recall: A review of the literature. *Frontiers in Psychology, 8*, https://doi.org/10.3389/fpsyg.2017.00663https://doi.org/10.3389/fpsyg.2017.00663.

Ebbinghaus, H. (1885/1964). *Memory: A Contribution to Experimental Psychology*. Translated by H. A. Ruger & C. E. Bussenius. New York: Dover.

Epstein, W. (1961). The influence of syntactical structure on learning. *The American Journal of Psychology, 74*(1), 80–85.

Ericsson, K. A., Chase, W. G., & Faloon, S. (1980). Acquisition of a memory skill. *Science, 208*, 1181–1182.

Estes, W. K. (1972). An associative basis for coding and organization in memory. In A. W. Melton & E. Martin (Eds.), *Coding Processes in Human Memory* (pp. 161–190). New York: Wiley.

Glanzer, M., & Cunitz, A. R. (1966). Two storage mechanisms in free recall. *Journal of Verbal Learning and Verbal Behavior, 5*, 351–360.

Gold, J. M., Murray, R. F., Sekuler, A. B., Bennett, P.J., & Sekuler, R. (2005). Visual memory decay is deterministic. *Psychological Science, 16*, 769–774.

Golomb, J. D., & Kanwisher, N. (2012). Retinotopic memory is more precise than spatiotopic memory. *Proceedings of the National Academy of Sciences, 109*(5), 1796–1801.

Grossenbacher, P. G., & Lovelace, C. T. (2001). Mechanisms of synesthesia: Cognitive and physiological constraints. *Trends in Cognitive Sciences, 5*(1), 36–41.

Hardt, O., Nader, K., & Nadel, L. (2013). Decay happens: The role of active forgetting in memory. *Trends in Cognitive Sciences, 17*(3), 111–120.

Henderson, J. M., & Anes, M. D. (1994). Roles of object-file review and type priming in visual identification within and across eye fixations. *Journal of Experimental Psychology: Human Perception and Performance, 20*, 826–839.

Henson, R. N. A. (1998). Short-term memory for serial order: The start-end model. *Cognitive Psychology, 36*, 73–137.

Hintzman, D. L. (2016). Is memory organized by temporal contiguity? *Memory & Cognition, 44*(3), 365–375.

Hochel, M., & Milán, E. G. (2008). Synaesthesia: The existing state of affairs. *Cognitive Neuropsychology, 25*, 93–117.

Hollingworth, A., & Henderson, J. M. (2003). Testing a conceptual locus for the inconsistent object change detection advantage in real-world scenes. *Memory & Cognition, 31*, 930–940.

Irwin, D. E. (1996). Integrating information across saccadic eye movements. *Current Directions in Psychological Science, 5*, 94–100.

Irwin, D. E., & Brockmole, J. R. (2000). Mental rotation is suppressed during saccadic eye movements. *Psychonomic Bulletin & Review, 7*, 654–661.

Irwin, D. E., Brown, J. S., & Sun, J-S. (1988). Visual masking and visual integration across saccadic eye movements. *Journal of Experimental Psychology: General, 117*, 276–287.

Irwin, D. E., & Robinson, M. M. (2016). Perceiving a continuous visual world across voluntary eye blinks. *Journal of Experimental Psychology: Human Perception and Performance, 42*(10), 1490–1496.

Irwin, D. E., Yantis, S., & Jonides, J. (1983). Evidence against visual integration across saccadic eye movements. *Perception & Psychophysics, 34*, 49–57.

Ishiguro, S., & Saito, S. (2019). Person-based organisation in working memory. *Quarterly Journal of Experimental Psychology, 72*(6), 1439–1452.

Johnson, A. J., Shaw, J., & Miles, C. (2016). Tactile order memory: Evidence for sequence learning phenomena found with other stimulus types. *Journal of Cognitive Psychology, 28*(6), 718–725.

Jones, T., & Farrell, S. (2018). Does syntax bias serial order reconstruction of verbal short-term memory? *Journal of Memory and Language, 100*, 98–122.

Kahneman, D., Treisman, A., and Gibbs, B. J. (1992). The reviewing of objects files: Object-specific integration of information. *Cognitive Psychology, 24*, 175–219.

Kanwisher, N. G. (1987). Repetition blindness: Type recognition without token individuation. *Cognition, 27*, 117–143.

Keppel, G., & Underwood, B. J. (1962). Proactive inhibition in short-term retention of single items. *Journal of Verbal Learning and Verbal Behavior, 1*, 153–161.

Levin, D. T., & Simons, D. J. (1997). Failure to detect changes to attended objects in motion pictures. *Psychonomic Bulletin & Review, 4*, 501–506.

Lewandowsky, S., & Murdock, B. B. (1989). Memory for serial order. *Psychological Review, 96*, 25–57.

Luria, A. R. (1968). *The Mind of a Mnemonist: A Little Book About a Vast Memory*. New York: Basic Books.

Madigan, S., & O'Hara, R. (1992). Short-term memory at the turn of the century: Mary Whiton Calkins's memory research. *American Psychologist, 47*, 170–174.

Mahrer, P., & Miles, C. (1999). Memorial and strategic determinants of tactile recency. *Journal of Experimental Psychology: Learning, Memory and Cognition, 25,* 630–643.

Marks, L. E., & Miller, G. A. (1964). The role of semantic and syntactic constraints in the memorization of English sentences. *Journal of Verbal Learning and Verbal Behavior, 3*(1), 1–5.

Marshuetz, C. (2005). Order information in working memory: An integrative review of evidence from brain and behavior. *Psychological bulletin, 131*(3), 323–339.

Maurer, D. (1997). Neonatal synaesthesia: Implications for the processing of speech and faces. In S. Baron-Cohen, & J. E. Harrison (Eds.), *Synaesthesia: Classic and Contemporary Readings* (pp. 224–242). Malden, MA: Blackwell.

Miles, C., & Hodder, K. (2005). Serial position effects in recognition memory for odors: A reexamination. *Memory & Cognition, 33,* 1303–1314.

Miller, G. A. (1956). The magical number seven, plus or minus two: Some limits on our capacity for processing information. *Psychological Review, 63,* 81–97.

Morton, J., Crowder, R. G., & Prussin, H. A. (1971). Experiments with the stimulus suffix effect. *Journal of Experimental Psychology: Monograph, 91,* 169–190.

Murdock, B. B. (1962). The serial position effect of free recall. *Journal of Experimental Psychology, 64,* 482–488.

Neath, I., Surprenant, A. M., & Crowder, R. G. (1993). The context-dependent stimulus suffix effect. *Journal of Experimental Psychology: Learning, Memory and Cognition, 19,* 698–703.

Norris, D. (2017). Short-term memory and long-term memory are still different. *Psychological Bulletin, 143*(9), 992–1009.

Norris, D., Kalm, K., & Hall, J. (2020). Chunking and redintegration in verbal short-term memory. *Journal of Experimental Psychology: Learning, Memory, and Cognition, 46*(5), 872–893.

Oberauer, K. (2002). Access to information in working memory: Exploring the focus of attention. *Journal of Experimental Psychology: Learning, Memory, and Cognition, 28*(3), 411–421.

O'Donnell, R. E., Clement, A., & Brockmole, J. R. (2018). Semantic and functional relationships among objects increase the capacity of visual working memory. *Journal of Experimental Psychology: Learning, Memory, and Cognition, 44*(7), 1151–1158.

Parmentier, F. B. R., Tremblay, S., & Jones, D. M. (2004). Exploring the suffix effect in serial visuospatial short-term memory. *Psychonomic Bulletin & Review, 11,* 289–295.

Perham, N., Marsh, J. E., & Jones, D. M. (2009). Syntax and serial recall: How language supports short-term memory for order. *Quarterly Journal of Experimental Psychology, 62,* 1285–1293.

Peterson, L. R., & Peterson, M. J. (1959). Short-term retention of individual verbal items. *Journal of Experimental Psychology, 58,* 193–198.

Portrat, S., Barrouillet, P., & Camos, V. (2008). Time-related decay or interference-based forgetting in working memory? *Journal of Experimental Psychology: Learning, Memory, and Cognition, 34,* 1561–1564.

Radvansky, G. A., Gibson, B. S., & McNerney, M. W. (2011). Synesthesia and memory: Color congruency, von Restorff, and false memory effects. *Journal of Experimental Psychology: Learning, Memory, and Cognition, 37*(1), 219.

Radvansky, G. A., Gibson, B. S., & McNerney, M. W. (2014). Working memory, situation models, and synesthesia. *American Journal of Psychology, 127*(3), 325–342.

Ricker, T. J., Sandry, J., Vergauwe, E., & Cowan, N. (2020). Do familiar memory items decay? *Journal of Experimental Psychology: Learning, Memory, and Cognition, 46*(1), 60–76.

Ricker, T. J., Vergauwe, E., & Cowan, N. (2016). Decay theory of immediate memory: From Brown (1958) to today (2014). *Quarterly Journal of Experimental Psychology, 69*(10), 1969–1995.

Rundus, D. (1971). Analysis of rehearsal processes in free recall. *Journal of Experimental Psychology, 89,* 63–77.

Schilling, R. F., & Weaver, G. E. (1983). Effect of extraneous verbal information on memory for telephone numbers. *Journal of Applied Psychology, 68*(4), 559–564.

Seiler, K. H., & Engelkamp, J. (2003). The role of item-specific information for the serial position curve in free recall. *Journal of Experimental Psychology: Learning, Memory, and Cognition, 29,* 954–964.

Simons, D. J., & Levin, D. T. (1998). Failure to detect changes to people during a real-world interaction. *Psychological Bulletin & Review, 5,* 644–649.

Smilek, D., Dixon, M. J., Cudahy, C., & Merikle, P.M. (2002). Synesthetic color experiences influence memory. *Psychological Science, 13*, 548–552.

Sperling, G. (1960). The information available in brief visual presentations. *Psychological Monographs: General and Applied, 74 (11)*, 1–29.

Sternberg, S. (1966). High-speed scanning in human memory. *Science, 153*, 652–654.

Sternberg, S. (1969). The discovery of processing stages: Extensions of Donders' method. *Acta Pscyhologica, 30*, 276–315.

Sternberg, S. (1975). Memory scanning: New findings and current controversies. *Quarterly Journal of Experimental Psychology, 27*, 1–32.

Sternberg, S. (2016). In defence of high-speed memory scanning. *Quarterly Journal of Experimental Psychology, 69*(10), 2020–2075.

Talmi, D., Grady, C. L., Goshen-Gottstein, Y., & Moscovitch, M. (2005). Neuroimaging the serial position curve: A test of single-store versus dual-store models. *Psychological Science, 16*, 716–723.

Thalmann, M., Souza, A. S., & Oberauer, K. (2019). How Does Chunking Help Working Memory? *Journal of Experimental Psychology: Learning, Memory, and Cognition, 45*(1), 37–55.

Theios, J., Smith, P. G., Haviland, S. E., Traupmann, J., & Moy, M. C. (1973). Memory scanning as a serial self-terminating process. *Journal of Experimental Psychology, 97*(3), 323–336.

Townsend, J. T. (1990). Serial vs. parallel processing: Sometimes they look like Tweedledum and Tweedledee but they can (and should) be distinguished. *Psychological Science, 1*, 46–54.

Van der Stigchel, S., & Hollingworth, A. (2018). Visuospatial working memory as a fundamental component of the eye movement system. *Current Directions in Psychological Science, 27*(2), 136–143.

Waugh, N. C., & Norman, D. A. (1965). Primary memory. *Psychological Review, 72*, 89–104.

Wegner, D. M. (1989). *White Bears and Other Unwanted Thoughts: Suppression, Obsession, and the Psychology of Mental Control*. New York: Viking.

Yaro, C., & Ward, J. (2007). Searching for Shereshevskii: What is superior about the memory of synaesthetes? *Quarterly Journal of Experimental Psychology, 60*, 681–695.

Zeamer, C., & Fox Tree, J. E. (2013). The process of auditory distraction: Disrupted attention and impaired recall in a simulated lecture environment. *Journal of Experimental Psychology: Learning, Memory, and Cognition, 39*(5), 1463–1472.

Zechmeister, E. B., & Nyberg, S. E. (1982). *Human Memory: An Introduction to Research and Theory*. Pacific Grove: Brook/Cole Publishing.

CHAPTER 5

Working Memory

The previous chapter dealt with the retention of information in the short term. We saw that short-term memory includes conscious experience. However, we do more than just retain information over time. We are constantly thinking about things. This "thinking" implies an active processing or manipulating of information. For example, when you are thinking about how to get to a store that you have never been to before, you combine various bits of knowledge that you already have: the layout of the city, information from a map, knowledge of traffic patterns in that area, and conversations with your friends about the location of the store. By actively using this information, you can determine the best route to take. This involves the controlled use of information in short-term memory. Because of the special nature of this kind of processing, this is called **working memory**. The phrase *short-term memory* is reserved more for the brief retention of information. In fact, some researchers consider working memory and short-term memory to be different psychological constructs (e.g., Cantor et al., 1991).

This chapter provides an overview of some of the major issues with working memory. We begin with one of the more popular theories of working memory, Baddeley's multicomponent model. We examine the role of each part of working memory from this perspective and some of the memory phenomena associated with it. Regardless of how working memory is best conceived, these sections highlight several things that working memory does well and poorly. After this, we consider other views of what working memory is and how it operates, including Cowan's embedded processes model and Engle's controlled attention theory. Finally, some applications of working memory to more complex levels of processing are considered.

BADDELEY'S MULTICOMPONENT MODEL

The best known (among memory researchers) theory of working memory is **Baddeley's multicomponent model** (Baddeley, 1986, 2000; Baddeley & Hitch, 1974). This model working memory is made up of several components: (1) the phonological loop, (2) the visuospatial sketchpad, (3) the episodic buffer, and (4) the central executive. An overview of the model is shown in Figure 5.1. The phonological loop, visuospatial sketchpad, and episodic buffer are subsystems under the control of a generalized **executive controller**, which runs the operation. The **phonological loop** is the part of working memory responsible for processing verbal and auditory information. The **visuospatial sketchpad** is responsible for processing visual and spatial knowledge. The **episodic buffer** is where multimodal information from different parts of working memory are combined or bound together. Note that there are some bits in gray in Figure 5.1 that are not formal parts of the model but which are likely to be involved at some level.

The phonological loop and visuospatial sketchpad are treated separately because of how different types of information tend not to influence one another. For example, if you are thinking about verbal information, such as reading a book, you are more likely to experience interference and distraction if you are exposed to other verbal or auditory information, such as people talking in the background. However, reading is relatively unaffected by spatial tasks, such as tapping out a beat with your hand. Conversely, visual–spatial tasks, such as tracing a route on a map, are disrupted by other visual–spatial tasks but not by verbal tasks (Baddeley & Andrade, 2000; but see Vergauwe et al., 2010). There is interference if two tasks use the same part of working memory. For example, people have difficulty detecting visual and auditory signals if they are maintaining visual and auditory images, respectively (Segal & Fusella, 1970; 1971). Cross-system deficits are observed when executive controller processes are affected, such as when tasks involve large memory loads (Morey & Cowan, 2005).

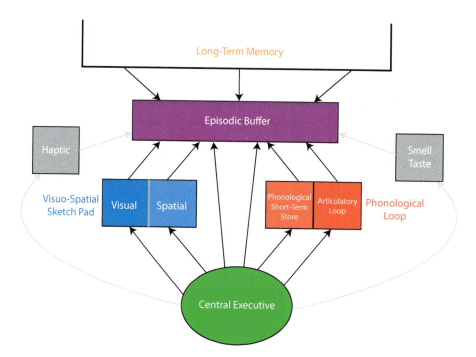

FIGURE 5.1 *An Expanded Version of the Baddeley Model of Working Memory*

Source: adapted and expanded on from Baddeley, A. D. (2000). The episodic buffer: A new component of working memory? *Trends in Cognitive Science, 4,* 417–423.

The episodic buffer helps *bind* information from different sources. The episodic buffer is also a limited capacity temporary storage system that brings together information from other parts of working memory as well as long-term memory. This binding creates a unified episodic memory of an experience that can then be stored in long-term memory. So, for example, your memory for an event will include how things looked, the sound of a person's voice, where things were, what they meant, and so on, all integrated into a single memory, such as an event model.

The central executive is the control center of Baddeley's model. Although each subsystem has some capacity, the central executive has additional capacity to devote to a subsystem if needed. For example, if you are thinking about a difficult problem while walking, you may stop because the visual–spatial part of working memory that helps you navigate has some of its resources taken away by the central executive to be used elsewhere. An important job of the central executive is to regulate the flow of information in the current stream of thought as a supervisory attentional system (Norman & Shallice, 1986).

Phonological Loop

Of the various working memory components, the phonological loop has received the most attention. Many of the studies of working memory follow from research in the verbal learning tradition, and the phonological loop is concerned with processing verbal items. Studies of the phonological loop focus on linguistic materials, which are either read or heard, although other acoustic items have been used. Thus, the parts of the brain often implicated in phonological loop processing include linguistic aspects of the temporal lobe (Jonides et al., 2005).

The phonological loop has two parts: the **phonological store** and the **articulatory loop** (see Figure 5.2). The phonological store is a temporary storehouse, whereas the

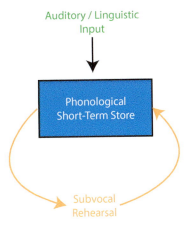

FIGURE 5.2 *The Phonological Loop, with the Phonological Store and the Articulatory Loop*

Source: adapted from Gathercole, S. E. (1997). Models of verbal short-term memory. In M. A. Conway (Ed.), *Cognitive Models of Memory*, pp. 13–45. Cambridge, MA: MIT Press.

articulatory loop is for active rehearsal. A helpful analogy is that the phonological store is an inner ear that listens to what we say to ourselves, and the articulatory loop is our inner voice that says what we are thinking. Information first enters the phonological store, but over time, this information may be interfered with (Oberauer, 2019) and can eventually become lost. To prevent this, the articulatory loop actively refreshes the information in the phonological store. The more information that is held in the phonological store, the harder the task of the articulatory loop, and the more likely information will be forgotten. Please note that while we are talking about a phonological loop here, this same basic process is thought to operate for language processing in general, including non-spoken languages, such as American Sign Language (Wilson & Fox, 2007).

To illustrate the role of the phonological loop let's look at some prominent effects that have been observed (Gathercole, 1997). These provide insight into characteristics of working memory. Along with the description of each of these is an explanation for why they occur.

The **word length effect** is the finding that people's word span is smaller for longer words than for shorter words. There are two types of word length effects. First, the *syllabic word length effect* is the finding that it is harder to remember words with more syllables than fewer syllables (Baddeley et al., 1975). This occurs because more time is needed to rehearse some items in a set, causing other items not to be refreshed, making it more likely they will be forgotten (Cowan et al., 2003).

A finding related to this is that Chinese speakers have larger digit spans than English speakers, who in turn have larger digit spans than Welsh speakers (Hoosain & Salili, 1988). In Chinese the digits are all monosyllables, whereas in English some digit names are multisyllabic, thereby lengthening articulation time. For example "seven" in English, is "qi" in Chinese. Welsh is even worse than English. The digit span of Chinese–English bilinguals varies, depending on which language they are speaking. Thus, Chinese speakers are fortunate enough to have a language with syllabically simpler words for digits.[1] A similar line of reasoning, in terms of "articulation time," explains the finding that memory spans are smaller with American Sign Language (ASL) than with spoken language (Wilson & Emmorey, 2006). The signs take longer to produce. That said, there have been some suggestions that this effect is not replicable (Guitard et al., 2018).

The second word length effect is the *articulatory word length effect* which is the idea that processing can be affected by articulation duration, apart from the number of syllables. The longer it takes to physically say the words, the fewer that can be recalled. Keeping the number of syllables constant, more short-duration words, such as "wicket" and "bishop," can be recalled relative to long-duration words, such as "harpoon" and "Friday." While there is evidence for the syllabic word length effect, it may not be replicable (e.g., Bireta et al., 2006; Hulme et al., 2004).

The **articulatory suppression** effect is a reduced verbal span when people speak while simultaneously trying to remember a set of items (Murray, 1967; Peterson & Johnson, 1971). For example, suppose you are given a set of words to hold in your

---

1 For a comparison of English, Spanish, Hebrew, and Arabic see Naveh-Benjamin and Ayes (1986).

phonological loop. While you get the words, you also say aloud some word over and over—for example, "the" (i.e., "the," "the," "the," etc.). This results in a reduced memory span. In other words, talking about one thing makes it difficult to remember something else. A more everyday example is when someone tells you his or her name and college major at a party while you are talking. Your talking impedes your ability to rehearse and remember the person's name and major. In some sense, this is the suffix effect run amok. What happens is that an articulatory suppression task takes up resources from the articulatory loop, even if what you are trying to remember is a melody and not verbal per se (Nees et al., 2017). As a result, information in the phonological store cannot be adequately refreshed, and so it is lost from working memory.

The **irrelevant speech effect** is the finding that the phonological loop is less efficient when there is irrelevant speech in the background, even if it is in a language people do not understand (Colle & Welsh, 1976). You may have had the experience of trying to read in a room where other people are talking. It is difficult to concentrate on your reading. This is because the background speech enters working memory and takes up some of the resources of the phonological loop, causing what you are reading to be harder to process and more likely to be forgotten.

This has implications for students (such as yourself) regarding the best way to study. Salamé and Baddeley (1989) had students try to learn information either in

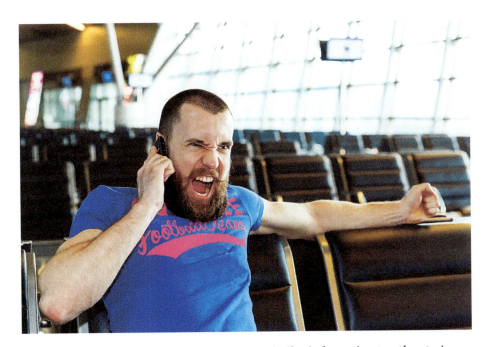

PHOTO 5.1 *Because working memory processes similar information together, trying to do one task, such as trying to read a book (which contains language) in an airport while some other loud person is talking on a cell phone (which also contains language) can disrupt performance. In this case, this is an illustration of the irrelevant speech effect*

Source: Mikhail Starodubov/Shutterstock.com

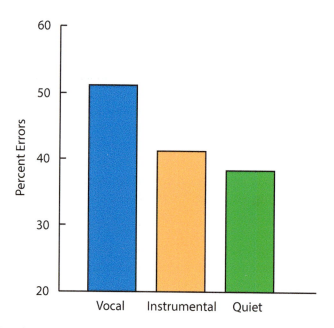

FIGURE 5.3 *Working Memory Performance with Different Types of Background Music*

Source: adapted from Salamé, P., & Baddeley, A. (1989). Effects of background music on phonological short-term memory. *Quarterly Journal of Experimental Psychology, 41A*, 107–122.

silence or while listening to either instrumental music or music with vocals. The results are shown in Figure 5.3. As you can see, memory was best when students were in quiet conditions. However, when there was background noise that involved language, such as music with vocals, memory was worse. Listening to instrumental music had a moderate effect. The linguistic nature of the vocals interfered with the operation of the phonological loop. So, when you study, it is best to do so under quiet conditions, if you can. If you must have background noise, choose instrumental music (Vasilev et al., 2018).

The **phonological similarity effect** is the finding that phonologically similar items are more likely to lead to errors (Baddeley, 1966; Conrad & Hull, 1964). That is, when the words share the same sounds (e.g., "whole," "bowl," "boat," "bone," and "phone") people forget more and make more errors than when the words do not (e.g., "whole," "line," "milk," "fire," and "hunt"). Performance is not as bad when the words in the list rhyme (share the same ending sound), worse when they are alliterative (share the same beginning sound), and is worst when both of these are present in a list (Gupta et al., 2005). Under these circumstances, people are likely to misremember a similar sounding word. For example, if one of the words was "bowl," people might misremember it as "roll," which sounds similar but looks different, but not "fowl," which looks similar but sounds different. As an everyday example, if you are busily working in the kitchen with someone and ask "Can you please pass me the bowl?" because their working memory is largely occupied by whatever it is that they are doing, they may pass you a roll instead of a bowl. This occurs because information degrades in the phonological store. When it is time for an item to be rehearsed, some reconstruction may be needed. Because phonological information is auditory, this reconstruction is based on the fragmentary phonological information that is available. When there are phonologically similar items, it is harder to keep track of which ones have and have not been rehearsed. This makes it more likely that an unrehearsed item is not refreshed, and forgetting occurs (Li et al., 2000).

It should be noted that none of these effects take into account knowledge in long-term memory that may be used to support working memory. Working memory is influenced by prior knowledge. For example, memory spans are larger for words than for nonwords. This is the **lexicality effect** (Hulme et al., 1991). People use long-term knowledge to support and reconstruct information in the phonological store. Information in long-term memory can even reverse some phonological loop effects. For example, for the phonological similarity effect, performance is worse when items are phonologically similar. However, if the words are embedded in the context of meaningful sentences, this effect reverses: performance is better for words that are phonologically similar rather than different (Copeland & Radvansky, 2001; Macnamara et al., 2011). This commonly occurs with poetry and song lyrics. People can draw on knowledge of the sentence along with memory of the rhyme scheme to come up with the appropriate response. For example, you could remember "pole" if you know that all of the words in a set rhyme with "hole" and the sentence was something like "The vaulter was surprised when he discovered that he had somehow broken his ____." Thus, people can use long-term knowledge to aid short-term recall.

TRY IT OUT

In this chapter, a straight-forward way to assess working memory is to look at aspects of the phonological loop which rely on verbal materials. In this section we look at two ways to manipulate phonological loop processing, namely, word length effect and articulatory suppression. Ideally you should have at least 24 participants for each of these tasks. Now, using these basic ground rules, here are some things you could do:

Word length effect. For this task, create two lists of eight words (nouns). One list of words should all be one syllable long. The other should all be three or four syllables long. For each person, pick out five of the words from one of the lists at random. Read them at the rate of one word per second. At the end of the list, have the person write down the words in the order that they heard them. After this, read the second list and have the person recall that one. Across your participants, half of the people get the short words list first, and the other half get the long words list first. Score performance on the two lists separately by counting up the number of words correctly recalled for each. If all goes well, most people should have better recall for the list of short words than for the list of long words (see Neath, 1998).

Articulatory suppression. For this task, create ten similar lists of five two-syllable words each. For each person, read a list of words at the rate of one per second. For five of the lists have people simply listen and then write down the words in the order that they heard them. For the other five lists have the people say the word "the" over and over from the time you start reading to the time they finish recalling the words. What you should find is that people remember fewer words when they were articulating than when they were not.

Stop and Review

Baddeley's multicomponent model is the dominant theory of working memory. It is made up of a phonological loop, a visuospatial sketchpad, an episodic buffer, and a central executive. The phonological loop is geared toward processing verbal and acoustic information. This is done using the phonological store, which is more passive, and the articulatory loop, which is more active. Evidence for the operation of the phonological loop comes from the word length effect, articulatory suppression, the irrelevant speech effect, the phonological similarity effect, and the lexicality effect. These effects are embodied in a sense that the phonological loop is treating the information as if it were spoken or heard, even when it is only visually read.

Visuospatial Sketchpad

Another working memory subsystem is the visuospatial sketchpad, which is responsible for visual information, such as size or color, and spatial information, such as the relative orientation, or spatially manipulating an object in your head. Although some people suggest that there are separate spatial and visual components (Darling et al., 2009; Klauer & Zhao, 2004), we treat them together here. As you read about different aspects of the visuospatial sketchpad, note how they involve some element of embodied cognition, as if working memory is simulating the world and how we interact with it.

Also, the visuospatial sketchpad involves more right than left hemisphere processing. This is consistent with the idea that the right hemisphere is dominant for spatial and holistic processing. Moreover, the premotor cortex (BA 6) is the part of the brain that is particularly important for the visuospatial sketchpad (Smith, 2000) as well as those portions of the parietal lobes involved in perception (Jonides et al., 2005).

One of the main tasks of the visuospatial sketchpad is the construction, maintenance, and manipulation of **mental images** that are isomorphically related to perceptual experience. Perception and mental imagery use a lot of the same neural processes (Dijkstra et al., 2019). As an example of the commonality of mental images with perception, mental images are sensitive to object size and viewer distance. People are better able to identify the components of an image if it is large or the viewing distance is close (Kosslyn, 1975). The more working memory capacity people have, the more accurate are visual characteristics such as color (Allen et al., 2011).

Mental images must be actively maintained or rehearsed in the visuospatial sketchpad, or they degrade. This is outlined in the CRT model of visual imagery (Kosslyn, 1975). When you watch television, the image you see on a screen (which used to be a cathode ray tube or CRT) is not presented all at once. Instead, it is continuously refreshed, with the image constantly scanning from top to bottom and then starting over again. The speed at which this is done is the refresh rate. Thus, even a static image is constantly decaying and being reconstructed. The CRT model of visual imagery assumes that a similar process occurs in the visuospatial sketchpad. A mental image is constantly decaying and being refreshed. This is like the operation of the articulatory loop as described earlier.

As with the word length effect, people find it harder to maintain complex rather than simple mental images (Kosslyn, 1975). The more components to an image, the more elements that need to be refreshed, and the more opportunity there is for forgetting.

How does the visuospatial sketchpad manipulate information and to what aim? One role is as a surrogate for physical reality. People might make decisions about objects at two different locations by **mental scanning** across their mental image. Mental scanning time increases with the distance that needs to be covered. In one study, Kosslyn and his colleagues had people memorize a map of an island, like the one in Figure 5.4. The task was to verify some aspect of one of the island locations. The results, shown in Figure 5.5, reveal that response time increased with

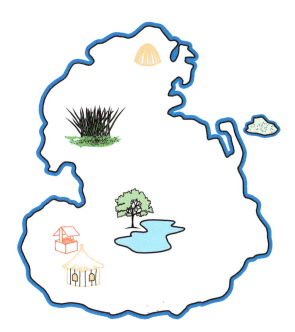

FIGURE 5.4 *Map of an Island Used in Kosslyn's Mental Scanning Experiments*

Source: adapted from Kosslyn, S. M., Ball, T. M., & Reiser, B. J. (1978). Visual images preserve metric spatial information: Evidence from studies of image scanning. *Journal of experimental psychology: Human Perception and Performance, 4*(1), 47–60

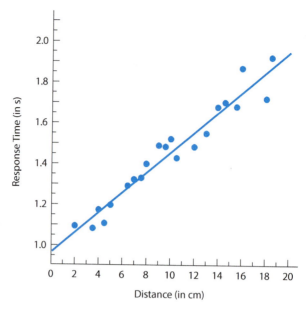

FIGURE 5.5 *Response Time in Kosslyn's Mental Scanning Study as a Function of Distance on the Island Map.*

Source: adapted from Kosslyn, S. M., Ball, T. M., & Reiser, B. J. (1978). Visual images preserve metric spatial information: Evidence from studies of image scanning. *Journal of Experimental Psychology: Human Perception and Performance, 4*(1), 47–60

the distance from one location to another. Mental imagery processes in working memory rely on similar visual and spatial processes as those used during perception, except that people produce the images themselves, rather than having them present in the environment (Kosslyn et al., 1978; Kosslyn & Pomerantz, 1977).

Processing information in the visuospatial sketchpad has isomorphic qualities similar to what it would be like in reality. A striking example of this is a study by Intons-Peterson and Roskos-Ewoldsen (1989) with students at Indiana University Bloomington. In this study, students did a mental scanning task, much like the Kosslyn study. However, rather than a map of an island, the students used their knowledge of the Bloomington campus. More importantly, students were asked to imagine themselves going from one location to another, carrying either a balloon or a load of bricks. In both cases, response time increased with greater distances. Moreover, the response time was greater when the students imagined they were carrying the heavy load rather than the light one. Thus, the operation of working memory captures various aspects of the world.

Another visuospatial working memory process is **mental rotation**, in which people need to mentally turn an object. This might be done so that they can make a decision, such as identifying the object. Imagine a sign that is upside down. You must mentally rotate the letters or numbers to decipher the message. Another possibility is that you may need to compare two objects for some purpose, such as working on a jigsaw puzzle. You mentally rotate the pieces to see if they fit together before picking them up and trying them out.

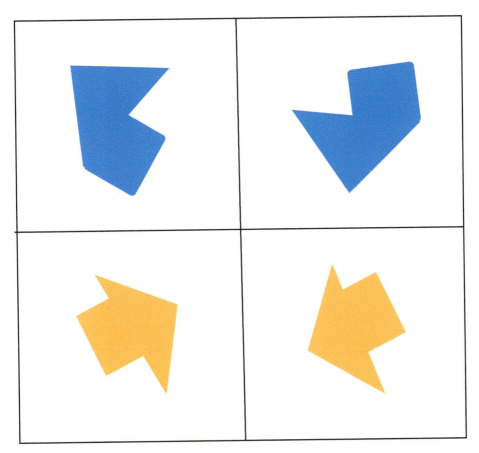

FIGURE 5.6 *Abstract Object Pairs that Could be Used in Mental Rotation Studies. The Top Pair are the Same, and the Bottom Pair are Different*

Source: adapted from Folk, M. D., & Luce, R. D. (1987). Effects of stimulus complexity on mental rotation rate of polygons. *Journal of Experimental Psychology: Human Perception and Performance, 13*(3), 395–404

Research has shown that, like visual scanning, mental rotation has characteristics that mimic physical rotation. The greater the degree of rotation, the longer it takes to do. In a seminal study by Shepard and Metzler (1971), students saw pairs of three-dimensional figures. They had to say whether the figures were the same or different. An example of an abstract figure that could be used for such a task is shown in Figure 5.6. The results from such a task, as seen in Figure 5.7, show that response time increased with the degree of mental rotation that was needed.

Mental rotation reflects embodied cognition. We mentally rotate as if we were actually turning an object (Gardony et al., 2013). This is reinforced by the finding that if there is unseen tactile feedback, such as feeling the actual object being turned in one's hand, then performance improves. This benefit is not observed if people simply feel the object and it is not rotated, if a different object is rotated in their hand, or if the rotation is in a different direction (Wraga et al., 2000; Wraga et al., 2008). Finally, mental rotation is easier if the object is easier to rotate in real life

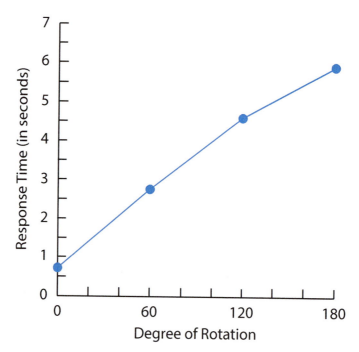

FIGURE 5.7 *Response Time Results from a Mental Rotation Task*

Source: created from data reported in Folk, M. D., & Luce, R. D. (1987). Effects of stimulus complexity on mental rotation rate of polygons. *Journal of Experimental Psychology: Human Perception and Performance, 13*(3), 395–404

(Flusberg & Boroditsky, 2011), again, even though all that is actually being rotated is a thought (and thoughts don't weigh anything).

In terms of the neurological underpinnings, the parietal lobes tend to be more involved, along with some coordinating support from the frontal lobes. Furthermore, if the mental rotation is demanding, there may be more involvement of the left hemisphere than the right, suggesting an increase in analytic processing (Just et al., 2001). It is difficult to clearly identify one type of processing with any one brain structure. Many visuospatial processes involve more right hemisphere activity when more holistic processing is needed. However, when more analytical processing is needed, there can be more left hemisphere dominance. Mental rotation is one cognitive task in which males tend to outperform females, with differences emerging in the teenage years (Voyer et al., 1995; 2017).

Visuospatial sketchpad processing is also observed in the phenomenon of **boundary extension** (Intraub & Richardson, 1989; for a review, see Hubbard et al., 2010), which is memory for details beyond what is seen (Intraub et al., 1992). As noted in the discussion of iconic memory in Chapter 4, when we view the world, we are only getting bits and pieces of it at a time. What gives us the experience of being in a world filled with more visual information than is available to us in the moment? In part, we fill in beyond the edges with what we *think* should be there. This is especially striking in memory of pictures, television shows, or movies. When you remember a movie, it is unlikely that your memory contains the experience of the edge of the screen and the theater beyond that. You remember more of the scene than you actually saw.

In studies of boundary extension, people might see a series of photos, such as those in Figure 5.8. Then, they would be given probe pictures with the task of

A

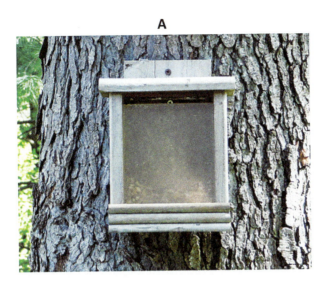

B

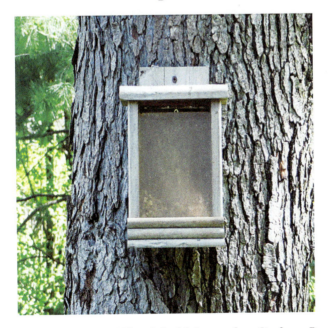

FIGURE 5.8 *Example of Pictures as They Would Appear for a Study on Boundary Extension. If People Saw the Picture A, There Was a Bias to Later Say That the Picture B Was Actually Seen Because the Boundaries of Picture A Were Expanded*

indicating whether each was seen before (old) or not (new). Some of these would be old, original versions. Some shots would be closer up, and others would be taken from further back (and thereby extending the boundary of the original). People make more errors by selecting more pictures that were taken from further out. Moreover, if they draw what they saw, their drawings tend to include information beyond the image boundaries. People fill in the surrounding space using the visuospatial sketchpad and then incorporate this extension into their memory of the scene. Boundary extension occurs even when images were viewed as briefly as 42 ms (Intraub & Dickinson, 2008).

Boundary extension is not automatic. For it to occur, people must think that what is being viewed is a scene. There must be some sort of background, even if it is only imagined. Pictures of objects without a background do not produce boundary extension (Gottesman & Intraub, 2002; Intraub et al., 1998). Thus, the operation of the visuospatial sketchpad depends on knowledge in long-term memory. If a picture does not activate this knowledge, then no boundary extension occurs.

There are other aspects of the visuospatial sketchpad that involve the interpretation of real or perceived motion. Because of this, it is called **dynamic memory** (Hubbard, 2005).

When we watch moving objects and blink or look away briefly, they often continue in motion. This continued motion is captured in the visuospatial sketchpad. **Representational momentum** is a bias for people to misremember the location or orientation of an object further along its path of travel than where it actually was the last time it was seen (Freyd, 1987; Freyd & Finke, 1984). It is as if people have difficulty stopping the object in their visuospatial sketchpad. An example of representational momentum is shown in Figure 5.9. Here, a box appears to be rotating across a series of displays. After the last display there is a delay, and

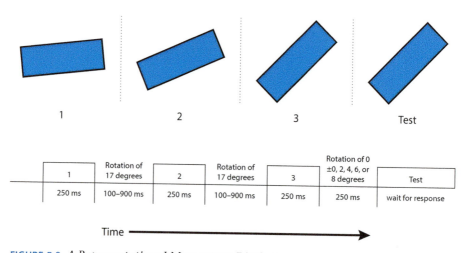

	1	Rotation of 17 degrees	2	Rotation of 17 degrees	3	Rotation of 0 ±0, 2, 4, 6, or 8 degrees	Test
	250 ms	100–900 ms	250 ms	100–900 ms	250 ms	250 ms	wait for response

Time ⟶

FIGURE 5.9 *A Representational Momentum Display*

Source: Freyd, J. J., & Finke, R. A. (1984). Representational momentum. *Journal of Experimental Psychology: Learning, Memory, and Cognition, 10*, 126–132

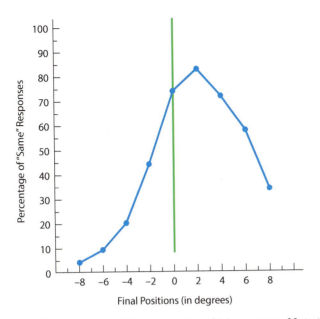

FIGURE 5.10 *Results from a Study of Representational Momentum. Note that estimates of final position are distorted in the direction of the object's motion*

Source: Freyd, J. J., & Finke, R. A. (1984). Representational momentum. *Journal of Experimental Psychology: Learning, Memory, and Cognition, 10,* 126–132

people are given a test display. The task is to say whether the object is in the same orientation as it was when it was last seen. These test objects can be the actual last display, a box rotated slightly backward, or a box rotated slightly forward. The results, shown in Figure 5.10, reveal a tendency for people to misremember the box as being further along in its rotation than it actually was.

Other studies have shown representational momentum along the path of an object's trajectory (Hubbard, 1990). For example, if you see a car moving along a street, and then it disappears behind a bush, you misremember it as being further along its path of travel than it actually was. Representational momentum is influenced by the speed of an object, with faster objects exhibiting more representational momentum (Hubbard & Bharucha, 1988). This takes into account regular properties of the world. For example, you may misremember a pendulum beginning its backswing when that has not yet occurred (Verfaillie & Y'dewalle, 1991) or remember a ball bouncing off a wall before it happens (Hubbard & Bharucha, 1988). Also, when the movement is perceived as a threat (using an axe against someone), then representational momentum effects are larger (Greenstein et al., 2016).

Representational momentum also reflects properties such as a centripetal force (Hubbard, 1996). This involves active processing in the visuospatial sketchpad because the amount of distortion is directly related to the speed of the mental rotation. The faster people mentally rotate, the greater the distortion (Munger et al., 1999). Representational momentum tends to follow medieval impetus theories of motion rather than Newtonian or other modern views. This is true even for physics experts (Kozhevnikov & Hegarty, 2001). Thus, this aspect of working memory has only a limited influence from knowledge in declarative long-term memory (but see Courtney & Hubbard, 2008). It is important to note that representational momentum influences are not limited to visuospatial memory as they are also observed with music pitches moving up or down (Kelly & Freyd, 1987).

Representational gravity is the finding that memory for object positions tends to be distorted toward the Earth (Freyd et al., 1988; Hubbard, 1995; 2020). An example is shown in Figure 5.11. Here, people viewed a plant that was initially on top of a table or suspended by a hook. Then, in a later display, the table or hook was absent. People were then tested for their memory of the plant's location. People tend to remember it as being lower than it actually was, consistent with the idea that representational gravity is influencing the visuospatial memory, moving the plant lower. Note that in this case, the image is not in motion. The motion is implied by an existing component of the world that interacts with the objects, namely gravity. In general, when static images convey likely interactions among objects, the visuospatial sketchpad infers some type of motion (Coventry et al., 2013).

Similarly, if a circle is seen on an incline, it is remembered as being further down the incline, as if it had rolled. The greater the incline, the greater the distortion. Objects moving along a trajectory may be remembered as being lower than they originally were, as if being pulled down by gravity (Hubbard, 1990). Visuospatial working memory takes into account physical principles to anticipate what will

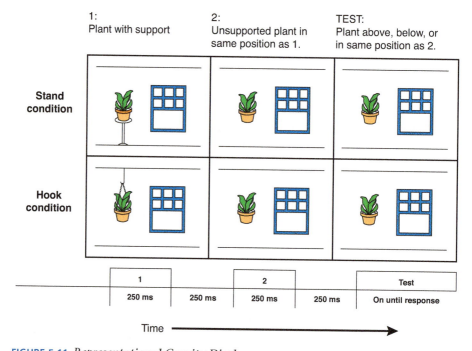

FIGURE 5.11 *Representational Gravity Display*

Source: Freyd, J. J., Pantzer, T. M., & Cheng, J. L. (1988). Representing statics as forces in equilibrium. *Journal of Experimental Psychology: General, 117*, 395–407.

happen next. If you see a paint can tipping off a ladder, you do not need to watch it fall to know that it is coming down, and you need to move out of the way. Note that our understanding of gravity appears to be adaptive to other gravitational experiences, such as what would be experienced on another planet, such as Mars (Torok et al., 2019).

Representational friction is the finding that moving objects slow down when moving along another object (such as the ground) that can produce friction (Hubbard, 1995). The greater the implied contact, the greater the implied friction. In some sense, representational friction puts the brakes on representational momentum. Overall, people are unconsciously predicting the outcome of events using the visuospatial sketchpad.

Stop and Review

The visuospatial sketchpad is dedicated to processing visual and spatial information. It captures many qualities of the world in an analog and isomorphic format. People treat mental images as if they were seeing actual images. These images can degrade and be lost if they are not refreshed. The operation of the visuospatial sketchpad reflects the manipulation of mental images as if people were actually interacting with things in the world. This is evidenced by mental scanning, mental rotation, and boundary extension effects. The dynamic operation of the visuospatial sketchpad on information in working memory is seen in effects such as representational momentum, gravity, and friction, to predict where things will be in the very near future.

Episodic Buffer

The episodic buffer is a more recent addition to Baddeley's multicomponent model, so there is less to say about it. The role of the episodic buffer is to bind together information from various sources in working memory and long-term memory. This process uses attention and can be disrupted by concurrent tasks (Elsley & Parmentier, 2009). Episodic buffer integration was shown in a study by Jefferies et al. (2004), in which people were given either lists of words or sentences with the task of recalling them later. While they were holding these items in working memory, people did a demanding distractor task that consumed central executive resources. What was found was that performance was disrupted on the sentence task, but not the word task. This is because sentences require people to bind together the words into a coherent whole. This is not needed in the word list task. With a heavier working memory load, people had difficulty doing this, and so performance was hampered.

Another example of the operation of the episodic buffer is a study by Darling and Havelka (2010) in which people had to remember digits. These digits were presented one at a time either (a) at a single position on a screen, (b) on a number line, or (c) arranged in a keyboard pattern (such as that found on a telephone). They found that memory was better in the third condition because for a keyboard layout, people could bind spatial information together with the digit information to better remember the sequence.

Central Executive

The final piece of Baddeley's multicomponent model is the **central executive**. This is involved in the allocation of attention (i.e., deciding what to and what not to think about), as well as the active processing of information that is not handled by the subsystems. Thus, the central executive is given the lion's share of what we consider "thinking." Some have even suggested that the range of processes attributed to the central executive is so vast, that the idea of a single central executive could be abandoned altogether (Logie, 2016). Researchers who study the central executive often tie it up to see what impact its absence has. This can be done by giving a task such as generating a list of random numbers (which is much harder than it sounds). This leads people to do more poorly on tasks that require active thinking in which control over the flow of information is at a premium.

In some sense, the central executive distributes memory resources. You can improve memory if there are more resources available. Activity that brings the body to a higher or optimal state of arousal has a positive effect on working memory. This is why you think more clearly when you have had enough sleep. Moreover, executive processing is resource consuming, and can show deficits when resources are low, such as when there are low levels of blood glucose and/or brain glycogen (Gailliot, 2008). Increasing physical activity increases working memory performance. That said, after high levels of aerobic activity, such as running a marathon, explicit memory may be compromised, although implicit memory is largely unaffected (Eich & Metcalfe, 2009).

The disruption of the central executive is seen when there has been brain damage, particularly the medial frontal lobes (BA 32), as revealed by EEG recordings (Gevins et al., 1997). This can result in a symptom known as **dysexecutive syndrome**, where people lose some central executive functions. With this syndrome, people may exhibit two types of behavior: perseveration and distraction. **Perseveration** is when people have been doing a task one way and need to do it another way, but the switch is not made. For example, if people are first asked to sort a deck of cards by suit, they could do so easily. But if they were then asked to then sort the cards by value, they would continue to sort them by suit. What is especially odd is that people can report what the correct sorting strategy should be and may admit they are not following the new strategy even as they continue to follow the old one. Relatedly, some behaviors exhibit elements of distraction. **Distraction** occurs when people are supposed to be attending to one task, but some elements of the environment take attention away from it. For example, if they are not currently processing information, attention might drift and become locked on some other stimulus in the environment.

Overall, the dysexecutive syndrome illustrates the attentional control that has been attributed to the central executive. When this component has been damaged, the flow of the stream of thought is disrupted, getting stuck on old processes, and drifting out to unrelated areas.

Stop and Review

The episodic buffer is where information is integrated from the other working memory subsystems and long-term memory to make new integrated episodic memories. In comparison, the central executive coordinates what is attended to and what is not. People with brain damage can have problems with the central executive, producing the dysexecutive syndrome. Dysexecutive syndrome can involve perseverations of no longer appropriate behaviors and distractions to irrelevant environmental stimuli.

COWAN'S EMBEDDED PROCESSES MODEL

Another conception of working memory is **Cowan's** (1988) **embedded processes model** (see Figure 5.12). Here, working memory is not a separate part of memory, apart from long-term memory. Instead, it is a portion of long-term memory that is in a currently activated state. Working memory is, more simply, that part of our knowledge (as well as incoming information from the environment) that is in a more accessible or active state.

Within working memory is the focus of attention composed of those elements to which attention is currently directed. Generally, information is in the focus of attention. However, when an event boundary occurs, such as when unexpected changes happen, attention shifts to a new event, and working memory must be updated (Ongchoco & Scholl, 2019; 2020). The focus of attention is about four items.

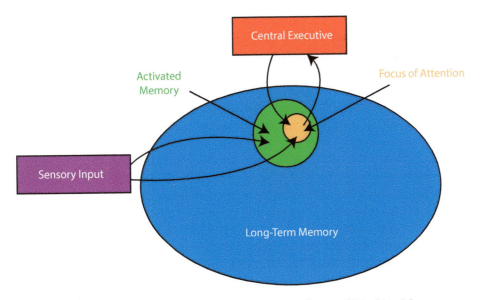

FIGURE 5.12 *Schematic of Cowan's Attentional Focus Theory of Working Memory*

Source: adapted from Cowan, N. (1988). Evolving conceptions of memory storage, selective attention, and their mutual constraints within the human information-processing system. *Psychological Bulletin, 104*(2), 163–191

Like Baddeley's model, there is a central executive that directs where the focus of attention is. Thus, overall, information in the focus of attention is what people are currently attending to and thinking about at the moment, and the larger portion of working memory contains information that is readily available to be brought into the focus of attention as needed.

This theory of working memory is related to the idea of a long-term working memory (Ericsson & Kintsch, 1995). **Long-term working memory** is a way to coordinate large amounts of information. Essentially, it is a set of retrieval cues held in working memory that reference information in long-term memory. By using these cues, people can quickly access to the information as needed.

In some ways this approach to working memory makes a lot of sense. Early theories of memory were based on the computer metaphor. In a computer, when information is actively processed, a copy of it is put into an active state, namely in Random Access Memory (RAM). Information enters RAM either through an input device or from permanent storage, such as a hard drive. It is moved from one part to another (RAM) where it can be actively worked on (via the CPU). The bits in RAM are flexible. Well, the human brain just does not work this way. While there are different parts of the brain that process information in different ways, there is not a separate part that brings in information from other parts to be actively processed. There is no part of the brain that is a separate working memory store. Instead, the patterns of neural firing are involved in representing the ideas that are active when we think about them. This is more in line with Cowan's embedded processes model.

ENGLE'S CONTROLLED ATTENTION MODEL

Another working memory theory is **Engle's controlled attention model** (Kane & Engle, 2002). Like the embedded process model, there is no separate working memory store per se. Instead, working memory contents are the information that is currently activated. An important idea here is that working memory is influenced by the effectiveness with which people control the contexts and processes of memory and cognition via attention; that is how much cognitive control one has. There are two components of control: (a) the scope of attention (how many things are captured by attention at a time) and (b) the control of attention (how effective is the control of where attention is directed) (Chow & Conway, 2015; Shipstead et al., 2015). This working memory control of attention involves the frontal lobes, particularly the prefrontal cortex (Kane & Engle, 2002), as well as the locus coeruleus in the pons of the brain stem (Unsworth & Robison, 2017). For this view, measures of working memory span (see the next section) reflect how much control people have in processing information in working memory.

This view can account for a broader range of findings, such as the fact that working memory is disrupted by irrelevant tactile stimulation (i.e., feeling something crawling on your skin that you do not expect) (Dalton et al., 2009). For Baddeley's multicomponent model there should be a separate system for tactile information, and this should not disrupt processing much in other systems. However, for Engle's view, the critical factor is how disruptive the processing is for the amount of attentional control it requires.

Another major influence of working memory is on long-term memory. Working memory capacity is related to long-term memory consolidation. People with larger working memory span scores benefit more from memory consolidation, especially during sleep (Fenn & Hambrick, 2015). Thus, people with greater working memory control are better at getting information into long-term memory.

Working memory ability is also related to how effectively people manage sources of interference to retrieve information from long-term memory. People with larger working memory capacities better retrieve memories than those with smaller capacities and show smaller fan effects (see Chapter 8) (Cantor & Engle, 1993; Radvansky & Copeland, 2006). Similarly, Kane and Engle (2000) found that people with larger working memory span scores showed less proactive interference. Put another way, people with smaller working memory capacities search through a larger set of information during memory retrieval, making retrieval less efficient (Unsworth, 2007). As an illustration, imagine that you are trying to remember the name of a historical figure (say, Tycho Brahe). When you try this, other memories of other similar historical figures can produce interference (e.g., Galileo Galilei, Isaac Newton, Johannes Kepler, and Nicholas Copernicus). Greater working memory control allows us to better select out which long-term memories are needed to do a task, thereby reducing effects of memory interference.

In addition, any activity in your environment can intrude on long-term memory search, such as seeing a picture of Francis Bacon in the book when you are trying to remember facts about Tycho Brahe. If you have better control over working memory, then this is easier compared to people whose memory search drifts more toward inappropriate memories and environmental stimuli. Overall, working memory is improved by removing visual distractions if you just close your eyes while thinking (Vredeveldt et al., 2011).

Another important part of working memory is knowing what *not* to attend to, or even to actively inhibit or suppress to keep out of the current stream of processing. Suppression is an attention process that memory can use to control what is being currently thought about. It keeps irrelevant information out of working memory or removes information that has become irrelevant or inappropriate (Conway & Engle, 1994). Thus, the suppression of irrelevant information is an important determinate to effective working memory processing (Kane et al., 2001). Memory suppression is closely tied to the prefrontal cortex (Kane & Engle, 2000).

The idea that different aspects of working memory are about the control of processing is supported by neuroimaging findings. Event Related Synchronization (ERS) and Event Related Desynchronization (ERD) analyses of EEG data reveal that different aspects of working memory are observed in different wavebands. Gamma-band synchronization reflects the maintenance of information, alpha-band synchronization reflects the control of attention and inhibitory processes, and theta-band activity reflects the sequencing of information (Roux & Uhlhaas, 2014). For example, when information is being maintained in working memory, there is increased alpha power over posterior brain regions that may be involved in the suppression of some sensory processing (Klimesch et al., 2007).

The suppression of information in working memory can create situations where performance is actually worse for things that were just thought about. This is seen in a study by Johnson et al. (2013). An outline of their procedure is shown in Figure 5.13. First, they showed 29 students from Yale University and the Ohio State University two words on a screen for 1.5 seconds. Then there was a blank screen for half a second followed by a screen, shown for 1.5 seconds, of an arrow that pointed to the location of one of the two words. The task was to say what the word at that location was. Then, after a delay, people were shown a target word that could be (a) the word just said (refreshed), (b) the other word from the display (unrefreshed), or (c) a new word (control). The task was to say that probe word as quickly as possible. There were 144 trials, with 48 trials in each of these three conditions.

The primary data of interest are the response times to say the word at the end of each trial. Because spoken responses were used, the researchers had to throw out trials where a person misspoke, stammered, spoke too quietly to trigger the device, or made nonspeech sounds (e.g., coughing). The data are shown in Figure 5.14. People were slower to say the target word if they had just said it in response to the arrow cue than if it was the other word (people were slowest in saying a new word). This suggests that when working memory processes something, and then moves on to the next task, it inhibits or suppresses the memory for what was just processed. This may occur because the just-processed information is typically not needed for a new task, and people are more effective if the newly irrelevant information is removed from working memory.

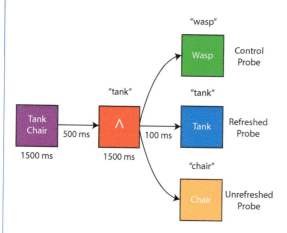

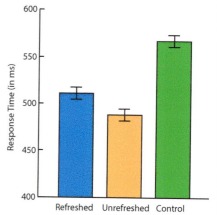

FIGURE 5.13 *Pattern of Vocal Response Times as a Function of Whether the Target Item Was Recently Refreshed or Not (Relative to an Unseen Control Condition)*

Source: adapted from Johnson, M. R., Higgins, J. A., Norman, K. A., Sederberg, P. B., Smith, T. A., & Johnson, M. K. (2013). Foraging for thought an inhibition-of-return-like effect resulting from directing attention within working memory. *Psychological Science, 24*(7), 1104–1112.

FIGURE 5.14 *Pattern of Response Times as a Function of Whether a Target Item Had Been Refreshed or Not*

Source: adapted from Johnson, M. R., Higgins, J. A., Norman, K. A., Sederberg, P. B., Smith, T. A., & Johnson, M. K. (2013). Foraging for thought: An inhibition-of-return-like effect resulting from directing attention within working memory. *Psychological Science, 24*(7), 1104–1112.

Stop and Review

Cowan's embedded processes model views working memory not as a separate store, but as those contents of long-term memory that are currently active. Moreover, this information can vary in terms of whether it is part of the central focus of attention. Alternatively, Engle's controlled attention model suggests working memory processing critically involves the controlled flow of the current stream of thought. This involves both the activation and maintenance of relevant information and the suppression of irrelevant information.

SPAN TESTS

In Chapter 4, we briefly examined measures of short-term memory span, including word span and digit span. These are **simple span** measures because people have to do one simple task—remember something for a brief period of time and then report it back. However, this is not a measure of working memory because people are not doing much mental work. To address this, several **complex span** tests have been developed (see Conway et al., 2005). A complex span test has at least two components. One is a retention component, such as the simple span measure, in which people retain a set of information for a time. The other is an active processing component, depending on the working memory process of interest. Overall, this approach better measures working memory than short-term memory.

Complex span tests are important because they are strongly related to measures of fluid intelligence (I.Q.) (Engle et al., 1999; Unsworth & Engle, 2006; but see Mogle et al., 2008), apart from things like levels of expertise (Hambrick & Meinz, 2011). They are even related to things such as decision making, with people scoring lower on complex span tests being more likely to make impulsive decisions (Hinson et al., 2003). Moreover, working memory processes may have a strong genetic component (Friedman et al., 2008). That said, working memory may be something different from fluid intelligence per se (Shipstead et al., 2016).

Reading Span

One of the first complex span tests is Daneman and Carpenter's (1980) **reading span** test. In this test, people read aloud sets of two to six sentences, such as "The taxi turned up Michigan Avenue, where they had a clear view of the lake." At the end of each set, people must recall the last word in each of the sentences of that set. The largest set of words that can all be accurately recalled is the reading span score. The retention component here is remembering the final words. The processing component is thinking about the sentence to read it effectively. Sentence span is a good predictor of language processing (Daneman & Merikle, 1996). Language processing requires an active manipulation of knowledge, much like the processing component of the reading span task, which is absent in the simple span tests.

Comprehension Span

Another example of verbal span tests are **comprehension span** tests (Waters & Caplan, 1996). Here, people read sentences and then recall the last word of each one in each set size from 2 to 6. Rather than read the sentences aloud, people make sensibility judgments. Some of the sentences are sensible, such as "It was the gangsters that broke into the warehouse," whereas others are not, such as "It was the warehouse that broke into the gangsters." These sensibility judgments require deeper thinking about the meaning of the sentences, providing a better measure of higher-level working memory processes, such as those operating at the mental model level (see Chapter 7).

Operation Span

A poplar measure of working memory is the **operation span** test (Turner & Engle, 1989). In this test, people read aloud a two-step math problem, such as $(2 \times 4) + 1 = 8$, and then indicate whether the solution is correct. After this, a word is presented. These math operation–word combinations are given in set sizes from 2 to 6. At the end of each set people recall as many words from that set as they can. The largest set size that can be accurately recalled is the operation span score. The retention component is remembering the words from each set, and the processing component is solving the math problems. The complex span test has been suggested to be a more domain-independent measure of working memory relative to reading span, which is more closely tied to language processing.

Spatial Span

One final complex span test discussed here is Shah and Miyake's (1996) **spatial span** test, which taps into spatial working memory (there are others, e.g., Woods et al., 2016). In this test, a series of letters are shown that have been rotated from the normal upright position. The initial task is to indicate whether the letters are normal, or mirror reversed. This is the active processing component. Then, after a set of letters, people indicate where the tops of the letters were in the set by pointing to a predetermined set of locations. This is the retention component. Visuospatial working memory ability has consequences for visuospatial tasks. For example, Du et al. (2015) found that variations in visuospatial working memory span predicted the ability to successfully dock a spacecraft.

n-Back Test

Another popular test of working memory, particularly in neuroscience, is Kirchner's (1958) **n -back test**. In this task, people view a series of items, such as letters, digits, pictures, etc. For each item, people must indicate "yes" or "no" whether the current item is the same as the one *n* items back. Typically, *n* is two, but other values have been used as well. People need to keep a certain number of items in

Improve Your Memory

One point that should be apparent is that working memory is very limited. There are only so many things you can think about at once. Thus, when you are learning something, you want to make some effort to allow working memory to focus on the information you are trying to process. Any distraction (other people talking, music playing, activity around you, etc.) will capture portions of working memory to process that other, irrelevant information. To improve your memory, you should try to study in places where such distractions are relatively minimized. A quiet library is a better place to study and learn than a crowded bus or a dorm room with videos and music playing.

Working memory can also be captured and drawn away by task-irrelevant thoughts that you may have. This could be things that you are concerned or worried about. When people are anxious, they think about whatever it is that is making them anxious. These task-irrelevant thoughts consume working memory resources, leaving less for whatever it is that they are supposed to be doing (e.g., studying, taking a test, or writing a paper) (Beilock, 2008). For example, people who are math anxious do worse on math problems that they would otherwise be able to solve because their working memory capacity is consumed with irrelevant anxious thoughts (Ashcraft, 2002; Ashcraft & Krause, 2007). Negative and irrelevant information clogs up working memory.

Students who engage in expressive writing to disclose personal emotions can increase working memory span (Klein & Boals, 2001). This benefit is observed even weeks after the disclosure. Apparently, this expression decreases the implicit need or desire to think about the anxiety provoking thoughts, so they intrude less. People who write about negative experiences showed a larger increase in working memory span than people who write about neutral or positive experiences. Thus, if you express thoughts about what is troubling you, it might help you increase your working memory capacity and improve your memory overall.

working memory to do this task. The processing component is the judgment about the current item, and the retention component is the number of items held in working memory. That said, there is some suggestion that the *n*-back test may be more like a simple span than a complex span task (Redick & Lindsey, 2013). This test, unlike the other complex span tasks, is a continuously running task, rather than being broken up into separate trials (for a meta-analysis and associated brain regions, see Owen et al., 2005).

The Influence of Video Games

There are a number of different measures of working memory. From these, we can estimate the resources people can bring to bear when they need to think. How fixed is this value? More importantly, can it be improved? Here we consider two lines of evidence suggesting that, to some degree, there can be improvements in working memory span.

The first of these is research on the influence of playing action video games (such as first person shooters) on visuospatial sketchpad processing. Some studies suggest that people who spend time playing these improve some visuospatial working memory abilities (Feng et al., 2007; see Bediou et al., 2018 for a review) and that brain areas such as the entorhinal cortex (BAs 28 & 34) (Kühn & Gallinat, 2013) and the hippocampus may be affected (West et al., 2017). That said, more complex abilities may be unaffected (Blacker et al., 2014). This is important because any enhanced visuospatial ability could spill over to more complex tasks that place an emphasis on these, such as science, technology, engineering, and math (STEM) fields (Sanchez, 2012; Uttal et al., 2013). Moreover, people who are better at spatial tasks, which involve perspective taking, are also better at some social skills that involve taking other people's point of view into consideration (Shelton et al., 2012).

However, the broad-based influence of video games on memory is not clear, and there is some suggestion that any influence may be minor at best (Sala et al., 2018; Unsworth et al., 2015). Also, there are costs of video games, such as decreases in sustained attention (Trisolini et al., 2018).

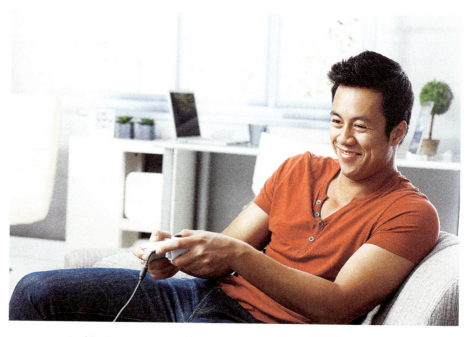

PHOTO 5.2 *A ubiquitous activity in modern culture is playing video games. While there is some evidence that this activity may actually improve some aspects of working memory processing, the evidence is equivocal*

Source: StockLite/Shutterstock.com

Working Memory Training

The work with video games suggests that there might be some aspects of working memory that can be facilitated, at least to a limited degree, with training. A bigger question is whether working memory overall can be improved. This is important because, as mentioned earlier, scores on working memory span tests are highly correlated with measures of intelligence. Is there some way to boost or improve working memory and thereby improve intelligence? There have been several efforts to address this. Some studies have shown that, with weeks of training, there can be moderate improvements on working memory span scores and measures of general intelligence (Au et al., 2015).

Other studies suggest otherwise. It is possible to improve performance on working memory span tests simply by having people practice taking them. This improvement is either very limited in its generalization (Waris et al., 2015) or does not generalize to other cognitive tasks at all, such as those reflecting general intelligence (e.g., Chooi, & Thompson, 2012; Melby-Lervåg et al., 2016; Redick, et al., 2013; Shipstead et al., 2012). Moreover, many studies reporting an improvement may be underpowered (not enough participants or observations) (Bogg & Lasecki, 2015), and so this limits the conclusions that can confidently be drawn. That said, some activities may boost cognition. For example, playing a musical instrument may do this (Gordon et al., 2015; Okada & Slevc, 2018), as well as formal education (Ritchie & Tucker-Drob, 2018). Working memory training, rather than providing a global benefit, may be limited to cases that use the same mental processes learned during training (Gathercole et al., 2019). That is, when training involves learning new working memory tools, then some transfer benefits may be seen.

Although greater working memory capacity is often desirable, there are cases when it is a disadvantage. In a study by Beilock and DeCaro (2007) students were given math problems that required a complex solution at first. However, later problems could be solved more efficiently with a simple solution.[2] People with greater working memory spans were more likely to miss the simpler solution and continued using a more complex formula. However, people with lower working memory spans, because they prefer simpler solutions (because of their smaller capacity), were more likely to notice and use the simpler solution. In essence, people with more working memory capacity were better able to construct complex solutions, but they continued to use them even when a simpler solution was possible.

Stop and Review

There are several ways to quantify working memory capacity. Word and digit spans are simple span tests that only measure retention. Complex span tests have both retention and processing components. Complex span tests include the reading span, comprehension span, operation span, spatial span, and *n*-back tests. Performance on complex span tests is related to other measures, such as general intelligence. There has been some effort to explore whether training can improve working

---

2 Some of you may remember this as the Luchin's water jug problem.

memory and, hence, intelligence. This includes playing action-based video games and tasks that emphasize working memory training in general. While working memory span scores can be improved, the reliability and generalizability of this evidence is uncertain.

PUTTING IT ALL TOGETHER

Memory is not just about holding onto information over time, it is also about doing something with it. This is working memory. There are different theories of just what working memory is, how it relates to other types of memory, and what it does for us. For Baddeley's multicomponent model there are different modules, each specialized for different types of information and processing. These include a phonological loop, a visuospatial sketchpad, an episodic buffer, and an executive controller. In comparison, Cowan's embedded processes and Engle's controlled attention models eschew the idea that working memory is a separate system. Instead, it is much more unitary and akin to theories of attention.

How does working memory relate to other aspects of memory? For Baddeley's multicomponent model, working memory is separate from long-term memory. Working memory uses knowledge recovered from long-term memory to create what will eventually be long-term memories. The different systems of working memory correspond to different brain areas. Verbal/acoustic information is processed by different brain areas than visuospatial information. The episodic buffer has processes ascribed to the hippocampus, and the central executive has characteristics associated with frontal lobe and attention control. Alternatively, the other theories integrate concepts of working memory with general principles of memory and cognition, such as long-term memory structure and processes, and attention. For Cowan's embedded processes model, working memory is part of long-term memory. It is just that part that you are currently using. These are the neural assemblies that are currently firing. This knowledge is limited in scope at any one time or is primed to become involved in whatever you may be thinking about at the time. For Engle's controlled attention model, working memory is the control of the flow of thought, both for what is currently being thought about, and what is retrieved and stored in long-term memory. Working memory is more what you can do, and how efficiently you do it, than what you have.

What does working memory do for you? For Baddeley's multiple component model, it allows you to maintain different types of content, manipulate it, and put it together to form new ideas and understandings. It holds onto ideas as they are being thought about, with multiple thoughts being handled by different parts of working memory. For Cowan's embedded processes model, working memory is a spotlight focusing your attention on this or that idea. It is the active use of knowledge either from the past (long-term memory) or the present (sensory inputs). Finally, for Engle's controlled attention model, working memory is what makes you intelligent. The better you control the flow of thoughts, the better you can think about things, and the more intelligent you are.

STUDY QUESTIONS

1. What are the primary components of the Baddeley's working memory theory?
2. What are the primary components of the phonological loop?
3. What are some of the major findings that support the idea of a phonological loop?
4. What is the nature of the information in the visuospatial sketchpad?
5. What is the evidence that the visuospatial sketchpad captures real-world, physical processes?
6. What is the purpose of the episodic buffer?
7. What is the role of the central executive in working memory?
8. What are the major features of Conway's embedded processes model? Compare and contrast this model of working memory with Baddeley's multicomponent model.
9. What are the major features of Engle's controlled attention model? Compare and contrast this model of working memory with other models of working memory.
10. What are the different types of span tests? What are the properties of each span test?
11. How effective are video games and working memory training tasks at improving memory and cognition?
12. What are some of the ways in which working memory capacity influences other types of thought?

KEY TERMS

- articulatory loop
- articulatory suppression
- Baddeley's multicomponent model
- boundary extension
- central executive
- complex span
- comprehension span
- Cowan's embedded processes model
- distraction
- dynamic memory
- dysexecutive syndrome
- Engle's controlled attention model
- episodic buffer
- executive controller
- irrelevant speech effect
- lexicality effect
- long-term working memory
- mental images
- mental rotation
- mental scanning
- *n*-back test
- operation span
- perseveration
- phonological loop
- phonological similarity effect
- phonological store
- reading span
- representational friction
- representational gravity
- representational momentum
- simple span
- spatial span
- visuospatial sketchpad
- word length effect
- working memory

EXPLORE MORE

Here are some additional readings for you to further explore issues of working memory.

Baddeley, A. D. (1986). *Working Memory*. Oxford: Oxford University Press.

Beilock, S. (2010). *Choke: What the Secrets of the Brain Reveal About Getting It Right when You Have to.* New York: Simon & Schuster.

Cowan, N. (2012). *Working Memory Capacity.* New York: Psychology Press.

Engle, R. W., Tuholski, S. W., Laughlin, J. E., & Conway, A. R. A. (1999). Working memory, short-term memory, and general fluid intelligence: A latent variable approach. *Journal of Experimental Psychology: General, 128*, 309–331.

Intraub, H., & Richardson, M. (1989). Wide-angle memories of close-up scenes. *Journal of Experimental Psychology: Learning, Memory, and Cognition, 15*, 179–187.

Kosslyn, S. M., Ball, T. M., & Reiser, B. J. (1978). Visual images preserve metric spatial information: Evidence from studies of image scanning. *Journal of Experimental Psychology: Human Perception and Performance, 4*(1), 47–60.

Shepard, R. N., & Metzler, J. (1971). Mental rotation of three-dimensional objects. *Science, 171*, 701–703.

REFERENCES

Allen, E. C., Beilock, S. L., & Shevell, S. K. (2011). Working memory is related to perceptual processing: A case from color perception. *Journal of Experimental Psychology: Learning, Memory, and Cognition, 37*(4), 1014–1021.

Ashcraft, M. H. (2002). Math anxiety: Personal, educational, and cognitive consequences. *Current Directions in Psychological Science, 11*, 181–185.

Ashcraft, M. H., & Krause, J. A. (2007). Working memory, math performance, and math anxiety. *Psychonomic Bulletin & Review, 14*, 243–248.

Au, J., Sheehan, E., Tsai, N., Duncan, G. J., Buschkuehl, M., & Jaeggi, S. M. (2015). Improving fluid intelligence with training on working memory: A meta-analysis. *Psychonomic Bulletin & Review, 22*(2), 366–377.

Baddeley, A. D. (1966). Short-term memory for word sequences as a function of acoustic, semantic, and formal similarity. *Quarterly Journal of Experimental Psychology, 18*, 302–309.

Baddeley, A. D. (1986). *Working Memory*. Oxford: Oxford University Press.

Baddeley, A. D. (2000). The episodic buffer: A new component of working memory? *Trends in Cognitive Science, 4*, 417–423.

Baddeley, A. D., & Andrade, J. (2000). Working memory and the vividness of imagery. *Journal of Experimental Psychology: General, 129*, 126–145.

Baddeley, A. D., & Hitch, G. (1974). Working memory. *Psychology of Learning and Motivation, 8*, 47–89.

Baddeley, A. D., Thomson, N., & Buchanan, M. (1975). Word length and the structure of short-term memory. *Journal of Verbal Learning and Verbal Behavior, 14*, 575–589.

Bediou, B., Adams, D. M., Mayer, R. E., Tipton, E., Green, C. S., & Bavelier, D. (2018). Meta-analysis of action video game impact on perceptual, attentional, and cognitive skills. *Psychological Bulletin, 144*(1), 77–110.

Beilock, S. L. (2008). Math performance in stressful situations. *Current Directions in Psychological Science, 17*, 339–343.

Beilock, S. L., & DeCaro, M. S. (2007). From poor performance to success under stress: Working memory, strategy selection, and mathematical problem solving under pressure. *Journal of Experimental Psychology: Learning, Memory, and Cognition, 33*, 983–998.

Bireta, T. J., Neath, I., & Surprenant, A. M. (2006). The syllable-based word length effect and stimulus set specificity. *Psychonomic Bulletin & Review, 13*, 434–438.

Blacker, K. J., Curby, K. M., Klobusicky, E., & Chein, J. M. (2014). Effects of action video game training on visual working memory. *Journal of Experimental Psychology: Human Perception and Performance, 40*(5), 1992.

Bogg, T., & Lasecki, L. (2015). Reliable gains? Evidence for substantially underpowered designs in studies of working memory training transfer to fluid intelligence. *Frontiers in Psychology, 5*, 1589.

Cantor, J., & Engle, R. W. (1993). Working-memory capacity as long-term memory activation: An individual differences approach. *Journal of Experimental Psychology: Learning, Memory, and Cognition, 19*, 1101–1114.

Cantor, J., Engle, R. W., & Hamilton, G. (1991). Short-term memory, working memory, and verbal abilities: How do they relate? *Intelligence, 15*, 229–246.

Chooi, W-T., & Thompson, L. A. (2012). Working memory training does not improve intelligence in heathy young adults. *Intelligence, 40*, 531–542.

Chow, M., & Conway, A. R. (2015). The scope and control of attention: Sources of variance in working memory capacity. *Memory & Cognition, 43*(3), 325–339.

Colle, H. A., & Welsh, A. (1976). Acoustic masking in primary memory. *Journal of Verbal Learning and Verbal Behavior, 15*, 17–32.

Conrad, R., & Hull, A. (1964). Information, acoustic confusion, and memory span. *British Journal of Experimental Psychology, 55*, 75–84.

Conway, A. R. A., & Engle, R. W. (1994). Working memory and retrieval: A resource-dependent inhibition model. *Journal of Experimental Psychology: General, 123*, 354–373.

Conway, A. R. A., Kane, M. J., Bunting, M. F., Hambrick, D. Z., Wilhelm, O., & Engle, R. W. (2005). Working memory span tasks: A methodological review and user's guide. *Psychonomic Bulletin & Review, 12*, 769–786.

Copeland, D. E., & Radvansky, G. A. (2001). Phonological similarity in working memory. *Memory & Cognition, 29*, 774–776.

Courtney, J. R., & Hubbard, T. L. (2008). Spatial memory and explicit knowledge: An effect of instruction on representational momentum. *Quarterly Journal of Experimental Psychology, 61*, 1778–1784.

Coventry, K. R., Christophel, T. B., Fehr, T., Valdés-Conroy, B., & Herrmann, M. (2013). Multiple routes to mental animation: Language and functional relations drive motion processing for static images. *Psychological Science, 24*(8), 1379–1388.

Cowan, N. (1988). Evolving conceptions of memory storage, selective attention, and their mutual constraints within the human information-processing system. *Psychological Bulletin, 104*(2), 163–191.

Cowan, N., Baddeley, A. D., Elliott, E. M., & Norris, J. (2003). List composition and the word length effect in immediate recall: A comparison of localist and globalist assumptions. *Psychonomic Bulletin & Review, 10*, 74–79.

Dalton, P., Lavie, N., & Spence, C. (2009). The role of working memory in tactile selective attention. *Quarterly Journal of Experimental Psychology, 62*, 635–644.

Daneman, M., & Carpenter, P. A. (1980). Individual differences in working memory and reading. *Journal of Verbal Learning and Verbal Behavior, 19*, 430–466.

Daneman, M., & Merikle, P. M. (1996). Working memory and language comprehension: A meta-analysis. *Psychonomic Bulletin and Review, 3*, 422–433.

Darling, S., Della Sala, S., & Logie, R. H. (2009). Dissociation between appearance and location within visuo-spatial working memory. *Quarterly Journal of Experimental Psychology, 62*, 417–425.

Darling, S., & Havelka, J. (2010). Visuospatial bootstrapping: Evidence for binding of verbal and spatial information in working memory. *Quarterly Journal of Experimental Psychology, 63*(2), 239–245.

Dijkstra, N., Bosch, S. E., & van Gerven, M. A. (2019). Shared neural mechanisms of visual perception and imagery. *Trends in Cognitive Sciences, 23*(5), 423–434.

Du, X., Zhang, Y., Tian, Y., Huang, W., Wu, B., & Zhang, J. (2015). The influence of spatial ability and experience on performance during spaceship rendezvous and docking. *Frontiers in Psychology, 6*, 955.

Eich, T. S., & Metcalfe, J. (2009). Effects of the stress of marathon running on implicit and explicit memory. *Psychonomic Bulletin & Review, 16*, 475–479.

Elsley, J. V., & Parmentier, F. B. R. (2009). Is visual-spatial binding in working memory impaired by a concurrent memory load? *Quarterly Journal of Experimental Psychology, 62*, 1696–1705.

Engle, R. W., Tuholski, S. W., Laughlin, J. E., & Conway, A. R. A. (1999). Working memory, short-term memory, and general fluid intelligence: A latent-variable approach. *Journal of Experimental Psychology: General, 128*, 309–331.

Ericsson, K. A., & Kintsch, W. (1995). Long-term working memory. *Psychological Review, 102*, 211–245.

Feng, J., Spence, I., & Pratt, J. (2007). Playing an action video game reduces gender differences in spatial cognition. *Psychological Science, 18*(10), 850–855.

Fenn, K. M., & Hambrick, D. Z. (2015). General intelligence predicts memory change across sleep. *Psychonomic Bulletin & Review, 22*(3), 791–799.

Flusberg, S. J., & Boroditsky, L. (2011). Are things that are hard to physically move also hard to imagine moving? *Psychonomic Bulletin & Review, 18*(1), 158–164.

Folk, M. D., & Luce, R. D. (1987). Effects of stimulus complexity on mental rotation rate of polygons. *Journal of Experimental Psychology: Human Perception and Performance, 13*(3), 395–404.

Freyd, J. J. (1987). Dynamic mental representations. *Psychological Review, 94*, 427–438.

Freyd, J. J., & Finke, R. A. (1984). Representational momentum. *Journal of Experimental Psychology: Learning, Memory, and Cognition, 10*, 126–132.

Freyd, J. J., Pantzer, T. M., & Cheng, J. L. (1988). Representing statics as forces in equilibrium. *Journal of Experimental Psychology: General, 117*, 395–407.

Friedman, N. P., Miyake, A., Young, S. E., DeFries, J. C., Corley, R. P., & Hewitt, J. K. (2008). Individual differences in executive functions are almost entirely genetic in origin. *Journal of Experimental Psychology: General, 137*(2), 201–225.

Gailliot, M. T. (2008). Unlocking the energy dynamics of executive functioning: Linking executive functioning to brain glycogen. *Perspectives on Psychological Science, 3*, 245–263.

Gardony, A. L., Taylor, H. A., & Brunyé, T. T. (2013). What does physical rotation reveal about mental rotation? *Psychological Science, 25*(2), 605–612.

Gathercole, S. E. (1997). Models of verbal short-term memory. In M. A. Conway (Ed.), *Cognitive Models of Memory* (pp. 13–45). Cambridge, MA: MIT Press.

Gathercole, S. E., Dunning, D. L., Holmes, J., & Norris, D. (2019). Working memory training involves learning new skills. *Journal of Memory and Language, 105*, 19–42.

Gevins, A., Smith, M. E., McEvoy, L, & Yu, D. (1997). High-resolution EEG mapping of cortical activation related to working memory: Effects of task difficulty, type of processing, and practice. *Cerebral Cortex, 7*, 374–385.

Gordon, R. L., Fehd, H. M., & McCandliss, B. D. (2015). Does music training enhance literacy skills? A meta-analysis. *Frontiers in Psychology, 6*, 1777.

Gottesman, C. V., & Intraub, H. (2002). Surface construal and the mental representation of scenes. *Journal of Experimental Psychology: Human Perception and Performance, 28*, 589–599.

Greenstein, M., Franklin, N., Martins, M., Sewack, C., & Meier, M. A. (2016). When anticipation beats accuracy: Threat alters memory for dynamic scenes. *Memory & Cognition, 44*(4), 633–649.

Guitard, D., Gabel, A. J., Saint-Aubin, J., Surprenant, A. M., & Neath, I. (2018). Word length, set size, and lexical factors: Re-examining what causes the word length effect. *Journal of Experimental Psychology: Learning, Memory, and Cognition, 44*(11), 1824–1844.

Gupta, P., Lipinski, J., & Aktunc, E. (2005). Reexamining the phonological similarity effect in immediate serial recall: The roles of type of similarity, category cuing, and item recall. *Memory & Cognition, 33*, 1001–1016.

Hambrick, D. Z., & Meinz, E. J. (2011). Limits on the predictive power of domain-specific experience and knowledge in skilled performance. *Current Directions in Psychological Science, 20*(5), 275–279.

Hinson, J. M., Jameson, T. L., & Whitney, P. (2003). Impulsive decision making and working memory. *Journal of Experimental Psychology: Learning, Memory, and Cognition, 29*, 298–306.

Hoosain, R., & Salili, F. (1988). Language differences, working memory, and mathematical ability. In M. M. Gruneberg, P. E. Morris, & R. N. Sykes (Eds.), *Practical Aspects of Memory: Current Research and Issues* (pp. 512–517). Chichester, UK: Wiley.

Hubbard, T. L. (1990). Cognitive representation of linear motion: Possible direction and gravity effects in judged displacement. *Memory & Cognition, 18*, 299–309.

Hubbard, T. L. (1995). Cognitive representation of motion: Evidence for friction and gravity analogues. *Journal of Experimental Psychology: Learning, Memory, and Cognition, 21*, 241–254.

Hubbard, T. L. (1996). Representational momentum, centripetal force, and curvilinear impetus. *Journal of Experimental Psychology: Learning, Memory, and Cognition, 22*, 1049–1060.

Hubbard, T. L. (2005). Representational momentum and related displacements in spatial memory: A review of the findings. *Psychonomic Bulletin & Review, 12*, 822–851.

Hubbard, T. L. (2020). Representational gravity: Empirical findings and theoretical implications. *Psychonomic Bulletin & Review, 27*(1), 36–55.

Hubbard, T. L., & Bharucha, J. J. (1988). Judged displacement in apparent vertical and horizontal motion. *Perception & Psychophysics, 44*, 211–221.

Hubbard, T. L., Hutchison, J. L., & Courtney, J. R. (2010). Boundary extension: Findings and theories. *Quarterly Journal of Experimental Psychology, 63*(8), 1467–1494.

Hulme, C. Maughan, S., & Brown, G. D. A. (1991). Memory for familiar and unfamiliar words: Evidence for a long-term memory contribution to short-term memory span. *Journal of Memory and Language, 30*, 685–701.

Hulme, C., Suprenant, A. M., Bireta, T. J., Stuart, G., & Neath, I. (2004). Abolishing the word-length effect. *Journal of Experimental Psychology: Learning, Memory, and Cognition, 30*, 98–106.

Intons-Peterson, M. J., & Roskos-Ewoldsen, B. B. (1989). Sensory-perceptual qualities of images. *Journal of Experimental Psychology: Learning, Memory, and Cognition, 15*, 188–199.

Intraub, H., Bender, R. S., & Mangels, J. A. (1992). Looking at pictures but remembering scenes. *Journal of Experimental Psychology: Learning, Memory, and Cognition, 18*, 180–191.

Intraub, H., & Dickinson, C. A. (2008). False memory 1/20th of a second later: What the early onset of boundary extension reveals about perception. *Psychological Science, 19*, 1007–1014.

Intraub, H., Gottesman, C. V., & Bills, A. J. (1998). Effects of perceiving and imagining scenes on memory for pictures. *Journal of Experimental Psychology: Learning, Memory, and Cognition, 24*, 186–201.

Intraub, H., & Richardson, M. (1989). Wide-angle memories of close-up scenes. *Journal of Experimental Psychology: Learning, Memory, and Cognition, 15*, 179–187.

Jefferies, E., Lambon Ralph, M. A., & Baddeley, A. D. (2004). Automatic and controlled processing in sentence recall: The role of long-term and working memory. *Journal of Memory and Language, 51*, 623v643.

Johnson, M. R., Higgins, J. A., Norman, K. A., Sederberg, P. B., Smith, T. A., & Johnson, M. K. (2013). Foraging for thought: An inhibition-of-return-like effect resulting from directing attention within working memory. *Psychological Science, 24*(7), 1104–1112.

Jonides, J., Lacy, S. C., & Nee, D. E. (2005). Processes of working memory in mind and brain. *Current Directions in Psychological Science, 14*, 2–5.

Just, M. A., Carpenter, P. A., Maguire, M., Diwadkar, V., & McMains, S. (2001). Mental rotation of objects retrieved from memory: A functional MRI study of spatial processing. *Journal of Experimental Psychology: General, 130*, 493–504.

Kane, M. J., Bleckley, M. K., Conway, A. R. A., & Engle, R. W. (2001). A controlled-attention view of working-memory capacity. *Journal of Experimental Psychology: General, 130*, 169–183.

Kane, M. J., & Engle, R. W. (2000). Working-memory capacity, proactive interference, and divided attention: Limits on long-term memory retrieval.

Journal of Experimental Psychology: Learning, Memory, and Cognition, 26, 336–358.

Kane, M. J., & Engle, R. W. (2002). The role of prefrontal cortex in working-memory capacity, executive attention, and general fluid intelligence: An individual-differences perspective. *Psychonomic Bulletin & Review, 9,* 637–671.

Kelly, M. H., & Freyd, J. J. (1987). Explorations of representational momentum. *Cognitive Psychology, 19,* 369–401.

Kirchner, W. K. (1958). Age differences in short-term retention of rapidly changing information. *Journal of Experimental Psychology, 55*(4), 352–358.

Klauer, K.C., & Zhao, Z. (2004). Double dissociations in visual and spatial short-term memory. *Journal of Experimental Psychology: General, 133,* 355–381.

Klein, K., & Boals, A. (2001). Expressive writing can increase working memory capacity. *Journal of Experimental Psychology: General, 130,* 520–533.

Klimesch, W., Sauseng, P., & Hanslmayr, S. (2007). EEG alpha oscillations: The inhibition–timing hypothesis. *Brain Research Reviews, 53*(1), 63–88.

Kosslyn, S. M. (1975). Information representation in visual images. *Cognitive Psychology, 7,* 341–370.

Kosslyn, S. M., Ball, T. M., & Reiser, B. J. (1978). Visual images preserve metric spatial information: Evidence from studies of image scanning. *Journal of Experimental Psychology: Human Perception and Performance, 4*(1), 47–60.

Kosslyn, S. M., & Pomerantz, J. R. (1977). Imagery, propositions, and the form of internal representations. *Cognitive Psychology, 9,* 52–76.

Kozhevnikov, M., & Hegarty, M. (2001). Impetus beliefs as default heuristics: Dissociation between explicit and implicit knowledge about motion. *Psychonomic Bulletin & Review, 8,* 439–453.

Kühn, S., & Gallinat, J. (2013). Amount of lifetime video gaming is positively associated with entorhinal, hippocampal and occipital volume. *Molecular Psychiatry, 19,* 842–847.

Li, X., Schweickert, R., & Gandour, J. (2000). The phonological similarity effect in immediate recall: Positions of shared phonemes. *Memory & Cognition, 28,* 1116–1125.

Logie, R. H. (2016). Retiring the central executive. *Quarterly Journal of Experimental Psychology, 69*(10), 2093–2109.

Macnamara, B. N., Moore, A. B., & Conway, A. R. (2011). Phonological similarity effects in simple and complex span tasks. *Memory & Cognition, 39*(7), 1174–1186.

Melby-Lervåg, M., Redick, T. S., & Hulme, C. (2016). Working memory training does not improve performance on measures of intelligence or other measures of "far transfer" evidence from a meta-analytic review. *Perspectives on Psychological Science, 11*(4), 512–534.

Mogle, J. A., Lovett, B. J., Stawski, R. S., & Sliwinski, M. J. (2008). What's so special about working memory? An examination of the relationships among working memory, secondary memory, and fluid intelligence. *Psychological Science, 19,* 1071–1077.

Morey, C. C., & Cowan, N. (2005). When do visual and verbal memories conflict? The importance of working memory load and retrieval. *Journal of Experimental Psychology: Learning, Memory, and Cognition, 31,* 703–713.

Munger, M. P., Solberg, J. L., & Horrocks, K. K. (1999). The relationship between mental rotation and representational momentum. *Journal of Experimental Psychology: Learning, Memory, and Cognition, 25,* 1557–1568.

Murray, D. J. (1967). The role of speech responses in short-term memory. *Canadian Journal of Psychology, 21,* 263–276.

Naveh-Benjamin, M., & Ayres, T. J. (1986). Digit span, reading rate, and linguistic relativity. *Quarterly Journal of Experimental Psychology, 38*(4), 739–751.

Neath, I. (1998). *Human Memory: An introduction to research, data, and theory.* Pacific Grove, CA: Thomson Brooks/Cole Publishing.

Nees, M. A., Corrini, E., Leong, P., & Harris, J. (2017). Maintenance of memory for melodies: Articulation or attentional refreshing? *Psychonomic Bulletin & Review, 24*(6), 1964–1970.

Norman, D. A., & Shallice, T. (1986). Attention to action. In R. J. Davison, G. E. Schwartz, & D. Shapiro (Eds.). *Consciousness and Self-Regulation* (pp. 1–18). New York: Plenum Press.

Oberauer, K. (2019). Is Rehearsal an Effective Maintenance Strategy for Working Memory? *Trends in Cognitive Sciences, 23*(9), 798–809.

Okada, B. M., & Slevc, L. R. (2018). Individual differences in musical training and executive functions: A latent variable approach. *Memory & Cognition, 46*(7), 1076–1092.

Ongchoco, J. D. K., & Scholl, B. J. (2019). Did that just happen? Event segmentation influences enumeration and working memory for simple overlapping visual events. *Cognition, 187,* 188–197.

Ongchoco, J. D. K., & Scholl, B. J. (2020). Enumeration in time is irresistibly event-based. *Psychonomic Bulletin & Review, 27,* 307–314.

Owen, A. M., McMillan, K. M., Laird, A. R., & Bullmore, E. (2005). N-back working memory paradigm: A meta analysis of normative functional neuroimaging studies. *Human Brain Mapping, 25*(1), 46–59.

Peterson, L. R., & Johnson, S. T. (1971). Some effects of minimizing articulation on short-term retention. *Journal of Verbal Learning and Verbal Behavior, 10,* 346–354.

Radvansky, G. A., & Copeland, D. E. (2006) Memory retrieval and interference: Working memory issues. *Journal of Memory and Language, 55,* 33–46.

Redick, T. S., & Lindsey, D. R. B. (2013). Complex span and *n*-back measures of working memory: A meta-analysis. *Psychonomic Bulletin & Review, 20*(6), 1102–1113.

Redick, T. S., Shipstead, Z., Harrison, T. L., Hicks, K. L., Fried, D. E., Hambrick, D. Z., Kane, M. J., & Engle, R. W. (2013). No evidence of intelligence improvement after working memory training: A randomized, placebo-controlled study. *Journal of Experimental Psychology: General, 142*(2), 359–379.

Ritchie, S. J., & Tucker-Drob, E. M. (2018). How much does education improve intelligence? A meta-analysis. *Psychological Science, 29*(8), 1358–1369.

Roux, F., & Uhlhaas, P. J. (2014). Working memory and neural oscillations: Alpha–gamma versus theta–gamma codes for distinct WM information? *Trends in Cognitive Sciences, 18*(1), 16–25.

Sala, G., Tatlidil, K. S., & Gobet, F. (2018). Video game training does not enhance cognitive ability: A comprehensive meta-analytic investigation. *Psychological Bulletin, 144*(2), 111–139.

Salamé, P., & Baddeley, A. (1989). Effects of background music on phonological short-term memory. *Quarterly Journal of Experimental Psychology, 41A,* 107–122.

Sanchez, C. A. (2012). Enhancing visuospatial performance through video game training to increase learning in visuospatial science domains. *Psychonomic Bulletin & Review, 19*(1), 58–65.

Segal, S. J., & Fusella, V. (1970). Influence of imaged pictures and sounds on detection of visual and auditory signals. *Journal of Experimental Psychology, 83*(3 pt. 1), 458–464.

Segal, S. J., & Fusella, V. (1971). Effect of images in six sense modalities on detection of visual signal from noise. *Psychonomic Science, 24,* 55–56.

Shah, P., & Miyake, A. (1996). The separability of working memory resources for spatial thinking and language processing: An individual differences approach. *Journal of Experimental Psychology: General, 125,* 4–27.

Shelton, A. L., Clements-Stephens, A. M., Lam, W. Y., Pak, D. M., & Murray, A. J. (2012). Should social savvy equal good spatial skills? The interaction of social skills with spatial perspective taking. *Journal of Experimental Psychology: General, 141*(2), 199–205.

Shepard, R. N., & Metzler, J. (1971). Mental rotation of three-dimensional objects. *Science, 171,* 701–703.

Shipstead, Z., Harrison, T. L., & Engle, R. W. (2015). Working memory capacity and the scope and control of attention. *Attention, Perception, & Psychophysics, 77*(6), 1863–1880.

Shipstead, Z., Harrison, T. L., & Engle, R. W. (2016). Working memory capacity and fluid intelligence: Maintenance and disengagement. *Perspectives on Psychological Science, 11*(6), 771–799.

Shipstead, Z., Redick, T. S., & Engle, R. W. (2012). Is working memory training effective? *Psychological Bulletin, 138*(4), 628–634.

Smith, E. E. (2000). Neural bases of human working memory. *Current Directions in Psychological Science, 9,* 45–49.

Torok, A., Gallagher, M., Lasbareilles, C., & Ferrè, E. R. (2019). Getting ready for Mars: How the brain perceives new simulated gravitational environments. *Quarterly Journal of Experimental Psychology, 72*(9), 2342–2349.

Trisolini, D. C., Petilli, M. A., & Daini, R. (2018). Is action video gaming related to sustained attention of adolescents? *Quarterly Journal of Experimental Psychology, 71*(5), 1033–1039.

Turner, M. L., & Engle, R. W. (1989). Is working memory capacity task dependent? *Journal of Memory and Language, 28,* 127–154.

Unsworth, N. (2007). Individual differences in working memory capacity and episodic retrieval: Examining the dynamics of delayed and continuous distractor free recall. *Journal of Experimental Psychology: Learning, Memory, and Cognition, 33,* 1020–1034.

Unsworth, N., & Engle, R. W. (2006). Simple and complex memory spans and their relation to fluid abilities: Evidence from list-length effects. *Journal of Memory and Language, 54,* 68–80.

Unsworth, N., & Engle, R. W. (2007). The nature of individual differences in working memory capacity: Active maintenance in primary memory and controlled search from secondary memory. *Psychological Review, 114,* 104–132.

Unsworth, N., Redick, T. S., McMillan, B. D., Hambrick, D. Z., Kane, M. J., & Engle, R. W. (2015). Is playing video games related to cognitive abilities? *Psychological Science, 26*(6), 759–774.

Unsworth, N., & Robison, M. K. (2017). A locus coeruleus-norepinephrine account of individual differences in working memory capacity and attention control. *Psychonomic Bulletin & Review, 24*(4), 1282–1311.

Uttal, D. H., Miller, D. I., & Newcombe, N. S. (2013). Exploring and enhancing spatial thinking Links to achievement in science, technology, engineering, and mathematics? *Current Directions in Psychological Science, 22*(5), 367–373.

Vasilev, M. R., Kirkby, J. A., & Angele, B. (2018). Auditory distraction during reading: A Bayesian meta-analysis of a continuing controversy. *Perspectives on Psychological Science, 13*(5), 567–597.

Verfaillie, K., & Y'dewalle, G. (1991). Representational momentum and event course anticipation in the perception of implied periodic motions. *Journal of Experimental Psychology: Learning, Memory, and Cognition, 17,* 302–313.

Vergauwe, E., Barrouillet, P., & Camos, V. (2010). Do mental processes share a domain-general resource? *Psychological Science, 21*(3), 384–390.

Voyer, D., Voyer, S., & Bryden, M. P. (1995). Magnitude of sex differences in spatial abilities: A meta-analysis and consideration of critical variables. *Psychological Bulletin, 117,* 250–270.

Voyer, D., Voyer, S. D., & Saint-Aubin, J. (2017). Sex differences in visual-spatial working memory: A meta-analysis. *Psychonomic Bulletin & Review, 24*(2), 307–334.

Vredeveldt, A., Hitch, G. J., & Baddeley, A. D. (2011). Eyeclosure helps memory by reducing cognitive load and enhancing visualisation. *Memory & Cognition, 39*(7), 1253–1263.

Waris, O., Soveri, A., & Laine, M. (2015). Transfer after working memory updating training. *PLoS one, 10*(9), e0138734.

Waters, G. S., & Caplan, D. (1996). The measurement of verbal working memory capacity and its relation to reading comprehension. *Quarterly Journal of Experimental Psychology, 49A,* 51–79.

West, G. L., Konishi, K., & Bohbot, V. D. (2017). Video games and hippocampus-dependent learning. *Current Directions in Psychological Science, 26*(2), 152–158.

Wilson, M. & Emmorey, K. (2006). Comparing sign language and speech reveals a universal limit on short-term memory capacity. *Psychological Science, 17,* 682–683.

Wilson, M., & Fox, G. (2007). Working memory for language is not special: Evidence for an articulatory loop for novel stimuli. *Psychonomic Bulletin & Review, 14,* 470–473.

Woods, D. L., Wyma, J. M., Herron, T. J., & Yund, E. W. (2016). An improved spatial span test of visuospatial memory. *Memory, 24*(8), 1142–1155.

Wraga, M., Creem, S. H., & Proffitt, D. R. (2000). Updating displays after imagined object and viewer rotations. *Journal of Experimental Psychology: Learning, Memory, and Cognition, 26,* 151–168.

Wraga, M., Swaby, M., & Flynn, C. M. (2008). Passive tactile feedback facilitates mental rotation of handheld objects. *Memory & Cognition, 36,* 271–81.

CHAPTER 6

Nondeclarative Memory

When we think about "remembering," we usually think about times when we are consciously aware of using our memories, such as trying to remember a person's name, the answer to an exam question, or where we left the car keys. This conscious, explicit use of memory is readily understood and apparent. We are also painfully aware of when this conscious memory has failed and we forget something. It is not difficult to talk about such experiences, the content of these memories, and our awareness of them. This is what makes them declarative memories. However, as prominent as this type of memory is, much of human memory operates at an unconscious level. Some of these unconscious memories are so far removed from awareness that it is very difficult, if not impossible, to accurately talk about them. These are **nondeclarative memories**. An interesting thing about nondeclarative memories is that they are relatively spared in cases of amnesia, consistent with the idea that this is a distinctly different way of remembering.

This chapter covers several aspects of nondeclarative memory. We start with some basic forms of learning and memory. One is classical conditioning, in which an organism learns to respond to signals that are predictive of future outcomes. In a sense, the organism is showing memory for previous environmental contingencies. We also examine more "cognitive" sorts of nondeclarative memory, particularly procedural and implicit memories. These are memories we use for various tasks that influence our behaviors without conscious awareness.

CLASSICAL CONDITIONING

Classical conditioning is one of the simplest forms of learning. Its formal discovery is credited to Ivan Pavlov (1849–1936), a famous Russian physiologist (see Chapter 1). Thus, it is sometimes called **Pavlovian conditioning**. In classical conditioning, an organism learns that certain stimuli are reliable predictors of the imminent onset of other important stimuli (Pavlov, 1923). We examine classical conditioning in three forms: abstract; concrete, with the experimental situation used by Pavlov; and an example with human memory.

Learning Paradigm

The basic classical conditioning paradigm is shown in Figure 6.1. Classical conditioning starts with a stimulus that elicits a response. This is the unconditioned stimulus, or US, and the response it elicits is the unconditioned response, or UR. Both are unconditioned because no learning is needed. Another stimulus is introduced that elicits no response called a neutral stimulus, or NS. During learning, the NS is presented prior to the US in a reliable and consistent way. Over time, the organism associates the NS with the upcoming US. As a result, a preparatory response is made, as if the US were about to occur. The NS is now a conditioned stimulus, or CS, and the response that is made in the presence of a CS is the conditioned response, or CR.

As an example of classical conditioning, let us look at Pavlov's experiment. Pavlov received a Nobel Prize for his work on digestion. After getting his prize, he started researching the initial stage of digestion, salivation. Pavlov collected saliva from dogs by surgically inserting tubes into their mouths and feeding them. Pavlov found that the dogs sometimes salivated when they were not being fed. Pavlov noticed that this salivation occurred with some regularity: it often preceded the actual presentation of food by when the dogs first saw the person who fed them. Pavlov suspected that the dogs had made a mental connection between that person and the food. Thus, the dogs would salivate at the sight of that person. Pavlov decided to test his theory.

In his study, Pavlov used meat as the US and the dogs' salivation as the UR. As an NS, he used a bell. He rang the bell before he gave the meat. Over time, the dogs learned that the bell meant food. The dogs began to salivate when the bell rang but before they were fed. The bell was now a CS, and the salivation was a CR.

Another example of classical conditioning that relates more to human activity is the development of phobias. These are irrational fears people develop, such as a fear of elevators, open spaces, public speaking, and so on. These phobias can develop through a nondeclarative, classical conditioning process of which people are unaware. Specifically, people may have an initial negative experience with a situation that will come to elicit the phobia. For example, they may have a negative public speaking experience, the anxiety experienced prior to public speaking is classically conditioned, and people begin to avoid that situation, creating the

Basic Paradigm

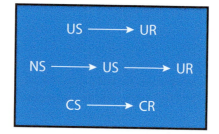

FIGURE 6.1 *The Basic Classical Conditioning Paradigm*

phobia. Thus, from a nondeclarative memory perspective, emotionally negative and unexpected events become strongly associated with information, leading them to be better remembered (Kalbe & Schwabe, 2020).

Happily, classical conditioning can also be used to get rid of phobias through a process known as **systematic desensitization** (Wolpe, 1958). In this clinical method, people first think of situations that are remote from the one that elicits the phobia. Over time, people are slowly brought closer and closer to the situation that produces the phobia. At each step people remain at that stage until they do not feel disturbed. When a feeling of calm is associated with the situation at each stage, people then move on to the next stage. This continues until they finally reach the phobia-inducing situation, which is then classically conditioned to a relaxed feeling. At this point the phobia is conquered.

Associative Structure

What kind of association is learned in classical conditioning? There are two general possibilities. The first is that the CS is directly associated with the CR. That is, the CS directly causes the CR to occur. This is a **stimulus–response association**. The other is that the CS is directly associated with a *memory* of the US, which leads to the production of the CR. In other words, the CS is predicting the onset of the US, so this elicits a CR in preparation for the US. This is a **stimulus–stimulus association**. In most cases, it is stimulus–stimulus associations that are learned. That is, the organism learns a predictive relationship.

Because of stimulus–stimulus associations, what is important in classical conditioning is not contiguity but contingency. **Contiguity learning** is the idea that learning occurs when an NS and a US occur near each other in time. However, while timing is influential, it is not the critical factor. Instead, learning is driven by deriving some cause–effect relationship (however primitive). **Contingency learning** involves a sensitivity to the underlying causal structure rather than simply relying on things that happen to occur together in time. The importance of establishing a contingency relationship is more likely to be important when there is awareness of the CS. When a CS is presented subliminally (e.g., 50 ms presentation), then unconscious conditioning occurs because the CS has been perceptually bound to the US (Greenwald & De Houwer, 2017).

Important Phenomenon

There are many important phenomena of classical conditioning. First, there is an acquisition period or **learning curve**. An association is not acquired immediately. This takes time. For example, it takes a while for a dog to learn that the sound of a bell is a signal for the presentation of food. This is because not all co-occurrences in the environment are meaningful but may be due to chance. By only encoding and using those relationships that are stable and meaningful, classical conditioning allows for a more direct way to prepare for events in the environment.

Of course, the environment is not always stable, and we need to adapt to change, not only by learning new associations, but also by ceasing to respond to associations that are no longer relevant. When a CS is repeatedly presented without a US, responding to that CS ceases. This type of forgetting is called **extinction**. For example, if a bell rings but no food is offered, the dog will no longer salivate when it hears the bell.

When extinction has occurred, forgetting is not complete. This is revealed by two phenomena. The first is **spontaneous recovery**. This occurs when, after extinction, there is a delay, and then the CS is presented again. The CR, which was extinct, reemerges, but it is not as strong as before. The organism remembers the original association with the CS and forgets that it is no longer predictive and useful. This may be advantageous because environmental conditions might be present that make the CS meaningful again after an absence. The other phenomenon is **savings**. This is similar to the savings derived by Ebbinghaus (see Chapter 3). Savings shows that after extinction, when relearning occurs, less time is required to learn than the first time. Thus, some memory for that association remains, even though it appears to be forgotten.

Unconscious classical conditioning processes can influence our preferences. The **mere exposure effect** (Zajonc, 1968; 2001) is the finding that people prefer things they have been exposed to before. When we encounter something, we register it, even if only at a subconscious level. As long as there are no negative connotations, a mild positive association is established. That is, the absence of negative associations in nondeclarative memory is interpreted, at some level, as something we have experienced that does not hurt us. For example, if you eat a new berry that you have never seen before, and you do not get sick, then you will prefer it to another new one that you have never tried. Thus, we prefer things we have been exposed to before, even if we do not consciously remember them.

The effects of mere exposure influence our lives and our culture. As an example, Cutting (2003) showed that the development of the standard Western canon of French Impressionist paintings (the set of works identified by experts as the core or most important ones) is highly related to exposure. Adults' preferences were related to frequency of exposure in the culture rather than to whether people consciously recognized the painting, the complexity of the painting, or its prototypicality. Importantly, children who have not had this exposure do not show this bias. Thus, there does not seem to be anything special about the paintings at the core of the canon. What puts them at the core is their frequency of exposure, which influences our preferences. A finding related to this is preferences for songs that make up the top 40. People are exposed to these songs more, and this is why they prefer them, even though there are others out there that they might like better. However, the lower level of exposure results in a reduced preference.

This influence of memory on preferences differs from explicit memory of whether something is old or new. Different parts of the brain are activated, depending on the judgments people make. The preference judgments that drive the mere exposure effect involve the right lateral frontal lobe, which is not observed with standard memory judgments (Elliot & Dolan, 1998).

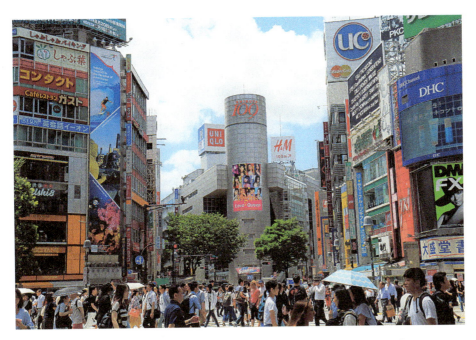

PHOTO 6.1 *Advertisers try to get your attention in part to make their product name familiar and, consistent with the mere exposure effect, cause you to like it more*

Source: TK Kurikawa/Shutterstock.com

The strength of the mere exposure effect can vary (Bornstein, 1989). It grows larger with more exposures, up to a point. With too many exposures, the effect starts to decline. The effect is also more likely to occur when something is presented in multiple contexts rather than the same context over and over. Similarly, the mere exposure effect is greater with a delay between the time when the information was received and when the preference ratings are given. Finally, there is an embodied aspect to mere exposure. If you are chewing gum when you are exposed to stimuli, you would show a mere exposure effect if the items are Chinese ideographs, but not for words (Topolinski & Strack, 2009a). This is because the words could be spoken, but the mental and neural machinery that would simulate this is taken up by the action of moving your mouth to chew the gum.

For the Representation-Mapping Model (Montoya et al., 2017), the mere exposure effect arises out of new exposures matching prior memories. This leads them to be favored and liked more. Over time, with more and more exposures, it becomes better learned, and ceases being interesting.

INSTRUMENTAL CONDITIONING

The other major tradition in conditioning research is **instrumental conditioning**, such as when you learn putting your finger in a light socket is a bad idea. Unlike classical conditioning where we learn to prepare for an upcoming event, in instrumental conditioning we are acting on the environment and then remembering and evaluating the consequences of those actions. Much of instrumental conditioning can be captured by Thorndike's Law of Effect. This states that the consequences of an action that have a positive outcome will be reinforced, whereas consequences that have a negative or neutral outcome will not be reinforced. Reinforced means that the behavior is more likely to occur in the future. Essentially, with the Law of Effect, the time and energy that we have available can be directed toward activities that benefit ourselves and away from activities that either provide no benefit or may actually cause harm.

The domain of instrumental conditioning is too extensive to be adequately covered here. However, it should be noted that we have many nondeclarative memories that have been brought about through instrumental conditioning. Often we are unaware that our behavior is being influenced by prior memories of both pleasant and unpleasant events. Instrumental conditioning is, in some cases, the use of unconscious memories to shape our behaviors and thoughts.

CAUSAL LEARNING

Work on conditioning has been extended to understanding human causal learning. That is, how do we figure out the cause and effect relations in the world? For example, how do we learn the causal relations that are needed to understand how technology works, what causes diseases, or how to find food. In essence, this is what goes on in conditioning. We learn which events predict other events (often some sort of causal relation) so that we can prepare for it. An example of two possible causal structures for the presence of a virus and two symptoms is shown in Figure 6.2 to give you an idea of what causal associations are. Many of the same principles that are observed in conditioning are also observed in causal learning (e.g., Mitchell

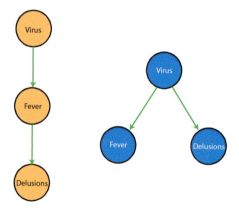

FIGURE 6.2 *Example of Two Different Causal Structures for a Virus and Two Symptoms. On the Left, the Virus Causes Fever, which then Causes Delusions. However, on the Right, the Virus Directly Causes Both Fever and Delusions*

et al., 2006). Read the Study In Depth box to get a better idea of the relationship between classical conditioning and studies of causal learning.

At this point it is unclear the extent to which the memory principles that underlie conditioning also drive causal learning. There are several theories that try to explain this type of memory (Perales & Shanks, 2007). Some of these are based on theories of conditioning, such as associative models (Shanks & Dickenson, 1987) that involve the Rescorla-Wagner (1972) model of classical conditioning. Others are based on normative information about event probabilities, such as the Power PC theory (Cheng, 1997). Still others assume a more rule-based approach using the idea that people are drawing inferences (Mitchell et al., 2005). There are also theories that take a Bayesian approach to causality understanding (Gerstenberg & Tenenbaum, 2017). It should be noted that causal learning is more effective when people have an opportunity to interact with a system, although it can occur through passive observation (Enkvist et al., 2006).

When doing causal learning, people often think about the underlying mechanisms of the situation rather than thinking more probabilistically and abstractly (which would give a better understanding) (Park & Sloman, 2013). This can be difficult because it is often the case that many things are varying at a time (Derringer & Rottman, 2018). For example, the proneness of people to a disease may be due to several factors, such as the amount of sleep they get, the cleanliness of the environment, their genetic makeup, and so on.

A study by Taylor and Ahn (2012) is an example of the correspondence between causal learning and traditional conditioning. In this study, for some conditions, Taylor and Ahn had 80 people participate in an internet study. The purported task was for people to understand how certain medical conditions might be related to one another.

People learned that sick patients who have an imaginary condition called Burlosis is associated with having another imaginary condition called Caprix. This was done by presenting descriptions of 20 "patients" who often showed evidence of these two conditions occurring together. This information was presented in a way to lead participants to conclude that Burlosis caused Caprix. Half of the people were only told about the co-occurrence of Burlosis and Caprix, whereas the other half were given additional information about the presence of some (again, imaginary) thing called Ablique. After reviewing the 20 cases, all participants were then told that scientists had discovered that Ablique was a new virus. The task at this point was to assess the cases again, this time with all participants being given information about the presence of the Ablique virus, to assess whether it caused Caprix in addition to Burlosis.

What was found was that people who did not receive information about the occurrence of Ablique from the beginning were much less likely to include this virus as a causal agent in the occurrence of Caprix compared to those who had information about the presence of Ablique from the beginning. The explanation was that, for those people who initially did not receive information about the presence of Ablique, there was a "causal imprinting" of the Burlosis–Caprix connection. The subsequent introduction of information about Ablique was disregarded in favor of the already held causal explanation.

This finding parallels work in classical conditioning on the phenomenon of **blocking** in which the prior learning of an association blocks the acquisition of any new associations for subsequent information that might occur at the same time (Kamin, 1969). More generally, this work suggests that once people have an idea for "why" something happens, it is difficult for them to change their minds and accept new ideas about other possible causes. There is a bias to fall back on prior causal understandings (see also the section on retraction in Chapter 8). This is less of a problem for people who have more complete information at the outset. This may be why, to some degree, people have difficulty with complicated and nuanced explanations, such as those developed more recently by science. They tend to continue to rely on their prior, simpler explanations.

Stop and Review

A fundamental form of nondeclarative memory is conditioning. This involves learning a predictive association between two stimuli, one that is already important and one that is learned as a predictor of the first. These associations take some time to be learned and can be forgotten through extinction. Phenomena like spontaneous recovery and savings illustrate that after extinction/forgetting has occurred, there is still some association deep in memory. An example of an effect of conditioning of this type in human memory is the mere exposure effect. More recent work in this area has investigated how people learn cause and effect relationships in the world.

PROCEDURAL AND MOTOR MEMORY

Knowledge of how to do things, such as play the piano, throw a ball, or walk, is an important part of nondeclarative memory. This is memory for skills, which is a form of nondeclarative memory. For example, just because people are skilled athletes does not *necessarily* mean that they will make a good coach. This is because much of the knowledge is unconscious and procedural. We now look at the acquisition of skills and the influence of expertise on procedural and motor memory.

Motor Memory

Motor memories, like other memories, once acquired need to go through a process of consolidation to make them more permanent and enduring. If this consolidation is disrupted, such as by learning new, similar motor memories soon after the original ones were learned, then consolidation is disrupted, and the new memories can be forgotten (Brashers-Krug et al., 1996). Motor memory consolidation is more likely to occur when people randomize their practice strategies and do not spend too much time practicing one aspect of a skill (Kim et al., 2016). Also, if declarative knowledge is acquired prior to learning a motor skill, this may delay the consolidation of the motor memory, making it more likely to be forgotten (Breton & Robertson, 2014). Motor memories, like other memories, benefit from a period of sleep in which consolidation can operate (Kempler & Richmond, 2012), and sleep deprivation can disrupt performance and memory gains (Stepan et al., 2019). The acquisition of new motor skills results in a near-term increase in the size of neural assemblies involved in the task, but after time, there is a renormalization to the prior size (Wenger et al., 2017).

Negative Transfer

Once a procedural or motor memory is created, it can impede the learning of new skills. With **negative transfer** prior procedural knowledge impedes the ability to learn new things (Anderson, 2000). For example, if people have learned to drive a manual transmission car and then drive one with an automatic transmission, there may be some negative transfer when they try to step on the clutch (which is not there). The amount of negative transfer experienced is a function of the degree of overlap between the old and new skills (Woltz et al., 2000).

Memory traces for older information are well established when new information is encountered. Because these older traces are stronger, they are activated when you try to learn something new. This activation blocks the acquisition of the new skill. Understanding negative transfer is important because when people try to learn a new way of doing a task, the recurrence of prior, and now inappropriate, procedural and motor memories can cause accidents, such as when a new task is learned in the workplace (Besnard & Cacitti, 2005).

Stages of Skill Acquisition

Many tasks improve with practice. These are **skills**. Some skills are activities where expertise is widely recognized, such as being able to play a sport, play a musical instrument, or craft a best-selling novel. Most skills, however, are very mundane, and you may not consider them "skills." These include things like walking, reading, riding a bicycle, driving a car, and having a conversation.

Although many skills are stored in nondeclarative memory, the process of skill development is similar to all of them. There are three **stages of skill acquisition**: the cognitive stage, the associative stage, and the autonomous stage (Fitts & Posner, 1967). These are shown in Figure 6.3. These stages reflect a transition from an arduous and clumsy execution of an activity to an easier and more fluid execution (Frank & Macnamara, 2017). Note that this does not mean we must necessarily be in one particular stage. It is possible for experts in a skill to spend most of their time at the autonomous stage but still have nondeclarative memory for the associative and cognitive stages. As skills develop, we make choices about which strategy to use (Bajic & Rickard, 2009).

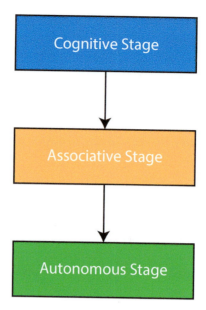

FIGURE 6.3 *The Three Stages of Skill Acquisition*

At the beginning of a skill is the **cognitive stage**. This is when we consciously and deliberately go about performing the actions of the task. For example, when learning to play chess, people exert a great deal of effort trying to consciously assess what is going on to keep the game progressing and either not get wiped out or, better yet, defeat the opponent. This often takes the form of comparing the current state with the desired state and taking whatever action brings one closer to the desired state.

After some time in the cognitive stage, we move on to the **associative stage**. At this stage we can more quickly retrieve the knowledge needed to do the task. That is, memories become directly associated with different aspects of the skill. The need to mentally think things through is less necessary. Information is quickly and easily retrieved, although some deliberate and conscious effort is still needed. For example, a chess player would directly retrieve information about what a set of moves would entail, and different alignments on the board begin to be viewed as offensive or defensive.

After more practice, we move to the final, **autonomous stage**. In this stage the execution of a skill has become more proceduralized and moves from involving consciousness to being largely unconscious. Memories and knowledge have moved from being dominated by declarative knowledge to being dominated by nondeclarative knowledge. This is the case when people learn a motor skill, such as playing a musical instrument. When people become experts, the execution of various components is done with little conscious involvement other than the desire to execute a particular series of moves. There is less overt, conscious involvement in the execution of the smaller steps of the skill.

Triarchic Theory of Skill Learning

Another theory is Chein and Schneider's (2012) **Triarchic theory of skill learning**. This view is grounded in neurophysiological evidence. As illustrated in Figure 6.4, the three types of skill processing in this model are (a) the metacognitive system, (b) the cognitive control network, and (c) the representation system. All systems are assumed to be engaged during skill execution, although the level of dominance of each system varies with skill level.

The **metacognitive system** is most engaged when we first learn a skill. This involves conscious deliberative thought and action and is devoted to processing information in more novel contexts, as is the case early on in skill acquisition. This system involves the anterior prefrontal cortex (BA 10) along with other brain areas, to reconfigure the pathways and processing in the brain to adapt to the new skill. This system can do what it needs to do quickly, although the results are not immediately long-lasting.

The **cognitive control network** becomes more engaged as people become more skilled. This system is devoted to managing the process of the skill and making its execution more automatic. This network is composed of several brain areas working together, particularly the dorsolateral prefrontal cortex (BAs 9 & 46), the anterior cingulate cortex (BAs 24, 32, & 33), the inferior frontal junction, and the posterior parietal cortex (BA 7). This network takes longer to develop than the metacognitive system, however it is more enduring.

Skill performance is dominated more by the **representation system** with further practice. As people practice a skill, the cell assemblies in whatever part of the brain that are relevant become increasingly wired together. The memory traces are the direct mental instructions for how to do the skill. Mediation from the other systems is less and less involved. Thus, the skill becomes more automatic. Because the parts

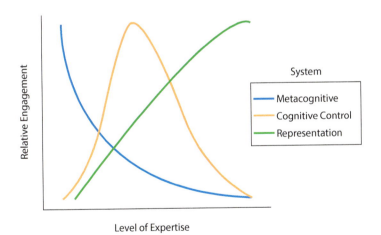

FIGURE 6.4 *The Relative Influence of the Three Neurological Systems in the Triarchic Theory of Skill Learning*

Source: adapted from Chein, J. M., & Schneider, W. (2012). The brain's learning and control architecture. *Current Directions in Psychological Science, 21*(2), 78–84

of the brain involved can vary depending on the nature of the skill, the whole brain needs to be considered as the site of this system. Also, in contrast to the cognitive control network, which is more domain independent, the representation system is domain dependent. That is, these skills are represented very specifically, and transfer to other domains is unlikely. For example, the skill that you developed in your automobile driving does not transfer over to your tennis swing. This network takes a very long time to develop, but its processes are extremely enduring.

Choking Under Pressure

Typically, the automation of skills in memory is helpful. However, there are cases where it can have the opposite effect. This occurs when people try to consciously think about what they are doing when the skill is highly automatized. An example of this is when players succumb to the pressure of the moment and do worse than they would otherwise. The athletes' conscious thoughts about what they are doing intrude on and conflict with the automatic processes from procedural memory (Beilock & Carr, 2001). This is known as **choking under pressure** because skilled experts often do not spend much effort consciously thinking about the mechanics of their skill. However, when in a high-pressure situation, they may start to do this, and these conscious thoughts compete with the nondeclarative ones. This competition reduces performance. At a low level of skill (novices), we perform better if we focus on accuracy, whereas at a high level of skill (experts), we do better if we focus on speed (Beilock et al., 2004). These performance differences between experts and novices are shown in Figure 6.5.

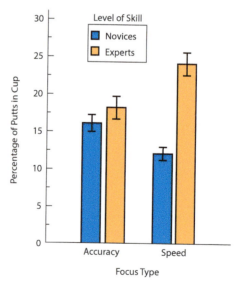

FIGURE 6.5 *Mean Percentage of Putts Made for Novices and Experts as a Function of Whether They Were Instructed to Focus on Accuracy or Speed*

Source: adapted from Beilock, S. L., Bertenthal, B. I., McCoy, A. M., & Carr, T. H. (2004). Haste does not always make waste: Expertise, direction of attention, and speed versus accuracy in performing sensorimotor skills. *Psychonomic Bulletin & Review, 11*, 373–379

It is important to note that not all forms of choking under pressure are the same (DeCaro et al., 2011). In the form discussed here, where the task primarily involves nondeclarative memory, such as putting a golf ball, people are more likely to experience choking under pressure when they have **monitoring pressure** that focuses on how they are doing the skill (e.g., knowing that you are being video-taped). Here there is a conflict between more conscious, deliberate declarative and more unconscious, automatic thoughts.

In comparison, there can be pressure for more declarative memory tasks. An example of this might be when people take a mathematics exam. Under this circumstance, people are more likely to choke under pressure when they have **outcome pressure** that focuses on the outcome of their performance (e.g., knowing that your GPA depends on how well you do on the exam). Here, people experience anxiety, and this anxiety fills working memory with irrelevant information (see Chapter 5). This reduces functional working memory span and compromises the ability to think effectively. As a result, people perform worse than their actual knowledge level.

Practice and the Nature of Expertise

Expertise at a task takes time to emerge. But is practice sufficient to become an expert? Does talent or some other predisposition also play a role? There is some ambiguity about this. There are some researchers who assert that practice is the primary contributor to expertise (Ericsson et al., 1993). That said, there may be differences in how people with higher and lower levels of expertise go about their practice. People who reach higher levels of expertise tend to spend more practice time on skills that they are weak at, whereas people who reach lower levels of expertise tend to spend more practice time on skills that they are already good at (Coughlan et al., 2014).

While extensive practice is necessary, there are other factors, such as a basic level of intelligence or genetic predispositions that can contribute to the achievement of high levels of expertise (Campitelli & Gobet, 2011; MacNamara et al., 2014). Thus, there is a mixture of nature and nurture when it comes to whether people achieve a high level of expertise in a skill. One view is the Multifactor Gene–Environment Interaction Model (MGIM) (Ullén et al., 2016). This view assumes that there are several factors influencing the achievement of expertise, including:

- Deliberate Practice
- Physical Traits (e.g., height for basketball players)
- Intelligence and Cognitive Abilities
- Personality (e.g., grit)
- Genetic Biases.

The combination of these factors is outlined in Figure 6.6. As can be seen, several factors work together to bring about the degree to which people are considered experts in a field, such as sports, music, dance, etc.

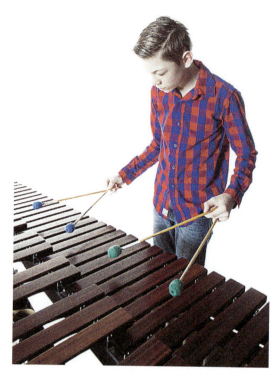

PHOTO 6.2 *High levels of skill with a task depend on our going through a process of moving our motor memories from a slow deliberate process, to a quicker, more automatic process*

Source: Anton Havelaar/Shutterstock.com

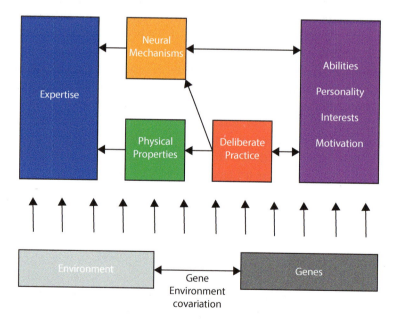

FIGURE 6.6 *The Multifactor Gene-Environment Model (MGIM)*

Source: adapted from Ullén, F., Hambrick, D. Z., & Mosing, M. A. (2016). Rethinking expertise: A multifactorial gene–environment interaction model of expert performance. *Psychological Bulletin, 142*(4), 427–446

Improve Your Memory

One thing that should be obvious at this point is that the more you practice something, the better your memory for it will be. This is just as true for nondeclarative memories, such as motor skills like playing a sport, as it is for declarative memories, such as remembering what you learned in class. However, a point that is often overlooked is that it takes time for the memories to seep in and become permanent. That is, all kinds of memories need some time to consolidate. So, when you are trying to learn something new, such as a skill, occasionally take a break from practice and allow the memories to become more permanent. These breaks can take the form of simply stepping away from the task for a few minutes or hours, taking a nap, or getting some sleep and practicing some more the next day. So, while practice does make perfect, it is better that you do not do it all at once. Take breaks and give your memories a chance to become permanent.

Stop and Review

Procedural memory is nondeclarative memory for how to do things. Some of this involves motor memory for how to execute physical tasks. The acquisition of such memories is harder if there exists a prior skill that is similar, thereby producing negative transfer. Skills start out as conscious, declarative memories, but with practice, they become more automatic procedural memories. People start at the cognitive stage, move to the associative stage, and finally reach the autonomous stage. The Triarchic theory is rooted in neuroscience and suggests that the three aspects of skills are the metacognitive system, cognitive control network, and the representation system. They are all always involved, but there are variations with which these systems dominate as skill level increases. At high levels of skill, conscious awareness can actually disrupt memory, leading one to choke under pressure. High levels of expertise are a result of extensive, appropriate practice, in conjunction with some innate traits.

IMPLICIT MEMORY

The last form of nondeclarative memory covered here is implicit memory. **Implicit memory** does not require consciousness and can operate without awareness that memory is being used. For example, some accounts of *déjà vu* attribute the odd feeling of familiarity one has with a new situation to unconscious, implicit memories of different, but similar experiences (Brown, 2003; Cleary, 2008). Also, the idea of *intuition* appears to rely on implicit memory because it is an unconscious feeling about something. For example, if people are given word triads, such as "dream," "ball," and "book" or "salt," "deep," and "foam," they intuitively know that the first three do not go together, but the second three do (they are related to a fourth concept: sea), even if they consciously do not know why (Topolinski & Strack, 2009b). As a general note, it is important to keep in mind that although some learning and memory may be implicit and unconscious, with extensive practice this knowledge may eventually bubble up to consciousness and become more explicit (Goujon et al., 2014).

In some sense, any form of nondeclarative memory can manifest as a type of implicit memory. For example, procedural memories can be implicit, such as knowledge of how to walk. The concept of *savings*, as originally described by Ebbinghaus, is a form of implicit memory in which we are unaware of how previous, unconscious memories influence later learning (Nelson, 1978). This section considers how knowledge gets into memory without awareness, how implicit memory is assessed using **indirect memory tasks**, the effects of data-driven and conceptually driven processes on implicit memory, and the unconscious learning of sequential orders.

Incidental Learning

We have already discussed implicit memory in Chapter 3. People learn things by either explicitly—intentionally trying to learn them—or implicitly—incidentally learning them. Incidental learning is a form of implicit memory because we are not consciously aware of knowledge being stored in memory. Although it is difficult to observe incidental learning as it happens (because it's incidental), neurological measures can provide some insight. EEG recordings show that information that is remembered later involves increased theta band and decreased alpha band synchronization (Klimesch et al., 1996). Moreover, people who remember more show more alpha band change in the lower half of the band, whereas people who remember less show more desynchronization in the upper alpha band.

Much of the tacitly acquired information from incidental learning makes up the contents of implicit memory. That is, the influences that are exerted on our thoughts and behaviors by implicit memory rely on knowledge that was unconsciously acquired. For example, people moving to a new part of the country may alter their speech patterns to conform to the local accent. This occurs without being explicitly aware that they are changing how they speak. You may have noticed this in your own experience. If you have gone away to college, you may find that how you speak when you are at school differs from how you speak at home.

Indirect Tests of Memory

It is difficult to clearly understand what implicit memory is and does because it is largely unconscious. To see its effects, people must show an influence of prior experience (memory) without an awareness of doing so. Thus, we need an indirect way to test memory. There are several indirect tests, some of which are examined here. Most of these focus on verbal memory. However, some nonverbal tasks are described as well.

An extensively used form of indirect memory testing is **priming**. Priming occurs when people are faster and/or more accurate at retrieving *target* information that has been facilitated by an earlier *prime* trial (Tulving & Schacter, 1990). There are different types of priming, but here we focus on the most basic: repetition priming. **Repetition priming** is when people better respond to an item that was encountered recently. This occurs even if we are unaware that we are using a memory. For example, if you saw the word "assassin" earlier, you will recognize it faster and more accurately when you see it again later. Repetition priming is larger when the information is presented in the same way it was encountered earlier. For example, people have a better memory for rotating objects if the objects are rotating in the same direction as the first time they saw them (Liu & Cooper, 2003). This suggests that even seemingly irrelevant details about things in the world can influence memory later.

The amount of benefit we get from repetition priming depends on how the information was learned in the first place. Let's look at memory for information read in a book (Raney, 2003). If repetition priming operates, we will show a benefit by reading the text faster the second time. However, the nature of this priming can vary. Suppose a reader is relying primarily on memory of the text itself (such as surface form or textbase memory). This can occur when people do not comprehend what they are reading and so do not build adequate mental models of the described events. Under these conditions, repetition priming is more likely to be affected by perceptual characteristics, such as handwriting, the font style, or the word order. In contrast, if readers understood what is being read and can build adequate mental models, repetition priming extends to other texts that refer to the same state of affairs. Moreover, this repetition priming is less influenced by perceptual properties.

Priming involves a decrease in neural activity in some brain areas (Schacter & Badgaiyan, 2001). Repetition priming is associated with decreased activity in the visual cortex, whereas semantic priming is associated with decreased activity in the frontal lobes. This decreased neural activity reflects the lower amount of work needing to be done because memory engrams are already at a heightened level of availability based on the recent experience.

Indirect memory tests, such as repetition priming, influence multiple levels of representation (see Chapter 7). For example, people respond faster to words that were seen in a word list than those seen in a paragraph. However, people read a passage of text faster if that same text has been read earlier, but not if they see the same words out of context, such as in a word list (Levy & Kirsner, 1989). This suggests that for repetition priming to occur, the appropriate level of representation needs to be retrieved. Retrieving the wrong kind of memory is less helpful.

Similarly, in a study by Oliphant (1983), the first occurrences of repeated target words were presented either in the context of the study (as is normally done), or as part of the instructions. Repetition priming was observed when a word was in the study itself (the standard condition) but not when it was in the instructions. This suggests that memory is compartmentalized. It may be influenced by how we parse up the world, even at an unconscious level. This suggests that some implicit memory processes, like priming, may not cross event boundaries. That said, this effect may be limited to common, high-frequency

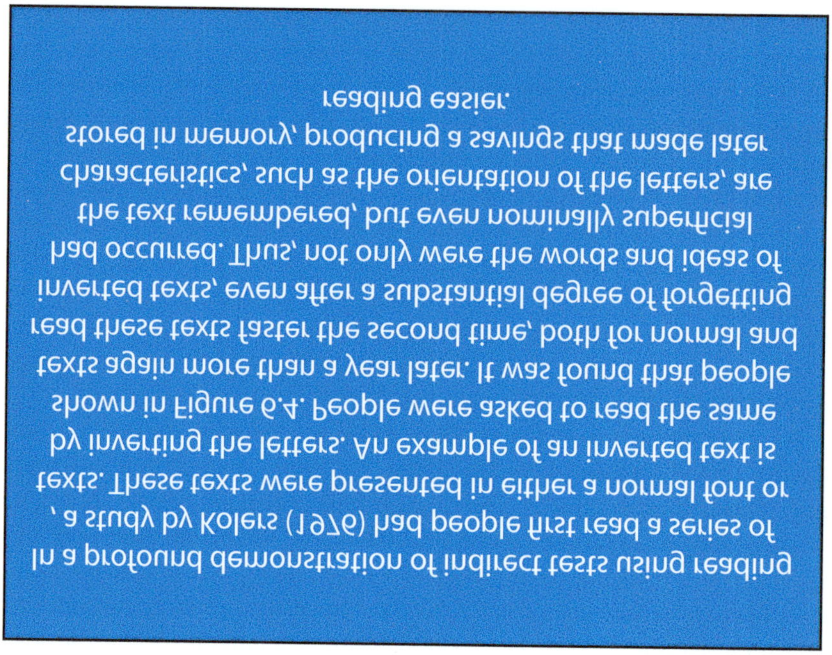

In a profound demonstration of indirect tests using reading, a study by Kolers (1976) had people first read a series of texts. These texts were presented in either a normal font or by inverting the letters. An example of an inverted text is shown in Figure 6.9. People were asked to read the same texts again more than a year later. It was found that people read these texts faster the second time, both for normal and inverted texts, even after a substantial degree of forgetting had occurred. Thus, not only were the words and ideas of the text remembered, but even nominally superficial characteristics, such as the orientation of the letters, are stored in memory, producing a savings that made later reading easier.

FIGURE 6.7 *Inverted Text*

Source: adapted from Kolers, P. A. (1976). Reading a year later. *Journal of Experimental Psychology: Human Learning and Memory, 2,* 554–565

elements of an experience, and may not apply to unusual, low-frequency elements (Coane & Balota, 2010).

In a profound demonstration of indirect tests, Kolers (1976) had people first read a series of texts presented either normally or by inverting the letters. An example of an inverted text is shown in Figure 6.7. People were asked to read the same texts again more than a year later. Kolers found that people read these texts faster the second time, both for normal and inverted texts, even after a substantial degree of forgetting had occurred. Thus, not only were the words and ideas of the text remembered, but even nominally superficial characteristics, such as the orientation of the letters, were stored in memory, producing a savings that made later reading easier.

Many indirect memory tasks involve having people reconstruct partial or degraded information in some way. The idea is that if this information is in memory, even at an unconscious level, it should be easier to do this reconstruction. One example is a **word-stem completion** task (Graf et al., 1982). In this task people are given the initial few letters of a word (the "stem"), with the task of completing it with the first word that comes to mind. We are more likely to complete these stems with words seen recently, even though we are unaware that we are using prior knowledge. This isolation of implicit memory can be shown by using methods such as the process-dissociation procedure (see Chapter 3) (Toth et al., 1994).

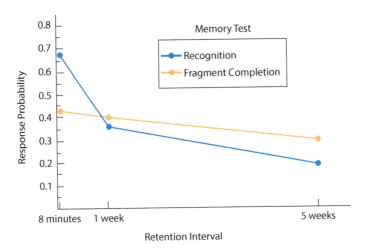

FIGURE 6.8 *The Enduring Influence of Implicit Memory (Word Fragment Completion) Relative to Explicit Memory (Recognition)*

Source: Tulving, E., Schacter, D. L., & Stark, H. A. (1982). Priming effects in word-fragment completion are independent of recognition memory. *Journal of Experimental Psychology: Learning, Memory and Cognition, 8,* 336–342

Another indirect memory task is **word fragment completion**. For this task people are given words with missing letters, such as A _ _ A _ _ IN, and are to complete them. Again, we do better if we saw the words recently (Tulving et al., 1982). Moreover, as shown in Figure 6.8, this ability remains stable even after a long delay, whereas more conscious and explicit recognition memory continues to decline over time. This illustrates the enduring influence of implicit memory processes on behavior. Also, note that the pattern of forgetting for the recognition data follows a power function, much like Ebbinghaus's (1885), but the word fragment completion data follows a linear function, further illustrating that these are different types of memory.

Another indirect memory test is anagram solution (Srivinas & Roediger, 1990) in which people are given anagrams, such as "tderhun" for the word "thunder." People are better at solving the anagrams if they were exposed to a word recently than if they were not. Again, people are not consciously using memory to help them solve the anagrams.

Finally, another verbal indirect memory task is **lexical decision** (Duchek & Neely, 1989). For this, people are given a string of letters with the task of indicating whether each is a word or not (hence the term *lexical decision*). What is of interest is how fast people respond to words depending on what occurred earlier. People respond faster when they were exposed to the word recently or to words that are related to ideas they were thinking about recently. Similar effects are observed with a **naming** task in which people simply name aloud, as quickly as possible, visually presented words (Hashtroudi et al., 1988). A more everyday influence of this is that you are more likely to say a word if you have heard it recently.

TRY IT OUT

For this Try it Out section, we focus on word fragment completion (see Neath, 1998). Ideally you should have at least 24 participants. This study is broken down into two parts. For the first part have half of the people go through a list of 20 words printed on index cards, whereas the rest do something unrelated. Below is a list of words used by Tulving et al. (1982). Pick 20 of these. Be sure to include all the letters in a word and not the underlining shown here. What your people should do is rate each word for pleasantness. That is, how pleasant the words are to them. After going through the entire list, have them spend 10 minutes doing a distractor task. This can be any task that does not refer to the words that they just rated (such as solving math problems, sorting decks of cards, circling the letter "h" in a page from an article, etc.).

The second half of the study involves both groups of people. Present them with a list of 60-word fragments. These are the words listed below. You should remove the letters that are underlined and replace them with blank spaces. The task is to complete those words. It is important that you *do not* tell the one group that these words are related to the ones that they rated earlier. These words should be presented in a random order, with the only constraint being that the 20 words used in the first half of the study are not in any of the first ten fragments. You should find that the people who originally rated the words for pleasantness should be more likely to complete those 20 fragments than the people who did not originally see those words.

AGNOSTIC	ANTENNA	ANTIQUE	ASSASSIN	BASILICA	BAYONET
BOURBON	BROCCOLI	CASHMERE	CHASSIS	CHIMNEY	CHIPMUNK
CONIFER	CUTLERY	DELIRIUM	DINOSAUR	ELECTRON	ELLIPSE
EPITAPH	FASCISM	GAZELLE	GRANARY	HAYLOFT	HORIZON
HYDRANT	INFERNO	ISTHMUS	JAMBOREE	KEROSENE	LACROSSE
LECTERN	LEPROSY	LETTUCE	LINEAGE	MARTINI	MASCARA
MYSTERY	NIRVANA	NOCTURNE	OBELISK	OCTOPUS	PARANOIA
PHOENIX	POLLIWOG	QUARTET	RAINBOW	RHOMBUS	ROTUNDA
SAPPHIRE	SEQUOIA	SHERIFF	SURGEON	THEOREM	TWILIGHT
UNIVERSE	VENDETTA	VERMOUTH	WARRANTY	YOGURT	ZEPPELIN

Indirect memory influences are also seen when perceptual clarity is compromised. For example, imagine that a word is presented for only a fraction of a second, such as for 35 ms. Under these conditions, it is difficult to consciously identify the word. However, if people previously saw it, then **perceptual identification** is enhanced (Jacoby & Dallas, 1981). That is, it is easier to identify what was seen if it was seen recently. This process can also be seen in pop music. Sometimes song lyrics are unclear, and you have to guess at them. However, if you *read* the lyrics first, you can easily follow them the next time you hear the song. Relatedly, it has been found that people find it easier to understand voices if they are from someone that they know as compared to a stranger (Holmes et al., 2018).

Although many of the indirect memory tasks use verbal materials, implicit memory is important for all types of information. An example of a nonverbal task is priming for pictures of possible and impossible objects (see Figure 6.9). First, people view a set of objects as part of some task, such as judging whether an object faces left or right. Then, they are asked to make *possible–impossible* decisions. Some of the objects in the second test are the same as those in the first test. The degree to which responses are faster and more accurate for old objects relative to new ones is an indicator of priming. Priming occurs only for possible objects and not

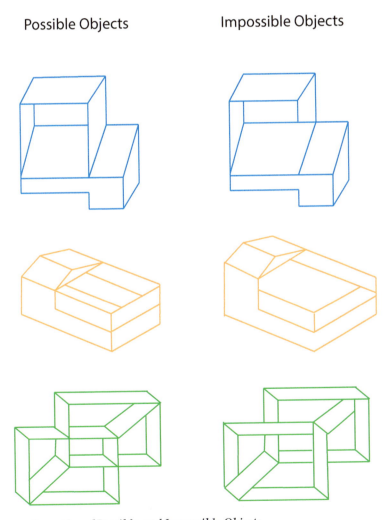

FIGURE 6.9 *Examples of Possible and Impossible Objects*

Source: Ratcliff, R., & McKoon, G. (1995). Bias in the priming of object decisions. *Journal of Experimental Psychology: Learning, Memory, and Cognition, 21*(3), 754

for impossible objects (Schacter et al., 1990). This suggests that memory takes into account an understanding of the object as a whole and not just the parts that make up an image.

The influence of implicit memory also occurs with odors. Holland et al. (2005) had students at Radboud University take a lexical decision task in a room either with a citrus-scented cleaner in a cupboard (out of sight) or with no cleaner (control). The odor prime led people to respond faster to cleaning related words (e.g., "poetsen," the Dutch word for "cleaning") on a lexical decision task. Thus, implicit memory has a multimodal and pervasive influence on how we think.

Implicit memory works on us in many ways, even for information for which we are unaware. For example, Kunst-Wilson and Zajonc (1980) subconsciously presented randomly generated geometric shapes for only 1 ms. Later, people were given a forced-choice recognition test to select which shapes were seen earlier. For a forced-choice recognition test people must pick one item from a set of two or more, much like a multiple-choice test. In this case, performance was above chance. That is, people selected the prior shapes more often than if they were just guessing. This is interesting because there is no conscious awareness of seeing the shapes before.

Data-Driven and Conceptually Driven Processes

Although the distinction between explicit and implicit memory is complex, some attempts have been made to describe the differences between them. One idea is that implicit memory tends to be driven more by the perceptual characteristics. This is referred to as *data-driven processing* because the mental activity is driven more by information in the environment (the data) than the contents of thought. In contrast, explicit memory is driven more by the mental characteristics. This is referred to as *conceptually driven processing* because the mental activity is driven more by prior knowledge, expectations, and goals. As an illustration, seeing a cloud in the sky as a cloud is an example of data-driven processing, but seeing shapes (such as a bunny) in the clouds is an example of conceptually driven processing.

Generally, implicit memory is more affected by how information was originally presented—for example, written or oral. Thus, implicit memory is more influenced by data-driven processing. In contrast, explicit memory is more affected by the amount of processing that was done during encoding, such as whether it was generated or not. Thus, explicit memory is more influenced by conceptually driven processing (Blaxton, 1989).

Sequence Learning

Another type of knowledge that is encoded into nondeclarative, implicit memory is the order of events. Nondeclarative memory is good at picking up on regularities in our experiences, a process called *statistical learning* (Santolin & Saffran, 2017). Regular repeating patterns may not reach conscious awareness, but our implicit memory is attuned to these. In a study by Nissen and Bullemer (1987; see also Abrahamse et al., 2010; Fu et al., 2008), students saw a row of four lights, with a button below each

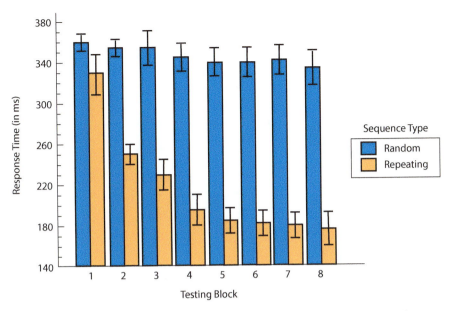

FIGURE 6.10 *Improvement on a Serial Order Task with Random and Repeating Sequences*

Source: adapted from Nissen, M. J., & Bullemer, P. (1987). Attentional requirements of learning: Evidence from performance measures. *Cognitive Psychology, 19*, 1–32

one. The task was to press the button below a light *after* it lit up. There were two groups in this study. In the random order, control group, the lights came on in a random order throughout the study. However, in the experimental group, the lights came on in a consistent ten-light sequence. The speed with which people pushed the buttons increased (i.e., response time decreased), with even a little exposure in the experimental group (see Figure 6.10). It is even possible to see eye movements anticipating the next item in a series (Tremblay & Saint-Aubin, 2009).

When people are asked to explicitly report the sequence, they cannot (but see Wilkinson & Shanks, 2004). People used memories for the sequence before they were consciously aware of doing so. Moreover, explicitly knowing that there will be a repeating sequence does not seem to help much, if at all (Sanchez & Reber, 2013). Similar results occur in visual search tasks (looking for an object in a display) when a response sequence is repeated (Jiménez & Vázquez, 2008). While this can occur in various modalities, such as touch and vision, it does not transfer across modalities, such as from visual to auditory, suggesting that there is a perceptual component—it is not simply action-based (Abrahamse et al., 2008).

Another, more complex, type of sequence learning involves the implicit learning of **artificial grammars** (Pothos, 2007). In some of these studies, people are given sequences of letters. These are created using an algorithm such as the one shown in Figure 6.11. For example, in this case, the sequences GKGKF, LZZLF, and GKKGF are valid or "grammatical" sequences, whereas ZLFKL, KKGGF, and FZZZL are not. During an initial learning phase, people are shown a series of letter strings that were generated using the algorithm and asked to copy them. Even in the absence

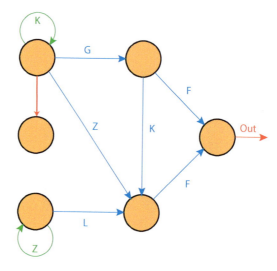

FIGURE 6.11 *Algorithm Used to Generate Artificial Grammar*

Source: adapted from Reber, A. S. (1967). Implicit learning of artificial grammars. *Journal of Verbal Learning and Verbal Behavior, 6*, 855–863

of explicit memorization, people learn not just the sequences that were seen, but the "grammar" or production algorithm used to generate them. Implicit memory shows itself in the ability to also accept (at above chance rates) valid sequences that were never seen before and to accept new sequences that used different letter sets but that followed the same rules (Reber, 1967; 1969; Vokey & Highham, 2005) and which even may affect visual dwell times (Silva et al., 2017).

That said, people may also develop expectations based on the structure of the individual items (Pothos, 2005). People may be learning bigram probabilities (i.e., the probability that a given letter will follow another) rather than an entire grammar (Poletiek & Wolters, 2009). It is likely that both "grammatical" rules and bigram memories are operating (Opitz & Hofmann, 2015). Not surprisingly, the extraction of an artificial grammar is aided by neurological processes operating during sleep (Neuwenhuis et al., 2013).

Artificial grammar learning is a general memory process that not only applies to sequences of letters, but also to varied types of information, such as sequences of dance movements (Opacic et al., 2009) or musical tones (Tillmann & Poulin-Charronnat, 2010). It should be noted that although this is a largely unconscious, implicit process, some conscious influences might also play a role if we become aware of the repetition (Dulany et al., 1984). That is, memory is better if people have conscious awareness of the overarching structure of the artificial grammar (Sallas et al., 2007).

Memory under Anesthesia

Most of what has been considered in this chapter are circumstances that involve memory for information presented when people are conscious. One way to study unconscious learning is to look at things encountered when people are under anesthesia. One purpose of anesthesia is to make sure people do not remember what happened during surgery (such as feeling the incision being made). However, the brain is not completely dormant under anesthesia. The question is whether it is active enough to learn new things.

In some cases, people are read to while they are anesthetized for surgery. It might be a list of words or sentences, or a story. After surgery, they are tested to see if they show memory for that material. Based on a review by Andrade (1995), there is some evidence of learning under anesthesia. This includes a greater likelihood of using words heard during anesthesia on a later implicit memory test. Some assessments have looked at more complex forms of learning, such as providing answers to general knowledge questions, false fame effects (Chapter 13), classical conditioning, behavioral suggestion (such as touching one's ear or chin), and therapeutic suggestions. In one study, Schwender et al. (1993) had 15 patients listen to *Robinson Crusoe* while they were anesthetized and undergoing surgery. After surgery, when asked to free associate to the word *Friday*, ten of these patients responded with "Robinson Crusoe," and five did not. In contrast, none of another group of 15 patients who did not hear the novel gave this response.

What people learn under anesthesia is important because this may influence recovery. It has been suggested that derogatory comments made about patients, such as commenting on an obese patient's weight, can lead them to recover more slowly. This is known as "fat lady syndrome." Some surgeons make a point of speaking about

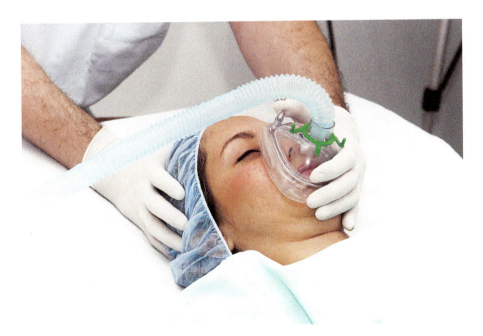

PHOTO 6.3 *One of the important reasons for anesthesia during surgery is so that we don't remember what happened. However, there is some evidence that our brains do process some information and we do remember some things, although not much*

Source: herjua/Shutterstock.com

how well things are going during the surgery, even if it is not completely true, to facilitate recovery. This is consistent with research showing that learning of things such as tone–odor pairs or new vocabulary learning can occur during sleep. This largely happens only during certain phases of slow wave sleep and has no impact on conscious, explicit memory (Ruch & Henke, 2020).

The effects of learning under anesthesia are at an unconscious, implicit level. However, it should also be noted that it has been difficult to replicate these findings. In almost every case where studies have found evidence of memory, there are similar ones that have not. There are many reasons for this. In some cases, it may be that the data just happened to fall in such a way that an effect was observed and reported. Researchers are less likely to report *not* finding an effect. Thus, researchers may have tested memory under anesthesia, not found any evidence for it, and therefore did not publish their findings. Alternatively, it could be that memory and amnesia effects are very weak and are difficult to measure in the first place. Work from neuroimaging studies has suggested that while basic auditory and other sensory processing continues while under anesthesia, more complex, interpretive processes are not functioning (MacDonald et al., 2015), including such fundamental aspects of thinking, such as the default mode network (DMN) (see Chapter 2) This calls into question any findings based on the meaningfulness of the material. Finally, it is difficult to control factors that could influence the observed results. These include the type of anesthesia used, how deeply the patients go under, the extent of the surgery, and so on. Thus, as it stands, there is the intriguing possibility that there may be some nondeclarative learning under anesthesia, but it is unclear when this happens and to what extent.

Stop and Review

Implicit memory is memory that is largely outside of conscious awareness, although we may be aware of its outcomes. Incidental learning is a form of implicit memory. To test implicit memory, indirect methods look at the influence of memory without making people aware that they are using their memories. Such tasks include priming, word stem completion, lexical decision, word naming, and perceptual identification tasks. All of these are founded on the idea that processing is biased toward recent experiences. The distinction between implicit and explicit memory can be thought of in terms of a difference between data-driven and conceptually driven processing. One form of implicit memory involves unconscious sequence learning, as well as the implicit acquisition of underlying grammatical structures. Finally, implicit memory may (or may not) be operating when people are under anesthesia.

PUTTING IT ALL TOGETHER

Not all memory is conscious. Most of it is unconscious. Because of this, it is difficult to articulate just what nondeclarative memory is doing. A primary reason for memory is to prepare you for the future. The idea of quick, efficient, and unconscious preparation for what is going to happen soon or next captures a lot of what nondeclarative memory does. You prefer things you have been exposed to before, even unconsciously. Also, the unconscious learning of sequences and artificial grammars is inherently predictive. Prediction is also seen in classically conditioned contingency relationships. Your skills, after sufficient practice, are often nondeclarative memories for how to execute large sets of motor movements at a high level of speed and accuracy. This would not be possible if you were to think about every little step you take next along the way. This includes both specialized skills, such as playing the English horn, as well as more mundane skills, like walking and chewing gum at the same time. This is done without using much, if any, conscious mental effort. Disrupting this unconscious flow can cause you to choke.

The other thing that nondeclarative memory does is allow you to pick up knowledge without explicitly trying to do so. Your brain is always tracking your experiences to try to understand the world. It does this without you having to devote conscious effort. Moreover, memory draws upon this knowledge and influences your behavior without bringing information into conscious awareness. This is the realm of implicit memory. You have all kinds of knowledge in nondeclarative memory that you are not aware of. Because these memories operate below the radar screen of awareness, several indirect methods are needed to assess how this important part of your memory is involved in your life. These include spontaneous recovery, savings, and negative transfer phenomena, as well as changes in performance on repetition priming, word-stem completion, word fragment completion, lexical decision, and perceptual identification tasks.

STUDY QUESTIONS

1. What are the primary components of classical conditioning, and how does learning occur?
2. What are some of the important phenomena of classical conditioning?
3. How is the mere exposure effect a nondeclarative memory phenomenon? How can it be viewed as a classical conditioning phenomenon?
4. In what way are studies of causal learning examples of nondeclarative memory?
5. People learn procedural tasks by learning new motor programs. How do these motor memories resemble or differ from declarative memories? How are they affected by negative transfer?
6. What are the stages that knowledge goes through to develop skilled procedural memories? How does Chein & Schneider's Triarchic theory map onto different brain networks?
7. Where does expertise at a skill come from? That is, what does a person need to have or do to become an expert at a skill?
8. What is implicit memory, and how is it measured?
9. What are some sorts of effects of implicit memory that can be observed?
10. What sort of knowledge can be learned and influence later behavior with implicit memory?
11. How is the operation of memory affected by anesthesia used in medicine?

KEY TERMS

- artificial grammars
- associative stage
- autonomous stage
- blocking
- choking under pressure
- classical conditioning
- cognitive control network
- cognitive stage
- contiguity learning
- contingency learning
- extinction
- implicit memory
- indirect memory tasks

- instrumental conditioning
- learning curve
- lexical decision
- mere exposure effect
- metacognitive system
- monitoring pressure
- naming
- negative transfer
- nondeclarative memory
- outcome pressure
- Pavlovian conditioning
- perceptual identification
- priming

- repetition priming
- representation system
- savings
- skills
- spontaneous recovery
- stages of skill acquisition
- stimulus–response association
- stimulus –stimulus association
- systematic desensitization
- Triarchic theory of skill learning
- word fragment completion
- word-stem completion

EXPLORE MORE

Here are some additional readings that you can explore to give you better insight into some of the principles of nondeclarative memory.

Andrade, J. (1995). Learning during anaesthesia: A review. *British Journal of Psychology, 86,* 479–506.

Beilock, S. (2015). *How the Body Knows Its Mind: The Surprising Power of the Physical Environment to Influence How You Think and Feel.* New York: Simon & Schuster.

Brown, A. S. (2003). A review of the déjà vu experience. *Psychological Bulletin, 129,* 394–413.

Campitelli, G., & Gobet, F. (2011). Deliberate practice: Necessary but not sufficient. *Current Directions in Psychological Science, 20*(5), 280–285.

Chein, J. M., & Schneider, W. (2012). The brain's learning and control architecture. *Current Directions in Psychological Science, 21*(2), 78–84.

Pothos, E. M. (2007). Theories of artificial grammar learning. *Psychological Bulletin, 133,* 227–244.

REFERENCES

Abrahamse, E. L., Jiménez, L., Verwey, W. B., & Clegg, B. A. (2010). Representing serial action and perception. *Psychonomic Bulletin & Review, 17*(5), 603–623.

Abrahamse, E. L., van der Lubbe, R. H. J., & Verway, W. B. (2008). Asymmetrical learning between a tactile and visual serial RT task. *Quarterly Journal of Experimental Psychology, 61,* 210–217.

Anderson, J. R. (2000). *Learning and Memory: An integrated approach.* New York: John Wiley. & Sons.

Andrade, J. (1995). Learning during anesthesia: A review. *British Journal of Psychology, 86,* 479–506.

Bajic, D., & Rickard, T. C. (2009). The temporal dynamics of strategy execution in cognitive skill learning. *Journal of Experimental Psychology, 35,*113–121.

Beilock, S. L., Bertenthal, B. I., McCoy, A. M., & Carr, T. H. (2004). Haste does not always make waste: Expertise, direction of attention, and speed versus accuracy in performing sensorimotor skills. *Psychonomic Bulletin & Review, 11,* 373–379.

Beilock, S. L., & Carr, T. H. (2001). On the fragility of skilled performance: What governs choking under pressure? *Journal of Experimental Psychology: General, 130,* 701–725.

Besnard, D., & Cacitti, L. (2005). Interface changes causing accidents. An empirical study of negative transfer. *International Journal of Human–Computer Studies, 62*(1), 105–125.

Blaxton, T. A. (1989). Investigating dissociations among memory measures: Support for a transfer-appropriate processing framework. *Journal of Experimental Psychology: Learning, Memory, and Cognition, 15,* 657–668.

Bornstein, R. F. (1989). Exposure and affect: Overview and meta-analysis of research, 1968–1987. *Psychological Bulletin, 106,* 265–289.

Brashers-Krug, T., Shadmehr, R., & Bizzi, E. (1996). Consolidation in human motor memory. *Nature, 382*(6588), 252–255.

Breton, J., & Robertson, E. M. (2014). Flipping the switch: Mechanisms that regulate memory consolidation. *Trends in Cognitive Sciences, 18*(12), 629–634.

Brown, A. S. (2003). A review of the déjà vu experience. *Psychological Bulletin, 129,* 394–413.

Campitelli, G., & Gobet, F. (2011). Deliberate practice: Necessary but not sufficient. *Current Directions in Psychological Science, 20*(5), 280–285.

Chein, J. M., & Schneider, W. (2012). The brain's learning and control architecture. *Current Directions in Psychological Science, 21*(2), 78–84.

Cheng, P. W. (1997). From covariation to causation: A causal power theory. *Psychological Review, 104,* 367–405.

Cleary, A. M. (2008). Recognition memory, familiarity, and déjà vu experiences. *Current Directions in Psychological Science, 17,* 353–357.

Coane, J. H., & Balota, D. A. (2010). Repetition priming across distinct contexts: Effects of lexical status, word frequency, and retrieval test. *Quarterly Journal of Experimental Psychology, 63*(12), 2376–2398.

Coughlan, E. K., Williams, A. M., McRobert, A. P., & Ford, P. R. (2014). How experts practice: A novel test of deliberate practice theory. *Journal of Experimental Psychology: Learning, Memory, and Cognition, 40*(2), 449.

Cutting, J. E. (2003). Gustave Caillebotte, French Impressionism, and mere exposure. *Psychonomic Bulletin & Review, 10,* 319–343.

DeCaro, M. S., Thomas, R. D., Albert, N. B., & Beilock, S. L. (2011). Choking under pressure: Multiple routes to skill failure. *Journal of Experimental Psychology: General, 140*(3), 390–406.

Derringer, C., & Rottman, B. M. (2018). How people learn about causal influence when there are many possible causes: A model based on informative transitions. *Cognitive Psychology, 102,* 41–71.

Duchek, J. M., & Neely, J. H. (1989). A dissociative word-frequency X levels-of-processing interaction in episodic recognition and lexical decision tasks. *Memory & Cognition, 17,* 148–162.

Dulany, D. E., Carlson, R. A., & Dewey, G. I. (1984). A case of syntactical learning and judgment: How conscious and how abstract? *Journal of Experimental Psychology: General, 113,* 541–555.

Ebbinghaus, H. (1885/1964). *Memory: A Contribution to Experimental Psychology*. Translated by H. A. Ruger & C. E. Bussenius. New York: Dover.

Elliott, R., & Dolan, R. J. (1998). Neural response during preference and memory judgments for subliminally presented stimuli: A functional neuroimaging study. *The Journal of Neuroscience, 18,* 4697–4704.

Enkvist, T., Newell, B., Juslin, P., & Olsson, H. (2006). On the role of causal intervention in multiple-cue judgment: Positive and negative effects on learning. *Journal of Experimental Psychology: Learning, Memory, and Cognition, 32,* 163–179.

Ericsson, K. A., Krampe, R. T., & Tesch-Römer, C. (1993). The role of deliberate practice in the acquisition of expert performance. *Psychological Review, 100,* 363–406.

Fitts, P. M., & Posner, M. I. (1967). *Human Performance*. Belmont, CA: Brooks/Cole.

Frank, D. J., & Macnamara, B. N. (2017). Does the acquisition of spatial skill involve a shift from algorithm to memory retrieval? *Journal of Experimental Psychology: Learning, Memory, and Cognition, 43*(12), 1845–1856.

Fu, Q., Fu, X., & Dienes, Z. (2008). Implicit sequence learning and conscious awareness. *Consciousness and Cognition, 17*, 185–202.

Gerstenberg, T., & Tenenbaum, J. B. (2017). Intuitive theories. In M. Waldman (Ed.), *Oxford Handbook of Causal Reasoning* (pp. 515–548). New York: Oxford University Press.

Goujon, A., Didierjean, A., & Poulet, S. (2014). The emergence of explicit knowledge from implicit learning. *Memory & Cognition, 42*(2), 225–236.

Graf, P., Mandler, G., & Haden, P. E. (1982). Simulating amnesic symptoms in normal subjects. *Science, 218*, 1243–1244.

Greenwald, A. G., & De Houwer, J. (2017). Unconscious conditioning: Demonstration of existence and difference from conscious conditioning. *Journal of Experimental Psychology: General, 146*(12), 1705–1721.

Hashtroudi, S., Ferguson, S. A., Rappold, V. A., & Chrosniak, L. D. (1988). Data-driven and conceptually driven processes in partial-word identification and recognition. *Journal of Experimental Psychology: Learning, Memory, and Cognition, 14*, 749–757.

Holland, R. W., Hendriks, M., & Aarts, H. (2005). Smells like clean spirit: Nonconscious effects of scent on cognition and behavior. *Psychological Science, 16*, 689–693.

Holmes, E., Domingo, Y., & Johnsrude, I. S. (2018). Familiar voices are more intelligible, even if they are not recognized as familiar. *Psychological Science, 29*(10), 1575–1583.

Jacoby, L. L., & Dallas, M. (1981). On the relationship between autobiographical memory and perceptual learning. *Journal of Experimental Psychology: General, 110*, 306–340.

Jiménez, L., & Vázquez, G. A. (2008). Implicit sequence learning in a search task. *Quarterly Journal of Experimental Psychology, 61*, 1650–1657.

Kalbe, F., & Schwabe, L. (2019). Beyond arousal: Prediction error related to aversive events promotes episodic memory formation. *Journal of Experimental Psychology: Learning, Memory, and Cognition, 46*(2), 234–246.

Kamin, L. J. (1969). Predictability, surprise, attention, and conditioning. *Punishment and Aversive Behavior*, 279–296.

Kempler, L., & Richmond, J. L. (2012). Effect of sleep on gross motor memory. *Memory, 20*(8), 907–914.

Kim, T., Rhee, J., & Wright, D. L. (2016). Allowing time to consolidate knowledge gained through random practice facilitates later novel motor sequence acquisition. *Acta Psychologica, 163*, 153–166.

Klimesch, W., Doppelmayr, M., Russegger, H., & Pachinger, T. (1996). Theta band power in the human scalp EEG and the encoding of new information. *Neuroreport, 7*, 1235–1240.

Kolers, P. A. (1976). Reading a year later. *Journal of Experimental Psychology: Human Learning and Memory, 2*, 554–565.

Kunst-Wilson, W. R., & Zajonc, R. B. (1980). Affective discrimination of stimuli that cannot be recognized. *Science, 207*, 557–558.

Levy, B. A., & Kirsner, K. (1989). Reprocessing text: Indirect measures of word and message level processes. *Journal of Experimental Psychology: Learning, Memory, and Cognition, 15*, 407–417.

Liu, T., & Cooper, L. A. (2003). Explicit and implicit memory for rotating objects. *Journal of Experimental Psychology: Learning, Memory, and Cognition, 29*, 554–562.

MacDonald, A. A., Naci, L., MacDonald, P. A., & Owen, A. M. (2015). Anesthesia and neuroimaging: Investigating the neural correlates of unconsciousness. *Trends in Cognitive Sciences, 19*(2), 100–107.

MacNamara, B. N., Hambrick, D. Z., & Oswald, F. L. (2014). Deliberate practice and performance in music, games, sports, education, and professions: A meta-analysis. *Psychological Science, 25*(8), 1608–1618.

Mitchell, C. J., Lovibond, P. F., & Gan, C. Y. (2005). A dissociation between causal judgment and outcome recall. *Psychonomic Bulletin & Review, 12*, 950–954.

Mitchell, C. J., Lovibond, P. F., Minard, E., & Lavis, Y. (2006). Forward blocking in human learning sometimes reflects the failure to encode a cue–outcome relationship. *Quarterly Journal of Experimental Psychology, 59*, 830–844.

Montoya, R. M., Horton, R. S., Vevea, J. L., Citkowicz, M., & Lauber, E. A. (2017). A re-examination of the mere exposure effect: The influence of repeated exposure on recognition, familiarity, and liking. *Psychological Bulletin, 143*(5), 459–498.

Neath, I. (1998). *Human Memory: An introduction to research, data, and theory*. Pacific Grove, CA: Thomson Brooks/Cole Publishing.

Nelson, T. O. (1978). Detecting small amounts of information in memory: Savings for nonrecognized items. *Journal of Experimental Psychology: Human Learning and Memory, 4*(5), 453–468.

Nieuwenhuis, I. L., Folia, V., Forkstam, C., Jensen, O., & Petersson, K. M. (2013). Sleep promotes the extraction of grammatical rules. *PloS one, 8*(6), e65046.

Nissen, M. J., & Bullemer, P. (1987). Attentional requirements of learning: Evidence from performance measures. *Cognitive Psychology, 19*, 1–32.

Oliphant, G. W. (1983). Repetition and recency effects in word recognition. *Australian Journal of Psychology, 35*, 393–403.

Opacic, T., Stevens, C., & Tillmann, B. (2009). Unspoken knowledge: Implicit learning of structured human dance movement. *Journal of Experimental Psychology: Learning, Memory, and Cognition, 35*, 1570–1577.

Opitz, B., & Hofmann, J. (2015). Concurrence of rule- and similarity-based mechanisms in artificial grammar learning. *Cognitive Psychology, 77*, 77–99.

Park, J., & Sloman, S. A. (2013). Mechanistic beliefs determine adherence to the Markov property in causal reasoning. *Cognitive Psychology, 67*(4), 186–216.

Pavlov, I. P. (1923). New researches on conditioned reflexes. *Science, 58*, 359–361.

Perales J. C., & Shanks, D. R. (2007). Models of covariation-based causal judgment: A review and synthesis. *Psychonomic Bulletin & Review, 14*, 577–596.

Poletiek, F. H., & Wolters, G. (2009). What is learned about fragments in artificial grammar learning? A transitional probabilities approach. *Quarterly Journal of Experimental Psychology, 62*, 868–876.

Pothos, E. M. (2005). Expectations about stimulus structure in implicit learning. *Memory & Cognition, 33*, 171–181.

Pothos, E. M. (2007). Theories of artificial grammar learning. *Psychological Bulletin, 133*, 227–244.

Raney, G. E. (2003). A context-dependent representation model for explaining text repetition effects. *Psychonomic Bulletin & Review, 10*, 15–28.

Ratcliff, R., & McKoon, G. (1995). Bias in the priming of object decisions. *Journal of Experimental Psychology: Learning, Memory, and Cognition, 21*(3), 754–767.

Reber, A. S. (1967). Implicit learning of artificial grammars. *Journal of Verbal Learning and Verbal Behavior, 6*, 855–863.

Reber, A. S. (1969). Transfer of syntactic structure in synthetic languages. *Journal of Experimental Psychology, 81*, 115–119.

Rescorla, R. A., & Wagner, A. R. (1972). A theory of Pavlovian conditioning: Variations of the effectiveness of reinforcement and nonreinforcement. In A. H. Black & W. F. Prokasy (Eds.), *Classical Conditioning II: Current Research and Theory* (pp. 64–99). New York: Appleton-Century-Crofts.

Ruch, S., & Henke, K. (2020). Learning during sleep: A dream comes true? *Trends in Cognitive Sciences, 24*(3), 170–172.

Sallas, B., Mathews, R. C., Lane, S. M., & Sun, R. (2007). Developing rich and quickly accessed knowledge of an artificial grammar. *Memory & Cognition, 35*, 2118–2133.

Sanchez, D. J., & Reber, P. J. (2013). Explicit pre-training instruction does not improve implicit perceptual-motor sequence learning. *Cognition, 126*(3), 341–351.

Santolin, C., & Saffran, J. R. (2018). Constraints on statistical learning across species. *Trends in Cognitive Sciences, 22*(1), 52–63.

Schacter, D. L., & Badgaiyan, R. D. (2001). Neuroimaging of priming: New perspectives on implicit and explicit memory. *Current Directions in Psychological Science, 10*, 1–4.

Schacter, D. L., Cooper, L. A., & Delaney, S. M. (1990). Implicit memory for unfamiliar objects depends on access to structural descriptions. *Journal of Experimental Psychology: General, 119*, 5–24.

Schwender, D., Kaiser, A., Klasing, S., Peter, K., & Pöppel, E. (1993). Explicit and implicit memory and mid-latency auditory evoked potentials during cardiac surgery. In B. Bonke (Ed.), *Memory and Awareness in Anesthesia* (pp. 85–98). Upper Saddle River, NJ: Prentice-Hall.

Shanks, D. R., & Dickinson, A. (1987). Associative accounts of causality judgment. *The Psychology of Learning and Motivation, 21*, 229–261.

Silva, S., Inácio, F., Folia, V., & Petersson, K. M. (2017). Eye movements in implicit artificial grammar learning. *Journal of Experimental Psychology: Learning, Memory, and Cognition, 43*(9), 1387–1402.

Srivinas, K., & Roediger, H. L. (1990). Classifying implicit memory tests: Category association and anagram solution. *Journal of Memory and Language, 29*, 389–412.

Stepan, M. E., Fenn, K. M., & Altmann, E. M. (2019). Effects of sleep deprivation on procedural errors. *Journal of Experimental Psychology: General, 148*(10), 1828–1833.

Taylor, E. G., & Ahn, W. K. (2012). Causal imprinting in causal structure learning. *Cognitive Psychology, 65*(3), 381–413.

Tillmann, B., & Poulin-Charronnat, B. (2010). Auditory expectations for newly acquired structures. *Quarterly Journal of Experimental Psychology, 63*(8), 1646–1664.

Topolinski, S., & Strack, F. (2009a). Motormouth: Mere exposure depends on stimulus-specific motor simulations. *Journal of Experimental Psychology: Learning, Memory, and Cognition, 35*, 423–433.

Topolinski, S., & Strack, F. (2009b). The architecture of intuition: Fluency and affect determine intuitive judgments of semantic and visual coherence and judgments of grammaticality in artificial grammar learning. *Journal of Experimental Psychology: General, 138*, 39–63.

Toth, J. P., Reingold, E. M., & Jacoby, L. L. (1994). Toward a redefinition of implicit memory: Process dissociations following elaborative processing and self-generation. *Journal of Experimental Psychology: Learning, Memory, and Cognition, 20*, 290–303.

Tremblay, S., & Saint-Aubin, J. (2009). Evidence of anticipatory eye movements in the spatial Hebb repetition effect: Insights for modeling sequence learning. *Journal of Experimental Psychology, Learning, Memory, and Cognition, 35*, 1256–1265.

Tulving, E., & Schacter, D. L. (1990). Priming in human memory systems. *Science, 247*, 301–306.

Tulving, E., Schacter, D. L., & Stark, H. A. (1982). Priming effects in word-fragment completion are independent of recognition memory. *Journal of Experimental Psychology: Learning, Memory and Cognition, 8*, 336–342.

Ullén, F., Hambrick, D. Z., & Mosing, M. A. (2016). Rethinking expertise: A multifactorial gene–environment interaction model of expert performance. *Psychological Bulletin, 142*(4), 427–446.

Vokey, J. R., & Higham, P. A. (2005). Abstract analogies and positive transfer in artificial grammar learning. *Canadian Journal of Experimental Psychology, 59*, 54–61.

Wenger, E., Brozzoli, C., Lindenberger, U., & Lövdén, M. (2017). Expansion and renormalization of human brain structure during skill acquisition. *Trends in Cognitive Sciences, 21*(12), 930–939.

Wilkinson, L., & Shanks, D. R. (2004). Intentional control and implicit sequence learning. *Journal of Experimental Psychology: Learning, Memory, and Cognition, 30*, 354–369.

Wolpe, J. (1958). *Psychotherapy by Reciprocal Inhibition.* Stanford, CA: Stanford University Press.

Woltz, D. J., Gardner, M. K., & Bell, B. G. (2000). Negative transfer errors in sequential cognitive skills: Strong-but-wrong sequence application. *Journal of Experimental Psychology: Learning, Memory, and Cognition, 26*(3), 601–625.

Zajonc, R. B. (1968). Attitudinal effects of mere exposure. *Journal of Personality and Social Psychology Monograph Supplement, 9*, 1–27.

Zajonc, R. B. (2001). Mere exposure: A gateway to the subliminal. *Current Directions in Psychological Science, 10*, 224–228.

CHAPTER 7

Episodic Memory: Past and Future

Memories help define who we are. Our opinions, attitudes, likes, and dislikes are a result of our experiences. Memory is the repository of those experiences and the shaper of our future actions. Thus, it is important to understand our memories for the events and episodes of our lives. Memories of experienced events are stored and remembered in ways that have unique characteristics. Memories for events that we experienced are **episodic memories**, whereas memories for general world knowledge are **semantic memories**. An example of this distinction is the difference between knowing the last movie you saw (episodic) versus knowing what a movie is (semantic). This chapter and the next largely cover episodic memories. Semantic memories are covered in Chapter 9.

Several aspects of episodic memory are covered here. We first look at characteristics of episodic memory. After that we consider the content of an episodic memory and how it can be used to cue retrieval. This is followed by a consideration of how context influences episodic memory. We also look at how different types of practice improve memory. We then cover how organization and distinctiveness can both improve episodic memory along with a consideration of the role of adaptive memory. Finally, we extend the idea of episodic memory to events that are likely to happen in the future.

MENTAL TIME TRAVEL

One of the hallmarks of episodic memory, for Tulving (1983; 2002), is the ability to engage in **mental time travel**, which is associated with his idea of autonoetic consciousness. Episodic memory allows us to mentally reinstate the context or circumstances of events and mentally relive or replay them. Neuroimaging evidence suggests that people and animals replay events from the past, such as the previous navigation of a maze (Wilson & McNaughton, 1994). Moreover, this is the type of thinking that we do when we are mind wandering (Corballis, 2013), and involves the operation of the default mode network (see Chapter 2).

The bulk of the research on episodic memory has focused on remembering events from the past. However, mental time travel also involves thinking about future events. In general, the neural systems for episodic memory, are also used in future thinking, navigation (which involves the context in which one finds oneself), theory of mind (considering people's perspectives), and imagining fictitious worlds (as when reading a novel) (Hassabis & Maguire, 2007).

Contents and Cuing

Like most memories, episodic memories are amalgams of different types of information. For example, when you remember a birthday party, you may recall the people, food, music, and gifts. Alternatively, you may remember a conversation you had with someone, but have no memory of songs that were sung, what other guests were wearing, or the party decorations. Our coverage starts with different kinds of information that are in episodic memory and how that information is used later during remembering.

Serial Position Effects

The discussion of short-term memory in Chapter 4 introduced the serial position curve, with superior memory for things at the beginning (primacy effect) and at the end of a sequence (recency effect). Serial position curves are also seen in long-term memory, such as memories of going to the theater (Sehulster, 1989). The explanation for episodic memory differs from that for short-term memory. Primacy and recency effects are attributed to the distinctiveness of those positions (Healy et al., 2000). In addition, the primacy effect reflects novelty. The first item is unusual relative to the context that preceded it, and so it is remembered better. The recency effect reflects a standard forgetting curve, with more recent events being remembered better than older events. Finally, events at the beginning and end of a sequence are less susceptible to interference (see Chapter 8).

Levels of Representation

When we experience an event, we process it at multiple levels. Each of these leaves a memory trace. An illustration of this is memory for text, where there are three levels of representation: the surface form, the textbase, and the mental model (van Dijk & Kintsch, 1983). The surface form captures the verbatim text. This is important initially but is quickly forgotten (Sachs, 1967). The textbase is an abstract representation of the text. For example, the sentences "The girl hit the boy" and "The boy was hit by the girl" have different surface forms but the same underlying meaning, which is captured by the textbase. At the highest level is the mental model (Johnson-Laird, 1983; Radvansky & Zacks, 2014; Zwaan & Radvansky, 1998), which represents the state of affairs described by the text, rather than the text itself (Glenberg et al., 1987). The mental model is a mental simulation of the described events. Another way to think of mental models is that they often contain the who, what, when, where, why, and how of an experience. The binding of information that makes up episodic memories occurs in the hippocampus. Thus, a mental model can include some perceptual, or other experiential, details.

In general, mental models are remembered over long periods of time. People use knowledge at this level to make memory decisions about what was encountered before (Bransford et al., 1972). For example, people who read "The turtles sat on a log, and the fish swam beneath them" are more likely to say later that they read the sentence "The turtles sat on a log, and the fish swam beneath it" because this sentence describes the same situation.

In a study by Fisher and Radvansky (2018), people read a text and then took a recognition test either immediately or up to three months later. The results are shown in Figure 7.1. As you can see, the surface form memory decays rapidly. Textbase memory, although initially better, shows a decline somewhere between one and seven days. However, memory for the mental model was relatively durable. As a real-life example, when you read a news article, you quickly forget the exact wording, but remember the basic ideas for a while. However, your memory for the described event (what the article was about) is more enduring and is what you remember over the long term.

Overall, episodic memories, including mental models, are supported by the posterior medial (PM) brain network (Ritchey & Cooper, 2020), including the parahippocampal cortex (BA 27), retrosplenial cortex (BAs 29 & 30) in the temporal

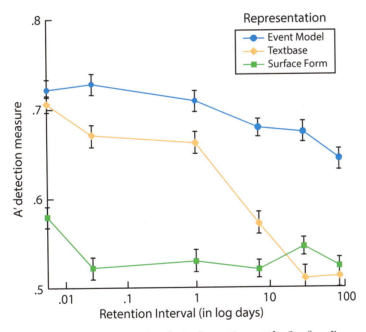

FIGURE 7.1 *Episodic Memory Retention for Information at the Surface Form, Textbase, and Mental Model Levels*

Source: adapted from Fisher, J. S., & Radvansky, G. A. (2018). Patterns of forgetting. *Journal of Memory and Language, 102*, 130–141

lobe, and the precuneus (BA 7), angular gyrus (BA 39), posterior cingulate cortex (BA 23 & 31) in the parietal lobe, and the medial prefrontal cortex (BAs 12, 24, 25, 32, & 33). Thus, there is integrating and coordinating of a large amount of information to make complex episodic memories. This gives episodic memory flexibility.

Cuing

When we recall an event, we may do so easily, but sometimes we need a prompt. This is **cuing**. For example, you may have trouble remembering someone's name because you cannot remember were you know them from. While talking to the person something is said about treating injuries and you remember that this is a medic who treated your friend for a small cut at the county fair. The detail of treating injuries served as a cue to help you to retrieve that memory. In general, memory cues improve retrieval (Tulving & Pearlstone, 1966) by accessing memory traces that contain the same information. Long-term memory is content addressable, so we can access information using the components that make it up.

If the term "cuing" makes you think of cued recall from Chapter 3, then you are correct in a broad sense. Something in the environment triggers memory retrieval. This is the cue. Episodic memory cuing progresses in a regular way. Based on EEG and MEG data, the process takes 1000 to 2000 ms (Staresina & Wimber, 2019). Sensory processing takes about 500 ms, followed by hippocampal and cortical processing, which is the next at 500 to 1500 ms.

There are two types of episodic retrieval cues: feature cues and context cues. Feature cues are discussed here and context cues next. Feature cues involve components of the memory itself. With our medic example, the treating of an injury is part of the memory. It is a feature of the previous event. Features are any component that can help access the sought-after memory. That said, some features are better cues than others.

One of the best feature cues is yourself. This is the **self-reference effect**. If you can relate things to aspects of who you are, then your memory will be better (Rogers et al., 1977; Symons & Johnson, 1997). This self-referencing is often spontaneous. For example, people are more inclined to remember other people's birthdays that are closer to their own (Kesebir & Oishi, 2010). We also better remember things that we think of as belonging to us in some way (van den Bos et al., 2010). Self-reference is also more likely to involve remembering emotional events (Gutchess & Kensinger, 2018).

Odors are powerful memory cues. Herz and Engen (1996) noted that the smell of things is a good memory cue because of the ease with which odors tap into emotional aspects of memories. This may be why some odors are strongly associated with certain emotions (think of flowers and perfumes). There is a strong neurological connection of olfactory parts of the cortex to the amygdala and hippocampus (only two or three synapses away).

It might be tempting to think that the more closely a cue matches the original memory, the better it will be. While this is true, in general, the degree of overlap is not what is most critical. What is more critical is how diagnostic a cue is. The

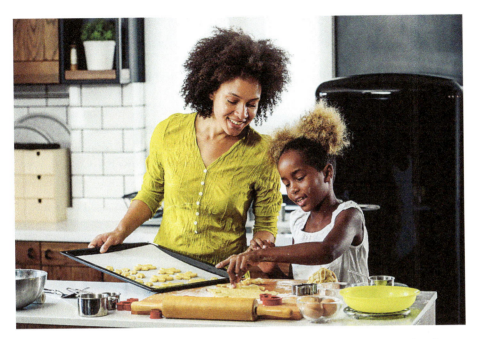

PHOTO 7.1 *Memories can be triggered by cues that are parts of those memories. Some of the most powerful episodic memory cues are odors of events from our past, such as smelling cookies and being reminded of times spent with your mother as a child*

Source: Lordn/Shutterstock.com

fewer memories a cue corresponds to, the more likely remembering will be successful (Nairne, 2002). For example, if you have lunch in the same place every day, someone trying to remind you of an event by cuing with that place is not going to be very helpful. This is because it is not diagnostic information. However, if you are cued with a place where you had lunch only once, this is going to select out just a single memory and will be more effective.

Another important role of cuing is to strengthen memories. This may occur subconsciously. For example, during sleep, if people hear sounds or smell odors that were present during learning, this cues rehearsals, thereby strengthening those memories (Hu et al., 2020; Paller, 2017).

Stop and Review

Episodic memory involves mental time travel for events that differ from the current moment, with a focus on individual experiences. Episodic memories are influenced by the order in which things were learned, showing a serial position curve. They also capture information at multiple levels of representation. Some of these are forgotten quickly (surface form and textbase), whereas others are retained longer (mental models). Episodic memory content can cue remembering by selecting out individual traces at retrieval. With the appropriate cues, otherwise forgotten memories can be retrieved.

TRY IT OUT

Here we consider a demonstration of the principle of cuing. This task requires at least 12 people.

To demonstrate episodic memory cuing, we will use a method developed by Bransford and Stein (1984). First, read the list of sentences below to a group of participants. Then, wait a minute, and have people try to recall as many as they can by writing the sentences down on a sheet of paper.

A brick can be used as a doorstop.
A wine bottle can be used as a candle holder.
A record can be used to serve potato chips.
A leaf can be used as a bookmark.
A newspaper can be used to swat flies.

A sheet can be used as a sail.
A bathtub can be used as a punch bowl.
A rock can be used as a paperweight.
A pen can be used as an arrow.
A rug can be used as a bedspread.

A scissors can be used to cut grass.
A balloon can be used as a pillow.
A dime can be used as a screwdriver.

A ladder can be used as a bookshelf.
A pan can be used as a drum.

A guitar can be used as a canoe paddle.

An orange can be used to play catch.
A TV antenna can be used as a clothes rack.

A boat can be used as a shelter.
A flashlight can be used to hold water.
A knife can be used to stir paint.
A barrel can be used as a chair.
A telephone can be used as an alarm clock.

A board can be used as a ruler.
A shoe can be used to pound nails.
A lampshade can be used as a hat.

When they are done, have them draw a line under the last one that they recalled. Then read the words below and ask people to write down any additional sentences they can recall. You should find that people can now remember more sentences. This is because the words below serve as retrieval cues and help people access otherwise forgotten memories.

Brick; Wine bottle; Record; Leaf; Newspaper; Sheet; Bathtub; Rock; Pen; Rug; Scissors; Balloon; Dime; Ladder; Pan; Guitar; Orange; TV antenna; Boat; Flashlight; Knife; Barrel; Telephone; Board; Shoe; Lampshade

CONTEXT

Another important part of episodic memories is the context in which information is learned. There are a variety of contexts. We start with the external contexts in which we find ourselves. One role of the hippocampus is to bind such information together to form episodic memories (Ranganath, 2010). If you remember, in Chapter 2 we discussed how the hippocampus integrates information from anterior and posterior inputs. The anterior inputs correspond more to content information and the posterior inputs more to contextual information.

Context is important for episodic memory because context changes can indicate new events (Ezzyat & Davachi, 2011), such as a shift in spatial location or temporal framework (e.g., a day later). Context is a powerful memory cue. The activation of context during memory retrieval is associated with activity in the parahippocampal cortex (Diana et al., 2013), part of the posterior input stream to the hippocampus.

Encoding Specificity

The influence of environmental context on memory is reflected in the **encoding specificity principle** (Thompson & Tulving, 1970). This is the superior ability to remember when the retrieval context matches the encoding context. For example, if you learn something in one room, it is easier to recall it when you are in the same room. It is not unusual to fail to remember something until you return to the room where you got the information in the first place. Smith (1988) provides a clear account of the power of encoding specificity.

> Having lived most of his life in St. Louis, Missouri, except for two years at the University of Texas at Austin, and four years in the military service during the Second World War, my father returned to Texas after 42 long years of forgetting. Although previously certain that he could recall only a few disembodied fragments of memories of his college days, he became increasingly amazed, upon his return, at the freshness and detail of his newly remembered experiences. Strolling along the streets of Austin, my father suddenly stopped and animatedly described the house in which he lived in a location now occupied by a parking lot. He recalled in vivid detail, for example, how an armadillo had climbed up the drainpipe one night and became his pet, and how the woman who had cooked for the residents of his house had informed them of the attack on Pearl Harbor, abruptly ending his college career. Not until he returned to the setting in which those long-past events had occurred had my father thought or spoken of them.
>
> (p. 13)

The encoding specificity principle is illustrated in a study in which scuba divers learned lists of words. Some were learned on land and others underwater. Later the divers were tested in either the same or a different context. As shown in Figure 7.2, memory was better when the words were recalled in the same context rather than in the different one (Godden & Baddeley, 1975).

For encoding specificity, the contexts at encoding and retrieval do not need to be identical, but only similar (Smith et al., 2014). Importantly, it is observed when an environment is either present or only thought about (Smith, 1979). Thinking about a prior context has behavioral manifestations. For example, people look to a place on a computer screen where something was previously seen, even if the screen is blank (Johansson & Johansson, 2013). Presumably, the context is a retrieval cue. Also, although encoding specificity is stronger with recall than recognition (Smith et al., 1978), it operates for both (Smith & Vela, 2001), and even indirect memory tests (Smith et al., 2018).

As a student, you may think that encoding specificity means that it is better to study in the same room where you will take an exam. However, this applies the encoding specificity principle in a suboptimal way. Memories are strongly associated with a context when the context is always the same. Something that is learned in different contexts—if you study in different places—does not exhibit strong encoding specificity. The information is more context independent (Smith et al., 1978). You can use the knowledge when you need it, not just when you happen to be in the right place. Thus, it is best to not study in the same place all the time. Mix it up.

State-Dependent Memory

Context may refer to external, environmental contexts, such as a room or to internal contexts. One internal context is our physiological state (e.g., being sleepy, drunk, or excited). Memory is better when we are in a similar physiological state during recall as we were during learning. This is **state-dependent memory**.

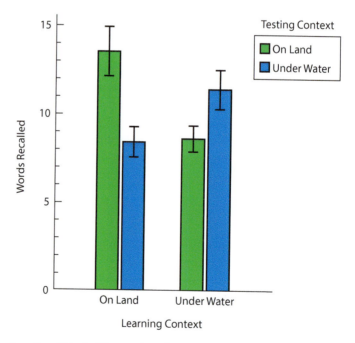

FIGURE 7.2 *Results of Study Illustrating the Effect of Encoding Specificity on Memory for Word Lists*

Source: adapted from Godden, D. B., & Baddeley, A. D. (1975). Context-dependent memory in two natural environments: On land and underwater. *British Journal of Psychology, 66*, 325–331

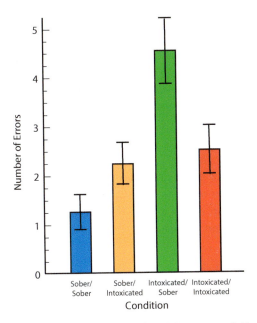

FIGURE 7.3 *Results of a Study on State-Dependent Memory and Alcohol Consumption*

Source: created from data reported in Goodwin D. W., Powell, B., Bremer, D., Hoine, H., & Stern, J. (1969). Alcohol and recall: State-dependent effects in man. *Science, 163,* 2358–2360

An example of state dependent memory is a study in which people learned while they were sober or drunk. They then had memory tested in either the same or a different state. As shown in Figure 7.3, memory was better when they were in the same state at both learning and test (Goodwin et al., 1969). If people studied drunk, they did better on the test if while drunk. (It is important to keep in mind that memory is worse overall if people are drunk during learning or testing.) Similar state-dependent memory effects occur with nicotine (Peters & McGee, 1982), marijuana (Eich et al., 1975), Ritalin (Swanson & Kinsbourne, 1976), and the physiological changes associated with aerobic exercise (Miles & Hardman, 1998).

Mood-Dependent Memory

Another internal context is mood or emotion. We are always in some mood. Emotional states are stored in memory, allowing for **mood-dependent memory**. Memory is better if we are in the same mood we were in when we learned the information as when we try to remember it (Blaney, 1986; Bower, 1981). For example, when you are happy, you remember things better that you learned when you were happy. Say you have a fight with your boyfriend/girlfriend. While you are angry, you think of reasons why he or she is such a jerk (They really are, aren't they?). Later, you calm down and think about his or her good qualities. You are happy and think of the reasons why he or she is so nice (They really are, aren't they?). When you have another fight weeks later, all the negative thoughts come back to mind more easily because you initially thought of them while you were angry.

A related concept is **mood-congruent memory**, which is the finding that it is easier to think of things that are consistent with one's current mood. For example, a depressed mood makes it more likely that depressing ideas are retrieved. Mood-congruent memory is supported by neurological work. Maratos et al. (2001) tested memory for words that were read in the context of emotionally positive, negative, or neutral sentences. Later, a recognition test was given during an fMRI scan. Words read in emotionally positive or negative contexts were accompanied by more activation in brain regions associated with emotion, such as the amygdala and orbitofrontal cortex (BA 11).

Overall, all kinds of contexts can influence episodic memory. As noted by Terry (2000), other types of context that influence memory include music, odors, temperature, time of day, body position (lying down or standing up), phone calls, and pain. Even the sound of a person's voice can be a context and can influence memory (Goh, 2005).

Transfer Appropriate Processing

Memory is also influenced by the context of our thoughts during learning. Memory is better when retrieval uses mental processes that are more in tune with those used at learning, a principle called **transfer appropriate processing** (Roediger & Blaxton, 1987; but see Mulligan & Lozito, 2006). As a simple example of this, bilinguals find it easier to remember things when the language used at encoding and retrieval are the same (Marian & Neisser, 2000). This is also related to the idea of depth of processing (see Chapter 3). When learning emphasizes meaning, this has a greater positive impact on direct memory tests such as recall or recognition. In contrast, when learning emphasizes shallow surface characteristics, this has a greater impact on indirect memory tests, possibly because similar neural structures are activated when transfer appropriate processing occurs (Schendan & Kutas, 2007).

An example of transfer appropriate processing is a study by Morris et al. (1977) in which students responded to words using either a meaning-based (deep-level) task, such as whether the word "plane" made sense in the sentence "The _____ had a silver engine" or a rhyme-based (shallow-level) task, such as whether the word "eagle" made sense in the sentence "_____ rhymes with legal." Later, students took either a standard recognition test (a direct memory test) or a rhyming recognition test (an indirect test) in which they indicated whether a new word rhymed with one that was heard earlier (e.g., "regal"). The results, shown in Figure 7.4, reveal that memory is better when the encoding and retrieval processes match than when they do not. Thus, depth of processing is not a clear guide to future memory. Instead, successful memory also depends on how people think about things.

Stop and Review

Episodic memories store information about the context in which events were experienced. Context can be the external environment or people's physiological or emotional states. For the encoding specificity principle, when the encoding and

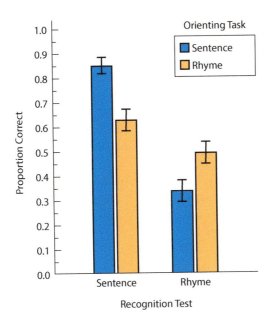

FIGURE 7.4 *Results of a Study of Transfer Appropriate Processing*

Source: created from data reported in Morris, C. D., Branstord, J. D., & Franks, J. J. (1977). Levels of processing versus transfer appropriate processing. *Journal of Verbal Learning and Verbal Behavior, 16,* 519–533

retrieval context match, there is a greater likelihood of remembering. However, when they differ, memory retrieval can be impaired. Finally, episodic memories also contain information about the mental processes used to create them, which can affect the transfer appropriate processing principle.

REPETITION AND PRACTICE

The more we are exposed to information, the more likely it will be remembered. This is the **repetition effect**. For example, information that is studied twice is more likely to be remembered than information studied only once. Having said that, repeated exposures vary in their effectiveness. How information is practiced has a profound impact on memory.

Massed and Distributed Practice

Practice can affect memory depending on whether repeated exposures are grouped together or spread out over time. This is a distinction between massed and distributed practice. **Massed practice** is when there is a single, lengthy study period. For example, if you spend five hours studying, massed practice would be a single five-hour session. In contrast, **distributed practice** (also called spaced practice) occurs when the effort is spread out across multiple study periods. An example of distributed practice is if you study for five hours by studying for one hour per day for five days. Massed practice is like cramming, and distributed practice is like consistently studying across a term. In general, memory is better following distributed practice than massed practice, and the longer the spacing between distributed practices, the better memory is (Glenberg & Lehmann, 1980).

An example of the difference between massed and distributed processing is shown in Figure 7.5. Memory improved more for distributed practice than massed practice. Distributed practice improves memory, even years later (Bahrick et al., 1993). What is odd is that people are largely unaware of the impact of these kinds of practice. Zechmeister and Shaughnessy (1980) found that students think that memory is better after massed than distributed practice. Reality tells a different story.

There are several explanations why distributed practice is better (Maddox, 2016). The first explanation is a **consolidation account** in which massed practice is inferior because consolidation has not run its course. With distributed practice, there is more consolidation, so memory is better (Landauer, 1969) and is less disrupted by other processes. Mass practice may overload the system, preventing some consolidation.

A second explanation is a **deficient-processing account** in which massed practice reflects a processing deficiency. There are two ways that this might happen. One is a habituation/attention problem in which we habituate to information during massed practice, and thus do not actively attend to it, leading to less improvement (Hintzman, 1974). Massed practice may also involve more mind wandering (Metcalfe & Xu, 2016). An accessibility/reconstruction variant is that massed practice is worse because less effort is needed to retrieve a memory because it is so fresh. As a result, we assume it is learned and do not devote the time and effort needed to actually learn it.

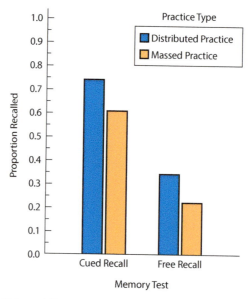

FIGURE 7.5 *Effects of Massed Versus Spaced Practice on Subsequent Memory (with a Constant Context)*

Source: adapted from Glenberg, A. M. (1979). Component-levels theory of the effects of spacing of repetitions on recall and recognition. *Memory & Cognition, 7,* 95–112

A third explanation is a **contextual variability account** in which differences in the variability of the contexts stored with the memories is what accounts for the differences in massed and distributed practice (Glenberg, 1976; 1979). For massed practice, the contexts are roughly the same. However, for distributed practice, the contexts (both internal and external) vary. A variety of contexts provides more retrieval pathways, making it more likely that the memory can be retrieved when needed. Moreover, sleeping between study sessions results in better memory (Bell et al., 2014). With study sessions on different days, there is a greater shift in context than if study sessions are separated within the same day, even if by 12 hours.

While the contextual variability account emphasizes differences between learning attempts (i.e., changes in context), a **study-phase retrieval account** emphasizes the similarities. When we have subsequent study sessions, this reminds us of prior sessions, allowing connections to be made between them (Benjamin & Tullis, 2010). Distributed practice reactivates prior memory traces, thereby strengthening them, and boosting resistance to forgetting. Also, the more connections between the information, the more elaborate the memory traces, and the better the information is remembered.

The interplay between context and practice is seen in a study by Verkoeijen et al. (2004). People were given either massed or distributed practice, with all the items shown on the same or a different background (context) each time. The results are shown in Figure 7.6. For massed practice, using different backgrounds helped memory because even though repetitions were close in time, each presentation was in a different context, thereby facilitating retrieval. In contrast, for distributed

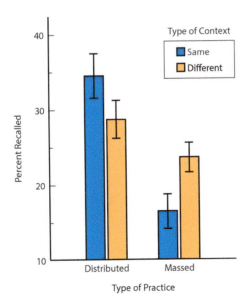

FIGURE 7.6 *Effects of Massed Versus Spaced Practice on Subsequent Memory (with Varying Context)*

Source: created from data reported in Verkoeijen, P. P. J. L., Rikers, R. M. J. P., & Schmidt, H. G. (2004). Detrimental influence of contextual change on spacing effects. *Journal of Experimental Psychology: Learning, Memory, and Cognition, 30*, 796–800

practice, the information was already distinct, so having each item on a different background actually made things worse. Changing the context made it harder to remember previous study experiences, and thus memory was poorer. However, when the background was the same in distributed practice, this reminded people of the previous experiences and helped memory.

Schedules of Practice

Another important issue to consider when thinking about memory and practice—particularly distributed practice—is the difference between uniform, expanding, and contracting **schedules of practice**. For a uniform schedule, there is a consistent delay between study periods (e.g., study every seven days), whereas for an expanding schedule, there are increasing delays (e.g., 1, 3, 6, 12 days, etc.), and for a contracting schedule there are decreasing delays (e.g., 7, 6, 5, 4 days, etc.).

Very few studies suggest that a contracting schedule produces better memory. For uniform and expanding schedules of practice, some studies have found no difference between them (Karpicke & Roediger, 2010). However, most of those studies manipulated the schedule of practice within a single session (Kang et al., 2014). Other studies have found that expanding schedules produce a greater memory benefit (Gerbier & Koenig, 2012), consistent with the contextual variability account. As delays grow larger, the contexts become more varied. Lindsey et al. (2014) describe a method where faster learning can occur using individualized schedules of rehearsal.

Overlearning and Permastore

If we continue to practice memorized information, then **overlearning** occurs (Driskell et al., 1992). As reported by Ebbinghaus (1885), overlearning strengthens memories and increases resistance to forgetting. Actors and musicians continue to rehearse their parts, even after they are flawless, to overlearn them. What about things that you learn in school? What is the fate of the information you are learning? What is the point of learning if you are only going to forget it all later? Well, although there is some forgetting, a great deal of what is learned in school is retained throughout life.

Harry Bahrick, at Ohio Wesleyan University, has addressed these issues. His method was to use alumni attending college reunions and test their memories for prior course material, such as Spanish, from three months to 50 years after graduation. He found that, although there is an initial period of forgetting for about three years, there is little forgetting after that (Bahrick, 1984). Similar effects have been found in actors' memory for play lines (Noice & Noice, 2002). These stabilized memories are described by being in **permastore**. Memories enter permastore after distributed practice and overlearning. The knowledge is so consolidated that it becomes resistant to forgetting.

It is important to note that forgetting occurs at similar rates for everyone. Even after the initial forgetting period, differences in knowledge persist. The people who got As always know more than the people who got Cs (Bahrick, 1984; Conway et al., 1991). So, study hard.

To Study or To Test

Now, consider another way to practice, namely by taking a test. Intuitively, it seems that studying should lead to better memory than testing. After all, studying is what gets material into memory in the first place. However, the opposite is true. People typically learn more, after an initial study period, by taking a test rather than doing further study (Gates, 1917; Glover, 1989; Roediger & Karpicke, 2006; Spitzer, 1939). This is the **testing effect** (see Rowland, 2014, for a meta-analysis). The critical point is the retrieval of the studied information. Thus, it is sometimes called the **retrieval practice effect** (Karpicke, 2012). One thing testing does is reduce the rate of forgetting. In a study by Roediger and Karpicke (2006) people who either studied further or took a test were assessed two minutes, two days, and one week later. The forgetting curves are shown in Figure 7.7. The forgetting curve is shallower for material that was tested as compared to when it was only studied.[1] This is consistent with the idea that testing increases memory consolidation (Antony et al., 2017). There are still some aspects of the testing effect that have not been accounted for. For example, it is does not occur for material that was heard (Wilkinson et al., 2019).

According to the *elaborative retrieval hypothesis*, the testing effect occurs because testing causes people to engage in deeper processing while taking the test (Carpenter, 2009). Testing increases the degree to which people organize information in memory,

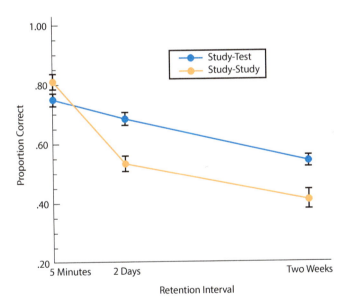

FIGURE 7.7 *Forgetting Curves as a Function of Whether People Simply Studied Material or Took a Test*

Source: adapted from Roediger, H. L., & Karpicke, J. D. (2006). Test-enhanced learning: Taking memory tests improves long-term retention. *Psychological Science*, *17*(5), 249–255

---

1 See Bäuml et al. (2014) and Racsmány et al. (2010) for evidence that the testing effect can sometimes be eliminated by sleep.

which boosts later retrieval (Zaromb & Roediger, 2010). In addition, testing reduces the effects of proactive interference (se Chapter 8) (Szpunar et al., 2008). That said, the testing effect may not be observed for complex materials (van Gog & Sweller, 2015). A similar idea is the *dual memory framework*, which suggests that memories generated during study differ from those generated during retrieval. Thus, people have more traces available to use at retrieval (Rickard & Pan, 2018).

Another theory of the retrieval practice effect is the *episodic context account* (Lehman et al., 2014). For this view, people encode the original context. During retrieval, people use this context as part of their memory search. If retrieval is successful, then there is also a memory with the new context that can be used to help later retrieval (Akan et al., 2018).

Yet another theory is the *relational processing hypothesis* (Rawson & Zamary, 2019). This builds on the finding that the testing effect is more likely, and is larger, for recall than for recognition during learning. Recall tests are more likely to emphasize relational processing, whereas recognition tests are more likely to emphasize item-specific processing (see the next section). Relational processing involves making connections, helping organize the material, and improving performance.

Improve Your Memory

As you read, memory is better if, after initially studying something, you take a test rather than continue to study more. You can use the testing effect to improve your memory for things that you are learning in school. What you should do is meet with some of your classmates on a regular basis to sit around and test each other. One person should have either the notes or the textbook (or both) and come up with questions for the others to answer. Being able to answer those questions will improve your memory more over that time than simply studying more. So, bottom line, a good way to improve memory for the material you are learning in your classes is to take quizzes and tests in a study group. Moreover, the act of thinking of such test questions also boosts memory because of the generation effect (see Chapter 3). Further still, not only does testing improve memory for the information that was tested, but it also aids any subsequent learning of new information that follows (Arnold & McDermott, 2013). This is a more effective use of your time. Be sure to take turns being the tester and the answerer. Because other classmates are not always available, find ways to test yourself. A simple way to do this is to make flashcards.

Stop and Review

Memory is better with distributed than massed practice. Massed practice may (a) not allow consolidation to complete, (b) promote less effort, (c) have reduced contextual variability, and (d) provide fewer opportunities to link the knowledge with prior memories. With distributed practice, memory is better with expanding schedules of practice. Continued practice can cause overlearning and permastore storage. Finally, the testing effect demonstrates better memory when practice takes the form of a test rather than additional studying.

ORGANIZATION AND DISTINCTIVENESS

Here we considered improvements in memory that come from organization (linking memories together) and distinctiveness (separating memories apart). We consider each of these, along with a consideration of why these seemingly opposite processes both enhance memory.

Organization

Episodic memory improves if people use **organization**. Figure 7.8 shows data for a study across several study sessions when a set of words was given in either an organized (i.e., based on categories) or random manner. Thus, chunking also works in long-term memory. An example of a pre-established structure that can aid memory is shown in Figure 7.9. Here, a hierarchical organization categorizes 17 words into groups of three or four items. Each of these sets is chunked, and the chunks are chunked.

The influence of organization and elaboration on memory is seen in actors' memories for scripts. Actors learn scripts really fast if they were simply rote learning a series of sentences. However, they are doing much more than this. They organize the material by creating integrated perceptual images, self-referencing the information by taking the perspective of the character, generating the lines themselves, as well as the way they are delivered, and generating emotional states to match the character's mood (Noice & Noice, 2006). All this organizes the material into a larger whole and allows it to be memorized faster.

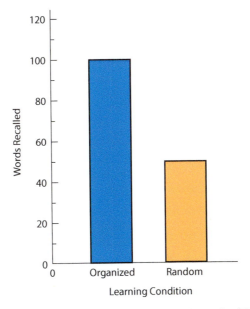

FIGURE 7.8 *The Influence of Studying Random Versus Organized Study Materials*

Source: adapted from Bower, G. H., Clark, M. C., Lesgold, A. M., & Winzenz, D. (1969). Hierarchical retrieval schemes in recall of categorized word lists. *Journal of Verbal Learning and Verbal Behavior, 8*, 323–343

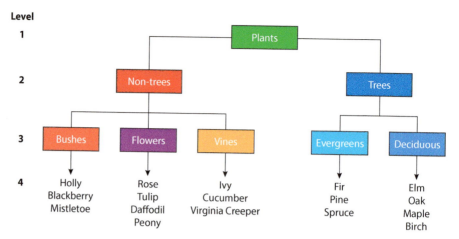

FIGURE 7.9 *Example of a Hierarchical Structure that Can Be Used to Help Organize Memory*

Source: adapted from Bower, G. H., Clark, M. C., Lesgold, A. M., & Winzenz, D. (1969). Hierarchical retrieval schemes in recall of categorized word lists. *Journal of Verbal Learning and Verbal Behavior, 8,* 323–343

Organization is also aided by the structure of events. As mentioned earlier, people create mental models to understand events. When people explicitly segment on-going activities into events, then memory is improved (Flores et al., 2017). Figure 7.10 shows that there is no real benefit immediately. However, over time, people remember segmented events better for at least a week, although this benefit appears to diminish by one month.

Organization, and hence memory, can be enhanced when people either do something with the information or expect to do something with it. In a study by Nestojko et al. (2014) people were given passages to read either with the expectation that they would be tested later or that they would teach the material to someone else. The expectation to teach led people to better structure and organize the information, which boosted memory.

Distinctiveness

Episodic memory can be enhanced when a memory is separated out from competing ones that produce interference (see Chapter 8). Thus, retrieval is better for information that is distinct. For example, if one word is printed in red in a list of black words, the red word is remembered better. Similarly, if the word "tulip" appears in a list of vehicle names, "tulip" is remembered better. This is called the **von Restorff effect**, after the woman who discovered it (Hunt, 1995; Schmidt & Schmidt, 2017). It is also called the **isolation effect** because distinctive information can be isolated from its contrasting context. It is more likely to be observed with recall than recognition (van Dam et al., 1974). This may be because recognition does not require a comparison with the other items in which a distinctive item was present. It is the setting or context that often makes something distinctive, not just the thing itself. This may be partially why emotional events are remembered better than neutral events (Talmi et al., 2007). Emotional events are distinct against a background of more common events.

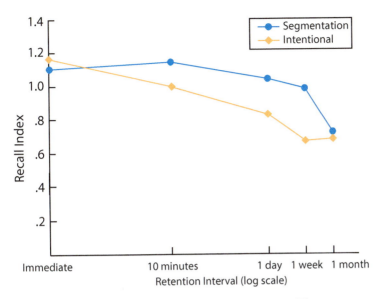

FIGURE 7.10 *The Influence of Event Structure on Memory over Time*

Source: created from data reported in Flores, S., Bailey, H. R., Eisenberg, M. L., & Zacks, J. M. (2017). Event segmentation improves event memory up to one month later. *Journal of Experimental Psychology: Learning, Memory, and Cognition, 43*(8), 1183–1202

An example of distinctive processing is the **bizarre imagery effect**. Here, people form mental images of what they are trying to remember. Forming a mental image involves some work, and so it improves memory (see Chapter 3). However, we can go a step further to create bizarre images. For example, to remember to buy ice cream, tomatoes, and carrots at the grocery store, you might imagine a bowl of ice cream with a face made with slices of tomatoes and carrots. Overall, people remember more when they use bizarre imagery (Einstein & McDaniel 1987). However, this only works when part of the information gets this treatment. If more than half or all the information is bizarre, none of the information is distinct, and memory is not improved (McDaniel & Einstein, 1986). The bizarre imagery effect, like the general isolation effect, reflects an influence on the ability to access the information at retrieval rather than different amounts of attention paid to information during learning (Riefer & Rouder, 1992).

Part of the impact of distinctive events on memory is that they are, in some way, unexpected. Unexpected events result in increased neural processing, such as in the hippocampus and the nucleus accumbens (BA 34) which enhances memory (Axmacher et al., 2010).

Relational and Item-Specific Processing

At this point there may seem to be a contradiction. On the one hand, organization helps memory, but on the other hand, distinctiveness helps memory. These processes seem to be opposites. The more organized information is, the less distinctive the elements are, because similarities are emphasized. Conversely, the more distinct information is, the less organized it is, because differences are emphasized. It is clear that both processes are at work (Hunt & McDaniel, 1993). **Relational processing** is helpful in generating a retrieval plan for later recall. **Item-specific processing** helps reduce sources of interference. The degree to which each of these aids memory is a function of the current set of information.

An illustration of the differential effects of relational and item-specific processing is a study by Hunt and Seta (1984) in which people learned items from categories of different sizes. This was done by emphasizing either relational processing (sorting items into categories) or item-specific processing (rating items for pleasantness). The results, shown in Figure 7.11, illustrate that memory was better for small categories for relational processing (helping identify interrelations among the few category members) but was better for larger categories for distinctiveness processing (helping people contend with larger amounts of interference).

The distinction between item-specific and relational processing has implications for learning. We do better if learning emphasizes the information for which memory is likely to be weak. This is the idea behind **material appropriate processing** (Einstein et al., 1990). For example, for descriptive texts, such as a college textbook, the emphasis is on sets of facts or item-specific information. Thus, memory is better if we engage in learning that emphasizes relational information. In contrast, with narrative texts, such as a novel, the emphasis is on the narrative flow and the interrelations among the events or relational information. Consequently, memory is better if we engage in learning that emphasizes item-specific information.

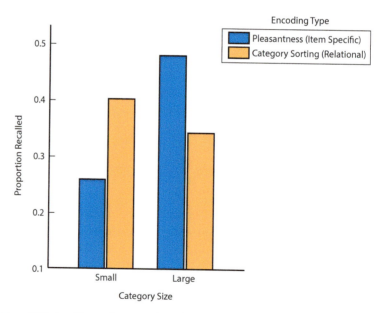

FIGURE 7.11 *Effects of Learning Emphasizing Distinctiveness and Relational Processing as a Function of Category Size*

Source: created from data reported in Hunt, R. R., & Seta, C. E. (1984). Category size effects in recall: The roles of relational and individual item information. *Journal of Experimental Psychology: Learning, Memory, and Cognition, 10*, 454–464

Fuzzy Trace Memory

As mentioned in Chapter 1, it is almost never the case that a single memory is involved. Different traces capture different information qualities. For example, one trace may have more detailed information, whereas another has more general information. During retrieval, these multiple traces work together to contribute to what is remembered. This is the idea behind **fuzzy trace theories** of memory (e.g., Brainerd & Reyna, 1990).

This is of interest for episodic memory because our experiences involve both details and gist. This was seen already with the coverage of different levels of episodic memory content and the distinction between item-specific and relational processing. Episodic memory is complex and interactive. This is supported by neuroimaging data. Detailed information is more supported by the parahippocampal gyrus and early visual cortex (BAs 17 & 18), whereas gist information is more supported by the inferior frontal gyrus (BA 47), and they all work together (Kim & Cabeza, 2007).

Adaptive Memory

One area of research on episodic memory has explored the influence of evolutionary pressures (Nairne & Pandeirada, 2008; 2016). The basic idea is that our memories evolved to serve particular environmental issues, perhaps those related to survival on the African savannah during the Pleistocene. Evolutionary pressures pushed us to be able to remember some things better than others (Scofield et al. (2018).

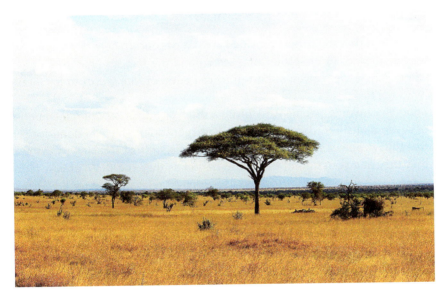

PHOTO 7.2 *According to the adaptive memory perspective, memory is better for information that is related to our survival. This builds on theories that memory evolved to remember those things that were more critical to survival in various environments, such as the African savannah*

Source: Maciej Czekajewski/Shutterstock.com

The idea that memory has evolved to accommodate environmental pressures is profound. A seminal study was done by Nairne and Pandeirada (2008). In one experiment, they tested 32 students from Purdue University. They had people go through a series of word lists from four categories: four-footed animals, weather phenomenon, vegetables, and types of human dwellings. There were eight words in each category. The words from a given category were presented together, although the order within a given category was randomized.

The important manipulation was whether a word was rated for (a) pleasantness (e.g., "How PLEASANT is this word?"), or survival (e.g., "How relevant is this word to the SURVIVAL situation?") on a 1 to 5 scale, with 1 indicating totally unpleasant/irrelevant and 5 indicating extremely pleasant/relevant. The instructions for the pleasantness ratings were:

In this task, we are going to show you a list of words, and we would like you to rate the pleasantness of each word. Some of the words may be pleasant and others may not—it's up to you to decide.

In comparison, the instructions for the survival situation were:

In this task we would like you to imagine that you are stranded in the grasslands of a foreign land, without any basic survival materials. Over the next few months, you will need to find steady supplies of food and water and protect yourself from predators. We are going to show you a list of words, and we would like you to rate how relevant each of these words would be for you in this survival situation. Some of the words may be relevant and others may not—it's up to you to decide.

The actual ratings that the people provided are not of concern here. Each word was presented for five seconds in the center of a screen and the response had to be given within that time. People were given a short practice period of four words to familiarize themselves with the task.

After rating all 32 words, people were given a short distractor task of remembering sequences of seven digits in order (a standard digit span task). This was done for two minutes. After this, people were given a surprise memory test of recalling as many of the words that they had seen during the rating period as they could. What was found was that people remembered the words rated for survival relevance better (66%) than those rated for pleasantness (55%). The explanation is that memory is more attuned to matters relating to personal survival.

People respond faster to words based on their subjective level of danger or usefulness (Wurm, 2007). The more dangerous or useful something is, the more likely it will be helpful to know about. Remembering this type of information is helpful to survival. Another important aspect of survival is knowing which places are dangerous and which are not. Thinking about the survival value of items helps us remember the locations where they were encountered (Nairne et al., 2012).

This bias for survival related information also plays into the fact that animate concepts (e.g., deer, dog, bird) are better remembered than inanimate ones (e.g., cloud, chair, ball). This is called the **animacy effect**. Animate entities are more likely to have implications for survival (Nairne et al., 2017; Nairne et al., 2013), and people are more likely to engage in elaborative processing with animate entities (Meinhardt et al., 2019).

Having people focus on survival value provides better memory compared to other ways of boosting memory. This includes creating mental images, generating information, and intentional learning (Nairne et al., 2008). Moreover, the effect persists for at least four days later (Clark & Bruno, 2016), although the nature of the forgetting curve is unknown at this point. Memory seems more attuned to grasslands survival than city survival (Weinstein et al., 2008), consistent with an evolutionary perspective. A survival effect is observed so long as there is a perceived threat (Olds et al., 2014). For example, it is observed when the threats are zombies (which are imaginary) (Soderstrom & McCabe, 2011). Even though zombies were not in the African savannah during the Pleistocene, they would still be predators, and so would threaten survival.

Relatedly, just thinking about your own death, such as being on death row, can produce a survival memory benefit (Hart & Burns, 2012). While thoughts of death improve memory, the benefits are not as great as those associated with a more general survival-based thinking (Klein, 2014).

Why do people have better memory for things related to their own survival? Some of this is a benefit from processes that are already known to boost memory, such as elaborative processing (Kroneisen & Erdfelder, 2011), increased item-specific and relational processing, relating information to yourself, and distinctive processing (Klein, 2012). A compelling argument has also been made that when you think about your survival, you think more about the usefulness of the items or information (Bell et al., 2015) and are engaging in more planning of what you will do to survive (Klein et al., 2011).

Stop and Review

Memory is improved by putting information into an organizational structure. It is also improved by making new information distinct. While these two seem to be at odds, both are effective under the right circumstances. Relational processing improves memory for information for which it is unclear how it relates to what is already known. Conversely, item-specific processing improves memory when people already have a well-developed organization, thereby helping make knowledge stand out and be less affected by interference. This is consistent with fuzzy trace theories of memory. Some work suggests that thinking about information within an adaptive, survival context can boost memory.

MEMORY FOR THE FUTURE

As noted at the beginning of the chapter, episodic memory involves mental time travel. Up to now we have been talking about travel backward in time. That is, episodic memory for what happened in the past. Here we consider mental time travel into the future. That is, episodic memory for what will happen. The primary reason we have memory is not so that we can think about the past but so that we can think about what we will do in the future (Klein, 2013a). After all, survival is more likely for creatures that have expectation, prediction, and planning ability. There are two types of future memories considered here. The first is remembering to do something in the future, which is prospective memory. The other is the ability to imagine how events will unfold in the future, which is episodic future thinking.

Prospective Memory

Prospective memory is remembering to do things in the future (Loftus, 1971). Remembering to give your roommate a message or to take the pizza out of the oven in 20 minutes are both examples of prospective memory. The (un)successful operation of prospective memory plays a critical role in the adherence of patients to their medication schedules (Zogg et al., 2012). Prospective memory can also be thought of as remembering to not do something that is normally done (Pink & Dodson, 2013), such as remembering not to back the car out of the garage after new cement has just been put down in the driveway. On average, we spontaneously engage in prospective memory about 15% of our waking time (Anderson & McDaniel, 2019).

Prospective memory has been tested many ways. Some are naturalistic, such as having people remember to call an experimenter at certain times (West, 1988). Others are laboratory-based, such as having people press a button when they see a certain word (Einstein & McDaniel, 1990) or after a certain amount of time has elapsed. Some studies have struck a middle ground and use virtual environments (Trawley et al., 2011). Performance under these conditions differs. For example, people tend to be under-confident for laboratory prospective memory tasks and over-confident in everyday life (Cauvin et al., 2019).

In general, the more important a prospective memory task is, the more likely it is to be done (Walter & Meier, 2014). Once a task is completed, although it is no longer as active in memory, it may be reactivated later, causing problems, such as doing a task again (see Möschl et al., 2020, for a review).

There are many differences between prospective and **retrospective memory** (memory for the past). Prospective memory has some components that are not found in retrospective memory. Prospective memory involves: (1) monitoring the environment for the cue to do something, (2) remembering what to do in the future, (3) retrieving the memory of what to do, and (4) actually doing it. Number 2 is like retrospective memory. Thus, prospective memory depends somewhat on retrospective memory but not vice versa. Prospective memory involves monitoring of the environment for a cue to remember, as well as the imagining of what will be done, a form of episodic future thinking (see next section) (Terrett et al., 2016). This is absent in retrospective memory.

Prospective memory requires control of thought, a frontal lobe function, and conscious experience to a greater degree. Thus, people are more aware of prospective than retrospective memory errors. People who complain about memory problems are more likely to have prospective memory problems (Mäntylä, 2003). Some prospective memory tasks requires a constant monitoring of the environment, much like a vigilance task. This may come at some cost as people have fewer resources for other tasks, especially if they have a large number of things that they need to remember to do (Hicks et al., 2005).

There are two traditional types of prospective memory: event-based and time-based (Einstein & McDaniel, 1990). **Event-based prospective memory** is a need to remember to do something when some event occurs—for example, remembering to give people a message when you see them. Event-based prospective memory is influenced by the relation between the event that is supposed to signal you to remember and the action to be done (McDaniel et al., 2004). When they are semantically related (e.g., write down the word "needle" when you hear the word "thread"), prospective memory is more automatic and is less influenced by things like divided attention. However, if they are not related (e.g., write down the word "needle" when you hear the word "parasol"), prospective memory is more deliberate and is more easily disrupted if attention is drawn elsewhere.

Event-based prospective memory also is harder when there are multiple cues as opposed to one and even more difficult if those cues are unrelated to one another (Marsh et al., 2003). Attention is drawn away from the prospective memory task when it is divided up among different things in the environment that we need to watch out for.

Time-based prospective memory is when people need to remember to do something at a certain time or after a certain time interval. Remembering to call home on Mother's Day or to take another pill in four hours are examples of time-based prospective memory. Time-based prospective memory is harder than event-based prospective memory (Einstein et al., 1995). With event-based prospective memory, there is something in the environment that reminds you to do something. With time-based prospective memory, it is up to you alone to remember. We can improve time-based prospective memory by making it more event-based. For example, you could set a timer and just wait for the buzzer to go off (an event) to remind you to take your pill.

With time-based prospective memory, people make more errors if the tasks are repetitive—for example, taking medications after certain intervals. The more people have done a task, the more likely an error will be made. Part of what is going on is that source monitoring errors occur (see Chapter 13), which then cause problems with prospective memory (Einstein et al., 1998). For example, we may be confused and think that we had just taken medication, when in fact we are remembering another time that we did so. This is a case in which doing something frequently actually makes memory worse, not better.

A third type of prospective memory that is not as well-researched is **activity-based prospective memory**. Here, people are asked to do something after another task has been completed (e.g., Kumar et al., 2008). For example, people might be asked to call their doctor after they are done watching a television show. Thus, prospective memory can guide action sequences.

Finally, there is **location-based prospective memory**. Here, people are to do something when they are in a particular place, such as when they are at a certain store in the mall (O'Rear & Radvansky, 2019). This may differ from other types of prospective memory because changes in location are a way to define new events.

Another issue is the relation between a prospective memory task and an on-going task in which it is embedded, particularly for event-based prospective memory. That is, whether the prospective memory task is focal or non-focal (McDaniel & Einstein, 2011). A prospective memory task is **focal** when it is part of the on-going task. For example, suppose that you see a list of animal names and you are to classify whether you would display them in a zoo (e.g., you would respond "yes" to "penguin", and "no" to "squirrel"). The prospective memory task might be pressing the space bar if you see the word "lion". This is a focal task because attention is already directed to the prospective memory cue as part of the on-going task.

A prospective memory task is **non-focal** when it is not part of the on-going task. For example, suppose during the animal classification task, instead of monitoring for the word "lion", you were to press the space bar whenever a small box in the upper left-hand corner of the screen flashed three times. When attention is divided, as it is with a non-focal task, prospective memory is worse, suggesting that some element of cognitive control is needed (Harrison et al., 2014).

The distinction between focal and non-focal tasks maps onto different neurological processes, as revealed by fMRI and MEG studies. On the one hand, focal tasks involve more working memory processes and are more likely to involve medial temporal lobe processes (McDaniel & Einstein, 2011) or posterior parietal lobe (Martin et al., 2007). However, non-focal tasks rely on more frontal lobe processes (Cockburn, 1995; Simons et al., 2006) because people need to disengage from the current task and attend to something else.

Episodic Future Thinking

Another way that episodic memory is involved in the future is when we imagine or plan for what may happen in the future. For example, thinking about how you will spend your afternoon today, how will you get that special someone to notice you, or what will happen if you drive in today's heavy snowfall. This is **episodic future thinking** (Atance & O'Neill, 2001; Szpunar, 2010) or **future-oriented mental time travel** (Klein, 2013b). Episodic future thinking allows us to predict and prepare for the future by planning how things may unfold over time (Klein et al., 2010). This is something that we do often, about every 15 minutes or so (D'Argembeau et al., 2011), and often involves our current concerns (Cole & Berntsen, 2016). Episodic future thinking is often correlated with prospective memory processes (e.g., Terrett et al., 2016).

Episodic future thinking uses many of the same neurological processes as episodic retrospective memory (Addis & Schacter, 2008), including the left hippocampus processing and posterior visual processing (Addis et al., 2007; Szpunar et al., 2007). The retention and projection of episodic memories and future thoughts follow similar gradients, such as the patterns shown in Figure 7.12. The distance into the past or the future engages the left posterior hippocampus (which is involved in contextual aspects of episodic memory) to similar degrees, regardless of the direction of time (Addis & Schacter, 2008; Spreng & Levine, 2006).

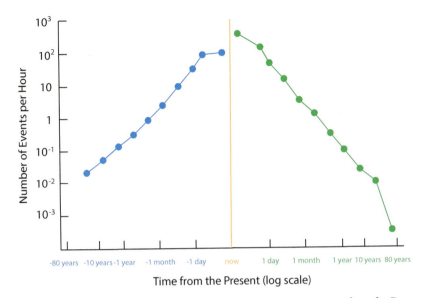

FIGURE 7.12 *Episodic Past and Future Thinking Functions Showing that the Pattern of Event Memories Reported Is Roughly Symmetrical for Various Distances from the Present*

Source: adapted from Spreng, R. N., & Levine, B. (2006). The temporal distribution of past and future autobiographical events across the lifespan. *Memory & Cognition, 34*(8), 1644–1651

When we think about the future, we use our prior episodic memories of similar experiences to guide what we imagine the future will be like (Szpunar & McDermott, 2008). This is the **constructive episodic simulation hypothesis** (Schacter & Addis, 2007). This is mental time travel because it feels as though we are pre-experiencing future events in much the same way that we are re-experiencing events from the past (D'Argembeau & Van der Linden, 2004). The more thoughts of the future conform to episodic experiences, the easier they are to construct (Szpunar & Schacter, 2013). For example, it is easier to imagine a future event involving yourself and two friends from school (because you have had experiences with them together in the past), than to imagine a future event involving yourself, a friend from school, and a friend from work (because these are different social circles, and so involve different events).

That said, there are differences in processing past and future events. In general, episodic future thinking is harder than remembering past events, is less vivid, more positive, and more important for your life story (we tend to think about the future in terms of how we would like life to unfold) (Anderson et al., 2012; Berntsen & Bohn, 2010). Neurologically, the anterior hippocampus, the right frontopolar cortex (BA 10), and the left ventromedial prefrontal cortex (BAs 14, 25 & 32) are more engaged for future events (Addis et al., 2007; Okuda et al., 2003). There is also some evidence that the left precuneus in the parietal lobe (BA 7) and parts of the right cerebellum are more active during episodic future thinking (Szpunar et al., 2007).

Stop and Review

Episodic memory is important for thinking about events of the future. Prospective memory is remembering to do something in the future. This can be event-based, time-based, or activity-based. Each has its own demands and challenges. Moreover, the ease with which a prospective memory is done is a consequence of whether it is focal or nonfocal. Another future-oriented use of memory is episodic future thinking. This draws on episodic memories of the past as a guide to thinking about the future, as well as using similar neurological structures. That said, episodic future thoughts being harder to create are also more positive and central to the life narrative.

PUTTING IT ALL TOGETHER

Episodic memory is your mental time travel device. Much of this is done using the integrative and binding abilities of the hippocampus. Episodic memories allow you to revisit prior experiences and events. You also use them to plan and prepare for the future. You integrate and interleave information with the current context. Your thought processes, emotions, and bodily states also serve as contexts. This includes transfer appropriate processing, mood dependent, and state dependent memory. To better remember something, you practice it. How well your practice improves memory reflects whether you practice the material all at once (bad) or distribute it (good); whether you continue to study or take a test; or other factors. With the right kind of practice, you can overlearn the information, consolidate it, and retain it for years. Finally, episodic memories give you the basis for thinking about what will happen in the future.

Episodic memory captures information at different levels of detail and gist. Knowledge of the context gets into your memories and plays an important role in the ability to remember, as with encoding specificity. This is as true for the spatial–temporal framework of your experiences as it is for the elements that make it up, such as the sights, sounds, and smells. These bits and pieces can then be used to cue yourself about what happened before. When learning, you improve your memory by emphasizing what is distinct, as well as linking and organizing it with other things. Which of these is better depends on what is lacking in the material itself. Finally, in terms of the future, episodic memory is important for planning how to interact with the world, as with prospective memory.

STUDY QUESTIONS

1. What is meant by the concept of mental time travel and why is this important for episodic memory?
2. What is the influence of the serial order of events on episodic memory?
3. What are the kinds of knowledge that are stored in episodic memories?
4. What kind of information can cue episodic memories? Are some cues better than others?

5. How does context influence episodic memory? What are the different types of contexts?
6. What does transfer appropriate processing tell us about what information is stored in episodic memory and how it is remembered later?
7. What are the different types of practice that we can engage in? Which of these is better for later memory retrieval?
8. What are the different explanations for why distributed practice is better than massed practice?
9. What are the different schedules of distributed practice, and which of these seems to serve as a better aid to memory over long periods of time?
10. What is overlearning, how does it come about, and what are the consequences for long-term memory?
11. What is the testing effect?
12. How does organization help episodic memory? How does distinctiveness help episodic memory? How are they opposites? How can this puzzle be resolved?
13. How does the distinction between item-specific and relational information influence later episodic memory?
14. How do fuzzy trace theories explain how our memories can be both accurate and general at the same time?
15. What is adaptive memory and how does it relate to the concept of evolution?
16. What is prospective memory? How does it compare to retrospective memory?
17. What are the different types of prospective memory? How is prospective memory affected by retention intervals?
18. What is episodic future thinking? How does this relate to episodic retroactive thinking?

KEY TERMS

- activity-based prospective memory
- animacy effect
- bizarre imagery effect
- consolidation account
- constructive episodic simulation hypothesis
- contextual variability account
- cuing, deficient-processing account
- distributed practice
- encoding specificity principle
- episodic future thinking
- episodic memories
- event-based prospective memory

- focal
- future-oriented mental time travel
- fuzzy trace theories
- isolation effect
- item-specific processing
- location-based prospective memory
- massed practice
- material appropriate processing
- mental time travel
- mood-congruent memory
- mood-dependent memory
- non-focal
- organization
- overlearning

- permastore
- relational processing
- repetition effect
- retrieval practice effect
- retrospective memory
- schedules of practice
- self-reference effect
- semantic memory
- state-dependent memory
- study-phase retrieval account
- testing effect
- time-based prospective memory
- transfer appropriate processing
- von Restorff effect

EXPLORE MORE

Here are some additional readings to allow you to explore more deeply issues involving episodic memory.

Bahrick, H. P. (1984). Semantic memory content in permastore: Fifty years of memory for Spanish learned in school. *Journal of Experimental Psychology: General, 113*(1), 1–29.

Hunt, R. R., & McDaniel, M. A. (1993). The enigma of organization and distinctiveness. *Journal of Memory and Language, 32*(4), 421–445.

Klein, S. B. (2013). The temporal orientation of memory: It's time for a change of direction. *Journal of Applied Research in Memory and Cognition, 2*(4), 222–234.

Smith, S. M., & Vela, E. (2001). Environmental context-dependent memory: A review and meta-analysis. *Psychonomic Bulletin & Review, 8,* 203–220.

Szpunar, K. K. (2010). Episodic future thought: An emerging concept. *Perspectives on Psychological Science, 5*(2), 142–162.

Tulving, E. (1983). *Elements of Episodic Memory.* New York: Oxford University Press.

REFERENCES

Addis, D. R., & Schacter, D. L. (2008). Constructive episodic simulation: Temporal distance and detail of past and future events modulate hippocampal engagement. *Hippocampus, 18*(2), 227–237.

Addis, D. R., Wong, A. T., & Schacter, D. L. (2007). Remembering the past and imagining the future: Common and distinct neural substrates during event construction and elaboration. *Neuropsychologia, 45*(7), 1363–1377.

Akan, M., Stanley, S. E., & Benjamin, A. S. (2018). Testing enhances memory for context. *Journal of Memory and Language, 103,* 19–27.

Anderson, F. T., & McDaniel, M. A. (2019). Hey buddy, why don't we take it outside: An experience sampling study of prospective memory. *Memory & Cognition, 47*(1), 47–62.

Anderson, R. J., Dewhurst, S. A., & Nash, R. A. (2012). Shared cognitive processes underlying past and future thinking: The impact of imagery and concurrent task demands on event specificity. *Journal of Experimental Psychology: Learning, Memory, and Cognition, 38*(2), 356–265.

Antony, J. W., Ferreira, C. S., Norman, K. A., & Wimber, M. (2017). Retrieval as a fast route to memory consolidation. *Trends in Cognitive Sciences, 21*(8), 573–576.

Arnold, K. M., & McDermott, K. B. (2013). Free recall enhances subsequent learning. *Psychonomic Bulletin & Review, 20*(3), 507–513.

Atance, C. M., & O'Neill, D. K. (2001). Episodic future thinking. *Trends in Cognitive Sciences, 5*(12), 533–539.

Axmacher, N., Cohen, M. X., Fell, J., Haupt, S., Dümpelmann, M., Elger, C. E., Schlaepfer, T. E., Lenartz, D., Sturm, V., & Ranganath, C. (2010). Intracranial EEG correlates of expectancy and memory formation in the human hippocampus and nucleus accumbens. *Neuron, 65*(4), 541–549.

Bahrick, H. P. (1984). Semantic memory content in permastore: Fifty years of memory for Spanish learned in school. *Journal of Experimental Psychology: General, 113*(1), 1–29.

Bahrick, H. P., Bahrick, L. E., Bahrick, A. S., & Bahrick, P. E. (1993). Maintenance of foreign language vocabulary and the spacing effect. *Psychological Science, 4*(5), 316–321.

Bäuml, K. H. T., Holterman, C., & Abel, M. (2014). Sleep can reduce the testing effect: It enhances recall of restudied items but can leave recall of retrieved items unaffected. *Journal of Experimental Psychology: Learning, Memory, and Cognition, 40*(6), 1568.

Bell, M. C., Kawadri, N., Simone, P. M., & Wiseheart, M. (2014). Long-term memory, sleep, and the spacing effect. *Memory, 22*(3), 276–283.

Bell, R., Röer, J. P., & Buchner, A. (2015). Adaptive memory: Thinking about function. *Journal of Experimental Psychology: Learning, Memory, and Cognition, 41*(4), 1038.

Benjamin, A. S., & Tullis, J. (2010). What makes distributed practice effective? *Cognitive Psychology, 61*(3), 228–247.

Berntsen, D., & Bohn, A. (2010). Remembering and forecasting: The relation between autobiographical memory and episodic future thinking. *Memory & Cognition, 38*(3), 265–278.

Blaney, P. H. (1986). Affect and memory: A review. *Psychological Bulletin, 99*, 229–246.

Bower, G. H. (1981). Mood and memory. *American Psychologist, 36*, 129–148.

Bower, G. H., Clark, M. C., Lesgold, A. M., & Winzenz, D. (1969). Hierarchical retrieval schemes in recall of categorized word lists. *Journal of Verbal Learning and Verbal Behavior, 8*, 323–343.

Brainerd, C. J., & Reyna, V. F. (1990). Gist is the grist: Fuzzy-trace theory and the new intuitionism. *Developmental Review, 10*(1), 3–47.

Bransford, J. D., Barclay, J. R., & Franks, J. J. (1972). Sentence memory: A constructive versus interpretive approach. *Cognitive Psychology, 3*, 193–209.

Bransford, J. D., & Stein, B. S. (1984). *The Ideal Problem Solver*. New York: Freeman.

Carpenter, S. K. (2009). Cue strength as a moderator of the testing effect: The benefits of elaborative retrieval. *Journal of Experimental Psychology: Learning, Memory, and Cognition, 35*(6), 1563–1569.

Cauvin, S., Moulin, C., Souchay, C., Schnitzspahn, K., & Kliegel, M. (2019). Laboratory vs. naturalistic prospective memory task predictions: Young adults are overconfident outside of the laboratory. *Memory, 27*(5), 592–602.

Clark, D. P. A., & Bruno, D. (2016). Fit to last: Exploring the longevity of the survival processing effect. *Quarterly Journal of Experimental Psychology, 69*(6), 1164–1178.

Cockburn, J. (1995). Task interruption in prospective memory: A frontal lobe function? *Cortex, 31*, 87–97.

Cole, S. N., & Berntsen, D. (2016). Do future thoughts reflect personal goals? Current concerns and mental time travel into the past and future. *Quarterly Journal of Experimental Psychology, 69*(2), 273–284.

Conway, M. A., Cohen, G., & Stanhope, N. (1991). On the very long-term retention of knowledge acquired through formal education: Twelve years of cognitive psychology. *Journal of Experimental Psychology: General, 120*(4), 395.

Corballis, M. C. (2013). Wandering tales: Evolutionary origins of mental time travel and language. *Frontiers in Psychology, 4*(485), 10–3389.

D'Argembeau, A., Renaud, O., & Van der Linden, M. (2011). Frequency, characteristics and functions of future-oriented thoughts in daily life. *Applied Cognitive Psychology, 25*(1), 96–103.

D'Argembeau, A., & Van der Linden, M. (2004). Phenomenal characteristics associated with projecting oneself back into the past and forward into the future: Influence of valence and temporal distance. *Consciousness and Cognition, 13*(4), 844–858.

Diana, R. A., Yonelinas, A. P., & Ranganath, C. (2013). Parahippocampal cortex activation during context reinstatement predicts item recollection. *Journal of Experimental Psychology: General, 142*(4), 1287–1297.

Driskell, J. E., Willis, R. P., & Copper, C. (1992). Effect of overlearning on retention. *Journal of Applied Psychology, 77*(5), 615–622.

Ebbinghaus, H. (1885). *Memory: A Contribution to Experimental Psychology* (H. A. Ruger & C. E. Bussenius, Trans.). New York: Teachers College, Columbia University.

Eich, J. E., Weingartner, H., Stillman, R. C., & Gillin, J. C. (1975). State-dependent accessibility of retrieval cues in the retention of a categorized list. *Journal of Verbal Learning and Verbal Behavior, 14*, 408–417.

Einstein, G. O., & McDaniel, M. A. (1987). Distinctiveness and the mnemonic benefits of bizarre imagery. In M. A. McDaniel & M. Pressley (Eds.), *Imagery and Related Mnemonic Processes: Theories, Individual Differences, and Applications* (pp. 78–102). New York: Springer.

Einstein, G. O., & McDaniel, M. A. (1990). Normal aging and prospective memory. *Journal of Experimental*

Psychology: Learning, Memory, and Cognition, 16(4), 717–726.

Einstein, G. O., McDaniel, M. A., Owen, P. D., & Coté, N. C. (1990). Encoding and recall of texts: The importance of material appropriate processing. *Journal of Memory and Language, 29*(5), 566–581.

Einstein, G. O., McDaniel, M. A., Richardson, S. L., Guynn, M. J., & Cunfer, A. R. (1995). Aging and prospective memory: Examining the influences of self-initiated retrieval processes. *Journal of Experimental Psychology: Learning, Memory, and Cognition, 21*(4), 996–1007.

Einstein, G. O., McDaniel, M. A., Smith, R., & Shaw, P. (1998). Habitual prospective memory and aging: Remembering intentions and forgetting actions. *Psychological Science, 9,* 284–288.

Ezzyat, Y., & Davachi, L. (2011). What constitutes an episode in episodic memory? *Psychological Science, 22*(2), 243–252.

Fisher, J. S., & Radvansky, G. A. (2018). Patterns of forgetting. *Journal of Memory and Language, 102,* 130–141.

Flores, S., Bailey, H. R., Eisenberg, M. L., & Zacks, J. M. (2017). Event segmentation improves event memory up to one month later. *Journal of Experimental Psychology: Learning, Memory, and Cognition, 43*(8), 1183–1202.

Gates, A. I. (1917). Recitation as a factor in memorizing. *Archives of Psychology, 6*(40).

Gerbier, E., & Koenig, O. (2012). Influence of multiple-day temporal distribution of repetitions on memory: A comparison of uniform, expanding, and contracting schedules. *Quarterly Journal of Experimental Psychology, 65*(3), 514–525.

Glenberg, A. M. (1976). Monotonic and nonmonotonic lag effects in paired-associate and recognition memory paradigms. *Journal of Verbal Learning and Verbal Behavior, 15*(1), 1–16.

Glenberg, A. M. (1979). Component-levels theory of the effects of spacing of repetitions on recall and recognition. *Memory & Cognition, 7*(2), 95–112.

Glenberg, A. M., & Lehmann, T. S. (1980). Spacing repetitions over 1 week. *Memory & Cognition, 8*(6), 528–538.

Glenberg, A. M., Meyer, M., & Lindem, K. (1987). Mental models contribute to foregrounding during text comprehension. *Journal of Memory and Language, 26,* 69–83.

Glover, J. A. (1989). The "testing" phenomenon: Not gone but nearly forgotten. *Journal of Educational Psychology, 81*(3), 392–399.

Godden, D. R., & Baddeley, A. D. (1975). Context-dependent memory in two natural environments: On land and underwater. *British Journal of Psychology, 66,* 325–331.

Goh, W. D. (2005). Talker variability and recognition memory: Instance-specific and voice-specific effects. *Journal of Experimental Psychology: Learning, Memory, and Cognition, 31*(1), 40–53.

Goodwin, D. W., Powell, B., Bremer, D., Hoine, H., & Stern, J. (1969). Alcohol and recall: State-dependent effects in man. *Science, 163,* 2358–2360.

Gutchess, A., & Kensinger, E. A. (2018). Shared mechanisms may support mnemonic benefits from self-referencing and emotion. *Trends in Cognitive Sciences, 22*(8), 712–724.

Harrison, T. L., Mullet, H. G., Whiffen, K. N., Ousterhout, H., & Einstein, G. O. (2014). Prospective memory: Effects of divided attention on spontaneous retrieval. *Memory & Cognition, 42*(2), 212–224.

Hart, J., & Burns, D. J. (2012). Nothing concentrates the mind: Thoughts of death improve recall. *Psychonomic Bulletin & Review, 19*(2), 264–269.

Hassabis, D., & Maguire, E. A. (2007). Deconstructing episodic memory with construction. *Trends in Cognitive Sciences, 11*(7), 299–306.

Healy, A. F., Havas, D. A., & Parker, J. T. (2000). Comparing serial position effects in semantic and episodic memory using reconstruction of order tasks. *Journal of Memory and Language, 42*(2), 147–167.

Herz, R. S., & Engen, T. (1996). Odor memory: Review and analysis. *Psychonomic Bulletin & Review, 3,* 300–313.

Hicks, J. L., Marsh, R. L., & Cook, G. I. (2005). Task interference in time-based, event-based, and dual intention prospective memory conditions. *Journal of Memory and Language, 53,* 430–444.

Hintzman, D. L. (1974). Theoretical implications of the spacing effect. In R. L. Solso (Ed.), *Theories in Cognitive Psychology: The Loyola Symposium* (pp. 77–99). Potomac, MD: Erlbaum.

Hu, X., Cheng, L. Y., Chiu, M. H., & Paller, K. A. (2020). Promoting memory consolidation during sleep: A meta-analysis of targeted memory reactivation. *Psychological Bulletin, 146*(3), 218–244.

Hunt, R. R. (1995). The subtlety of distinctiveness: What von Restorff really did. *Psychonomic Bulletin & Review, 2*(1), 105–112.

Hunt, R. R., & McDaniel, M. A. (1993). The enigma of organization and distinctiveness. *Journal of Memory and Language, 32*(4), 421–445.

Hunt, R. R., & Seta, C. E. (1984). Category size effects in recall: The roles of relational and individual item information. *Journal of Experimental Psychology: Learning, Memory, and Cognition, 10*(3), 454–464.

Johansson, R. & Johansson, M. (2013). Look here, eye movements play a functional role in memory retrieval. *Psychological Science, 25*(1), 236–242.

Johnson-Laird, P. N. (1983). *Mental Models*. Cambridge, MA: Harvard University Press.

Kang, S. H. K., Lindsey, R. V., Mozer, M. C., & Pashler, H. (2014). Retrieval practice over the long term: Should spacing be expanding or equal-interval? *Psychonomic Bulletin & Review, 21*(6), 1544–1550.

Karpicke, J. D. (2012). Retrieval-based learning: Active retrieval promotes meaningful learning. *Current Directions in Psychological Science, 21*(3), 157–163.

Karpicke, J. D., & Roediger, H. L. (2010). Is expanding retrieval a superior method for learning text materials? *Memory & Cognition, 38*(1), 116–124.

Kesebir, S., & Oishi, S. (2010). A spontaneous self-reference effect in memory: Why some birthdays are harder to remember than others. *Psychological Science, 21*(10), 1525–1531.

Kim, H., & Cabeza, R. (2007). Differential contributions of prefrontal, medial temporal, and sensory-perceptual regions to true and false memory formation. *Cerebral Cortex, 17*(9), 2143–2150.

Klein, S. B. (2012). A role for self-referential processing in tasks requiring participants to imagine survival on the savannah. *Journal of Experimental Psychology: Learning, Memory, and Cognition, 38*(5), 1234.

Klein, S. B. (2013a). The complex act of projecting oneself into the future. *Wiley Interdisciplinary Reviews: Cognitive Science, 4*(1), 63–79.

Klein, S. B. (2013b). The temporal orientation of memory: It's time for a change of direction. *Journal of Applied Research in Memory and Cognition, 2*(4), 222–234.

Klein, S. B. (2014). The effects of thoughts of survival and thoughts of death on recall in the adaptive memory paradigm. *Memory, 22*(1), 65–75.

Klein, S. B., Robertson, T. E., & Delton, A. W. (2010). Facing the future: Memory as an evolved system for planning future acts. *Memory & Cognition, 38*(1), 13–22.

Klein, S. B., Robertson, T. E., & Delton, A. W. (2011). The future-orientation of memory: Planning as a key component mediating the high levels of recall found with survival processing. *Memory, 19*(2), 121–139.

Kroneisen, M., & Erdfelder, E. (2011). On the plasticity of the survival processing effect. *Journal of Experimental Psychology: Learning, Memory, and Cognition, 37*(6), 1553.

Kumar, D., Nizamie, S. H., & Jahan, M. (2008). Activity-based prospective memory in schizophrenia. *The Clinical Neuropsychologist, 22*(3), 497–506.

Landauer, T. K. (1969). Reinforcement as consolidation. *Psychological Review, 76*(1), 82–96.

Lehman, M., Smith, M. A., & Karpicke, J. D. (2014). Toward an episodic context account of retrieval-based learning: Dissociating retrieval practice and elaboration. *Journal of Experimental Psychology: Learning, Memory, and Cognition, 40*, 1787–1794.

Lindsey, R. V., Shroyer, J. D., Pashler, H., & Mozer, M. C. (2014). Improving students' long-term knowledge retention through personalized review. *Psychological Science, 25*(3), 639–647.

Loftus, E. F. (1971). Memory for intentions: The effect of presence of a cue and interpolated activity. *Psychonomic Science, 23*, 315–316.

Maddox, G. B. (2016). Understanding the underlying mechanism of the spacing effect in verbal learning: A case for encoding variability and study-phase retrieval. *Journal of Cognitive Psychology, 28*(6), 684–706.

Mäntylä, T. (2003). Assessing absentmindedness: Prospective memory complaint and impairment in middle-aged adults. *Memory & Cognition, 31*, 15–25.

Maratos, E. J., Dolan, R. J., Morris, J. S., Henson, R. N. A., & Rugg, M. D. (2001). Neural activity associated with episodic memory for emotional context. *Neuropsychologia, 39*(9), 910–920.

Marian, V., & Neisser, U. (2000). Language-dependent recall of autobiographical memories. *Journal of Experimental Psychology: General, 129*(3), 361–368.

Martin, T., McDaniel, M. A., Guynn, M. J., Houck, J. M., Woodruff, C. C., Bish, J. P., Moses, S. N., Kičić, D., & Tesche, C. D. (2007). Brain regions and their dynamics in prospective memory retrieval: A MEG study. *International Journal of Psychophysiology, 64*(3), 247–258.

McDaniel, M. A., & Einstein, G. O. (1986). Bizarre imagery as an effective memory aid: The importance of distinctiveness. *Journal of Experimental Psychology: Learning, Memory, and Cognition, 12*(1), 54–65.

Marsh, R. L., Hicks, J. L., Cook, G. I., Hansen, J. S., & Pallos, A. L. (2003). Interference to ongoing activities covaries with the characteristics of an event-based intention. *Journal of Experimental Psychology: Learning, Memory, and Cognition, 29*(5), 861–870.

McDaniel, M. A., & Einstein, G. O. (2011). The neuropsychology of prospective memory in normal aging: A componential approach. *Neuropsychologia, 49*(8), 2147–2155.

McDaniel, M. A., Guynn, M. J., Einstein, G. O., & Breneiser, J. (2004). Cue-focused and reflexive-associative processes in prospective memory retrieval. *Journal of Experimental Psychology: Learning, Memory, and Cognition, 30*, 605–614.

Meinhardt, M. J., Bell, R., Buchner, A., & Röer, J. P. (2020). Adaptive memory: Is the animacy effect on memory due to richness of encoding? *Journal of Experimental Psychology: Learning, Memory, and Cognition, 46*(3), 416–426.

Metcalfe, J., & Xu, J. (2016). People mind wander more during massed than spaced inductive learning. *Journal of Experimental Psychology: Learning, Memory, and Cognition, 42*(6), 978–984.

Miles, C., & Hardman, E. (1998). State-dependent memory produced by aerobic exercise. *Ergonomics, 41*(1), 20–28.

Morris, C. D., Bransford, J. D., & Franks, J. J. (1977). Levels of processing versus transfer appropriate processing. *Journal of Verbal Learning and Verbal Behavior, 16*(5), 519–533.

Möschl, M., Fischer, R., Bugg, J. M., Scullin, M. K., Goschke, T., & Walser, M. (2020). Aftereffects and deactivation of completed prospective memory intentions: A systematic review. *Psychological Bulletin, 146*(3), 245–278.

Mulligan, N. W., & Lozito, J. P. (2006). An asymmetry between memory encoding and retrieval: Revelation, generation, and transfer-appropriate processing. *Psychological Science, 17*(1), 7–11.

Nairne, J. S. (2002). The myth of the encoding–retrieval match. *Memory, 10*, 389–395.

Nairne, J. S., & Pandeirada, J. N. S. (2008). Adaptive memory: Is survival processing special? *Journal of Memory and Language, 59*(3), 377–385.

Nairne, J. S., & Pandeirada, J. N. (2016). Adaptive memory: The evolutionary significance of survival processing. *Perspectives on Psychological Science, 11*(4), 496–511.

Nairne, J. S., Pandeirada, J. N. S., & Thompson, S. R. (2008). Adaptive memory: The comparative value of survival processing. *Psychological Science, 19*(2), 176–180.

Nairne, J. S., VanArsdall, J. E., & Cogdill, M. (2017). Remembering the living: Episodic memory is tuned to animacy. *Current Directions in Psychological Science, 26*(1), 22–27.

Nairne, J. S., VanArsdall, J. E., Pandeirada, J. N. S., & Blunt, J. R. (2012). Adaptive memory: Enhanced location memory after survival processing. *Journal of Experimental Psychology: Learning, Memory, and Cognition, 38*(2), 495.

Nairne, J. S., VanArsdall, J. E., Pandeirada, J. N. S., Cogdill, M., & LeBreton, J. M. (2013). Adaptive memory: The mnemonic value of animacy. *Psychological Science, 24*(10), 2099–2105.

Nestojko, J. F., Bui, D. C., Kornell, N., & Bjork, E. L. (2014). Expecting to teach enhances learning and organization of knowledge in free recall of text passages. *Memory & Cognition, 42*(7), 1038–1048.

Noice, H., & Noice, T. (2006). What studies of actors and acting can tell us about memory and cognitive functioning. *Current Directions in Psychological Science, 15*(1), 14–18.

Noice, T., & Noice, H. (2002). Very long term recall and recognition of well learned material. *Applied Cognitive Psychology*, *16*(3), 259–272.

Okuda, J., Fujii, T., Ohtake, H., Tsukiura, T., Tanji, K., Suzuki, K., Kawashima, R., Fukuda, H., Itoh, M., & Yamadori, A. (2003). Thinking of the future and past: The roles of the frontal pole and the medial temporal lobes. *Neuroimage*, *19*(4), 1369–1380.

Olds, J. M., Lanska, M., & Westerman, D. L. (2014). The role of perceived threat in the survival processing memory advantage. *Memory*, *22*(1), 26–35.

O'Rear, A. E., & Radvansky, G. A. (2019). Location-based prospective memory. *Quarterly Journal of Experimental Psychology*, *72*(3), 491–507.

Paller, K. A. (2017). Sleeping in a brave new world: Opportunities for improving learning and clinical outcomes through targeted memory reactivation. *Current Directions in Psychological Science*, *26*(6), 532–537.

Peters, R., & McGee, R. (1982). Cigarette smoking and state-dependent memory. *Psychopharmacology*, *76*, 232–235.

Pink, J. E., & Dodson, C. S. (2013). Negative prospective memory: Remembering *not* to perform an action. *Psychonomic Bulletin & Review*, *20*(1), 184–190.

Racsmány, M., Conway, M. A., & Demeter, G. (2010). Consolidation of episodic memories during sleep: Long-term effects of retrieval practice. *Psychological Science*, *21*(1), 80–85.

Radvansky, G. A., & Zacks, J. M. (2014). *Event Cognition*. Oxford University Press.

Ranganath, C. (2010). Binding items and contexts: The cognitive neuroscience of episodic memory. *Current Directions in Psychological Science*, *19*(3), 131–137.

Rawson, K. A., & Zamary, A. (2019). Why is free recall practice more effective than recognition practice for enhancing memory? Evaluating the relational processing hypothesis. *Journal of Memory and Language*, *105*, 141–152.

Rickard, T. C., & Pan, S. C. (2018). A dual memory theory of the testing effect. *Psychonomic Bulletin & Review*, *25*(3), 847–869.

Riefer, D. M., & Rouder, J. N. (1992). A multinomial modeling analysis of the mnemonic benefits of bizarre imagery. *Memory & Cognition*, *20*(6), 601–611.

Ritchey, M., & Cooper, R. A. (2020). Deconstructing the posterior medial episodic network. *Trends in Cognitive Sciences*, *24*(6), 451–465.

Roediger, H. L., & Blaxton, T. A. (1987). Effects of varying modality, surface features, and retention interval on priming in word-fragment completion. *Memory & Cognition*, *15*(5), 379–388.

Roediger, H. L., & Karpicke, J. D. (2006). The power of testing memory: Basic research and implications for educational practice. *Perspectives on Psychological Science*, *1*(3), 181–210.

Rogers, T. B., Kuiper, N. A., & Kirker, W. S. (1977). Self-reference and the encoding of personal information. *Journal of Personality and Social Psychology*, *35*(9), 677–688.

Rowland, C. A. (2014). The effect of testing versus restudy on retention: A meta-analytic review of the testing effect. *Psychological Bulletin*, *140*(6), 1432–1463.

Sachs, J. S. (1967). Recognition memory for syntactic and semantic aspects of connected discourse. *Perception & Psychophysics*, *2*(9), 437–442.

Schacter, D. L., & Addis, D. R. (2007). The cognitive neuroscience of constructive memory: Remembering the past and imagining the future. *Philosophical Transactions of the Royal Society of London B: Biological Sciences*, *362*(1481), 773–786.

Schendan, H. E., & Kutas, M. (2007). Neurophysiological evidence for the time course of activation of global shape, part, and local contour representations during visual object categorization and memory. *Journal of Cognitive Neuroscience*, *19*(5), 734–749.

Schmidt, S. R., & Schmidt, C. R. (2017). Revisiting von Restorff's early isolation effect. *Memory & Cognition*, *45*(2), 194–207.

Scofield, J. E., Buchanan, E. M., & Kostic, B. (2018). A meta-analysis of the survival-processing advantage in memory. *Psychonomic Bulletin & Review*, *25*(3), 997–1012.

Sehulster, J. R. (1989). Content and temporal structure of autobiographical knowledge: Remembering twenty-five seasons at the Metropolitan Opera. *Memory & Cognition*, *17*, 590–606.

Simons, J. S., Schölvinck, M. L., Gilbert, S. J., Frith, C. D., & Burgess, P. W. (2006). Differential components of prospective memory?: Evidence from fMRI. *Neuropsychologia, 44*(8), 1388–1397.

Smith, S. M., (1979). Remembering in and out of context. *Journal of Experimental Psychology: Human Learning and Memory, 5,* 460–471.

Smith, S. M., (1988). Environmental context–dependent memory. In G. M. Davies & D. M. Thomas (Eds.), *Memory in Context: Context in memory* (pp. 13–34). New York: Wiley.

Smith, S. M., Glenberg, A., & Bjork, R. A. (1978). Environmental context and human memory. *Memory & Cognition, 6,* 342–353.

Smith, S. M., Handy, J. D., Angello, G., & Manzano, I. (2014). Effects of similarity on environmental context cueing. *Memory, 22*(5), 493–508.

Smith, S. M., Handy, J. D., Hernandez, A., & Jacoby, L. L. (2018). Context specificity of automatic influences of memory. *Journal of Experimental Psychology: Learning, Memory, and Cognition, 44*(10), 1501–1513.

Smith, S. M., & Vela, E. (2001). Environmental context-dependent memory: A review and meta-analysis. *Psychonomic Bulletin & Review, 8,* 203–220.

Soderstrom, N. C., & McCabe, D. P. (2011). Are survival processing memory advantages based on ancestral priorities? *Psychonomic Bulletin & Review, 18*(3), 564–569.

Spitzer, H. F. (1939). Studies in retention. *Journal of Educational Psychology, 30*(9), 641.

Spreng, R. N., & Levine, B. (2006). The temporal distribution of past and future autobiographical events across the lifespan. *Memory & Cognition, 34*(8), 1644–1651.

Staresina, B. P., & Wimber, M. (2019). A neural chronometry of memory recall. *Trends in Cognitive Sciences, 23*(12) 1071–1085.

Swanson, J. M., & Kinsbourne, M. (1976). Stimulant-related state-dependent learning in hyperactive children. *Science, 192,* 1354–1356.

Symons, C. S., & Johnson, B. T. (1997). The self-reference effect in memory: A meta-analysis. *Psychological Bulletin, 121,* 371–394.

Szpunar, K. K. (2010). Episodic future thought: An emerging concept. *Perspectives on Psychological Science, 5*(2), 142–162.

Szpunar, K. K., & McDermott, K. B. (2008). Episodic future thought and its relation to remembering: Evidence from ratings of subjective experience. *Consciousness and Cognition, 17*(1), 330–334.

Szpunar, K. K., McDermott, K. B., & Roediger III, H. L. (2008). Testing during study insulates against the buildup of proactive interference. *Journal of Experimental Psychology: Learning, Memory, and Cognition, 34*(6), 1392–1399.

Szpunar, K. K., & Schacter, D. L. (2013). Get real: Effects of repeated simulation and emotion on the perceived plausibility of future experiences. *Journal of Experimental Psychology: General, 142*(2), 323–327.

Szpunar, K. K., Watson, J. M., & McDermott, K. B. (2007). Neural substrates of envisioning the future. *Proceedings of the National Academy of Sciences, 104*(2), 642–647.

Talmi, D., Luk, B. T. C., McGarry, L. M., & Moscovitch, M. (2007). The contribution of relatedness and distinctiveness to emotionally-enhanced memory. *Journal of Memory and Language, 56,* 555–574.

Terrett, G., Rose, N. S., Henry, J. D., Bailey, P. E., Altgassen, M., Phillips, L. H., Kliegel, M., & Rendell, P. G. (2016). The relationship between prospective memory and episodic future thinking in younger and older adulthood. *Quarterly Journal of Experimental Psychology, 69(2)*, 310–323.

Terry, W. S. (2000). *Learning and Memory: Basic Principles, Processes, and Procedures.* Boston, MA: Allyn & Bacon.

Thompson, D. M., & Tulving, E. (1970). Associative encoding and retrieval: Weak and strong cues. *Journal of Experimental Psychology, 86,* 255–262.

Trawley, S. L., Law, A. S., & Logie, R. H. (2011). Event-based prospective remembering in a virtual world. *Quarterly Journal of Experimental Psychology, 64*(11), 2181–2193.

Tulving, E. (1983). *Elements of Episodic Memory.* New York: Oxford University Press.

Tulving, E. (2002). Episodic memory: From mind to brain. *Annual Review of Psychology, 53,* 1–25.

Tulving, E., & Pearlstone, Z. (1966). Availability versus accessibility of information in memory for words. *Journal of Verbal Learning and Verbal Behavior, 5,* 381–391.

Van Dam, G., Peeck, J., Brinkerink, M., & Gorter, U. (1974). The isolation effect in free recall and recognition. *The American Journal of Psychology*, 87(3), 497–504.

van den Bos, M., Cunningham, S. J., Conway, M. A., & Turk, D. J. (2010). Mine to remember: The impact of ownership on recollective experience. *The Quarterly Journal of Experimental Psychology*, 63(6), 1065–1071.

van Dijk, T. A., & Kintsch, W. (1983). *Strategies of Discourse Comprehension*. New York: Academic Press.

Van Gog, T., & Sweller, J. (2015). Not new, but nearly forgotten: The testing effect decreases or even disappears as the complexity of learning materials increases. *Educational Psychology Review*, 27(2), 247–264.

Verkoeijen, P. P. J. L., Rikers, R. M. J. P., & Schmidt, H. G. (2004). Detrimental influence of contextual change on spacing effects in free recall. *Journal of Experimental Psychology: Learning, Memory, and Cognition*, 30(4), 796.

Walter, S., & Meier, B. (2014). How important is importance for prospective memory? A review. *Frontiers in Psychology*, 5(657), 10–3389.

Weinstein, Y., Bugg, J. M., & Roediger, H. L. (2008). Can the survival recall advantage be explained by basic memory processes? *Memory & Cognition*, 36(5), 913–919.

West, R. L. (1988). Prospective memory and aging. In M. M. Grunebberg, P. E. Morris, & R. N. Sykes (Eds.), *Practical Aspects of Memory: Current research and issues: Vol. 2. Clinical and educational implications* (pp. 119–125). New York: Wiley.

Wilkinson, A. M., Hall, A. C. G., & Hogan, E. E. (2019). Effects of retrieval practice and presentation modality on verbal learning: Testing the limits of the testing effect. *Memory*, 27(8), 1144–1157.

Wilson, M. A., & McNaughton, B. L. (1994). Reactivation of hippocampal ensemble memories during sleep. *Science*, 265(5172), 676–679.

Wurm, L. H. (2007). Danger and usefulness: An alternative framework for understanding rapid evaluation effects in perception? *Psychonomic Bulletin & Review*, 14(6), 1218–1225.

Zaromb, F. M., & Roediger, H. L. (2010). The testing effect in free recall is associated with enhanced organizational processes. *Memory & Cognition*, 38(8), 995–1008.

Zechmeister, E. B., & Shaughnessy, J. J. (1980). When you know that you know and when you think that you know but you don't. *Bulletin of the Psychonomic Society*, 15(1), 41–44.

Zogg, J. B., Woods, S. P., Sauceda, J. A., Wiebe, J. S., & Simoni, J. M. (2012). The role of prospective memory in medication adherence: A review of an emerging literature. *Journal of Behavioral Medicine*, 35(1), 47–62.

Zwaan, R. A., & Radvansky, G. A. (1998). Situation models in comprehension and memory. *Psychological Bulletin*, 123, 162–185.

CHAPTER 8

Forgetting

When our memories are working well and we can retrieve the knowledge that we need, we do not typically notice it. However, when our memory fails us, and we forget things, we are much more aware of its limitations. In general, when people take an interest in memory, the focus is not on remembering, but on the failure to remember, namely forgetting and how to avoid it. The type of forgetting that is of concern here is the normal, standard, everyday kind of forgetting that we experience in our lives. When the loss of information in memory exceeds this expected amount, it is no longer normal forgetting, and it crosses over into a catastrophic memory loss that is amnesia, which is the topic of Chapter 10. Often that kind of forgetting is due to some sort of trauma. Normal forgetting is not due to something wrong with the mind or brain but, instead, is a consequence of the normal operation of memory and how it manages information.

In our consideration of forgetting, and the idea that forgetting is something bad, we begin with Schacter's Seven Sins of Memory, along with a consideration of why these sins may actually be virtues. This is followed by coverage of the viability of decay, or the passage of time, as a mechanism of forgetting. After that, we consider one of the primary mechanisms of forgetting, namely interference. This is followed by a discussion of inhibition, which is used to regulate the influence of interference. After this we consider when people deliberately seek to forget information with directed forgetting and the management of knowledge that has been explicitly retracted. Then, we consider two aspects of experience that can influence the rate of forgetting, namely the collaborative forgetting that can occur when you try to remember things along with other people, and the influence of drugs and alcohol on forgetting.

THE SEVEN SINS OF MEMORY

In his book *The Seven Sins of Memory*, Schacter (2001) laid out memory problems as if they were seven sins. His seven sins of memory are: (1) transience, (2) absent-mindedness, (3) blocking, (4) misattribution, (5) suggestibility, (6) bias, and (7) persistence. An overview of each of these is presented here, followed by reasons why these seven sins may be virtues. Keep these in mind when you consider both parts of this chapter and other parts of this book.

Transience

The first sin of memory is transience. This is the idea that memories are forgotten with the passage of time. This is reflected in the Ebbinghaus forgetting curve introduced in Chapter 3. As a reminder, the more time that passes, the more likely that information is forgotten, with forgetting being more rapid early on and then slowing down as time progresses. Keep in mind that not all aspects of a memory are forgotten at once. Memories may still be present but become fragmented. The gaps in these memory fragments may be filled in with general knowledge (see Chapter 9). Thus, memory can go from being reproductive, in which the prior knowledge is brought back into working memory, to being reconstructive, in which people fill in the gaps that are created by forgetting. Alternatively, people may remember different features of objects or events but not remember to which they belong (Utochkin & Brady, 2020). For example, people may remember seeing two boxes and that one was open, but not remember which.

Absent-Mindedness

The second sin of memory is absent-mindedness. This is the idea that people are not paying attention when information is first encountered (and so it is never encoded into memory). As an example, Henkel (2014) had students at Fairfield University visit a museum. While there, they just looked at some objects and took photos of others. What she found was that when people took photographs, they remembered less than when they simply looked at the object. This happened because the act of taking a picture takes your attention away from what is going on, so you remember it less well.

Alternatively, absent-mindedness could occur if information makes it into memory, but people somehow fail to retrieve it. This reflects the distinction between availability and accessibility. Availability is whether a trace is even present somewhere in memory. It may not be available either because it was never encoded, or it was permanently lost. In comparison, accessibility is the idea that the trace is somewhere in memory, but the issue is whether people can successfully get to it. Sometimes forgetting occurs when a memory is available, but not accessible. Failure of accessibility can sometimes be overcome, as with cuing, or with the phenomena of reminiscence and hypermnesia, discussed in Chapter 3, in which previously forgotten information is remembered later. These memories were available but not accessible until later.

Another issue that absent-mindedness is relevant for is how does having attention divided among multiple tasks then influence later memory? Divided attention during learning clearly disrupts encoding, so we will not go too much into that here.[1] Of more interest is whether dividing attention during retrieval disrupts performance (Baddeley et al., 1984; Rohrer & Pashler, 2003). Distraction during

---

1 Multitasking while trying to learn is a very bad idea.

retrieval can slow the rate at which information is remembered, but overall accuracy is less affected, if at all. That said, divided attention can disrupt memory retrieval when the distracting task uses the same cognitive/neural systems (Fernandes & Moscovitch, 2000); for example, if you were trying to recall a list of words while at the same time listening to another set of words to assess whether any were repeated three times in a row. There may actually be some benefits for divided attention during retrieval. Kessler et al. (2014) found that dividing attention at retrieval can boost later memory, particularly if there is a 24-hour delay between learning and the first memory test. The effort needed to compensate for the retrieval difficulty on the first test boosts the memory, making it better retained and remembered.

Blocking

The third sin of memory is blocking. This is the idea that people have trouble accessing a desired memory because others get in the way. That is, these other memories block access to the desired one. For example, you may try to think of a person's name, but other, similar names keep popping up in your mind. This is the sin of memory that gets the most attention in this chapter when we discuss interference and inhibition. An idea that fits well with the blocking principle is the concept of cue overload in which the more things that are associated with a memory cue (i.e., the more memory traces that share that element), the less effective that cue is. The more memory traces associated with a cue, the more these other traces interfere with or block access to the desired memory. This harkens back to the idea discussed in Chapter 7 that the best memory cues are the ones that are most diagnostic. Diagnostic cues have low cue overload.

Misattribution

The fourth sin of memory is misattribution. This is the idea that people can remember something but misattribute where it came from. This is a forgetting of the nature of a memory, not its content. For example, you may mistakenly remember something about President Lincoln from a textbook you read, when in fact it was in a fictional movie that you saw. Misattribution can be striking, such as a feeling of déjà vu, or the more mundane experience of simply thinking that you remember information coming from one source, when in fact it came from somewhere else. Issues of source monitoring are covered in detail in Chapter 13. Moreover, Chapter 14 covers how misattribution can influence legal issues.

Suggestibility

The fifth sin of memory is suggestibility. This is when memories are implanted from outside sources, possibly causing correct information to be forgotten. This incorrect information may be introduced either explicitly or implicitly and may be done intentionally or unintentionally. Regardless of the circumstances, incorrect knowledge disrupts the memory. Issues of suggestibility are discussed in Chapter 13 where issues of memory and reality are brought into focus, as well as Chapter 14 in terms of incorrect information being suggested to witnesses.

Bias

The sixth sin of memory is bias. This is the idea that memory can be distorted toward what is currently known. For example, bias occurs if there is a forgetting of events or knowledge of your prior mental states, as a function of what is currently known. This was briefly covered in Chapter 3's discussion of the hindsight bias, and these memory biases are discussed in more detail in Chapter 15.

Persistence

The seventh sin of memory is persistence. This is when memory is compromised by incorrect knowledge that should be forgotten, but it is not. In other words, a failure to forget can be a problem. This incorrect information continues to infiltrate our stream of thought and distort memory, decision making, and thinking in general. The avoidance of persistence is covered in this chapter in the sections on directed forgetting and retraction.

The Virtues of Forgetting

The seven sins of memory can also be virtues. They occur for a reason and have some adaptive value. Transience and absent-mindedness are helpful because information that is not needed over long periods of time, perhaps because it is no longer relevant, falls out of accessible memory and does not clutter up processing. The shift from reproductive to reconstructive processes is helpful when we need to abstract generalities across a wide range of situations, rather than dealing with each new event from scratch. While blocking can occur because we may know so much and have so many experiences, the inhibition that can follow from the management of it helps streamline our thought and makes it more effective and efficient.

Misattribution and suggestibility are consequences of general memory processes that are clearly beneficial. While some things in the world are stable and consistent, others are in flux and change. This process allows these needed memory changes to be made. Alternatively, if we learn that our understanding of the world is incorrect, we need to modify our memory. For example, as a young child (like many children) you may have known that the Earth is round but thought that it is round like a plate. Or, perhaps, you knew that it is round like a ball but thought that we live on the inside of the ball. What you needed to do was alter your memory to contain the newer, correct information to update and improve your understanding. These processes are helpful. However, they are problematic when we update memory with information that is incorrect. Finally, the persistence of memories reflects the otherwise desired ability to hold onto information that might be useful in the future. This is only a problem when we retain information that is troubling or incorrect.

As you will see, one benefit of forgetting is that it causes memories that produce interference to be taken out of the current stream of processing, and thereby be less disruptive. Thus, while the inhibition of memories may seem like a negative consequence, it can actually be a benefit (Storm, 2011). Forgetting has also been suggested by Nørby (2015) to be helpful and adaptive for emotion regulation (it keeps us from dwelling on experiences that swing our emotions too far to the extremes), helping us to be more positive and forgiving. It also allows us to abstract away from the details to conceive of generalities, and it helps us disengage from the past, allowing us to focus on the present and the future.

Stop and Review

Forgetting is a big challenge to memory. Schacter has outlined his seven sins of memory, namely transience, absent-mindedness, blocking, misattribution, suggestibility, bias, and persistence. While these are described as sins, they also reflect more general memory processes that serve as virtues. Overall, forgetting likely exists because it is more efficient to lose some information rather than maintain all of it all, most of which may become irrelevant or inappropriate.

THE FORGETTING CURVE

A described in Chapter 3, importantly Ebbinghaus (1885) showed that memory changes over time, and this change is a regular negatively accelerating function (see Figure 3.8). Forgetting curves can help identify neurological disorders. For example, forgetting is more rapid in people who have neurological diseases, such as Alzheimer's Dementia, epilepsy, and traumatic brain injury (van der Werf et al., 2016). This rapid loss of memories, known as accelerated long-term forgetting, involves cases in which memory appears similar in impaired and normal people soon after learning, but differences emerge over time (e.g., weeks or months) (Elliott et al., 2014).

The negatively accelerating forgetting pattern has been widely observed (Rubin & Wenzel, 1996). However, Fisher and Radvansky (2019) reported that under some circumstances the pattern of forgetting is linear. To illustrate this difference, Figure 8.1 shows Ebbinghaus's data (top) plotted with a linear scale (left) and a logarithmic scale (right). The Fisher and Radvansky data (below) are similarly plotted. As you can see, a negatively accelerating pattern does not capture all the data very well. This is important because while a negatively accelerating pattern conveys a constant loss in the *proportion* of memories over time, a linear pattern of forgetting conveys a constant loss in the *amount* of information. That is, there is an *increase* in the proportion lost over time.

Why does linear forgetting occur? For Fisher and Radvansky (2019), this occurs if some criteria are met. First, the memories have many components or features. These features are forgotten following a standard Ebbinghaus pattern. Thus, during retrieval, there is only partial information available. However, we can

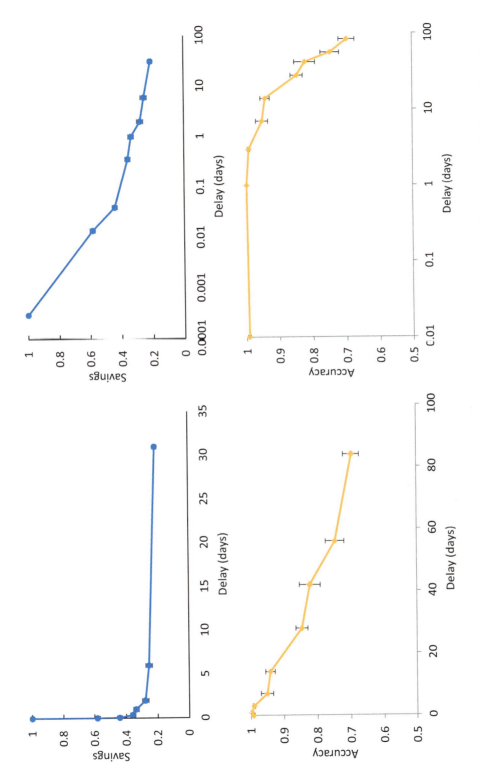

FIGURE 8.1 *Results of the Ebbinghaus (1885) (top) and Fisher and Radvansky (2019) Studies (Below). These Data Are Plotted with a Linear X-Axis (Left) and a Logarithmic X-Axis (Right)*

Source: created from data reported in Ebbinghaus, H. (1885/1964). *Memory: A Contribution to Experimental Psychology*. Translated by H. A. Ruger & C. E. Bussenius. New York: Dover; and Fisher, J. S., & Radvansky, G. A. (2019). Linear forgetting. *Journal of Memory and Language, 108*, 104035

reconstruct memories from these partial traces, and then give an accurate response, provided a sufficient portion of the memory is still accessible. Linear forgetting reflects a kind of averaging across traces along with memory reconstruction. Linear forgetting is more likely to be observed for complex memories (e.g., mental models) where there are many parts to a memory, allowing reconstruction to be more successful.

Stop and Review

The pattern of forgetting can be regular and stable. Science should allow us to predict what will be remembered in the future, to a reasonable degree. By knowing the pattern of forgetting, we can predict how much a person will likely remember after a given period of time.

FORGETTING THROUGH DECAY AND DISUSE

An intuitive account of forgetting is that as more time passes without a memory being used, it decays away and is eventually forgotten. This is the Law of Disuse (Thorndike, 1914). Although this idea is accepted by some neuroscientists (e.g., Hardt et al., 2013), the idea of forgetting caused by decay and disuse was rejected by psychologists after a brutal critique by McGeoch (1932). McGeoch argued that the passage of time causes nothing by itself. There must be some process that is correlated with time to cause forgetting. An analogy used by McGeoch is the phenomenon of rust. While the amount of rust increases with time, the mere passage of time does not cause rust. Instead it is the oxidation of the metal over time that causes rust. Thus, the idea that forgetting is a loss of memories over time explains nothing. It is only a description of the phenomenon. For McGeoch, events that occur between learning and testing (i.e., interference) are what causes forgetting. These processes are discussed in detail later.

New Theory of Disuse

After languishing for decades, the idea that decay and disuse play a role in forgetting was reconsidered in the New Theory of Disuse (Bjork & Bjork, 1992; 2006). This view does not assume that memories simply decay over time. It acknowledges that the more time that has passed since information was used, the less accessible it becomes, presumably because it is no longer needed. For example, if you move, your previous address becomes harder to remember, even though it was very well-known at one point.

An important distinction for the New Theory of Disuse is between storage strength and retrieval strength. Storage strength is how well a memory is encoded. The more practice you have with information, the greater the storage strength. In comparison, retrieval strength is the ease with which information is retrieved from memory. This distinction between storage strength and retrieval strength is

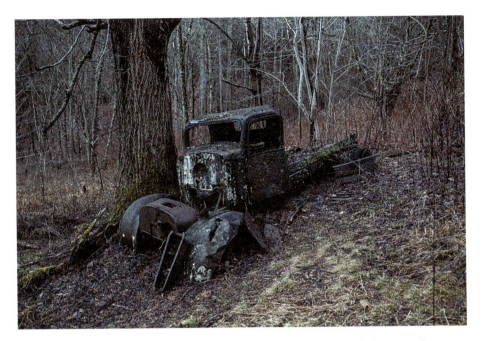

PHOTO 8.1. *After a period of time in which memories are not used, they may be forgotten to the point where they are not recognized or recoverable*

Source: Adam Patyk/Shutterstock.com

analogous to the concepts of habit strength and reaction potential in the behaviorist literature (Hull, 1943). Retrieval strength is strongest just after learning and can increase with practice. However, it weakens as new information is encountered, interfering with it. Thus, this is not a decay process, but a reflection of disuse. The passage of time corresponds to encountering other information, and the ability to access well-known but unused memories declines.

One study supporting the New Theory of Disuse was by Smith and Handy (2014). They had students at Texas A & M University memorize materials with either a constant context or varied contexts. They then gave memory tests immediately and days later. While immediate memory was worse in the varied context condition, it was better days later. Why? The explanation was that with varied contexts, this mismatch (following the encoding specificity principle) impairs the ability to develop retrieval strength because each experience is different. Thus, memories are not effectively cued early on, and performance was worse. However, each experience adds to the storage strength. These more challenging learning conditions give storage strength a boost, improving performance days later. This lends further support to the idea that when you study, it is to your benefit to do so in different places at different times of the day.

This view readily explains some memory phenomena. As one example, if people have acquired a skill to a high degree, such as a golf swing, and then learn a new swing, the newer learning will initially overpower the original and dominate performance. However, if the new skill is not continually practiced, the old one will re-emerge, causing a regression to prior ways of behaving. When you try to change a bad habit, you may be successful immediately, but over time, if you do not continue to focus on changing your ways, the old habit will re-emerge. As a more memory-based example, when people learn new information, this can produce retroactive interference (detailed below) in which the new memories impede the retrieval of older memories. However, retroactive interference weakens over time and the older memories play a larger role. Proactive interference effects, in which the older memories disrupt access to the newer ones, grow stronger (Briggs, 1954; Postman et al., 1968). The storage strength of an older, well-engrained memory is greater than that for a new memory. As the retrieval strength of newer memories weakens, the greater storage strength of older memories comes to dominate.

Stop and Review

Early ideas about forgetting suggested that memory traces decay over time. However, this has been rejected in favor of mechanisms of interference and inhibition. The New Theory of Disuse preserves the idea that disuse leads to poorer performance and couches this in a framework that incorporates interference and inhibition.

FORGETTING THROUGH INTERFERENCE

Each experience we have alters memory. Even the act of remembering alters memory because the *experience* of remembering gets stored. One consequence of this is that memories compete with one another. This competition is interference. Interference is a primary mechanism of forgetting. When two or more traces have overlapping information, and you only want one of them, interference occurs. Suppose you are trying to remember your friend Mary's phone number. You remember getting the number from Mary when you met her for lunch, but Susan was there, too, and you also got her number. These two memories compete because they both contain phone numbers and the element of having lunch, thereby producing interference. Here, several kinds of interference are covered, including proactive interference, retroactive interference, associative interference, and general interference.

Proactive Interference

Proactive interference occurs when older memories impair the retrieval of newer memories (Underwood, 1957). For example, if people study psychology and then study sociology, there is greater forgetting and worse performance on a subsequent sociology test. The degree of proactive interference experienced depends on the overlap between sets of information, not on how much was learned (Postman & Keppel, 1977). If it is difficult to differentiate between memory traces because of their content, then proactive interference is experienced. This is why sociology and psychology interfere with one another. Any effort that you can make to distinguish and differentiate sets of information reduces interference, and memory improves. Proactive interference is resolved by processes in the left lateral prefrontal cortex (BA 46), although the right dorsolateral prefrontal cortex (BA 8) and parietal regions (BA 7) may also be involved (Nee & Jonides, 2008).

The influence of trace relatedness on proactive interference has been studied extensively. When too much information of a similar type is encountered close in time, more proactive interference is experienced. When there is a break in similar types of information, memory improves, and there is a release from proactive interference. An example of release from proactive interference is a study by Wickens (1970; 1972) in which people were given lists of words to remember (see Table 8.1). The words in the first three lists were all fruits. If the fourth list were fruits again, then memory continued to decline, as shown in Figure 8.2. However, if the words belonged to a new category, release from proactive interference occurred. Moreover, the greater the difference, the greater the release. For example, vegetables are different from fruits, but they still have some features in common, whereas professions are quite distinct from fruits. The build-up and release from proactive interference occurs for real-world materials, such as televised new stories (Gunter et al., 1980). As people read more stories on a topic (e.g., politics), memory for each one declines, until there is a switch to a different topic (e.g., sports).

The build-up in proactive interference can be because of the continued, unsegmented learning of similar types of information. If people get information with

TABLE 8.1 *Stimulus Lists from Proactive Interference Study*

Condition	Trial 1	Trial 2	Trial 3	Trial 4
Fruits (control)	banana	plum	melon	orange
	peach	apricot	lemon	cherry
	apple	lime	grape	pineapple
Vegetables	banana	plum	melon	onion
	peach	apricot	lemon	radish
	apple	lime	grape	potato
Flowers	banana	plum	melon	daisy
	peach	apricot	lemon	violet
	apple	lime	grape	tulip
Meats	banana	plum	melon	salami
	peach	apricot	lemon	bacon
	apple	lime	grape	hamburger
Professions	banana	plum	melon	doctor
	peach	apricot	lemon	teacher
	apple	lime	grape	lawyer

Source: Wickens, 1972

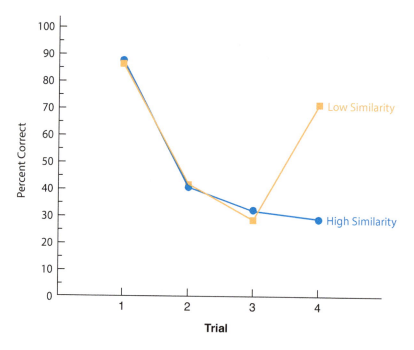

FIGURE 8.2 *Results from a Study of Release from Proactive Interference*

Source: adapted from Wickens, D. D. (1972). Characteristics of word encoding. In A. W. Melton & E. Martin (Eds.) *Coding Processes in Human Memory*, pp. 191–215. New York: Wiley

topics interleaved, rather than in blocks of related knowledge, then less proactive interference occurs (Del Missier et al., 2018). This difference between blocked and interleaved presentation is shown in Figure 8.3, along with some hypothetical data. Thus, given this, you may want to break up your studying from time to time to boost your retention.

Another way to segregate information, leading to a release from proactive interference, is by testing people prior to learning new information (Szpunar et al., 2008). Testing causes a shift in the perceived context, which leads to less interference (Pastötter et al., 2011), either because the memories may become more integrated, resulting in fewer competitor traces, reducing interference (Wahlheim, 2015), or because we are better able to monitor what we report as being part of the most recent information set (Pierce et al., 2017).

Proactive interference is also reduced by sleep. Abel and Bäuml (2014) had people learn two sets of information that overlapped in content and which produced proactive interference. This was evident for people tested immediately after learning. However, when tested 12 hours later, people who slept (learning in the evening, testing the next morning) exhibited less proactive interference compared to another group that was awake during the 12 hours (learning in the morning, testing later that evening). Consolidation served to separate out and distinguish the memory traces from one another, thereby reducing proactive interference.

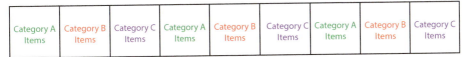

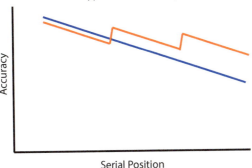

FIGURE 8.3 *Difference between Clock and Interleaved Presentation, along with a Hypothetical Pattern of Data*

Source: adapted from Del Missier, F., Sassano, A., Coni, V., Salomonsson, M., & Mäntylä, T. (2018). Blocked vs. interleaved presentation and proactive interference in episodic memory. *Memory, 26*(5), 697–711

TRY IT OUT

To illustrate proactive interference, and the subsequent release from it, we use the example illustrated in Table 8.1. For this project you should have at least 12 people in each group.

Give two or more groups of people the lists of fruit names. Have them recall the words at the end of each list. For all groups, the first three lists should be the same. However, on the fourth list, vary the nature of the list depending on what condition people are in. For one group, give them another list of fruit names. However, for other groups, give them lists of words that are further and further removed from fruits, namely vegetables, flowers, meats, and professions. You do not need all these groups to do this demonstration, but you need at least the first group and one other.

After people finish recalling, collect their responses and tabulate the number of correct recalls for each list. You should find that everyone gets worse from list 1 to 3, and that at list 4, the fruit group continues to get worse, but the other groups get better, with the amount of improvement being related to how different the words are from fruits.

Retroactive Interference

Retroactive interference is when newer memories make it harder to remember older memories (Melton & Irwin, 1940). A classic demonstration of this is a study by Jenkins and Dallenbach (1924) in which students at Cornell University learned lists of ten nonsense syllables. They were then tested one, two, four, and eight hours later. What is important is what they did during these intervals. They were given the lists either early in the day, so they were awake the whole time, or at night, so they were asleep during the retention period. The results in Figure 8.4 show less forgetting when the students slept than when they were awake. When we are awake, there is a continuous stream of new information (including thoughts). This produces retroactive interference, making the older information harder to remember. However, if we sleep, there is not as much new information, so there is less retroactive interference and forgetting. The degree to which retroactive interference benefits from sleep is like that observed with proactive interference (Abel & Bäuml, 2014).

With retroactive interference, newer experiences make it harder to remember older, similar experiences (Postman & Stark, 1969). For example, if you study psychology and then study sociology, you forget some of the psychology because the newer sociology memories interfere with the retrieval of older psychology knowledge. Retroactive interference is more pronounced with recall than with recognition. During recall people try to sort through many competing memory traces, allowing interference to occur. However, during recognition there are fewer traces involved because a more direct match can be made between the recognition probe and a memory trace. Thus, less interference occurs.

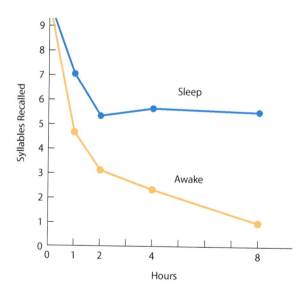

FIGURE 8.4 *Results from a Study of Long-Term Memory Interference*

Source: Created from data reported in Jenkins, J. G., & Dallenbach, K. M. (1924). Oblivescence during sleep and waking. *American Journal of Psychology, 35*, 605–622

In the verbal learning era, retroactive interference was thought of as a form of extinction, known as the unlearning of prior associations (Barnes & Underwood, 1959; Melton & Irwin, 1940). The idea was that new information causes older information to be lost or disrupted. However, this "unlearning" idea is not completely correct. Retroactive interference can subsequently be reduced or eliminated, suggesting that the original memories are still there, even if they are difficult to access. Thus, retroactive interference may only involve a disruption of the retrieval, not storage. If people are given the appropriate cues, retroactive interference is attenuated or eliminated (Tulving & Psotka, 1971).

Associative Interference

Associative interference reflects the complexity of newly learned information. The disruption of memory is not based on temporal order (as it is with proactive and retroactive interference), but on the number of associations with a concept. For example, if you have just learned five things about Jenny, you will be slower to verify any one of these than if you had learned only one thing. Associative interference can be described in terms of the fan effect. The term fan effect assumes that information is stored in a propositional memory network with nodes representing individual concepts and links representing the associations among them (see Chapter 18). During retrieval, the more links "fanning" off of a concept, the greater the interference from the competing associations, and retrieval time increases accordingly.

In one study, Anderson (1974) gave students at Stanford University lists of sentences to memorize, such as "The doctor is in the park" or "The lawyer is in the museum." The number of associations with the person and location concepts (e.g., doctor or park) was varied from one to three. Thus, there were one to three places that a person could be in and one to three people in a location. After memorization, a recognition test was given. The results, shown in Figure 8.5, were that as the number of associations with a concept increased, response time also increased.

A worrisome implication is that the more you know, the harder it should be to remember. However, experts have more information than novices with no deficit in the speed of remembering. This is the "the paradox of the expert" (Smith et al., 1978). A way out of this is to use chunking. Information that is integrated into a common memory trace reduces the amount of interference because there are fewer traces to compete with one another (Radvansky & Zacks, 1991).

Let us look at chunking in more detail. Suppose people memorize sentences about objects in locations. For some sentences, one object is in several locations, such as "The potted palm is in the hotel," "The potted palm is in the barbershop," and "The potted palm is in the airport." In these cases, multiple mental models are created, because each sentence refers to a different situation. Thus, there are three memory traces that can compete at retrieval. In contrast, for other sentences, multiple objects are in one location, such as "The pay phone is in the laundromat," "The oak counter is in the laundromat," and "The ceiling fan is in the laundromat." Here, a single mental model can include all this information because it all refers to a single event. As such, there is only one memory trace, and thus no interference (Radvansky & Zacks, 1991). These differential fan effects are shown in Figure 8.6, and this basic pattern of memory retrieval persists, even weeks later (Radvansky et al., 2017).

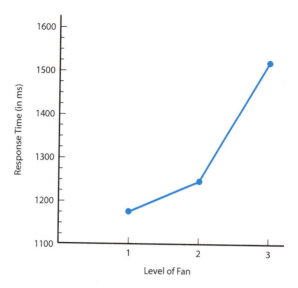

FIGURE 8.5 *Results from a Study of Associative Interference Producing a Fan Effect*

Source: created from data reported in Anderson, J. R. (1974). Retrieval of propositional information from long-term memory. *Cognitive Psychology, 6,* 451–474

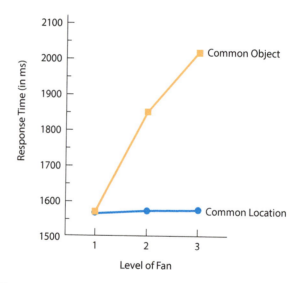

FIGURE 8.6 *Differential Interference Effects When Information Can and Cannot Be Integrated into Mental Models*

Source: Radvansky, G. A., Spieler, D. H., & Zacks, R. T. (1993). Mental model organization. *Journal of Experimental Psychology: Learning, Memory, and Cognition, 19,* 95–114

Walking Through Doorways Causes Forgetting

Forgetting and interference not only come from knowledge stored in memory, but also come from our interaction with events. When we move from one event to another, in the real or a fictional world, there is an event boundary (Radvansky &

Zacks, 2011). This can be a change in location, a jump in time, a change in activity, and so on. Encountering an event boundary leads us to set up a mental model of the new event. Importantly, the mental model for the old event is moved out of working memory to make way for the new one. This is supported by research showing that when event boundaries are encountered, hippocampal and related brain areas respond to these changes with increased activity (Brunec et al., 2018). This results in a remapping of cells to accommodate the new event. Event boundaries are regularly and easily identified by people (Newtson, 1973; Zacks et al., 2009). The organization of information into mental models has consequences for memory. To ease exposition, we focus on changes in spatial location.

When mental models are stored in memory, and they have shared elements, such as an object, if people need to retrieve one of them then the related but irrelevant models produce interference (cf. differential fan effects). This interference does not need to involve memorizing lists of sentences. Just walking through doorways can cause forgetting. Radvansky and Copeland (2006; Pettijohn & Radvansky, 2018) had people move from room to room in a virtual environment, moving objects from one place to the next. When people walked from one room to another, memory for the objects they were carrying was worse compared to if they had just walked across a large room. In other words, the event boundary disrupted memory. This is also observed with real and imagined environments (Lawrence & Peterson, 2016; Radvansky et al., 2010) and disrupts both relational and item information (Horner et al., 2016). In general, when there have been shifts from one event to another, people have difficulty accessing information in memory that is tied to prior events (Swallow et al., 2009; Zwaan, 1996).

At first blush this might seem like a context effect; an instance of encoding specificity (see Chapter 7). When the encoding context does not match the retrieval context, memory is worse. However, there is more going on here. If it were, then when people return to a prior room, memory should improve, but it does not. Moreover, if people walk through two doorways, then memory is even worse (Radvansky et al., 2011). The explanation is that each room people are in is a different event memory. When people pick up an object and move across a room, the object is in just one mental model, so there is no interference. However, when they walk into a new room, the object is now in two mental models. These memories compete during retrieval, producing interference. When people walk through two doorways there are three mental models, and things are even worse.

General Interference and Consolidation

As noted earlier, the more information overlaps in content, the greater the interference. However, there is more to interference than just overlapping content. Think back to the study by Jenkins and Dallenbach (1924). When people were awake, they experienced more interference. However, the information they learned was nonsense syllables. It is unlikely that they encountered many other nonsense syllables during the day. What is going on is that there is general interference that occurs when people process lots of different types of information in their daily activities.

Memories are first held in a limited memory system, such as the hippocampus. When new information is learned, this results in the formation of new memories, which displaces some older ones. This is why there is less retroactive interference following sleep. In general, the older a memory is, the more consolidated it is, and the less likely it will be susceptible to general interference. If the formation of new memories is prevented, retroactive facilitation can occur in which older memories are remembered better.

Avoiding Interference Through Resting

As you have seen, encountering information prior to, after, or overlapping with a memory trace you want to retrieve can produce interference. Also, sleep can often aid in segregating information during consolidation, thereby reducing interference. That said, one does not need to sleep to reduce interference. Taking some time to simply rest after learning can also accomplish this. For example, a study by Dewar et al. (2012; see also Martini et al., 2018) found that resting ten minutes in between reading two narrative texts boosted memory, both immediately and a week later.

Improve Your Memory

There is no question that interference is a major contributor to forgetting in memory. Anything that can minimize interference helps in reducing forgetting. One way to do this is to make information more distinct in some way, such as using bizarre imagery, different contexts, and so on. Many of these ideas were suggested in Chapter 7. As noted here, and hinted at in other chapters, interference and disruptions of memory that can lead to forgetting is less of an issue for memories that are more consolidated. Anything that can be done to facilitate consolidation should reduce forgetting. This is why taking breaks from studying and doing some quiet resting can improve memory. These rest periods allow knowledge that you have learned to be consolidated, causing forgetting from interference to be reduced.

Stop and Review

Some forgetting is caused by interference from competing memory traces. This interference may come in the form of proactive interference in which older memories impair the ability to access newer memories, or retroactive interference in which new memories impair the ability to access older memories. Interference can also be defined in terms of a general overlap among memory traces, as with associative interference. If memories are given time to consolidate, perhaps through a period of quiet resting, there is reduced forgetting from retrieval interference.

FORGETTING AND INHIBITION

Interference in memory is a problem if you want to remember accurately and quickly. One way to reduce and control interference is by using inhibition to actively reduce the activation of interfering memories. There are several examples of inhibition influences on memory (Anderson, 2003). That said, inhibiting related but irrelevant memories can also bring about forgetting.

Part-Set Cuing

As you learned in Chapter 7, retrieval cues can aid memory. However, there are exceptions. If we try to remember a set of things, such as the names of sports teams, the probability of recalling any one of them is higher if a simple recall test is used than if some of the names are given as cues to help us get started. This counterintuitive finding of poorer memory when provided with partial information is part-set cuing (Slamecka, 1968). This effect is generally greater when people are given items that they were more likely to recall than forget (Kroeger et al., 2019). There are three mechanisms that can influence part-set cuing (Bäuml & Aslan, 2006; Kroeger, et al., 2019). One is that giving people part of the set disrupts their retrieval plan (Basden et al., 1977), similar to the collaborative inhibition discussed later in this chapter.

A second mechanism is retrieval competition (Rundus, 1973). When people are given part-set cues, the activation level of those memories becomes higher. As a result, they are more likely to be accessed during a memory search. This then serves to reduce or block the retrieval of the other, noncued memories.

Another mechanism involves inhibition (Aslan et al., 2007). When people recall an item from a set, it has a higher activation than the rest. As a result, it blocks access to the others (Roediger et al., 1977). To reduce the interference, they are inhibited (Anderson & Neely, 1996). As people get further and further into the set, the unrecalled traces get more and more inhibited, making it harder to remember them (Oswald et al., 2006). Thus, for part-set cuing, providing people with part of a set leads them to inhibit memories that might otherwise be more available.

TRY IT OUT

A forgetting phenomenon that you can demonstrate is part-set cuing. For this you need two groups of at least 12 people each. First, for both groups, read everyone a list of 20 words. These words should be read at a rate of about one word per second. Then, after reading all the words, have people recall them. For the control group, just have the people try to recall all 20 words. However, for the experimental group, first give these people ten of the words from the original list. Then have them try to recall the other ten. When you are done, collect the response sheets, and score the recall performance of both groups only for the ten words that were not provided to the experimental group. What you should find is that the rate of recalling these ten words will be worse for the experimental group than the control group.

Negative Priming

Inhibition is also observed with associative interference. By focusing on memories that compete and produce interference, we can assess inhibition. If people are probed for interfering memories immediately after they have been inhibited, the memories are less available (Radvansky, 1999). The decreased availability of memory traces that were recently inhibited is negative priming. It is the opposite of normal (positive) priming, in which related information becomes more available. This is a case of retrieval-induced forgetting because remembering one thing makes remembering related things harder. In other words, remembering causes forgetting.

Retrieval Practice

Finally, inhibition occurs when people repeatedly retrieve part of a set of items (Anderson et al., 1994; but see Jonker et al., 2013). Repeated retrieval causes competing but unretrieved traces to be inhibited. As a result, the probability of recalling those nonpracticed memories decreases (Tulving & Hastie, 1972) and people forget that information faster. This retrieval-induced forgetting for related but unpracticed memories is the retrieval practice effect (Anderson & Spellman, 1995; see Murayama et al., 2014, for a meta-analysis). The study of the retrieval practice effect is detailed in the Study In Depth box.

STUDY IN DEPTH

The retrieval practice paradigm is a method for assessing retrieval inhibition. To better understand this paradigm, let us look at a study by Anderson and Spellman (1995). For this work each person received eight lists of words. Four of these were experimental lists, and four were untested filler lists. Each experimental list had six words in it, and all of the words in a list were members of the same category. For example, one person might see words in the categories listed below. Note that some of the items from one category could also be placed in another category. For example, there are some things that are both red and food. The categorized nature of these lists is important here.

RED	FOOD	FLY	LOUD
blood	bread	kite	thunder
fire	crackers	glider	yell
sunburn	peas	frisbee	traffic
apple	ketchup	butterfly	lawnmower
cherry	radish	eagle	sandblaster
tomato	strawberry	ladybug	compressor

For this study, 48 students from the University of California Los Angeles were tested. At the beginning there was an initial learning phase, in which people were shown all of the words in all of the lists. These lists were presented one category-word pair at a time, such as RED-blood, for five seconds each. The point was to set up the category-word associations in memory.

After the initial learning phase, the experiment went into the retrieval practice phase. Here, people were given a cued recall test in which they saw a category name and the first two letters of the target word, such as RED-bl_____. The task was to complete the target word. People were given ten seconds for each word. Importantly, not all of the categories were tested. Moreover, only half of the items from a practice category were actually practiced. Thus, there were only six items from the list of 24 that actually received retrieval practice, and these items were practiced twice. In addition, all of the words from the four filler lists were practiced once.

To better understand the logic of the retrieval practice phase, use Figure 8.7 as a guide. There were four conditions in the study. Assume that people practiced the first three words in the RED category and three from the FLY category. Those practiced items, such as RED-blood, are the **RP+ items**. These were words from a category that was practiced, and these were the words that were actually practiced. The words that were from the same category as the practice words, but were *not* actually ever practiced, such as "tomato," were the **RP-items**. That is, these were words from the category that was practiced, but the specific words were never actually practiced. The third condition were words from a non-practiced category that overlapped words in the practice category, such as "strawberry," the **NRP-similar items**, were words from a non-practiced category that overlapped words in the practice category, such as "strawberry." That is, these items were from a category that was not practiced, but were similar to items from a category that was practiced. Finally, for the fourth condition, words from a non-practiced category that did not overlap with a practiced category, such as "crackers" were the **NRP-dissimilar items**. These items served as the control condition to assess the influences of retrieval practice and inhibition.

The logic behind the study is that, first, words that were practiced will be recalled more later. This is hardly surprising. If you spend more time practicing something, you are going to remember it better. Second, and of primary importance, is what happens with the RP-items. Because they are in the same category as the practice items, they are related

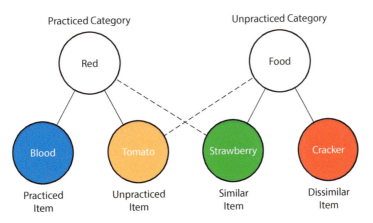

FIGURE 8.7 *Operation of Retrieval-Induced Inhibition in a Repeated Practice Paradigm*

Source: Anderson, M. C., & Spellman, B. A. (1995). On the status of inhibitory mechanisms in cognition: Memory retrieval as a model case. *Psychological Review, 102,* 68–100

and irrelevant. Thus, they are sources of interference at retrieval during retrieval practice, and so are actively inhibited. They will be recalled less often later. That is, people will have worse memories because they were inhibited. Third, and of secondary importance, is what happens to the NRP-similar items. Because they are from a non-practiced category, memory for them is worse than for those that were actually practiced. However, because they are also similar to the practiced category, there is some spill-over inhibition to these items, and they are remembered worse than the control items.

After going through retrieval practice, people were given a distractor task for 20 minutes to encourage some forgetting (we would not learn much if people recalled most or all of the words). After this distractor task, people took a cued recall test. For each category, they were given the category names (e.g., RED) and were to recall as many members of that category as they could. They were given 30 seconds for each category. The results, shown in Figure 8.8, show that, relative to the NRP-dissimilar condition, recalled words more often in the RP+ condition, consistent with the idea that practice improves memory. Importantly, for the RP-condition, people recalled those words at a *lower* rate, consistent with the idea that they were inhibited, making their retrieval more difficult. Finally, also, for the NRP-similar condition, people recalled these words less often, again showing evidence of retrieval inhibition.

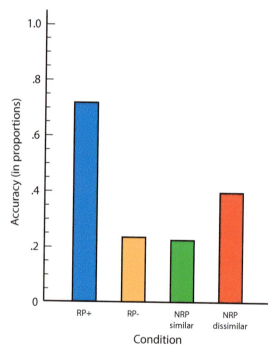

FIGURE 8.8 *Pattern of Recall Rates in Anderson and Spellman's (1995) Retrieval Practice Paradigm*

Source: created from data reported in Anderson, M. C., & Spellman, B. A. (1995). On the status of inhibitory mechanisms in cognition: Memory retrieval as a model case. *Psychological Review, 102*, 68–100

The repeated practice effect is observed with both recall and recognition (Hicks & Starns 2004), as well as indirect memory tests (Camp et al., 2005). It not only occurs for categorized lists of words, but also for sentences with similar concepts (Anderson & Bell, 2001), experienced events (Cinel et al., 2018), autobiographical memories via episodic future thinking (Ditta & Storm, 2016) and prospective memory (Utsumi & Saito, 2016), or even elements of prose (Saunders & MacLeod, 2006). Thus, it is pervasive.

It is important to keep in mind that the retrieval practice effect occurs only when there is some interference present during retrieval for the inhibition to counteract (Anderson et al., 2000). Merely exposing people to information is insufficient (Ciranni & Shimamura, 1999). This is supported by neuroimaging data that shows an increase in theta band activity in EEG recordings in cases where there is retrieval interference during a retrieval practice resulting in inhibition (Staudigl et al., 2010).

The retrieval practice effect can be modified depending on how people think about information. If we can integrate a set of information, then the effect is reduced or eliminated (Anderson & McCulloch, 1999). This is because there are fewer competitors, no interference, and therefore no need for inhibition. Alternatively, if memory traces are more distinct from one another, this can also reduce the effect by reducing interference (Anderson et al., 2000). Finally, consistent with the idea that inhibition is only temporarily used to manage retrieval interference, retrieval practice effects are reduced or eliminated after delays (e.g., a day later) when the inhibition has dissipated (Abel & Bäuml, 2012).

Stop and Review

Interference experienced during retrieval disrupts memory. Interference is reduced through inhibition, thereby facilitating the retrieval of target memories. However, this also makes the retrieval of inhibited memories harder. This is retrieval-induced forgetting. This is seen in part-set cuing, in which people who are given part of a set of information find it harder to retrieve the rest of the set, compared to if no cue is provided. Similarly, with negative priming, memories that were just previously sources of interference are responded to more slowly. Finally, the retrieval practice paradigm shows that repeatedly retrieving part of a set of items can make the rest of a set harder to recall later.

INTENTIONAL FORGETTING

Most studies of forgetting focus on how we forget things that we want to remember. However, there are times when we want to forget. An everyday example of this would be if someone were telling you their phone number and then realized they gave you the wrong one and said, "Oh, wait, that's not the number, the number is ..." Clearly you would want to forget the incorrect information. Here we cover two lines of research involving intentional forgetting: directed forgetting and retraction.

Directed Forgetting

The first type of intentional forgetting is when people are told to forget some things and to remember others. This is directed forgetting (Bjork, 1970). The effectiveness of directed forgetting is assessed on a final memory test in which people are told to retrieve all of the prior information, both things that they were told to remember, as well as the things that they were told to forget. There are two hallmarks of directed forgetting (relative to a control condition in which people are told to remember everything). The first is that the to-be-forgotten (TBF) information is remembered worse. The second is that the to-be-remembered (TBR) information is remembered better. There are three methods for studying directed forgetting: the item, list, and selective directed forgetting methods. Each of these is considered in turn.

For item method directed forgetting people are given a set of items, and after each one, they are explicitly told either to remember (TBR) or forget it (TBF). An everyday example of this is when we offload information, such as making a note, or saving a bookmark on a computer. When we do this, we do not feel a need to commit the information to memory. The consequences of this are like directed forgetting (Sparrow et al., 2011).

The explanation for forgetting here is that when people are told to forget an item, they stop rehearsing it, thus it is not stored in memory. In the absence of rehearsal, fewer TBF items are retrieved on a final memory test relative to the TBR items that were rehearsed more (Basden et al., 1993; Fawcett et al., 2016). It has been found that people look away from the spatial location of an item after a forget cue, and the iris expands, indicating some element of mental effort (Lee, 2018). This mental effort can be disrupted if TMS is applied to the dorsolateral prefrontal cortex (Xie et al., 2020).

For list method directed forgetting people are given a list of items. Then, they are either told to remember (control) or to forget (experimental) the list. Afterward, people are given a second list. Here, people need to rehearse all the first list items prior to the forget instruction, because they do not know that they will be told to forget it. Then people inhibit the TBF information in memory (Basden et al., 1993; Bjork, 1989). This inhibition is effortful. If people are disrupted by a secondary task, the inhibition of TBF information is reduced or eliminated (Conway et al., 2000). Moreover, like item method directed forgetting, this can be disrupted if TMS is applied to the dorsolateral prefrontal cortex (Hanslmayr, et al., 2012).

List-based directed forgetting is alleviated by a night's sleep (Abel & Bäuml, 2012 or even wakeful resting (Schlichting & Bäuml, 2017). Memory consolidation during sleep causes a lifting of the inhibition of memory traces. Also, forgetting is hindered if people have engaged in retrieval practice during learning (as opposed to simply studying) (Abel & Bäuml, 2016).

The inhibition of the TBF information is pervasive. It occurs both for direct memory tests, like recognition and recall, as well as indirect tests, like word fragment completion (MacCleod, 1989). Directed forgetting can occur for your autobiographical memories (Barnier et al., 2007). Directed forgetting is reduced if TBF items are meaningfully (semantically) related to the TBR items (Conway et al.,

2000). Presumably, the automatic priming of TBF items by TBR items keeps them from being effectively forgotten.

Note than while the inhibition account is the dominant explanation, directed forgetting can also be brought about by changes in (mental) context (Sahakyan & Kelley, 2002; but see Abel & Bäuml, 2017b). When you are told to forget something, this sets up a change in the mental context. This mismatch in mental context impairs the ability to access information in memory, much as is seen with encoding specificity (see Chapter 7).

For selective directed forgetting people are given a set of information and then are told to forget only part of it based on some criterion. For example, you might be told a bunch of facts about Tom and Bill in a random order. Then you are told to forget everything about Bill. After this, you then learn a bunch of facts about Steve. This is selective directed forgetting because people are not told to selectively edit memory based on some common concept, such as a person.

Selective directed forgetting is absent if the materials are highly integrated, perhaps because the various components of the materials continue to prime and activate information that was marked as TBF. As a result, materials continue to be remembered rather than forgotten (Delaney et al., 2009). It should be noted that selective directed forgetting is difficult to replicate (Akan & Sahakyan, 2018; Storm et al., 2013). Thus, while selective directed forgetting seems like it should be possible, and feels like something we do regularly, our understanding of how we actually go about it is not well understood at this time.

Retraction

Related to directed forgetting is the idea that sometimes we learn things and then we later find out that those things are incorrect. Information that we encounter is first treated as accurate until we have motivation to think otherwise (Gilbert et al., 1990). When information is then marked as incorrect it is said to be retracted. In general, while retraction does influence memory, people do have some difficulty altering their knowledge and understanding.

In an early study by Kay (1955) students at Cambridgeshire Technical College were given two stories to read for later recall. They then recalled the stories immediately and then five more times over the next four months. Importantly, people were given an opportunity to reread the stories after each recall attempt. What was striking was that when people made an error in the recall of the story, the error often persisted throughout the additional attempts, even though there was an opportunity to correct the mistake after each rereading. Given this resistance to modifying our understanding, it is best to try to understand something correctly the first time, to as great a degree as possible. This reflects the memory sin of persistence and is the general principle of memory. Even well-learned semantic knowledge held by experts shows some resistance to change. For example, even experts in astronomy are slower to verify the statement "The Earth revolves around the Sun" than "The Moon revolves around the Earth." This is because the first is inconsistent with our early held understanding of everyday experience, where the latter is not, even when people know very well that these statements are true (Shtulman & Valcarcel, 2012).

An interesting thing about retracted information is that it continues to influence our thinking. Thus, it is called the continued influence effect (CIE) (Wilkes & Leatherbarrow, 1988). For example, if people are told that a traffic accident involved older adults, and later this information is retracted, people may continue to make age-related inferences about the injured, such as suggesting that the family members who would need to be contacted would be their children (with no mention of other possibilities, such as parents). As a real-world example, during the 2003 Iraq War misinformation was sometimes reported by news outlets, such as a report that Iraqi forces were executing coalition prisoners of war. Afterward this misinformation was denied or corrected by news agencies. However, some people continued to use it (Lewandowsky et al., 2005). As another example, Greitemeyer (2014) found that some scientists continue to believe results that had been retracted (e.g., if it was found that someone faked the data).

The CIE is robust. It not influenced by whether the retraction is given immediately or after a short delay (Johnson & Seifert, 1994). That said, the CIE does require that the retracted information be part of the larger event. It is not observed if it was merely mentioned in passing (Johnson & Seifert, 1994). Further, the magnitude of the CIE can be reduced if people are given an alternative causal explanation (Ecker et al., 2011), such as being told that the injured in an accident were not older adults, but were patients at a local rehabilitation center. That said, it may also be the case that people will not believe and accept the correction (O'Rear & Radvansky, 2020), and there may even be a *backfire effect* in which they cling more strongly to the original, incorrect information (Nyhan & Reifler, 2010).

One theory of memory change in the face of explicit refutation is the Knowledge Revision Components framework (KReC) (Kendeou & O'Brien, 2014). This theory assumes that there are five mental processes that can affect memory change. The first is that information that is encoded into long-term memory is permanent regardless of whether it was later corrected. The second is that memories are passively activated when new, related information is encountered as a result of our trying to understand the events that we come across. This is a form of implicit priming. The third is that in order for a misunderstanding to be corrected, people need to reactivate the older incorrect memory along with the newer correct information. This is related to the idea of reconsolidation where older memories can be changed if they are reactivated. The fourth is that the new knowledge is integrated with older knowledge of the incorrect information. Again, this is part of a reconsolidation process. Finally, over time, as people retrieve and remember the newer correct information, it gains memory strength and dominates thinking over the older incorrect knowledge. Thus, over time, and with some appropriate effort, our misunderstandings can be corrected.

Stop and Review

Not all types of forgetting are bad. Sometimes we have good reason to forget. For directed forgetting, people are told to forget things, and they do so. This can also increase memory for other information. This can be done on either an item-by-item basis, resulting in differential rehearsal, or on a list-based basis, resulting in the inhibition of to-be-forgotten information. We also seem to have the ability to selectively forget information, but how this is done is not well understood. Other times, we need to forget things that turn out to be wrong and were retracted, but we are only partially successful at doing this.

SOCIAL INFLUENCES

Many of the studies discussed here have a person largely remembering alone. However, in our everyday lives, we are often in social situations, interacting with others. These other people can influence our memory. For example, people remember events differently depending on who they are with (who they are telling their story to), which can then bias later memories (Tversky & Marsh, 2000). Moreover, people who work with high-performing individuals recall more than people who work with low-performing individuals (Reysen, 2003). Finally, people remember information better if they think it comes from another person as compared to a computer (Reysen & Adair, 2008). Even how well we remember someone's face depends on social influences. People remember faces better when the person in the picture is looking at them versus when they are looking away (Mason et al., 2004). Thus, memory is influenced by other people. Here we look at how interacting with other people can cause forgetting, as well as some evidence that it can have the opposite effect.

Collaborative Inhibition

When people in groups try to recall something, they typically recall less than if they were separated, asked to recall information, and had their individual efforts pooled (Weldon & Bellinger, 1997). This decline in memory when working in a group is collaborative inhibition. In other words, overall, people are recalling less in a group than as individuals. This occurs for both retrospective and prospective memory tasks (Browning et al., 2018).

Collaborative inhibition is not a result of social loafing. Instead, people are encountering different ways that others have structured the information. Each person's recall is based on his or her own retrieval plan. When confronted with an organization that is different from one's own retrieval plan, recall becomes disrupted, and performance declines (Weldon et al., 2000). This is related to the part-set cuing phenomenon (but see Kelley et al., 2014). Not only is some information forgotten when it is recalled in groups, but a shared memory of an event becomes more homogeneous across the group members, both in terms of its content and its organization (Congleton & Rajaram, 2014).

People can insulate themselves against collaborative inhibition if they first retrieve information on their own, prior to being in a group setting. That is, the testing effect (Chapter 7) may guard against collaborative inhibition (Congleton & Rajaram, 2011). It should be noted that although people recall more alone than in groups, group recall does increase the accuracy of what is actually recalled (Harris

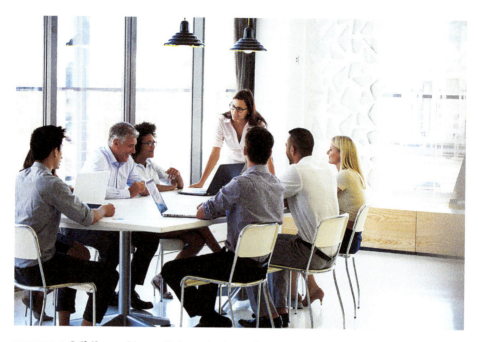

PHOTO 8.2 *While working collaboratively with others can often be beneficial, there is some evidence that collaborative memory retrieval can actually be worse (something called collaborative inhibition) than working alone and summing the groups' efforts*

Source: Monkey Business Images/Shutterstock.com

et al., 2012; Vollrath et al., 1989). It should also be noted that the collaborative inhibition effect dissipates over time (such as a day later) (Abel & Bäuml, 2017a). After forgetting occurs, hearing other people recall information may then serve as a trigger for remembering otherwise forgotten information.

When people recall events together, this can result in the inhibition of unrecalled memories. In other words, this is a retrieval practice effect both for the people who originally spoke, as well as the people who were only listening (Cuc et al., 2007). Thus, the same memory processes that lead to forgetting in an individual can be triggered just by listening to other people.

Collaborative inhibition not only applies when we try to retrieve information either alone or in a group, it can also occur when we learn information (Barber et al., 2010). This is even true if the same people are present at learning and retrieval (so, it is not poorer memory because of a change in social context). Different people create and use different retrieval cues from each other. When people study together, they do not develop retrieval cues that would be most helpful for their recall of the information. This is also the reason why we do not learn as well by using other people's class notes (Annis & Davis, 1975). That said, it should also be noted that it is possible for collaborative encoding to mitigate effects of collaborative inhibition at retrieval; in some sense shifting where the memory problems are originating from (Harris et al., 2012).

Collaborative Facilitation

Working with groups is not all bad and does not always lead to forgetting. Although recall memory is worse in groups than alone, the opposite is true for recognition (Vollrath et al., 1989). This is collaborative facilitation. In recall, the retrieval plan plays an important role in performance. In contrast, for recognition there is no retrieval plan. Memory only requires that something seem familiar, and anything more is a bonus. When people do recognition in groups, they can pool their resources to arrive at a consensus about what happened, although this is more effective at accepting old items than rejecting new ones (Clark et al., 2000).

Other People's Memories

From time to time we may be asked to evaluate the quality of other people's memories. While we can do this to some degree, there are some biases that can creep up. One is the *consensus bias* (Ross et al., 1977), which is the idea that we often assume that other people know what we know. Thus, if we have an idea, we implicitly expect other people to know this as well.

Another bias is that people expect others to do better when the pressure is on to remember. While motivation to remember can help when we first encode something, it does not help much, if at all, during retrieval. However, we often expect other people to remember more when they are motivated at retrieval (Kassam et al., 2009). Imagine a high-profile court case in which people are strongly motivated to remember something accurately. If they were trying to commit things to memory at the time the event occurred, then memory is better. However, if they were only motivated in hindsight to retrieve something that did not seem particularly important at the time, then memory is relatively poor regardless of the desire to remember. Despite this, we often expect other people to remember better because of a lack of insight we have into how memory works.

Stop and Review

Interacting with other people can also cause forgetting. This collaborative inhibition occurs when people recall less in groups. This may be a result of retrieval plan disruptions and the inhibition caused by socially induced retrieval practice. That said, collaborative facilitation can happen, as with recognition. Another problem that can arise is our blindness to other people's memories. People often cannot remember more just by trying harder, even at our (incorrect) insistence.

DRUGS AND ALCOHOL

Forgetting can also occur as a result of chemicals that we put into our bodies. In this section we look at the influence of drugs and alcohol and how they change memory and forgetting.

Drugs

One class of drugs that has a strong influence on memory is benzodiazepines (e.g., Valium and Halcion), which are depressants. These drugs influence memory by increasing GABA-related processes, which inhibit neural firing. Because of this suppressed neural activity, people taking these drugs have difficulty acquiring new memories. In a sense, this is a drug-induced form of anterograde amnesia, similar to what is seen in Korsakoff's patients (Curran, 1991). In other words, these drugs cause forgetting by impairing the ability to encode new knowledge. In addition, although memory is typically better for emotional information, people taking benzodiazepines do not show this benefit, suggesting that the drugs are also disrupting amygdala processing (Buchanan et al., 2003).

Benzodiazepines primarily compromise declarative rather than nondeclarative memory (Reder et al., 2006), with PET scans in one study showing suppressed processing in the right prefrontal cortex (BA 9), left parahippocampal gyrus (BA 35), and left anterior cingulated cortex (BA 32) (Mintzer et al., 2006).

A beneficial consequence of drug-induced anterograde amnesia is that retroactive interference effects are diminished. Memory for information learned prior to taking the drug is better than it would be otherwise (Fillmore et al., 2001). Because new memories are not created, they cannot interfere backward in time to cause retroactive interference. The better memory is retroactive facilitation.

Alcohol

Another substance that can influence memory is alcohol. While alcohol can have several effects, the focus here is on the consequences of individual episodes of drinking. In general, memory is worse for things learned under the influence of alcohol, although this may be primarily for peripheral and secondary information (Schreiber et al., 2011). Alcohol affects a broad range of memory processes (Maylor & Rabbitt, 1993), including executive working memory function (Saults et al., 2007), prospective memory (Leitz et al., 2009), and producing overconfidence in metamemory judgments (Nelson et al., 1986). Work using the process dissociation procedure has shown that alcohol's influence is more pronounced for explicit, declarative knowledge than for implicit, nondeclarative knowledge (e.g., Kirchner & Sayette, 2003). Part of the problem is that alcohol, as EEG recordings show, disrupts event-related synchronization and desynchronization (see Chapter 2) in the cortex in the theta and alpha band levels (Krause et al., 2002). Thus, the brain cannot coordinate processing as effectively after alcohol consumption. At high enough levels, people can experience blackouts during which there is no memory for any of the events of that time. This is a sign of a serious drinking problem.

In addition to the negative effects of alcohol on memory, there are some positive effects as well. Specifically, information is remembered better if people consume alcohol immediately afterward than if they do not (Moulton et al., 2005). This is another example of retroactive facilitation. Because information is so poorly encoded when one is under the influence of alcohol there are fewer new memory traces to produce retroactive interference. Also, alcohol may facilitate consolidation of the earlier memory traces, perhaps because of increased glucose levels (Scholey & Fowles, 2002).

Alcohol can even influence memory when it is not actually present, but it is just suggested to people that they have consumed alcohol. Assefi and Garry (2003) had students at Victoria University of Wellington watch a slide show of a man shoplifting at a bookstore. Later, people were given misleading post-event information (see Chapter 14). Even though all the students drank tonic water, half of them were told that it also contained vodka (the glasses were rimmed with vodka). Students who thought that they drank alcohol were more susceptible to misleading information and were more confident in their responses. This is a pattern consistent with actual alcohol consumption. Thus, just the thought of drinking alcohol can influence how people use their memories and what they forget.

Stop and Review

Forgetting can be caused by external influences. Some drugs, such as benzodiazepines, block normal operations of the nervous system resulting in a drug-induced amnesia. Alcohol can also disrupt the formation of new memories. In both cases, the blocked formation of new memories reduces retroactive interference, allowing for retroactive facilitation.

PUTTING IT ALL TOGETHER

The opposite of remembering is forgetting. Forgetting is often viewed negatively, almost like a sin. Forgetting is more likely when there is competition among memories, producing interference during retrieval. This can happen proactively, retroactively, associatively, and generally. Inference can cause you further difficulties when the process of inhibition is involved, causing some memories to be even harder to retrieve than before as they are pushed below their prior levels of accessibility. This is seen with part-set cuing, negative priming, and retrieval practice effects.

However, forgetting also allows some control over your thoughts, keeping them from being clogged with irrelevant information. In this case, a sin may be a virtue. When knowledge ceases to be relevant, forgetting causes it to become extinct through disuse. Here, forgetting comes about as interference keeps old and unwanted information at bay. While interfering memories that have been inhibited are harder to access, this inhibition is helpful in controlling the negative effects of interference. Inhibition can be deliberately used to keep incorrect and irrelevant knowledge out of mind, as with directed forgetting and retraction. The net result is that forgetting keeps out unwanted knowledge and promotes the remembering of wanted knowledge. Forgetting is everywhere, taking out the garbage and keeping things fresh.

Most of the forgetting considered here derives from the normal use of memory. Forgetting is just something that happens. However, forgetting can also happen when you interact with other people, as with collaborative inhibition, and when you take certain drugs and alcohol. Even walking through a doorway can cause forgetting. Overall, forgetting is not just a part of yourself, but is also part of how you interact with the world.

STUDY QUESTIONS

1. What are Schacter's seven sins of memory? How might these actually be virtues?
2. How does the passage of time influence forgetting? What is the Law of Disuse?
3. What is Bjork's New Theory of Disuse, and what are its core principles?
4. What is proactive interference, and how is it an interference theory of forgetting? How does proactive interference differ from negative transfer?
5. What is the release from proactive interference, and how can it be brought about?
6. What is retroactive interference, and how is it an interference theory of forgetting?
7. What is associative interface, and how does it produce the fan effect? How does the integration of information in memory cause a reduction in associative interference?
8. What is the role of inhibition in memory retrieval? How does this manage interference? How does this cause forgetting?
9. What are some of the effects that are produced by the operation of inhibition?
10. Under what circumstances do people intentionally forget information?
11. What is directed forgetting? What are the different ways of bringing this about? What is the cause of directed forgetting in each of these circumstances?
12. What does it mean for information to be retracted, and how well does memory handle retracted information?
13. What are ways in which social settings can promote forgetting? What are ways in which it promotes remembering? How well do we understand other people's memories?
14. What are the influences of drugs, such as benzodiazepines and alcohol, on remembering and forgetting?

KEY TERMS

- absent-mindedness
- accelerated long-term forgetting
- accessibility
- alcohol
- associative interference
- availability
- benzodiazepines
- bias
- blocking
- collaborative facilitation
- collaborative inhibition
- continued influence effect (CIE)
- cue overload
- directed forgetting
- event boundary
- event model
- fan effect
- forgetting
- inhibition

- interference
- item method directed forgetting
- Jost's Law
- Knowledge Revision Components framework (KReC)
- Law of Disuse
- list method directed forgetting
- misattribution
- negative priming

- New Theory of Disuse
- NRP-dissimilar items
- NRP-similar items persistence
- part-set cuing, persistence
- proactive interference
- reconstructive
- release from proactive interference
- reproductive
- retracted
- retrieval-induced forgetting

- retrieval practice effect
- retrieval strength
- retrieval-induced forgetting
- retroactive facilitation
- retroactive interference
- RP+ items, RP– items
- selective directed forgetting
- seven sins of memory
- storage strength
- suggestibility
- transience
- unlearning

EXPLORE MORE

Here are some additional readings for you to explore to get a deeper understanding of the issues involved in long-term memory forgetting.

Bjork, R. A., & Bjork, E. L. (1992). A new theory of disuse and an old theory of stimulus fluctuation. In A. Healy, S. Kosslyn, & R. Shiffrin (Eds.), *From Learning Processes to Cognitive Processes: Essays in Honor of William K. Estes* (pp. 35–67). Hillsdale, NJ: Erlbaum.

Della Sala, S. (2010). *Forgetting*. New York: Psychology Press.

Golding, J. M., & MacLeod, C. M. (2013). *Intentional Forgetting: Interdisciplinary Approaches*. New York: Psychology Press.

McGeoch, J. A. (1932). Forgetting and the law of disuse. *Psychological Review, 39,* 352–370.

Schacter, D. L. (2001). *The Seven Sins of Memory: How the Mind Forgets and Remembers*. Boston, MA: Haughton Mifflin.

REFERENCES

Abel, M., & Bäuml, K-H. T. (2012). Retrieval-induced forgetting, delay, and sleep. *Memory, 20*(5), 420–428.

Abel, M., & Bäuml, K-H. T. (2014). The roles of delay and retroactive interference in retrieval-induced forgetting. *Memory & Cognition, 42*(1), 141–150.

Abel, M., & Bäuml, K-H. T. (2016). Retrieval practice can eliminate list method directed forgetting. *Memory & Cognition, 44*(1), 15–23.

Abel, M., & Bäuml, K. H. T. (2017a). Collaborative remembering revisited: Study context access modulates collaborative inhibition and later benefits for individual memory. *Memory & cognition, 45*(8), 1319–1334.

Abel, M., & Bäuml, K. H. T. (2017b). Testing the context-change account of list-method directed forgetting: The role of retention interval. *Journal of Memory and Language, 92,* 170–182.

Akan, M., & Sahakyan, L. (2018). Repeated failures to obtain selective directed forgetting in lab and online samples and variations in stimuli. *Memory, 26*(3), 294–305.

Anderson, J. R. (1974). Retrieval of propositional information from long-term memory. *Cognitive Psychology, 6*(4), 451–474.

Anderson, M. C. (2003). Rethinking interference theory: Executive control and the mechanisms of forgetting. *Journal of Memory and Language, 49,* 415–455.

Anderson, M. C., & Bell, T. (2001). Forgetting our facts: The role of inhibitory processes in the loss of prepositional knowledge. *Journal of Experimental Psychology: General, 130,* 544–570.

Anderson, M. C., Bjork, R. A., & Bjork, E. L. (1994). Remembering can cause forgetting: Retrieval dynamics in long-term memory. *Journal of Experimental Psychology: Learning, Memory, and Cognition, 20,* 1063–1087.

Anderson, M. C., Green, C., & McCulloch, K. C. (2000). Similarity and inhibition in long-term memory: Evidence for a two-factor theory. *Journal of Experimental Psychology: Learning, Memory, and Cognition, 26,* 1141–1159.

Anderson, M. C., & McCulloch, K. C. (1999). Integration as a general boundary condition on retrieval-induced forgetting. *Journal of Experimental Psychology: Learning, Memory, and Cognition, 25,* 608–629.

Anderson, M. C., & Neely, J. H. (1996). Interference and inhibition in memory retrieval. In E. L. Bjork & R. A. Bjork (Eds.), *Memory: Handbook of Perception and Cognition* (pp. 237–313). San Diego, CA: Academic Press.

Anderson, M. C., & Spellman, B. A. (1995). On the status of inhibitory mechanisms in cognition: Memory retrieval as a model case. *Psychological Review, 102,* 68–100.

Annis, L., & Davis, J. K. (1975). The effect of encoding and an external memory device on note taking. *The Journal of Experimental Education, 44*(2), 44–46.

Aslan, A., Bäuml, K-H. T., & Grundgeiger, T. (2007). The role of inhibitory processes in part-list cuing. *Journal of Experimental Psychology: Learning, Memory, and Cognition, 33,* 335–341.

Assefi, S. L., & Garry, M. (2003). Absolut® memory distortions: Alcohol placebos influence the misinformation effect. *Psychological Science, 14*(1), 77–80.

Baddeley, A., Lewis, V., Eldridge, M., & Thomson, N. (1984). Attention and retrieval from long-term memory. *Journal of Experimental Psychology: General, 113*(4), 518.

Barber, S. J., Rajaram, S., & Aron, A. (2010). When two is too many: Collaborative encoding impairs memory. *Memory & Cognition, 38*(3), 255–264.

Barnes, J. M., & Underwood, B. J. (1959). "Fate" of first-list associations in transfer theory. *Journal of Experimental Psychology, 58*(2), 97–107.

Barnier, A. J., Conway, M. A., Mayoh, L., Speyer, J., Avizmil, O., & Harris, C. B. (2007). Directed forgetting of recently recalled autobiographical memories. *Journal of Experimental Psychology: General, 136,* 301–322.

Basden, B. H., Basden, D. R., & Gargano, G. J. (1993). Directed forgetting in implicit and explicit memory tests: A comparison of methods. *Journal of Experimental Psychology: Learning, Memory, and Cognition, 19*(3), 603–616.

Basden, D. R., Basden, B. H., & Galloway, B. C. (1977). Inhibition with part-list cuing: Some tests of the item strength hypothesis. *Journal of Experimental Psychology: Human Learning and Memory, 3,* 100–108.

Bäuml, K-H. T., & Aslan, A. (2006). Part-list cuing can be transient and lasting: The role of encoding. *Journal of Experimental Psychology: Learning, Memory, and Cognition, 32,* 33–43.

Bjork, R. A. (1970). Positive forgetting: The noninterference of items intentionally forgotten. *Journal of Verbal Learning and Verbal Behavior, 9*(3), 255–268.

Bjork, R. A. (1989). Retrieval inhibition as an adaptive mechanism in human memory. In H. L. Roediger & F. I. M. Craik (Eds.), *Varieties of Memory and Consciousness* (pp. 309–330). Hillsdale, NJ: Erlbaum.

Bjork, R. A., & Bjork, E. L. (1992). A new theory of disuse and an old theory of stimulus fluctuation. In A. Healy, S. Kosslyn, & R. Shiffrin (Eds.), *From Learning Processes to Cognitive Processes: Essays in Honor of William K. Estes* (pp. 35–67). Hillsdale, NJ: Erlbaum.

Bjork, R. A., & Bjork, E. L. (2006). Optimizing treatment and instruction: Implications of a new theory of disuse. In L-G. Nilsson, N. Ohta (Eds.), *Memory and Society: Psychological Perspectives* (pp. 116–140). New York: Psychology Press.

Briggs, G. E. (1954). Acquisition, extinction, and recovery functions in retroactive inhibition. *Journal of Experimental Psychology, 47*(5), 285–293.

Browning, C. A., Harris, C. B., Van Bergen, P., Barnier, A. J., & Rendell, P. G. (2018). Collaboration and prospective memory: Comparing nominal and collaborative group performance in strangers and couples. *Memory, 26*(9), 1206–1219.

Brunec, I. K., Moscovitch, M., & Barense, M. D. (2018). Boundaries shape cognitive representations of spaces and events. *Trends in Cognitive Sciences, 22*(7), 637–650.

Buchanan, T. W., Karafin, M. S., & Adolphs, R. (2003). Selective effects of triazolam on memory for emotional, relative to neutral, stimuli: Differential effects on gist versus detail. *Behavioral Neuroscience, 117*, 517–525.

Camp, G., Pecher, D., & Schmidt, H. G. (2005). Retrieval-induced forgetting in implicit memory tests: The role of test awareness. *Psychonomic Bulletin & Review, 12*, 490–494.

Cinel, C., Cortis Mack, C., & Ward, G. (2018). Towards augmented human memory: Retrieval-induced forgetting and retrieval practice in an interactive, end-of-day review. *Journal of Experimental Psychology: General, 147*(5), 632–661.

Ciranni, M. A., & Shimamura, A. P. (1999). Retrieval-induced forgetting in episodic memory. *Journal of Experimental Psychology: Learning, Memory, and Cognition, 25*, 1403–1414.

Clark, S. E., Hori, A., Putnam, A., & Martin, T. P. (2000). Group collaboration in recognition memory. *Journal of Experimental Psychology: Learning, Memory, and Cognition, 26*, 1578–1588.

Congleton, A. R., & Rajaram, S. (2011). The influence of learning methods on collaboration: Prior repeated retrieval enhances retrieval organization, abolishes collaborative inhibition, and promotes post-collaborative memory. *Journal of Experimental Psychology: General, 140*(4), 535–551.

Congleton, A. R., & Rajaram, S. (2014). Collaboration changes both the content and the structure of memory: Building the architecture of shared representations. *Journal of Experimental Psychology: General, 143*(4), 1570–1584.

Conway, M. A., Harries, K., Noyes, J., Racsmány, M., & Frankish, C. R. (2000). The disruption and dissolution of directed forgetting: Inhibitory control of memory. *Journal of Memory and Language, 43*, 409–430.

Cuc, A., Koppel, J., & Hirst, W. (2007). Silence is not golden: A case for socially shared retrieval-induced forgetting. *Psychological Science, 18*, 727–733.

Curran, H. V. (1991). Benzodiazepines, memory, and mood: A review. *Psychopharmacology, 105*, 1–8.

Delaney, P. F., Nghiem, K. N., & Waldum, E. R. (2009). The selective directed forgetting effect: Can people forget only part of a text? *Quarterly Journal of Experimental Psychology, 62*, 1542–1550.

Del Missier, F., Sassano, A., Coni, V., Salomonsson, M., & Mäntylä, T. (2018). Blocked vs. interleaved presentation and proactive interference in episodic memory. *Memory, 26*(5), 697–711.

Dewar, M., Alber, J., Butler, C., Cowan, N., & Della Sala, S. (2012). Brief wakeful resting boosts new memories over the long term. *Psychological Science, 23*(9), 955–960.

Ditta, A. S., & Storm, B. C. (2016). Thinking about the future can cause forgetting of the past. *Quarterly Journal of Experimental Psychology, 69*(2), 339–350.

Ebbinghaus, H. (1885). *Memory: A Contribution to Experimental Psychology* (H. A. Ruger & C. E. Bussenius, Trans.). New York: Teachers College, Columbia University.

Ecker, U. K. H., Lewandowsky, S., & Apai, J. (2011). Terrorists brought down the plane!—No, actually it was a technical fault: Processing corrections of emotive information. *The Quarterly Journal of Experimental Psychology, 64*(2), 283–310.

Elliott, G., Isaac, C. L., & Muhlert, N. (2014). Measuring forgetting: A critical review of accelerated long-term forgetting studies. *Cortex, 54*, 16–32.

Fawcett, J. M., Lawrence, M. A., & Taylor, T. L. (2016). The representational consequences of intentional forgetting: Impairments to both the probability and fidelity of long-term memory. *Journal of Experimental Psychology: General, 145*(1), 56–81.

Fernandes, M. A., & Moscovitch, M. (2000). Divided attention and memory: Evidence of substantial interference effects at retrieval and encoding. *Journal of Experimental Psychology: General, 129*(2), 155–176.

Fillmore, M. T., Kelly, T. H., Rush, C. R., & Hays, L. (2001). Retrograde facilitation of memory by triazolam: Effects on automatic processes. *Psychopharmacology, 158*, 314–321.

Fisher, J. S., & Radvansky, G. A. (2019). Linear forgetting. *Journal of Memory and Language, 108*, 104035.

Gilbert, D. T., Krull, D. S., & Malone, P. S. (1990). Unbelieving the unbelievable: Some problems in the rejection of false information. *Journal of Personality and Social Psychology, 59*(4), 601–613.

Greitemeyer, T. (2014). Article retracted, but the message lives on. *Psychonomic Bulletin & Review, 21*(2), 557–561.

Gunter, B., Clifford, B. R., & Berry, C. (1980). Release from proactive interference with television news items: Evidence for encoding dimensions within televised news. *Journal of Experimental Psychology: Human Learning and Memory, 6*(2), 216–223.

Hanslmayr, S., Volberg, G., Wimber, M., Oehler, N., Staudigl, T., Hartmann, T., ... & Bäuml, K. H. T. (2012). Prefrontally driven downregulation of neural synchrony mediates goal-directed forgetting. *Journal of Neuroscience, 32*(42), 14742–14751.

Hardt, O., Nader, K., & Nadel, L. (2013). Decay happens: The role of active forgetting in memory. *Trends in Cognitive Sciences, 17*(3), 111–120.

Harris, C. B., Barnier, A. J., & Sutton, J. (2012). Consensus collaboration enhances group and individual recall accuracy. *Quarterly Journal of Experimental Psychology, 65*(1), 179–194.

Henkel, L. A. (2014). Point-and-shoot memories: The influence of taking photos on memory for a museum tour. *Psychological Science, 25*(2), 396–402.

Hicks, J. L., & Starns, J. J. (2004). Retrieval-induced forgetting occurs in tests of item recognition. *Psychonomic Bulletin & Review, 11*, 125–130.

Horner, A. J., Bisby, J. A., Wang, A., Bogus, K., & Burgess, N. (2016). The role of spatial boundaries in shaping long-term event representations. *Cognition, 154*, 151–164.

Hull, C. L. (1943). *The Principles of Behavior*. New York: Appleton-Century-Crofts.

Jenkins, J. G., & Dallenbach, K. M. (1924). Obliviscence during sleep and waking. *The American Journal of Psychology, 35*(4), 605–612.

Johnson, H. M., & Seifert, C. M. (1994). Sources of the continued influence effect: When misinformation in memory affects later inferences. *Journal of Experimental Psychology: Learning, Memory, and Cognition, 20*(6), 1420–1436.

Jonker, T. R., Seli, P., & MacLeod, C. M. (2013). Putting retrieval-induced forgetting in context: An inhibition-free, context-based account. *Psychological Review, 120*(4), 852–872.

Kassam, K. S., Gilbert, D. T., Swencionis, J. K., & Wilson, T. D. (2009). Misconceptions of memory: The Scooter Libby effect. *Psychological Science, 20*, 551–552.

Kay, H. (1955). Learning and retaining verbal material. *British Journal of Psychology, 46*, 81–100.

Kelley, M. R., Pentz, C., & Reysen, M. B. (2014). The joint influence of collaboration and part-set cueing. *Quarterly Journal of Experimental Psychology, 67*(10), 1977–1985.

Kendeou, P., & O'Brien, E. J. (2014). The knowledge revision components (KReC) framework: Processes and mechanisms. In D. Rapp & J. Braasch (Eds.), *Processing Inaccurate Information: Theoretical and Applied Perspectives from Cognitive Science and the Educational Sciences* (pp. 353–377). Cambridge, MA: MIT Press.

Kessler, Y., Vandermorris, S., Gopie, N., Daros, A., Winocur, G., & Moscovitch, M. (2014). Divided attention improves delayed, but not immediate retrieval of a consolidated memory. *PloS one, 9*(3), e91309.

Kirchner, T. R., & Sayette, M. A. (2003). Effects of alcohol on controlled and automatic memory processes. *Experimental and Clinical Psychopharmacology, 11*, 167–175.

Krause, C. M., Aromäki, A., Sillanmäki, L., Åström, T., Alanko, K., Salonen, E., & Peltola, O. (2002). Alcohol-induced alterations in ERD/ERS during an auditory memory task. *Alcohol, 26*, 145–153.

Kroeger, M. E., Hueng, N. L., Curry, S. D., Copeland, M. B., & Kelley, M. R. (2019). On the composition of part-set cues. *Quarterly Journal of Experimental Psychology, 72*(10), 2365–2370.

Lawrence, Z., & Peterson, D. (2016). Mentally walking through doorways causes forgetting: The location updating effect and imagination. *Memory, 24*(1), 12–20.

Lee, Y. S. (2018). Withdrawal of spatial overt attention following intentional forgetting: Evidence from eye movements. *Memory, 26*(4), 503–513.

Leitz, J. R., Morgan, C., J. A., Bisby, J. A., Rendell, P. G., & Curran, H. V. (2009). Global impairment of prospective memory following acute alcohol. *Psychopharmacology, 205*, 379–387.

Lewandowsky, S., Stritzke, W. G. K., Oberauer, K., & Morales, M. (2005). Memory for fact, fiction, and misinformation: The Iraq war 2003. *Psychological Science, 16*, 190–195.

MacLeod, C. M. (1989). Directed forgetting affects both direct and indirect tests of memory. *Journal of Experimental Psychology: Learning, Memory, and Cognition, 15*, 13–21.

Martini, M., Martini, C., Maran, T., & Sachse, P. (2018). Effects of post-encoding wakeful rest and study time on long-term memory performance. *Journal of Cognitive Psychology, 30*(5–6), 558–569.

Mason, M. F., Hood, B. M., & Macrae, C. N. (2004). Look into my eyes: Gaze direction and person memory. *Memory, 12*, 637–643.

Maylor, E. A., & Rabbitt, P. M. A. (1993). Alcohol, reaction time and memory: A meta-analysis. *British Journal of Psychology, 84*, 301–317.

McGeoch, J. A. (1932). Forgetting and the law of disuse. *Psychological Review, 39*, 352–370.

Melton, A. W., & Irwin, J. M. Q., (1940). The influence of degree of interpolated learning on retroactive inhibition and the overt transfer of specific responses. *American Journal of Psychology, 53*, 173–203.

Mintzer, M. Z., Kuwabara, H., Alexander, M., Brasic, J. R., Ye, W., Ernst, M., Griffiths, R. R., & Wong, D. F. (2006). Dose effects of triazolam on brain activity during episodic memory encoding: A PET study. *Psychopharmacology, 188*, 445–461.

Moulton, P. L., Petros, T. V., Apostal, K. J., Park, R. V., Ronning, E. A., King, B. M., & Penland, J. G. (2005). Alcohol-induced impairment and enhancement

of memory: A test of the interference theory. *Physiology & Behavior, 85*, 240–245.

Murayama, K., Miyatsu, T., Buchli, D., & Storm, B. C. (2014). Forgetting as a consequence of retrieval: A meta-analytic review of retrieval-induced forgetting. *Psychological Bulletin, 140*(5), 1383–1409.

Nee, D. E., & Jonides, J. (2008). Dissociable interference-control processes in perception and memory. *Psychological Science, 19*, 490–500.

Nelson, T. O., McSpadden, M., Fromme, K., & Marlatt, G. A. (1986). Effects of alcohol intoxication on metamemory and on retrieval from long-term memory. *Journal of Experimental Psychology: General, 115*, 247–254.

Newtson, D. (1973). Attribution and the unit of perception of ongoing behavior. *Journal of Personality and Social Psychology, 28*(1), 28–38.

Nørby, S. (2015). Why forget? On the adaptive value of memory loss. *Perspectives on Psychological Science, 10*(5), 551–578.

Nyhan, B., & Reifler, J. (2010). When corrections fail: The persistence of political misperceptions. *Political Behavior, 32*(2), 303–330.

O'Rear, A. E., & Radvansky, G. A. (2020). Failure to accept retractions: A contribution to the continued influence effect. *Memory & Cognition, 48*(1), 127–144.

Oswald, K. M., Serra, M., & Krishna, A. (2006). Part-list cuing in speeded recognition and free recall. *Memory & Cognition, 34*, 518–526.

Pastötter, B., Schicker, S., Niedernhuber, J., & Bäuml, K.-H. T. (2011). Retrieval during learning facilitates subsequent memory encoding. *Journal of Experimental Psychology: Learning, Memory, and Cognition, 37*, 287–297.

Pettijohn, K. A., & Radvansky, G. A. (2018). Walking through doorways causes forgetting: Recall. *Memory, 26*(10), 1430–1435.

Pierce, B. H., Gallo, D. A., & McCain, J. L. (2017). Reduced interference from memory testing: A postretrieval monitoring account. *Journal of Experimental Psychology: Learning, Memory, and Cognition, 43*(7), 1063–1072.

Postman, L., & Keppel, G. (1977). Conditions of cumulative proactive inhibition. *Journal of Experimental Psychology: General, 106*, 376–403.

Postman, L., & Stark, K. (1969). Role of response availability in transfer and interference. *Journal of Experimental Psychology, 79*, 168–177.

Postman, L., Stark, K., & Fraser, J. (1968). Temporal changes in interference. *Journal of Verbal Learning and Verbal Behavior, 7*(3), 672–694.

Radvansky, G. A. (1999). Memory retrieval and suppression: The inhibition of situation models. *Journal of Experimental Psychology: General, 128*, 563–579.

Radvansky, G. A., & Copeland, D. E. (2006). Walking through doorways causes forgetting: Situation models and experienced space. *Memory & Cognition, 34*(5), 1150–1156.

Radvansky, G. A., Krawietz, S. A., & Tamplin, A. K. (2011). Walking through doorways causes forgetting: Further explorations. *Quarterly Journal of Experimental Psychology, 64*(8), 1632–1645.

Radvansky, G. A., O'Rear A. E., & Fisher, J. S. (2017). Event models and the fan effect. *Memory & Cognition, 45*(6), 1028–1044.

Radvansky, G. A., Spieler, D. H., & Zacks, R. T. (1993). Mental model organization. *Journal of Experimental Psychology: Learning, Memory, and Cognition, 19*, 95–114.

Radvansky, G. A., Tamplin, A. K., & Krawietz, S. A. (2010). Walking through doorways causes forgetting: Environmental integration. *Psychonomic Bulletin & Review, 17*(6), 900–904.

Radvansky, G. A., & Zacks, J. M. (2011). Event perception. *Wiley Interdisciplinary Reviews: Cognitive Science, 2*(6), 608–620.

Radvansky, G. A., & Zacks, R. T. (1991). Mental models and the fan effect. *Journal of Experimental Psychology: Learning, Memory, and Cognition, 17*, 940–953.

Reder, L. M., Oates, J. M., Thornton. E. R., Quinlan, J. J., Kaufer, A., & Sauer, J. (2006). Drug-induced amnesia hurts recognition, but only for memories that can be unitized. *Psychological Science, 17*, 562–567.

Reysen, M. B. (2003). The effects of social pressure on group recall. *Memory & Cognition, 31*, 1163–1168.

Reysen, M. B., & Adair, S. A. (2008). Social processing improves recall performance. *Psychonomic Bulletin & Review, 15*, 197–201.

Roediger, H. L., Stellon, C. C., & Tulving, E. (1977). Inhibition from part-list cues and rate of recall. *Journal of Experimental Psychology: Human Learning and Memory, 3*, 174–188.

Rohrer, D., & Pashler, H. E. (2003). Concurrent task effects on memory retrieval. *Psychonomic Bulletin & Review, 10*(1), 96–103.

Ross, L., Greene, D., & House, P. (1977). The "false consensus effect": An egocentric bias in social perception and attribution processes. *Journal of Experimental Social Psychology, 13*, 279–301.

Rubin, D. C., & Wenzel, A. E. (1996). One hundred years of forgetting: A quantitative description of retention. *Psychological Review, 103*(4), 734–760.

Rundus, D. (1973). Negative effects of using list items as recall cues. *Journal of Verbal Learning and Verbal Behavior, 12*, 43–50.

Sahakyan, L., & Kelley, C. M. (2002). A contextual change account of the directed forgetting effect. *Journal of Experimental Psychology: Learning, Memory, and Cognition, 28*(6), 1064–1072.

Saults, J. S., Cowan, N., Sher, K. J., & Moreno, M. V. (2007). Differential effects of alcohol on working memory: Distinguishing multiple processes. *Experimental and Clinical Psychopharmacology, 15*, 576–587.

Saunders, J. O., & MacLeod, M. D. (2006). Can inhibition resolve retrieval competition through the control of spreading activation? *Memory & Cognition, 34*(2), 307–322.

Schacter, D. L. (2001). *The Seven Sins of Memory: How the Mind Forgets and Remembers.* Boston, MA: Haughton Mifflin.

Schlichting, A., & Bäuml, K-H. T. (2017). Brief wakeful resting can eliminate directed forgetting. *Memory, 25*(2), 254–260.

Scholey, A. B., & Fowles, K. A. (2002). Retrograde enhancement of kinesthetic memory by alcohol and by glucose. *Neurobiology of Learning and Memory, 78*, 477–483.

Schreiber Compo, N., Evans, J. R., Carol, R. N., Kemp, D., Villalba, D., Ham, L. S., & Rose, S. (2011). Alcohol intoxication and memory for events: A snapshot of alcohol myopia in a real-world drinking scenario. *Memory, 19*(2), 202–210.

Shtulman, A., & Valcarcel, J. (2012). Scientific knowledge suppresses but does not supplant earlier intuitions. *Cognition, 124*(2), 209–215.

Slamecka, N. J. (1968). An examination of trace storage in free recall. *Journal of Experimental Psychology, 4,* 504–513.

Smith. E. E., Adams, N., & Schorr, D. (1978). Fact retrieval and the paradox of interference. *Cognitive Psychology, 10,* 438–464.

Smith, S. M., & Handy, J. D. (2014). Effects of varied and constant environmental contexts on acquisition and retention. *Journal of Experimental Psychology: Learning, Memory, and Cognition, 40*(6), 1582–1593.

Sparrow, B., Liu, J., & Wegner, D. M. (2011). Google effects on memory: Cognitive consequences of having information at our fingertips. *Science, 333*(6043), 776–778.

Staudigl, T., Hanslmayr, S., & Bäuml, K-H. T. (2010). Theta oscillations reflect the dynamics of interference in episodic memory retrieval. *Journal of Neuroscience, 30*(34), 11356–11362.

Storm, B. C. (2011). The benefit of forgetting in thinking and remembering. *Current Directions in Psychological Science, 20*(5), 291–295.

Storm, B. C., Koppel, R. H., & Wilson, B. M. (2013). Selective cues can fail to cause forgetting. *Quarterly Journal of Experimental Psychology, 66*(1), 29–36.

Swallow, K. M., Zacks, J. M., & Abrams, R. A. (2009). Event boundaries in perception affect memory encoding and updating. *Journal of Experimental Psychology: General, 138*(2), 236.

Szpunar, K. K., McDermott, K. B., & Roediger, H. L. (2008). Testing during study insulates against the buildup of proactive interference. *Journal of Experimental Psychology: Learning, Memory, and Cognition, 34,* 1392–1399.

Thorndike, E. L. (1914). *The Psychology of Learning.* New York: Teachers College, Columbia University.

Tulving. E., & Hastie, R. (1972). Inhibition effects of intralist repetition in free recall. *Journal of Experimental Psychology, 92,* 297–304.

Tulving, E., & Psotka, J. (1971). Retroactive inhibition in free recall: Inaccessibility of information available

in the memory store. *Journal of Experimental Psychology, 87,* 1–8.

Tversky, B., & Marsh, E. J. (2000). Biased retellings of events yield biased memories. *Cognitive Psychology, 40,* 1–38.

Underwood, B. J. (1957). Interference and forgetting. *Psychological Review, 64,* 49–60.

Utochkin, I. S., & Brady, T. F. (2019). Independent storage of different features of real-world objects in long-term memory. *Journal of Experimental Psychology: General, 149*(3), 530–549.

Utsumi, K., & Saito, S. (2016). When remembering the past suppresses memory for future actions. *Memory, 24*(4), 437–443.

van der Werf, S. P., Geurts, S., & de Werd, M. M. (2016). Subjective memory ability and long-term forgetting in patients referred for neuropsychological assessment. *Frontiers in Psychology, 7,* 605.

Vollrath, D. A., Sheppard, B. H., Hinsz, V. B., & Davis, J. H. (1989). Memory performance by decision-making groups and individuals. *Organizational Behavior and Human Decision Processes, 43,* 289–300.

Wahlheim, C. N. (2015). Testing can counteract proactive interference by integrating competing information. *Memory & Cognition, 43*(1), 27–38.

Weldon, M. S., & Bellinger, K. D. (1997). Collective memory: Collaborative and individual processes in remembering. *Journal of Experimental Psychology: Learning, Memory, and Cognition, 23,* 1160–1175.

Weldon, M. S., Blair, C., & Huebsch, P. D. (2000). Group remembering: Does social loafing underlie collaborative inhibition? *Journal of Experimental Psychology: Learning, Memory, and Cognition, 26,* 1568–1577.

Wickens, D. D. (1970). Encoding categories of words: An empirical approach to meaning. *Psychological Review, 77*(1), 1–15.

Wickens, D. D. (1972). Characteristics of word encoding. In A. W. Melton & E. Martin (Eds.), *Coding Processes in Human Memory* (pp. 191–215). New York: Wiley.

Wilkes, A. L., & Leatherbarrow, M. (1988). Editing episodic memory following the identification of error. *Quarterly Journal of Experimental Psychology,* *40*(2), 361–387.

Xie, H., Chen, Y., Lin, Y., Hu, X., & Zhang, D. (2020). Can't forget: Disruption of the right prefrontal cortex impairs voluntary forgetting in a recognition test. *Memory, 28*(1), 60–69.

Zacks, J. M., Speer, N. K., & Reynolds, J. R. (2009). Segmentation in reading and film comprehension. *Journal of Experimental Psychology: General, 138*(2), 307.

Zwaan, R. A. (1996). Processing narrative time shifts. *Journal of Experimental Psychology: Learning, Memory, and Cognition, 22*(5), 1196–1207.

CHAPTER 9

Semantic Memory

Sometimes our memories do not refer to specific events but are more encyclopedic. This general knowledge is **semantic memory**. Semantic memory allows us to take advantage of regularities in the world to make more accurate predictions about what will happen next. For example, if all you had to go on were episodic memories of specific instances, then every time you encountered a dog you would need to start all over again figuring out how you should react. Every time you saw a new chair, you would need to determine what its purpose was. Every time you went to a new restaurant, you would have to learn how to get some food. Semantic memories are generalizations that apply to a variety of similar circumstances.

In this chapter we cover several aspects of semantic memory. We first address the issue of semantic memory organization and how it provides not only the information we may need in the moment, but also other related information that is likely to be relevant. This is semantic priming. We then examine two classes of semantic memories and how we use them to understand our world. One is how categories are structured and used. We also consider how ordered relations are represented and influence memory. Another type of semantic memory is scripts and schemas for commonly experienced aspects of life. Finally, we look at cases where semantic memory falls short.

SEMANTIC PRIMING

A salient characteristic of semantic memory is its organization and structure. Remembering one **concept** makes related ideas more available. This facilitation of related ideas is **priming** (Meyer & Schvaneveldt, 1971). Semantic memory is structured based on meaning (Thompson-Schill et al., 1998) and similar concepts are metaphorically stored closer together. When a concept is activated, this activation spreads to related concepts. Because they are more activated, if there is then a need to use them, they can be used more readily. Note that concepts do not need to be abstract , but can be anything people are thinking about, including their emotional state. For example, people respond faster to happy words such as "peace" when in a happy mood and faster to sad words such as "die" when in a sad mood (Olafson & Ferraro, 2001).

A typical priming paradigm involves lexical decision. That is, people are given strings of letters and asked to indicate whether they are words. For example, "doctor" is a word, but "dohter" is not. In these studies, there are pairs of words: a critical item, called a **prime**, is followed by a **target**. What is of interest is how fast people respond to the target. If the prime is unrelated to the target, this is a baseline, *control* condition (e.g., "potato" followed by "doctor"). If the prime is semantically related to the target, this is the *experimental* condition (e.g., "nurse" followed by "doctor"). People respond faster to a target in the experimental condition relative to the control. Priming is observed in ERPs as early as 250 ms after a target is presented (Bentin et al., 1985). It is easier for the brain to activate that information, so it does not need to work as hard.

Semantic priming occurs because concepts are not understood in isolation but in terms of how they relate to each other. By activating related concepts, people bring to bear a larger set of knowledge to help them understand and think. For example, when you listen to a lecture, you need a broad understanding of what is being discussed. You do not just narrowly think about the specific words being said.

Priming helps us detect inconsistencies. When we encounter semantically anomalous information, such as hearing the sentence "The doctor listened with his carrot," ERP data show an increased negativity around 400 ms after first hearing it (Kutas & Hillyard, 1980). This is called the N400. That is, when memory is surprised by the anomalous information, it works harder to figure out what is going on.

STUDY IN DEPTH

Priming is a largely automatic, implicit process. Still, it is possible for it to be affected by conscious effort. This was shown in a study by James Neely (1977). In this study, 122 students at Yale University were given a series of category names followed by a lexical decision task. That is, people saw a category label, such as BIRD, followed by a string of letters, such as "bluejay," with the task of indicating whether that string was a word. These probes came 250, 400, or 700 ms after the category label. This difference between the onset of the category and the lexical decision probe is the stimulus onset asynchrony, or SOA.

There were five conditions in his study. The pattern of results for each of these is shown in Figure 9.1. The first condition was *Nonshift–Expected–Related* in which people expected that if a word followed the category name, it would be a member of that category, and it was—for example, seeing the category BIRD followed by the word "robin." As can be seen in Figure 9.1, consistent positive priming was observed at all SOAs.

A second condition was *Nonshift–Unexpected–Unrelated*, in which people expected that if a word followed the category name, it would be a member of that category, but it was not—for example, seeing BIRD followed by "arm." Looking at Figure 9.1, there is initially no effect on response time, but later people are slower to respond because the activation has all been directed to the BIRD portion of semantic memory. Thus, it takes time to disengage and move to another part of semantic memory.

The third condition was *Shift–Expected–Unrelated*, in which people were told to expect that when a word followed a category name, it would be a member of a certain unrelated category, and it was. An example of this would be seeing BODY followed by

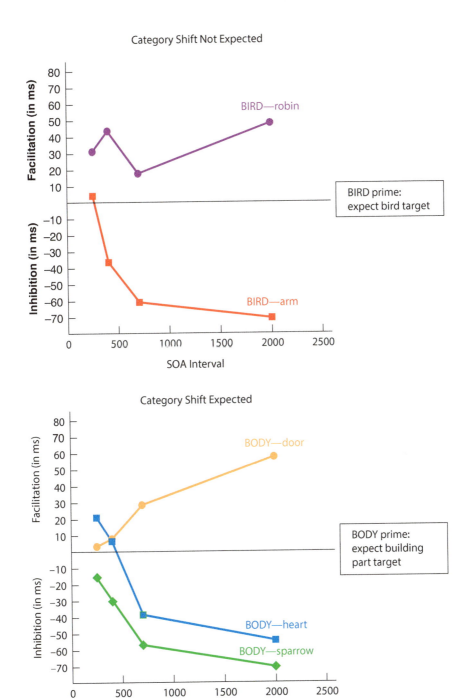

FIGURE 9.1 *Automatic and Controlled Priming in Semantic Memory*

Source: Neely, J. H. (1977). Semantic priming and retrieval from lexical memory: Roles of inhibitionless spreading activation and limited-capacity attention. *Journal of Experimental Psychology: General, 106,* 226–254

"door" when people were told that a building part was expected. As shown in Figure 9.1, priming develops over time. If people expect a building part when they get BODY, they can activate that part of semantic memory, but this takes time.

The fourth condition, *Shift–Unexpected–Unrelated*, was like the third, except the word was a member of an unrelated category—for example, seeing BODY followed by "sparrow." In Figure 9.1 there is initially some negative priming, and this gets larger over time. Because people expect a building part when they get BODY, they consciously activate the building portion of semantic memory. It requires effort to disengage this activation and move it.

The fifth condition was *Shift–Unexpected–Related*, which is like the previous two, except that the word was a member of the same category as the prime—for example, seeing BODY followed by "heart". In Figure 9.1, initially there is some positive priming. An automatic process activates the part of semantic memory associated with the category name. However, people shift activation to another part of semantic memory. Thus, some effort is needed to disengage from what is expected and move back to the original portion. This pattern of response times is supported by EEG recordings that show that the automatic activation of information emphasizes the parieto-temporal cortex, whereas the conscious evaluation emphasizes the frontal lobes (Krause et al., 1998).

Mediated Priming

The theory behind semantic priming is that when a concept is activated, this activation spreads to related concepts. How far does this spread go? Do only those concepts that are directly related to the first one get the spreading activation, or does it go beyond that? For example, when the concept "lion" is activated it is likely that "tiger" is activated because these are both large, predatory cats. If "tiger" is primed, are concepts related to it also activated, such as "stripes"? This is **mediated priming** because the connection between "lion" and "stripes" is mediated by "tiger."

In general, mediated priming does occur (Balota & Lorch, 1986), as shown using both response times and ERP data (Hill et al., 2002). However, mediated priming is more fragile than direct priming. The priming is smaller in magnitude, and it is sometimes not observed (De Groot, 1983).

Semantic Interconnectivity

In episodic memory, more associations with a concept can slow down retrieval, as in the fan effect. Semantic memory is made up of very large numbers of associations among concepts. This interconnectivity is a complex network of concepts and associations (see Chapter 18). Thus, based on the fan effect, we would expect that it should be difficult to retrieve semantic information. However, the opposite is true: concepts in semantic memory that have more interconnections are retrieved faster (Ashcraft, 1978a; Kroll & Klimesch, 1992).

In semantic memory these associations provide both direct and indirect connections among concepts. Two concepts might be directly associated and share several intermediate concepts, which increases the number of retrieval pathways between them. As a result, there are many ways that concepts can prime one another. The more indirect connections there are, the more likely any one of those pathways will be activated after a given time. Think of this as a horse race. If there are more horses running, the race will likely be over faster than if only a few horses are racing because it is more likely that there will be a fast horse in the bunch.

Inhibition

Like episodic memory, **inhibition** can help narrow a semantic memory search by suppressing related concepts during retrieval. For example, people retrieve the concept "salmon" for the category FISH slower if they had recently retrieved several other examples of fish. This inhibition occurs only if people actively retrieve information, not if they are passively reading (Blaxton & Neely, 1983). The need to select a specific semantic memory can cause the inhibition of related competitors that could otherwise produce interference.

Nature of Semantic Information

One generalization about semantic memory is the difference between taxonomic and thematic semantic relations. **Taxonomic relations** refer to shared features, such as knowing that "horse" and "cow" are both farm animals. In comparison, **thematic relations** refer to co-occurrence, such as knowing that "dog" and "leash" go together (Mirman et al., 2017). These types of semantic memory are activated at different rates (Kalénine et al., 2012), with thematic relations typically being retrieved faster than taxonomic relations. Importantly, it is possible to neurologically disrupt one type of knowledge and leave the other intact (e.g., Merck et al. 2014), suggesting that these are distinct types of semantic memory.

Although some theories give the impression that semantic memory has a clear structure, like a computer database, keep in mind that this is a memory system with a human face. Semantic memory certainly captures such distributional information (how often things occur), but it also captures more experiential, embodied aspects (Andrews et al., 2009). As an example, right-handers tend to associate positive concepts with the right half of space, whereas left-handers do the opposite (Casasanto, 2009). Another example is that information retrieval reflects perceptual qualities (Solomon & Barsalou, 2004), such as the amount of visual area taken up by a property. For example, for the concept *fish*, the property *scales* is relatively easy to retrieve compared to the property *eye*.

For abstract concepts (e.g., *barrier*) we tend to rely more on thematic relations (what tends to occur together), but for concrete concepts (e.g., *mushroom*) we rely more on taxonomic relations (Crutch et al., 2009). That said, it may be that even abstract concepts have an embodied element. Concepts, such as *horror* and *beauty*, have an emotional element, and the bodily experience of emotion may be tied, in some way, to some abstract concepts (Kousta et al., 2011). Moreover, even simple things like how we represent nouns and verbs reflect different aspects of semantic memory. ERP recordings show that nouns, particularly concrete nouns, tend to activate more of the sensory cortex (BAs 1, 2, & 3), whereas verbs of action tend to activate the motor cortex (BA 4) (Andres et al., 2008; Pulvermüller et al., 1999).

In a compelling demonstration of embodied semantic memory, Pecher et al. (2003) gave students a property identification task in which they were shown pairs of words, such as "BLENDER–loud." The task was to indicate whether the second word was a property of the first. Students were faster when the property was from the same sensory modality as the previous trial. For example, people were faster to respond to "BLENDER–loud" if it immediately followed "LEAVES–rustling" (which also involves sound) than if it followed "CRANBERRIES–tart" (which involves taste). This suggests that semantic knowledge, although abstract, is still influenced by how we physically interact with the world.

Finally, the concepts that we have in semantic memories are not stable and fixed. They are fluid and dynamic. Semantic memories are emergent and contextualized (Yee & Thompson-Schill, 2016). That is, they are (a) the sum of our long-term experiences (e.g., all of your encounters with lemons), (b) biased by our recent experiences (e.g., using lemons to make lemonade), (c) the context and the current task (finding lemons in the grocery store), and (d) your current mental state (e.g., what was recently primed in semantic memory). Thus, while semantic memories are often depicted as stable and enduring, it still experiences a great deal of flux.

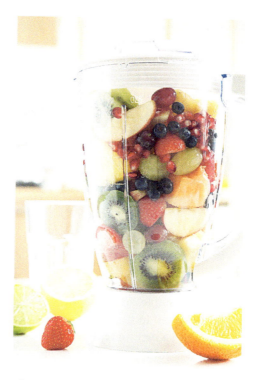

PHOTO 9.1 *When people access information in semantic memory, embodied influences, such as how a blender sounds, or how fruit tastes, can influence the availability of other information along that same sensory modality*

Source: sirtravelalot/Shutterstock.com

Stop and Review

The activation of knowledge in semantic memory causes the priming of related concepts. The more related the concepts are, the more they prime each other. After an initial, automatic process, people may also engage in a more consciously controlled search of semantic memory. Priming can extend beyond immediately related concepts to more distant concepts (albeit more weakly), as with mediated priming. Semantic memory retrieval, more generally, is facilitated by more connections among concepts. This contrasts with episodic memory, in which more associations impede retrieval. Finally, semantic information, although seemingly abstract, clearly captures embodied qualities of thought.

CATEGORIES

Rather than remembering lots of bits and pieces of information, we group knowledge together. This similarity-based grouping is **categorization**, in which two or more entities are treated as though they are equivalent. Categorization allows us to draw on prior experience in a regular and reliable fashion in new situations. We can assume that some of the elements of the new situation will be like previous ones. For example, having the category "dog" allows us to treat members of that category as more or less the same, such as knowing that all dogs eat dog food, may bite, and like to run. In this section we look at how semantic memory categorizes information. We first look at some properties of human categories, followed by some theories of categorization (Medin, 1989). After this, we look at cases of categorization in social situations, namely stereotypes and prejudice.

Properties of Categories

Mental categories are complex, with the various members relating to a category in different ways. One characteristic is the three **levels of categorization**: basic, subordinate, and superordinate (Rosch & Mervis, 1975). The basic level is the one at which we operate at most often. At this level categories are defined by features with enough detail to allow us to treat different members as similar but without more detail than is necessary. Examples of basic level categories are *saw, dog, chair*, or *drum*. The subordinate level provides detailed information about specific portions of a basic category. Examples of subordinate level categories are *camping saw, miniature poodle, leather recliner*, and *kettle drum*. Finally, the superordinate level provides very general information that captures a range of basic level categories. Examples of superordinate categories are *tool, pet, furniture*, and *musical instrument*.

These levels reflect how people use categories. In general, basic level category information is retrieved better than the others (Rosch et al., 1976). People retrieve more attributes and names for basic level categories (Tversky & Hemenway, 1984). This difference in retrieval speed is shown in Figure 9.2 and suggests that the basic level has some importance to semantic memory.

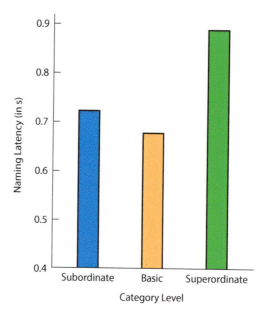

FIGURE 9.2 *Naming Time for Concepts at Different Category Levels*

Source: Tversky, B., & Hemenway, K. (1984). Objects, parts, and categories. *Journal of Experimental Psychology: General, 113*, 169–193

Categories have many members. Their combined influence manifests itself in several ways. First, categories exhibit a **central tendency** or averaged category ideal. This is important when we discuss category prototypes. Second, categories have **graded membership**. Mentally, some members are better members of the category than others. For example, *robin* is often thought of as being a better member of the category *bird* than is *penguin*. Alternatively, some things are ambiguous category members that may be marked with linguistic hedges—for example, statements like "technically, a tomato is a fruit" or "loosely speaking, a bat is a bird."

Finally, category members might not be defined by a single set of features. Different features may be shared among several instances. This is **family resemblance** (Rosch & Mervis, 1975). An example of this is the category *furniture*. Many types of furniture have legs, are made of wood, are intended to be used indoors, but this is not true of all types of furniture. People are sensitive to the correlations among features that define categories—for example, the idea that flying tends to go with birds and tires tend to go with bicycles. This is true both in terms of how categories are distinguished from one another, as well as the features that create a family resemblance within categories (Chin-Parker & Ross, 2002).

An important distinction is between **artifact categories** (things that people make) and **natural kind categories** (things that are found in nature). These are served by different brain regions (Martin & Chao, 2001). First, like most semantic memories, the left hemisphere tends to be more involved than the right. Natural kinds, such as animals, tend to involve more of the *medial* fusiform gyrus (BA 37) and superior temporal gyrus (BA 41). In comparison, artifacts involve more of the *lateral* fusiform gyrus (BA 37) and the posterior middle temporal gyrus (BA 21), near brain regions important for verbs and action (consistent with an embodied cognition view that artifacts are defined by how we use them). While both classes of categories show graded membership, this is more evident in artifact categories (Estes, 2004). We have more certainty about natural kinds (e.g., what makes something a bird) and have more ambiguity about artifacts (e.g., what makes something a tool). Also, we make perceptual decisions faster when comparing members of natural kind categories (what something looks like tells you what it is) but make manipulability (how you use it) decisions faster when comparing members of artifact categories (Kalénine & Bonthoux, 2008).

Classical Theory of Categorization

When you think of categories, you might think that we use rules to define them—for example, knowing that a *bachelor* is an unmarried adult male, that an *even number* is divisible by two, and that *speeding* is going faster than the posted limit. The idea that categories are defined by necessary and sufficient features is the **classical view of categorization**. They are *necessary* in that those features must be present, and they are *sufficient* in that if they are present, something is a member of a category. Any additional features are irrelevant. For instance, the number of teeth people have is additional information that has no bearing on whether they are bachelors.

A study by Bruner et al. (1956) assessed the classical view. In this study, people were shown items like those in Figure 9.3. These items are identified

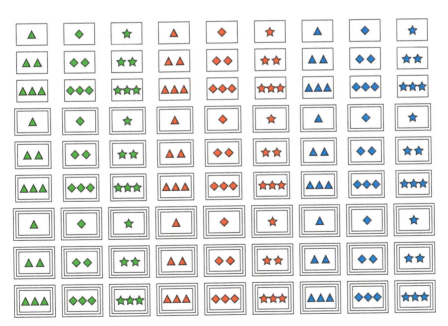

FIGURE 9.3 *Set of Stimuli Used to Illustrate the Classical View of Categorization*

Source: adapted from Bruner, J. S., Goodnow, J. J., & Austin, G. A. (1956). *A Study of Thinking*. Oxford, England: Wiley

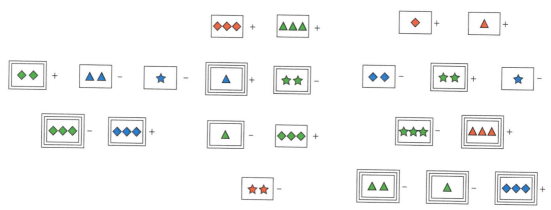

FIGURE 9.4 *Simple Set of Items Used to Derive a Category*

FIGURE 9.5 *Moderately Complex Set of Items Used to Derive a Category*

FIGURE 9.6 *More Complex Set of Items Used to Derive a Category*

along four dimensions: the type of objects, their number, their color, and the number of borders. People were given subsets of items, along with an indication of whether each was a member of a category. People could readily derive the category rules. Three category derivation examples are given in Figures 9.4, 9.5, and 9.6.

However, this is not how we typically use mental categories. The classical view cannot explain central tendency, graded membership, and family resemblance. For this view, something either satisfies the rules or it does not. Graded membership and such are irrelevant. However, the brain does not work on an either/or principle like a computer. Instead, it makes judgments based on loose and shifting collections of cell assemblies, giving our judgments a fuzzier quality (Lupyan, 2013). Keep in mind that the elements, features, or properties that define categories vary in their importance (Ashcraft, 1978b). More specifically, rarer features are more diagnostic than common features for defining a category (Mirman & Magnuson, 2009). For example, "has a trunk" is more defining of an elephant than is "breathes," although both are needed.

The shortfall of the classical view is also seen when we look at categories that have simple and clearly defined rules, such as the categories *even number* and *odd number*. However, they show graded membership (Armstrong et al., 1983). In the data, shown in Figure 9.7, "4" is rated as a better example of the category *even number* than is "106," even though they are both equally acceptable members of this category. In a similar study by Lupyan (2013), people were more willing to call equilateral triangles "triangles" compared to right, scalene, and isosceles triangles, even though they are all *triangles*. Similarly, people were more willing to call a woman a "grandmother" the older she was and the more grandchildren she had. Moreover, some people were willing to call a woman a "grandmother" if she was old and had children but no grandchildren. So, the big message here is that we play faster and looser with our mental categories than we sometimes might want to admit.

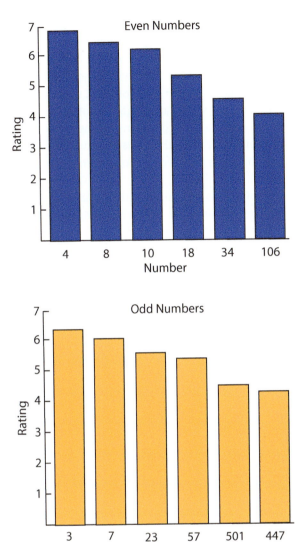

FIGURE 9.7 *Ratings of Items (Out of 6) for a Well-Defined Category—in this Case, Odd and Even Numbers*

Source: created from data reported in Armstrong, S. L., Gleitman, L. R., & Gleitman, H. (1983). What some concepts might not be. *Cognition, 13*(3), 263–308

Prototype Theory

Categories are organized, in part, using unconscious mental statistics. One idea of how this is done is the **prototype model**. For this view, categories are defined by a mental representation that is an average of all category members. This averaged representation is a *prototype* (Rosch, 1975), which may or may not correspond to an actual entity in the world. For example, the prototype for *dog* would be an average of all dogs ever encountered and may not correspond to any particular dog.

An example of prototype extraction using dot patterns is shown in Figure 9.8. The prototypes for the two categories are shown at the left. When people first learned the categories, they were shown deviations from the prototypes, such as those on the right. The prototypes were never shown during learning. However, when people were later asked to sort both old and new patterns, the prototypes were identified and correctly sorted at a high rate of accuracy. This suggests that they were derived and used to make decisions (Posner & Keele, 1968; 1970). If we can readily derive prototypes from things as meaningless as dot patterns, surely the same mental mechanisms are involved for deriving categories of our everyday experiences.

This use of prototypes is also seen with meaningful stimuli. For example, if photographs of faces are used for preference judgments along with morphed composites of faces, people rate the composite faces which are closer to a prototype face as being more attractive (Langlois & Roggman, 1990; but see Alley & Cunningham, 1991). That is, people prefer faces that are averages of others. Because they are averages, they have fewer unusual and distinguishing characteristics, and are easier to mentally process (Winkielman et al., 2006). A pretty face is a boring face. This is also part of the reason why attractive faces are harder to remember (Light et al., 1981). High attractiveness for more prototypical instances is also observed for dogs, cats, birds, fish, watches, and automobiles (Halberstadt & Rhodes, 2003).

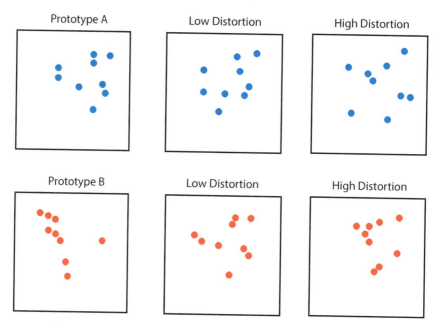

FIGURE 9.8 *Two Category Prototypes and Some Distortions*

Source: created from a description provided in Posner, M. I., & Keele, S. W. (1968). On the genesis of abstract ideas. *Journal of Experimental Psychology, 77,* 353–363

A nice thing about prototypes is that they provide a clear explanation for the central tendencies of categories (which is the prototype itself) and a graded category structure. The closer an instance is to the prototype, the better a member of the category it is. However, there are important aspects not accounted for. For example, people are often aware of a category size —that is, about how many different members are in the category. For example, we know that *insect types* is a large category, but *elephant types* is a small one. Prototypes convey no information about this variability. Also, a caricature (a category member with exaggerated features) is thought to better represent a category than a prototype when a category is considered in the context of other, related categories (Goldstone et al., 2003). That is because the caricature captures distinctive features and emphasizes them. This helps distinguish one category from other, similar categories.

Exemplar Theory

Another theory of categorization is **exemplar theory** (Medin & Schaffer, 1978; Nosofsky, 1988). In this view, people use all category members to make decisions. This captures central tendency, graded membership, and family resemblance, as well as information about category size, variability, correlated attributes, and any new information about the category. Because categorization is always using all the memory traces, new experiences have more influence. Exemplar theories can also explain the context sensitivity of categories. For example, the color gray is more similar to white in the context of hair color but is more similar to black in the context of clouds (Medin & Shoben, 1988).

Exemplar models have been developed into sophisticated mathematical models, such as the Generalized Context Model (Nosofsky, 1986; 2011). More recently, neural network models (see Chapter 18), based on neurobiological structures and principles, such as the COVIS model (Ashby et al., 1998; 2011; Ashby & Rosedahl, 2017) have also been successful. This approach assumes that category formation involves adjusting connections between the striatum (in the basal ganglia) and sensory association cortex.

While exemplar theory has successfully accounted for some categorization processes , it does not account for semantic memory more generally (Murphy, 2016). For example, exemplar theory does not explain levels of categorization (e.g., basic, superordinate, and subordinate), nor the explanations people generate to account for categories (see the next section).

A serious problem with both prototype and exemplar theories is an inherent circularity. Specifically, categories are defined by experiences with members of that category. That is, the members of the category all contribute to defining it. However, the memory traces that are selected are those that conform to the criteria of the category. In short, how can memory traces be selected to define a category if the category is needed to select them in the first place?

TRY IT OUT

Here is a study that illustrates the influence of human categories on thought (see Neath, 1998). For this task, you need to use this list of eight animals, namely, goose, duck, robin, sparrow, hawk, eagle, ostrich, and bat. This will serve as a basis for people making judgments.

For this project, you will need 36 people in six groups. Give people this list of animal names, preferably in a different random order for each person. Tell your participants to assume that these animals live near one another, such as on an island. Then ask people to estimate how many animals of the other species are infected given that a particular animal has a certain disease. Tell each group that the infected species is either the goose, duck, robin, sparrow, hawk, or eagle (leave out ostrich and bat), depending on the group, and have them estimate what percentage of the other animals are likely to be infected as well.

After people have made their estimates, gather the data together and calculate the average estimates for each of the different infected species. What you should find is that the more typical the infected animal is of the category *bird*, the higher the percentage of other animals infected, and the less typical the animal, the lower the percentage.

Explanation-Based Theory

Another view of categorization is that people try to have reasons for why things should be grouped together. For **explanation-based views**, categories are theories or explanations. For example, feathers and wings tend to go together because feathers are suited for flying. People use their knowledge to understand how the members of a category form a coherent group (Rehder & Ross, 2001). Examples of this are social groups, political events (e.g., revolutions), and social institutions (e.g., governments). These do not share physical features but overlap thematically (Goldwater et al., 2016). In general, when we create reasons for the categories that we use, we rely more on contrastive information (Chin-Parker & Cantelon, 2017).

In general, people place an emphasis on causes rather than effects (Ahn et al., 2000), consistent with the idea that they are using explanations for what makes something a category. For example, knowing that an animal swims is a more fundamental characteristic than knowing that it has webbed feet (presumably webbed feet help swimming). Also, categories are defined, in part, by how we interact with things (Markman & Ross, 2003), not just statistical regularities. What makes something a chair has more to do with your sitting in it than with the materials used to make it. Causal relations help define semantic memories (Fenker et al., 2005).

Importantly, people can make new categories on the fly. These are **ad hoc categories** (Barsalou, 1983). For example, coffee, perfume, leather, and skunks are all members of the category *things with a distinctive smell*. Ad hoc categories are interesting because people generate them off the cuff, but they still have many of the same properties as standard categories: central tendency, graded structures, and family resemblance. Thus, some semantic memory structures are generated spontaneously. This raises questions about the stability of semantic memory in general.

Consistent with the idea that we create categories as explanations is **psychological essentialism**, the idea that members of a category share an underlying essence, of which we may or may not be aware. This usually applies to natural kind categories, which can be defined by chemical structure or DNA, such as *water* or *skunk*. That said, some artifact categories, such as *scientific instruments*, are treated as though they have essential qualities, and some natural kind categories, like *humans*, are not (Kalish, 2002). People create categories pragmatically, as needed, to serve a purpose. The degree to which members fit a category is a function of how well they fulfill that purpose.

Stereotypes and Prejudice

There is no question that categorization, overall, is a valuable part of semantic memory. However, it can cause problems, such as when we engage in stereotyping. Stereotypes are categories for groups of people. When you stereotype people, you are treating them as if they are essentially the same as other members of that group. These stereotypes are activated automatically (Oakhill ct al., 2005). We use this semantic knowledge to make assumptions about people and are surprised when those assumptions are violated (Duffy & Keir, 2004). When a stereotype leads one person to treat another inappropriately, this is prejudice. So, while categories are generally useful, we must be careful with the categories we form about people.

Stop and Review

A central job of semantic memory is to create categories. Our categories are oriented around a basic level and show evidence of central tendency and graded membership, with family resemblance among the members. Mental categories typically do not follow the necessary and sufficient rules of classical categorization. Instead, they use probabilistic information, as in prototype and exemplar theories. Moreover, they also exhibit characteristics of problem solving, as with explanation-based categories. Overall, human categorization reflects both environmental (probabilistic theories) and goal-oriented (explanation-based theories) influences (Love, 2005; Rouder & Ratcliff, 2006).

ORDERED RELATIONS

Semantic memory can be influenced by knowledge that is ordered along some dimension, such as size, intelligence, or age. These are linear order effects (Banks, 1977). We first cover some classic order relations effects and then go over some embodied influences.

Classic Ordering Effects

One ordering effect is the **semantic distance effect** in which people make faster judgments about the order of two concepts as the distance between them increases (Rips et al., 1973). For example, it is easier to judge that an elephant is bigger than a rabbit than to judge that a dog is bigger than a rabbit. The farther apart two concepts are along a dimension, the easier it is to discriminate between them and so, people process this information quickly. As another example, people are more likely to confuse adjacent days of the week rather than days that are separated from one another (Ellis et al., 2015). As an embodied illustration, people find it easier to make memory responses on a computer keyboard if the response keys are far from one another, such as "A" and "L," than if they are adjacent, such as "K" and "L" (Lakens et al., 2011). Concepts that are close in semantic memory are harder to discriminate, so judgments that require people to distinguish between them are slower and more error prone.

For the **semantic congruity effect** people are faster to judge the relationship between two items if the comparison term matches the end of the dimension that they are on (Banks et al., 1975). For example, it is easier to judge that Jefferson was president before Monroe than it is to judge that Monroe was president *after* Jefferson because both are at the "early" end of the timeline. Dimensional information is stored in semantic memory with the concepts. Jefferson and Monroe are both marked as early U.S. presidents, so the attribute "early" is stored with them. When this knowledge is needed, if the attributes match the judgment, people respond faster than if there is a mismatch. With a mismatch, people need to think more to get the information lined up properly.

Finally, for the **serial position effect** people are faster to make judgments about two or more concepts at the extremes of a dimension than those in the middle (Shoben et al., 1989). For example, it is easier to judge that Rhode Island is smaller than Connecticut than to judge that Indiana is smaller than Ohio. Concepts that are at the ends of a dimension are more distinct and, so, are easier to discriminate, and semantic decisions can be made quickly.

More generally, serial position effects, like those observed in short-term memory (see Chapter 4), are also observed in semantic memory. An example of this would be memories for U.S. presidents (Roediger & Crowder, 1976) and church hymns

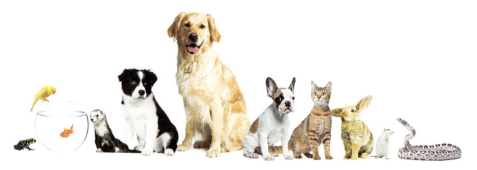

PHOTO 9.2 *When we judge information that is stored in semantic memory that varies along a dimension, such as size, the relative sizes of the items can influence the ease with which those semantic judgments are made*

Source: Eric Isselee/Shutterstock.com

(Maylor, 2002). These serial position curves are due to the frequency of exposure to information, with people encountering the names of the very early and recent presidents more so than others (Healy et al., 2000). This also accounts for the fact that Lincoln is remembered much better than he should be based on his serial position.

Embodied Influences on Ordered Relations

How we use our bodies to interact with the world can influence semantic order knowledge. One example of this is the Spatial-Numerical Association of Response Codes or **SNARC effect** (Dehaene et al., 1993). When people made judgments about numbers, such as whether they were odd or even, judgments about smaller numbers were made faster with the left hand. The reverse was true for the larger numbers. The SNARC effect is consistent with the idea that people have a mental number line in semantic memory going from left to right with small numbers on the left and large numbers appearing as one moves to the right (but see, Santens & Gevers, 2008), although this may be due to relative, rather than absolute, magnitudes (Nathan et al., 2009).

The SNARC effect reflects embodied experience in that it is more prominent in people who speak languages that are read left to right rather than right to left (Dehaene et al., 1993; Shaki & Fischer, 2008). However, it is also found in blind people (Castronovo & Seron, 2007), suggesting that it is not strictly visual. Moreover, the SNARC effect is not limited to numbers. Lidji et al. (2007) found a similar pattern with musical pitches. People respond faster to lower tones with the left hand and higher tones with the right, like the arrangement of notes on a piano or guitar string.[1]

Other examples of embodied influences on semantic memory include the findings that people are faster to identify words that refer to large objects (e.g., bookcase) than to small objects (e.g., teaspoon) (Sereno et al., 2009). Furthermore, the closer an object is to you, in space, time, or social relations, the more effectively it is processed. Although knowledge of an object could be abstract, it turns out that the more likely we are to interact with it, the more accessible it is in memory (Amit, et al., 2009). Semantic magnitudes can also influence our actions. For example, if people are asked to draw a line between two numbers, they draw it faster if the numbers are larger than smaller, even though the number magnitude is irrelevant (Girelli et al., 2016). Presumably, larger numbers convey a larger distance, which would require a faster speed to go from one to another in time. Thus, we incorporate embodied processing in abstract conceptual knowledge.

Stop and Review

Semantic memories capture ordered relations in the world, with the availability of knowledge being influenced by relative positions in those orders. The classic serial ordering effects are the semantic distance, the semantic congruity, and the serial order effects. In addition, ordered information can show embodied influences as exemplified by the SNARC effect.

---

1 See also Gevers et al. (2004) for a day of the week effect, and Prado et al. (2008) for a linear order effect.

SCHEMAS AND SCRIPTS

In life, there are many situations that are fairly regular in how they unfold and operate and how we react to them. That is, common experiences shared some framework that unites them. For example, your experiences of college lecture classes are similar and have a lot of commonalities. We can capitalize on this to help us understand new situations, much as we use categories to understand new objects or creatures. A semantic memory that captures commonly encountered aspects of life is called a **schema**. This idea was originally developed by Bartlett (1932).[2] Schemas contain basic information about the components of a certain aspect of life and how these parts interact with one another. A schema can be thought of as a blueprint for events that people draw upon to understand a specific case. In some sense, schemas are types of theory-based categories. The use of schemas in memory processing also involves, in various ways, the ventromedial prefrontal cortex (BA 10, 14, 25, & 32), the hippocampus, the angular gyrus (BA 39), and the unimodal associative cortices (depending on the modality) (for a review, see Gilboa & Marlatte, 2017). As you will see, schemas can be used to help memory, but they can also hurt memory.

Primary Schema Processes

There are five primary schema processes (Alba & Hasher, 1983). These are selection, abstraction, interpretation, integration, and reconstruction. The first four are for encoding new information, and the fifth is important for retrieval.

If people have a schema, they can use the process of **selection** to sort out which things are likely to be central and which are peripheral. That is, schemas select out those elements that are important. For example, when watching a football game, it is important to understand how much time has elapsed. Your schema tells you to pay attention to the clock. In contrast, if you were watching a baseball game, the amount of time that has elapsed is of considerably less importance. Thus, your schema for baseball would select out information about the time. Information that is important in schemas is more likely to be encoded and remembered.

Knowing which schema is relevant can influence performance. In a study by Bransford and Johnson (1972), people read an ambiguous passage (see Table 9.1). If people are told ahead of time that the passage is entitled "Washing Clothes," then they remember more of it later. The title allowed them to activate the appropriate schema and they could then select what was relevant in the passage and interpret it. This occurs during encoding because this title benefit is only seen when it is given *before* reading (Summers et al., 1985).

Abstraction involves converting the surface form of information (e.g., verbatim wording) into a more abstract representation that captures the underlying meaning (Burgoon et al., 2013). For example, when we hear sentences and comprehend

---

2 If you have more than one schema, they are called either schemas or schemata. Both plurals are acceptable.

TABLE 9.1 *Ambiguous Passage that Is Clarified by Activating the Appropriate Schema*

The procedure is actually quite simple. First arrange items into different groups. Of course one pile may be sufficient depending on how much there is to do. If you have to go somewhere else due to a lack of facilities, that is the next step; otherwise, you are pretty well set. It is important not to overdo things. That is, it is better to do too few things at once than too many. In the short run this may not seem important, but complications can easily arise. A mistake can be expensive as well. At first, the whole procedure will seem complicated. Soon, however, it will become just another facet of life. It is difficult to foresee any end to necessity for this task in the immediate future, but then, one never can tell. After the procedure is completed one arranges the material into different groups again. Then they can be put into their appropriate places. Eventually they will be used once more and the whole cycle will then have to be repeated. However, that is part of life.

Source: Bransford & Johnson, 1972

them, within a few minutes we are not able to distinguish verbatim sentences from paraphrases (Sachs, 1967; 1974). Similarly, if we see a picture, we are less likely to notice a change, such as adding or subtracting elements, rearranging entities in the scene, or changing the orientation of entities in the picture, if the rearranged picture fits the abstract, schematic memory of what we saw (Mandler & Ritchey, 1977).

This effect of schemas is not always in the direction of making things more general. Sometimes it can be the opposite if we go from a superordinate to a basic level category (Pansky & Koriat, 2004). For example, if one person hears "vehicle" (superordinate) and another hears "sports car" (subordinate), both will abstract this information to the basic level "car." Keep in mind that we are likely to notice changes that alter the meaning of what we saw or heard.

An example of abstraction is shown in Figure 9.9. In a study by Carmichael et al. (1932), people saw the line drawings in the middle column with one of two labels. Each of these labels is placed next to the drawing. After a time, people were asked to draw what they remembered seeing. Examples of the types of drawings that were made are on the right and left sides of Figure 9.8. People tended to distort their drawings to conform to the label that was provided. People used their schemas to abstract away and lose the ambiguous information. Thus, what is remembered is more schema consistent.

The schema process of **interpretation** allows people to fill in the gaps for things that were missed. When we read a book, watch television, or even experience events, there is a lot that we miss. For example, when you see a movie, many things happen off-camera. Still, you have no troubling inferring what they are. If you watch a film in which a person is boarding an airplane one moment and getting off the next, you do not think that the person got onto the plane and then immediately turned around and got off. Instead, you infer that there was a flight in between, although only a few seconds have elapsed in reality.

Original

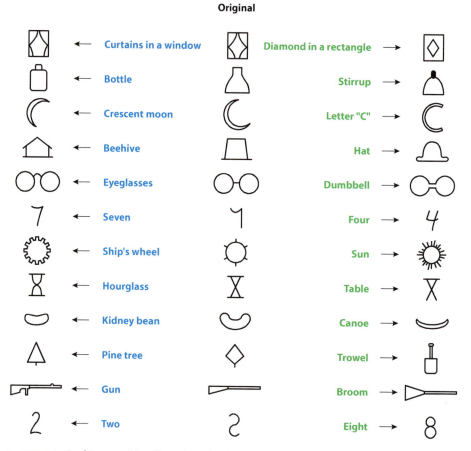

FIGURE 9.9 *Ambiguous Line Drawings in the Middle Were Given One of Two Labels. Later Reproductions by People, on the Left and Right, Conform to the Schema Activated by the Label*

Source: Carmichael, L., Hogan, H. P., & Walter, A. A. (1932). An experimental study of the effect of language on the reproductions of visually perceived forms. *Journal of Experimental Psychology, 15*, 73–86

Interpretation strongly influences memory. People may misremember having encountered things that they only inferred using a schema. For example, people who view a sequence of events in which they see an effect or outcome are likely to mistakenly claim to remember seeing a schema-consistent cause (Hannigan & Reinitz, 2001; Ianì et al., 2018). For example, people who saw a picture of a person pulling an orange out from the bottom of a pile (cause) are less likely to misremember seeing the pile fall (effect), but people who saw a picture of the oranges on the floor (effect) are more likely to misremember seeing an orange being pulled out of the bottom of the pile (cause).

In life we sometimes come across event descriptions that are given out piecemeal, and we need the schema process of **integration** to guide us in putting these pieces together into a coherent whole. For example, when reading a mystery novel, the author may give different aspects of the murder at different points in the story.

If you have any hope of figuring out what happened and who the guilty party is before being spoon-fed this information at the end, these pieces must be integrated into a common mental representation of the event. This is done using schemas.

Up to now we have seen how schemas influence encoding. However, schemas can also affect retrieval. Memories are not complete records of the past. They are fragmentary. Only bits and pieces of the original experience make it into consciousness. Sometimes there are a lot of fragments, enough to recover almost the entire memory, whereas in other cases the fragments are few and far between. Thus, some **reconstruction** is needed. With reconstruction, we fill in the gaps. This is like a paleontologist reconstructing an entire creature from fossilized bits and pieces.

Some evidence for reconstruction comes from Bartlett's (1932) work. In one set of experiments he gave British Cambridge University students a Native American folktale to read called "The War of the Ghosts." This tale is shown in Table 9.2. Sometime after reading—often several days, weeks, or months later—people were asked to recall the tale. People not only forgot parts of the story, but they added

TABLE 9.2 *"The War of the Ghosts," a Native American Folktale*

One night two young men from Egulac went down to the river to hunt seals, and while they were there it became foggy and calm. Then they heard war-cries, and they thought: "Maybe this is a war party." They escaped to the shore, and hid behind a log. Now canoes came up, and they heard the noise of paddles, and saw one canoe coming up to them. There were five men in the canoe, and they said:

"What do you think? We wish to take you along. We are going up the river to make war on the people."

One of the young men said: "I have no arrows."

"Arrows are in the canoe," they said.

"I will not go along. I might be killed. My relatives do not know where I have gone. But you," he said turning to the other, "may go with them."

So one of the young men went, but the other returned home.

And the warriors went on up the river to a town on the other side of Kalama. The people came down to the water, and they began to fight, and many were killed. But presently the young man heard one of the warriors say: "Quick, let us go home: that Indian has been hit." Now he thought: "Oh, they are ghosts." He did not feel sick, but they said he had been shot.

So the canoes went back to Egulac, and the young man went ashore to his house, and made a fire. And he told everybody and said: "Behold I accompanied the ghosts, and we went to fight. Many of our fellows were killed, and many of those who attacked us were killed. They said I was hit, and I did not feel sick."

He told it all, and then he became quiet. When the sun rose he fell down. Something black came out of his mouth. His face became contorted. The people jumped up and cried.

He was dead.

Source: Bartlett, 1932

TABLE 9.3 *Recall Attempt for "The War of the Ghosts" Four Months Later*

There were two men in a boat, sailing toward an island. When they approached the island, some natives came running toward them, and informed them that there was fighting going on the island, and invited them to join. One said to the other, "You had better go. I cannot very well, because I have relatives expecting me, and they will not know what has happened to me. But you have no one expecting you." So one accompanied the natives, but the other returned.

Here there is a part I can't remember. What I don't know is how the man got to the fight. However, anyhow the man was in the midst of the fighting, and was wounded. The natives endeavored to persuade the man to return, but he assured them that he had not been wounded.

I have an idea that his fighting won the admiration of the natives.

The wounded man ultimately fell unconscious. He was taken from the fighting by the natives.

Then, I think it is, the natives described what happened, and they seem to have imagined seeing a ghost coming out of his mouth. Really it was a kind of materialization of his breath. I know this phrase was not in the story, but that is the idea I have. Ultimately the man dies at dawn the next day.

Source: Bartlett, 1932

new elements. Often this new information was less consistent with the original story but more consistent with typical English folktales. One recall is shown in Table 9.3. Schema-based reconstruction is reflected in the idea that if the warrior had been shot, he would have fallen unconscious and been carried off the battlefield. However, this was not in the original story.

People also show schematic reconstruction with nonverbal information. In a study by Brewer and Treyens (1981), students at the University of Illinois at Urbana-Champaign were asked to wait in a graduate student's office before the experiment began. However, what they did not realize was that the experiment had already begun. After spending a few minutes in the "office," they were taken to another room, where their memory for the office was tested. What was found was that people tended to misremember items as being in the room when they were not. These were articles that were consistent with an office schema. For example, many people remembered seeing books, when there were none. Consistent with fuzzy trace theory, people use a combination of detailed memories and schemas to remember. Forgetting leads people to make judgments based on schemas rather than memories of particular instances (Gilovich, 1981). Memory reports become more schematic over time.

As a practical example of how schemas influence memory, take clinicians' memories of client cases. Description of client symptoms are not always clear cut in terms of how they fit with various diagnoses. There can be ambiguities. What clinicians may do is it take ambiguous information from a case and assign a clinical classification. Then, the clinician may use that classification as a schema and misremember the case as being more causally coherent than it was (Weine & Kim, 2019).

TRY IT OUT

Here is a study that can illustrate the influence of schemas (Zechmeister & Nyberg, 1982). You will need two passages. One should be the *washing clothes* passage in Table 9.1. The other is a passage about running a pizza parlor and is listed below.

You should have at least 12 people for this study. For each person, read them one of the passages with the title and the other without. If you test people individually, try to counterbalance the order in which they get the passages and the order in which they either do or do not get the titles. After reading each passage, have people write down as much as they can remember.

Then, score their recalls for how many basic ideas from the passages appear in their reports. What you should find is that people remember more from the passage for which you provided the title. The title activates the appropriate schema, making it easier to remember.

"Generally the atmosphere is not conducive to street clothing. Proper attire lessens the worry. It may also facilitate dexterity. Awe-filled spectators surely provide extra motivation. Hopefully, they don't cause distractions. Finesse and enthusiasm add a lot to the performance; however, the final results constitute the true measure of achievement. Experiment with ways of throwing. Making the thick pellets into thin skins is the aim. You usually cannot select all the constituents. Customers choose much themselves. Your task is to integrate the raw material. Careful engineering of embellishment placement guarantees consistency of quality. Once heated, no changes can be made. Consumption is imminent. Quantity ultimately secures survival."

Scripts

When knowledge refers to a sequence of events that occurs in a stereotyped fashion, this is a particular type of schema. **Scripts** are temporally ordered schemas that are structured according to the major components of the event (Abbott et al., 1985), with a preference for using script information in a forward order (Haberlandt & Bingham, 1984), although more central components may be more available (Galambos & Rips, 1982). People have good memories for the order of events for common aspects of life. When people are asked to list the components of a script, such as what happens at a restaurant, many of the lists have the same entries (Bower et al., 1979), suggesting that there is a great deal of regularity for this type of semantic memory. A typical list for what to do in a restaurant is shown in Figure 9.10.

Scripts influence how information is retrieved and used. For example, when people read a text of a scripted event, they take longer to read a sentence when the action is further along in the script from the prior sentence than if it is closer (Bower et al., 1979). For a story about going to a restaurant, if people had just read a sentence about waiting to be seated, they would read the next sentence faster if it was about looking at the menu than if it was about finishing the meal. People scan

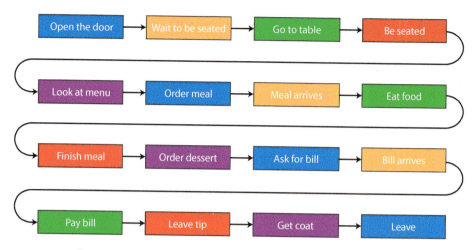

FIGURE 9.10 *Example of a Script for What to Do at a Restaurant*

Source: adapted from Bower, G. H., Black, J. B., & Turner, T. J. (1979). Scripts in memory for text. *Cognitive Psychology*, *11*, 117–220

their scripts to help make sense of what they are reading. When the information is close in the script, less effort is required. However, when the information is far in the script, more effort is needed because more of the script needs to be scanned to bring the person up to date. More knowledge must be inferred.

The influence of scripts is also seen when people are given information about a scripted event in a random order. During later recall, there is a tendency to report those fragments in an order that more closely approximates the script (Bower et al., 1979). Moreover, if people provide summaries of normal and scrambled texts, their summaries are similar (Kintsch et al., 1977). Thus, we use scripts to organize information to help us both understand it and remember it better.

Limits on Schema Usage

While schemas and scripts have a large influence on memory, they are not always used. For example, people are likely to make causal inferences because understanding causal relations is important for understanding how the world is structured and operates. However, when given partial information about a cause-and-effect sequence, people do not always make these inferences. There is a bias to infer causes but not effects because people can easily infer how they may have gotten to a current point in time (what caused this) if they access the appropriate schema. However, knowing what will happen next (what effects to predict) is more difficult because in many cases any number of possible outcomes could exist. This is not to say that people never use schemas to make predictions about the future—only that they are much less likely to do so.

It is possible to get people to disregard schema-generated information when the schema has been discredited. This was done in a study by Hasher and Griffin (1978; see also Anderson & Pichert, 1978), where students were given ambiguous texts, such

TABLE 9.4 *Ambiguous Story Consistent with Two Schemas—an Escaped Convict or a Deer Hunter*

The man walked carefully through the forest. Several times he looked over his shoulder and scrutinized the woods behind him. He trod carefully, trying to avoid snapping twigs and small branches that lay in his path, for he did not want to create excess noise. The chirping of the birds in the trees almost annoyed him, their loud calls serving to distract him. He did not want to confuse those sounds with the type he was listening for.

Source: Hasher & Griffin, 1978

TABLE 9.5 *Influence of a Schema Shift on Later Memory for Schema Consistent Inferences. The Data Are for the Percentage of Idea Units Recalled from an Ambiguous Story and the Number of Intrusions Based on the Initial Theme, the Alternate Theme, or Some Other Theme*

Condition	Idea Units	First Theme	Second Theme	Neutral
Same schema	35%	2.58	0.17	0.92
Schema shift	35%	0.54	0.08	1.33

Source: Hasher & Griffin, 1978

as the one in Table 9.4. It is ambiguous because it could be either about an escaped convict or a deer hunter. Students were first asked to read this text from one perspective. After a delay, the students were asked to recall the story. Some did this from the same perspective as they read it. In contrast, others were led to believe that the experimenter had given them the wrong title initially. They were then given the "correct" other title. The results are shown in Table 9.5. When there was a title switch, people recalled the same amount of information as when there was no switch. However, there were important differences. When there was a title switch, people made fewer intrusions, whereas those who did not have the switch made many schema-consistent intrusions. Thus, people can disregard schemas and use more detailed, verbatim memories.

Stop and Review

Semantic memories for commonly experienced aspects of life are schemas. During learning, schemas can be used in several ways. They can select out those aspects of an event that are more relevant and important, abstract away the critical ideas, help draw inferences through a process of interpretation, allow missing information and gaps to be filled, and facilitate the integration of otherwise separate bits of information into a single coherent memory. During retrieval, schemas can help reconstruct details that were forgotten. For standard sequences of events, people can use scripts. These provide a guide for people to know what the correct order of events should be. While schemas and scripts have powerful influences on memory, they do not always

> ## *Improve Your Memory*
>
> Semantic memory is our knowledge of the world. It is what we draw upon when we are trying to learn and understand new things. Semantic memory can help learning. When you encounter new materials in your classes or at work, it is rare that what you will learn bears almost no relation to what you already know. There is going to be some overlap. If you can activate or prime this knowledge prior to learning, this will help you better encode the new material. There are lots of ways to do this. Prior to reading a textbook, you can scan a chapter or section to see what the section titles are and if there are any terms in bold. This can activate the knowledge in semantic memory that will help you structure the new information. Also, to get more out of a lecture, read the syllabus to see what topics will be relevant that day. Reading the book ahead of class also provides semantic knowledge that will increase the amount of new material you will learn during a lecture (that you will hear only once).

dominate. Under the right circumstances, people can disregard their schemas and scripts and more accurately remember the details that were actually encountered.

PROBLEMS WITH SEMANTIC MEMORY

Semantic memories capture regularities about the world. Thus, they are useful in predicting new situations. They are reasonably accurate, as far they go, but are not perfect. They can sometimes lead us to make errors. Here we discuss two types of errors: semantic illusions and naïve physics.

Semantic Illusions

How many animals of each kind did Moses take on the ark? Many people respond with "two," but this is incorrect. Moses did not take any animals on the ark, Noah did. In the first study of this memory error, Erickson and Mattson (1981) found that 81% of students at the University of California, San Diego, responded with "two" even though they all knew the correct answer. Thus, this semantic memory error is called the **Moses Illusion**. Why do so many people make this mistake? Semantic memory, like other types of memory, is prone to error. In addition to general forgetting, errors can involve the inappropriate retrieval of information.

This illusion does not appear to be due to people mentally correcting the question or making rushed responses (Reder & Kusbit, 1991). It also occurs when there is overlapping lexical information, such as a similar name. An example of this would be when people give an inappropriate response to the question "What was the famous line uttered by Louis Armstrong when he first set foot on the moon?" (Büttner, 2007; Shafto & MacKay, 2000). Similarly, people are more likely to make a memory error when the people mentioned in the question look similar, even though no pictures are actually seen (Davis & Abrams, 2016). It is even shown by experts in a field of study, although to a smaller degree (Cantor & Marsh, 2017).

There are three theories of the Moses Illusion. First, semantic processing is very general unless people focus on the information of interest (Erickson & Mattson, 1981). That is, we only do a cursory check of semantic memory to see if the information is broadly consistent. Second, people do only a partial assessment of semantic information (Reder & Kusbit, 1991). That is, we retrieve some of the information from semantic memory, and, so long as it is a close fit, we go with it. Third, similar language elements, such as a similar name, can inappropriately activate information in semantic memory, giving the illusion that it is known (Shafto & MacKay, 2000). In other words, if it sounds close, we are often willing to disregard smaller inconsistencies. Overall, information in semantic memory is accessed in an imprecise way and can lead to errors.

Naïve Physics

Semantic memory illusions also apply to nonverbal knowledge. As discussed in Chapter 5, memory can incorporate physical principles of the world, such as gravity and friction. Some **naïve physics** knowledge is stored in semantic memory. However, when we consciously try to apply this knowledge, while we are accurate about some aspects of physics (e.g., Masin, 2016), misunderstandings can be revealed. In one study, students at Johns Hopkins University were given diagrams, such as those shown in Figure 9.11. The task was to indicate (1) the trajectory of a ball shot out of the tube, (2) the trajectory of the ball when the string broke, and (3) the path of the bomb when the plane dropped it. The responses are shown in Figure 9.12.

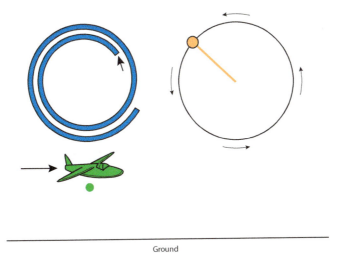

Ground

FIGURE 9.11 *Stimuli Used to Illustrate Principles of Naïve Physics. A Person's Task Is to Show the Path of the Ball Once It Leaves the Tube or Is Released*

Source: McCloskey, M. (1983). Naïve theories of motion. In D. Gentner & A. L. Stevens (Eds.), *Mental Models* (pp. 299–324). Hillsdale, NJ: Erlbaum

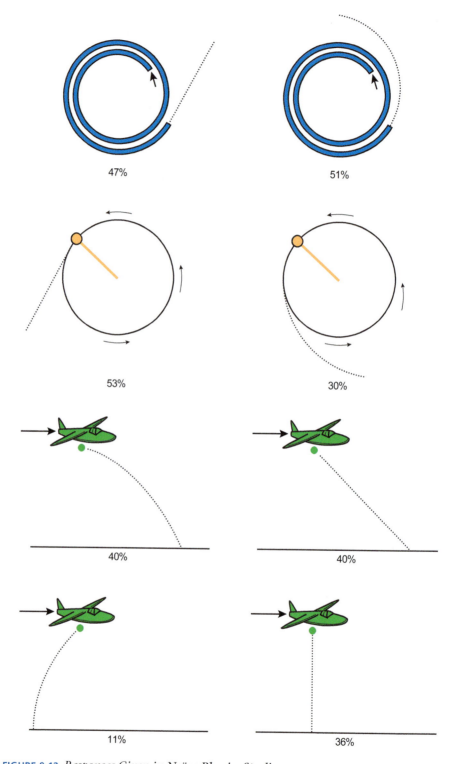

FIGURE 9.12 *Responses Given in Naïve Physics Studies*

Source: McCloskey, M. (1983). Naïve theories of motion. In D. Gentner & A. L. Stevens (Eds.), *Mental models* (pp. 299–324). Hillsdale, NJ: Erlbaum

Although people do sometimes give correct responses, they also give incorrect responses using incorrect semantic knowledge (McCloskey et al., 1980). What is interesting is that people respond as if they had medieval impetus theories of motion (but see Cooke & Breedin, 1994). This is more likely when people use static diagrams rather than moving displays (Kaiser et al., 1985; McCloskey & Kohl, 1983), although not always (Rohrer, 2003).

With education, we can overcome our naïve beliefs of motion. That said, they never seem to go away completely. For example, if people are asked to verify statements that are inconsistent with early childhood beliefs, such as the idea that the Earth goes around the Sun, people respond more slowly compared to statements that are consistent with early beliefs, such as the idea that the Moon goes around the Earth (Shtulman & Valcarcel, 2012). There is interference from older, incorrect knowledge. While education can improve memory (Donley & Ashcraft, 1992), it can also get in the way. Oberle et al. (2005) reported what they called the *Galileo bias* in which people mistakenly believe that if two balls of different weights dropped from 10 meters, they will hit the ground simultaneously. However, this does not take into account wind resistance. Even with extensive practice at dropping balls, students at Arizona State University continued to make errors based on semantic knowledge of what they had learned in elementary school about Galileo and gravity.

Incorrect understanding can be extended to semantic models of devices. For example, many people treat a thermostat not as a device for setting the ideal temperature (when the furnace should stop heating the house), but as a heat accelerator, setting the temperature much higher than the desired temperature in the mistaken belief that the house will get warmer faster (it will not).

Another source of misinformation in semantic memory is the understanding of how vision works. Vision works by light entering the eye and being absorbed by the photoreceptors (rods and cones) in the retina. However, a large number (33 to 86%, depending on the measure) of college-educated people mistakenly believe that vision involves something coming out of the eye (Winer et al., 2002). This extramission view of vision is reflected in people's responses when talking about or creating depictions of how vision works. This can include imagining rays coming out of the eyes or the belief that you can "feel it" when a person behind you is looking at you. This semantic misunderstanding of an intimate part of our experience illustrates the degree to which our knowledge may be erroneous.

Stop and Review

Our semantic memory is only as accurate as the information in it and how we use it. Breakdowns occur when knowledge is superficially accessed, as in the Moses Illusion or when semantic memories, although based on experience, have somehow been stored incorrectly, such as the errors people make on naïve physics tasks.

PUTTING IT ALL TOGETHER

This chapter looked at how you store and retrieve general world knowledge in semantic memory. Semantic memory is highly structured, and this reveals itself in several ways. It is reflected in the ease with which information is retrieved (as in priming) the organization of knowledge into categories, schemas, scripts, and ordered relations. Semantic memory is not a passive accumulation of knowledge and experiences. It is actively interpreting, abstracting, organizing, and structuring what you have perceived and thought. The mind abhors randomness and seeks structure. Semantic memory is the derivation and imposition of structure onto our storehouse of experience. Sometimes the structure of semantic memory is accurate and tells you how the world is, and sometimes it gets things wrong, and you misunderstand.

The organization of semantic memory reflects regularities in the world, both real and self-imposed. These regularities occur when semantic memory abstracts across experiences to derive a general understanding. Sometimes your semantic memory reflects this abstraction in the processing of knowledge apart from sensory-motor experiences. This is exemplified in several ways, such as with the priming of concepts, the derivation of rules, prototypes, and averages with categorization, and the construction of schematic knowledge apart from individual events and their details. That said, semantic memory breathes, blinks, tastes, pushes, pulls, grabs, and moves. It is alive. It reflects how you perceive the world and interact with it. It is embodied. Your embodied semantic memory is reflected in how things are primed, how you see natural kinds, how you use tools and artifacts, even how you use abstract ideas, like the number line.

STUDY QUESTIONS

1. What is semantic priming? What sort of information gets primed? How far does it extend?
2. How long does it take for information to be established in semantic memory?
3. To what degree can semantic priming be consciously controlled? When are semantic memories inhibited?
4. How does the interconnectivity of information influence the ease with which it is remembered?
5. What are the basic properties of categories formed in semantic memory?
6. What are some of the major theories of how people form categories?
7. What is the classical view of human categorization, and what are some of its major flaws?
8. What are the major types of probabilistic theories of categorization? What are their advantages and disadvantages?
9. What are explanation-based theories of categorization? How are they influenced by the concept of psychological essentialism?
10. How is semantic memory retrieval affected by the order of information along a dimension?
11. What is the SNARC effect and what does it reveal about how some information is stored in semantic memory?

12. What are the primary ways that schemas influence memory at encoding? At retrieval?
13. What are schemas for sequential event knowledge called? How do they operate?
14. How can people avoid the influence of schemas and remember more accurately?
15. What sorts of problems can occur when semantic memory is used? How do these errors arise?
16. How is semantic memory influence by embodied/perceptual aspects of experience?

KEY TERMS

- abstraction
- ad hoc categories
- artifact categories
- categorization
- central tendency
- classical view of categorization
- concept
- exemplar theory
- explanation-based views
- family resemblance
- graded membership
- inhibition
- integration
- interpretation
- levels of categorization
- mediated priming
- Moses Illusion
- naïve physics
- natural kind categories
- prime
- priming
- prototype model
- psychological essentialism
- reconstruction
- schema
- scripts
- selection
- semantic congruity effect
- semantic distance effect
- semantic memory
- serial position effect
- SNARC effect
- target
- taxonomic relations
- thematic relations

EXPLORE MORE

Here are some additional readings that can allow you to more deeply explore some of the basic principles of semantic memory.

Bartlett, F. C. (1932). *Remembering: A Study in Experimental and Social Psychology.* Cambridge, UK: Cambridge University Press.

Dehaene, S., Bossini, S., & Giraux, P. (1993). The mental representation of parity and number magnitude. *Journal of Experimental Psychology: General, 122,* 371–396.

Estes, W. K. (1994). *Classification and Cognition.* Oxford, UK: Oxford University Press.

Mandler, J. M. (2014). *Stories, Scripts, and Scenes: Aspects of Schema Theory.* New York: Psychology Press.

Winer, G. A., Cottrell, J E., Gregg, V., Fournier, J. S., & Bica, L. A. (2002). Fundamentally misunderstanding visual perception: Adults' belief in visual emissions. *American Psychologist, 57,* 417–424.

REFERENCES

Abbott, V., Black, J. B., & Smith, E. E. (1985). The representation of scripts in memory. *Journal of Memory and Language, 24,* 179–199.

Ahn, W-K., Kim, N. S., Lassaline, M. E., & Dennis, M. J. (2000). Causal status as a determinant of feature centrality. *Cognitive Psychology, 41,* 361–416.

Alba, J. W., & Hasher, L. (1983). Is memory schematic? *Psychological Bulletin, 93,* 203–231.

Alley, T. R., & Cunningham, M. R. (1991). Averaged faces are attractive, but very attractive faces are not average. *Psychological Science, 2,* 123–125.

Amit, E., Algom, D., & Trope, Y. (2009). Distance-dependent processing of pictures and words. *Journal of Experimental Psychology: General, 138,* 400–415.

Anderson, R. C., & Pichert, J. W. (1978). Recall of previously unrecallable information following a shift in perspective. *Journal of Verbal Learning and Verbal Behavior, 17,* 1–12.

Andres, M., Olivier, E., & Badets, A. (2008). Actions, words, and numbers: A motor contribution to semantic processing? *Current Directions in Psychological Science, 17,* 313–317.

Andrews, M., Vigliocco, G., & Vinson, D. (2009). Integrating experiential and distributional data to learn semantic representations. *Psychological Review, 116,* 463–498.

Armstrong, S. L., Gleitman, L. R., & Gleitman, H. (1983). What some concepts might not be. *Cognition, 13,* 263–308.

Ashby, F. G., Alfonso-Reese, L. A., & Waldron, E. M. (1998). A neuropsychological theory of multiple systems in category learning. *Psychological Review, 105*(3), 442.

Ashby, F. G., Paul, E. J., & Maddox, W. T. (2011). COVIS. In E. M. Pothos & A. Wills (Eds.), *Formal Approaches in Categorization* (pp. 65–87). New York: Cambridge University Press.

Ashby, F. G., & Rosedahl, L. (2017). A neural interpretation of exemplar theory. *Psychological Review, 124*(4), 472.

Ashcraft, M. H. (1978a). Property dominance and typicality effects in property statement verification. *Journal of Verbal Learning and Verbal Behavior, 17,* 155–164.

Ashcraft, M. H. (1978b). Property norms for typical and atypical items from 17 categories: A description and discussion. *Memory & Cognition, 6,* 227–232.

Balota, D. A., & Lorch, R. F. (1986). Depth of automatic spreading activation: Mediated priming effects in pronunciation but not in lexical decisions. *Journal of Experimental Psychology: Learning, Memory, and Cognition, 12,* 336–345.

Banks, W. P. (1977). Encoding and processing of symbolic information in comparative judgments. *The Psychology of Learning and Motivation, 11,* 101–159.

Banks, W. P., Clark, H. H., & Lucy, P. (1975). The locus of the semantic congruity effect in comparative judgments. *Journal of Experimental Psychology: Human Perception and Performance, 104,* 35–47.

Barsalou, L. W. (1983). Ad hoc categories. *Memory & Cognition, 11,* 211–227.

Bartlett, F. C. (1932). *Remembering: A Study in Experimental and Social Psychology.* Cambridge, UK: Cambridge University Press.

Bentin, S., McCarthy, G., & Wood, C. C. (1985). Event-related potentials, lexical decision and semantic memory. *Electroencephalography and Clinical Neurophysiology, 60,* 343–355.

Blaxton, T. A., & Neely, J. H. (1983). Inhibition from semantically related primes: Evidence of a category-specific inhibition. *Memory & Cognition, 11,* 500–510.

Bower, G. H., Black, J. B., & Turner, T. J. (1979). Scripts in memory for text. *Cognitive Psychology, 11,* 117–220.

Bransford, J. D., & Johnson, M. K. (1972). Contextual prerequisites for understanding: Some investigations of comprehension and recall. *Journal of Verbal Learning and Verbal Behavior, 11,* 717–726.

Brewer, W. F., & Treyens, J. C. (1981). Role of schemata in memory for places. *Cognitive Psychology, 13,* 207–230.

Bruner, J. S., Goodnow, J. J., & Austin, G. A. (1956). *A Study of Thinking.* Oxford, UK: Wiley.

Burgoon, E. M., Henderson, M. D., & Markman, A. B. (2013). There are many ways to see the forest for the trees: A tour guide for abstraction. *Perspectives on Psychological Science, 8*(5), 501–520.

Büttner, A. C. (2007). Questions versus statements: Challenging an assumption about semantic illusions. *Quarterly Journal of Experimental Psychology, 60*, 779–789.

Cantor, A. D., & Marsh, E. J. (2017). Expertise effects in the Moses illusion: Detecting contradictions with stored knowledge. *Memory, 25*(2), 220–230.

Carmichael, L., Hogan, H. P., & Walter, A. A. (1932). An experimental study of the effect of language on the reproductions of visually perceived forms. *Journal of Experimental Psychology, 15*, 73–86.

Casasanto, D. (2009). Embodiment of abstract concepts: Good and bad in right- and left-handers. *Journal of Experimental Psychology: General, 138*, 351–367.

Castronovo, J., & Seron, X. (2007). Semantic numerical representation in blind subjects: The role of vision in the spatial format of the mental number line. *Quarterly Journal of Experimental Psychology, 60*, 101–119.

Chin-Parker, S., & Cantelon, J. (2017). Contrastive constraints guide explanation-based category learning. *Cognitive Science, 41*(6), 1645–1655.

Chin-Parker, S., & Ross, B. H. (2002). The effect of category learning on sensitivity to within-category correlations. *Memory & Cognition, 30*, 353–362.

Cooke, N. J., & Breedin, S. D. (1994). Constructing naïve theories of motion on the fly. *Memory & Cognition, 22*, 474–493.

Crutch, S. J., Connell, S., & Warrington, E. K. (2009). The different representational frameworks underpinning abstract and concrete knowledge: Evidence from odd-one-out judgements. *Quarterly Journal of Experimental Psychology, 62*, 1377–1390.

Davis, D. K., & Abrams, L. (2016). Here's looking at you: Visual similarity exacerbates the Moses illusion for semantically similar celebrities. *Journal of Experimental Psychology: Learning, Memory, and Cognition, 42*(1), 75–90.

De Groot, A. M. B. (1983). The range of automatic spreading activation in word priming. *Journal of Verbal Learning and Verbal Behavior, 22*, 417–436.

Dehaene, S., Bossini, S., & Giraux, P. (1993). The mental representation of parity and number magnitude. *Journal of Experimental Psychology: General, 122*, 371–396.

Donley, R. D., & Ashcraft, M. H. (1992). The methodology of testing naïve beliefs in the physics classroom. *Memory & Cognition, 20*, 381–391.

Duffy, S. A., & Keir, J. A. (2004). Violating stereotypes: Eye movements and comprehension processes when text conflicts with world knowledge. *Memory & Cognition, 32*, 551–559.

Ellis, D. A., Wiseman, R., & Jenkins, R. (2015). Mental representations of weekdays. *PloS one, 10*(8), e0134555.

Erickson, T. D., & Mattson, M. E. (1981). From words to meaning: A semantic illusion. *Journal of Verbal Learning and Verbal Behavior, 20*, 540–551.

Estes, Z. (2004). Confidence and gradedness in semantic categorization: Definitely somewhat artifactual, maybe absolutely natural. *Psychonomic Bulletin & Review, 11*, 1041–1047.

Fenker, D. B., Waldmann, M. R., & Holyoak, K. J. (2005). Accessing causal relations in semantic memory. *Memory & Cognition, 33*, 1036–1046.

Galambos, J. A., & Rips, L. J. (1982). Memory for routines. *Journal of Verbal Learning and Verbal Behavior, 21*, 260–281.

Gevers, W., Reynvoet, B., & Fias, W. (2004). The mental representation of ordinal sequences is spatially organised: Evidence from days of the week. *Cortex, 40*, 171–172.

Gilboa, A., & Marlatte, H. (2017). Neurobiology of schemas and schema–mediated memory. *Trends in Cognitive Sciences, 21*(8), 618–631.

Gilovich, T. (1981). Seeing the past in the present: The effect of associations to familiar events on judgments and decisions. *Journal of Personality and Social Psychology, 40*, 797–808.

Girelli, L., Perrone, G., Croccolo, F., Roman, E. H., Bricolo, E., Mancin, M., & Rinaldi, L. (2016). Manual actions cover symbolic distances at different speed. *Acta Psychologica, 169*, 56–60.

Goldstone, R. L., Steyvers, M., & Rogosky, B. J. (2003). Conceptual interrelatedness and caricatures. *Memory & Cognition, 31*, 169–180.

Goldwater, M. B., Bainbridge, R., & Murphy, G. L. (2016). Learning of role-governed and thematic categories. *Acta Psychologica, 164*, 112–126.

Haberlandt, K., & Bingham, G. (1984). The effect of input direction on the processing of script statements. *Journal of Verbal Learning and Verbal Behavior, 23*, 162–177.

Halberstadt, J., & Rhodes, G. (2003). It's not just average faces that are attractive: Computer-manipulated averageness makes birds, fish, and automobiles attractive. *Psychonomic Bulletin & Review, 10*, 149–156.

Hannigan, S. L., & Reinitz, M. T. (2001). A demonstration and comparison of two types of inference-based memory errors. *Journal of Experimental Psychology: Learning, Memory, and Cognition, 27*, 931–940.

Hasher, L., & Griffin, M. (1978). Reconstructive and reproductive processes in memory. *Journal of Experimental Psychology: Human Learning and Memory, 4*, 318–330.

Healy, A. F., Havas D. A., & Parker, J. T. (2000). Comparing serial position effects in semantic and episodic memory using reconstruction of order tasks. *Journal of Memory and Language, 42*, 147–167.

Hill, H., Strube, M., Roesch-Ely, D., & Weisbrod, M. (2002). Automatic vs. controlled processes in semantic priming: Differentiation by event-related potentials. *International Journal of Psychophysiology, 44*, 197–218.

Ianì, F., Mazzoni, G., & Bucciarelli, M. (2018). The role of kinematic mental simulation in creating false memories. *Journal of Cognitive Psychology, 30*(3), 292–306.

Kaiser, M. K., Proffitt, D. R., & Anderson, K. (1985). Judgments of natural and anomalous trajectories in the presence and absence of motion. *Journal of Experimental Psychology: Learning, Memory, and Cognition, 11*, 795–803.

Kalénine, S., & Bonthoux, F. (2008). Object manipulability affects children's and adults' conceptual processing. *Psychonomic Bulletin & Review, 15*, 667–672.

Kalénine, S., Mirman, D., Middleton, E. L., & Buxbaum, L. J. (2012). Temporal dynamics of activation of thematic and functional knowledge during conceptual processing of manipulable artifacts. *Journal of Experimental Psychology: Learning, Memory, and Cognition, 38*(5), 1274–1295.

Kalish, C. W. (2002). Essentialist to some degree: Beliefs about the structure of natural kind categories. *Memory & Cognition, 30*, 340–352.

Kintsch, W., Mandel, T. S., & Kozminsky, E. (1977). Summarizing scrambled stories. *Memory & Cognition, 5*, 547–552.

Kousta, S-T., Vigliocco, G., Vinson, D. P., Andrews, M., & Del Campo, E. (2011). The representation of abstract words: Why emotion matters. *Journal of Experimental Psychology: General, 140*(1), 14–34.

Krause, W., Gibbons, H., & Schack, B. (1998). Concept activation and coordination of activation procedure require two different networks. *Neuroreport, 9*, 1649–1653.

Kroll, N. E. A., & Klimesch, W. (1992). Semantic memory: Complexity or connectivity? *Memory & Cognition, 20*, 192–210.

Kutas, M., & Hillyard, S. A. (1980). Reading senseless sentences: Brain potentials reflect semantic incongruity. *Science, 207*, 203–205.

Lakens, D., Schneider, I. K., Jostmann, N. B., & Schubert, T. W. (2011). Telling things apart: The distance between response keys influences categorization times. *Psychological Science, 22*(7), 887–890.

Langlois, J. H., & Roggman, L. A. (1990). Attractive faces are only average. *Psychological Science, 1*, 115–121.

Lidji, P., Kolinsky, R., Lochy, A., & Morais, J. (2007). Spatial associations for musical stimuli: A piano in the head? *Journal of Experimental Psychology: Human Perception and Performance, 33*, 1189–1207.

Light, L. L., Hollander, S., & Kayra-Stuart, F. (1981). Why attractive people are harder to remember. *Personality and Social Psychology Bulletin, 7*, 269–276.

Love, B. C. (2005). Environment and goals jointly direct category acquisition. *Current Directions in Psychological Science, 14*, 195–199.

Lupyan, G. (2013). The difficulties of executing simple algorithms: Why brains make mistakes computers don't. *Cognition, 129*(3), 615–636.

Mandler, J. M., & Ritchey, G. H. (1977). Long-term memory for pictures. *Journal of Experimental Psychology: Human Learning and Memory, 3*, 386–396.

Markman, A. B., & Ross, B. H. (2003). Category use and category learning. *Psychological Bulletin, 129*, 592–613.

Martin, A., & Chao, L. L. (2001). Semantic memory and the brain: Structure and processes. *Current Opinion in Neurobiology, 11*, 194–201.

Masin, S. C. (2016). The cognitive and perceptual laws of the inclined plane. *American Journal of Psychology, 129*(3), 221–234.

Maylor, E. A. (2002). Serial position effects in semantic memory: Reconstructing the order of verses of hymns. *Psychonomic Bulletin & Review, 9*, 816–820.

McCloskey, M. (1983). Naïve theories of motion. In D. Gentner & A. L. Stevens (Eds.), *Mental Models* (pp. 299–324). Hillsdale, NJ: Erlbaum.

McCloskey, M., Caramazza, A., & Green, B. (1980). Curvilinear motion in the absence of external forces: Naïve beliefs about the motion of objects. *Science, 210*, 1139–1141.

McCloskey, M., & Kohl, D. (1983). Naïve physics: The curvilinear impetus principle and its role in interactions with moving objects. *Journal of Experimental Psychology: Learning, Memory, and Cognition, 9*, 146–156.

Medin, D. L. (1989). Concepts and conceptual structure. *American Psychologist, 44*, 1469–1481.

Medin, D. L., & Schaffer, M. M. (1978). Context theory of classification learning. *Psychological Review, 85*, 207–238.

Medin, D. L., & Shoben, E. J. (1988). Context and structure in conceptual combination. *Cognitive Psychology, 20*, 158–190.

Merck, C., Jonin, P. Y., Laisney, M., Vichard, H., & Belliard, S. (2014). When the zebra loses its stripes but is still in the savannah: Results from a semantic priming paradigm in semantic dementia. Neuropsychologia, 53, 221–232.

Meyer, D. E., & Schvaneveldt, R. W. (1971). Facilitation in recognizing pairs of words: Evidence of a dependence between retrieval operations. *Journal of Experimental Psychology, 90*(2), 227–234.

Mirman, D., Landrigan, J. F., & Britt, A. E. (2017). Taxonomic and thematic semantic systems. Psychological bulletin, 143(5), 499–520.

Mirman, D., & Magnuson, J. S. (2009). The effect of frequency of shared features on judgments of semantic similarity. *Psychonomic Bulletin & Review, 16*, 671–677.

Murphy, G. L. (2016). Is there an exemplar theory of concepts? *Psychonomic Bulletin & Review, 23*(4), 1035–1042.

Nathan, M. B., Shaki, S., Salti, M., & Algom, D. (2009). Numbers and space: Associations and dissociations. *Psychonomic Bulletin & Review, 16*, 578–582.

Neath, I. (1998). *Human Memory: An introduction to research, data, and theory*. Belmont, CA: Thomson Brooks/Cole Publishing.

Neely, J. H. (1977). Semantic priming and retrieval from lexical memory: Roles of inhibitionless spreading activation and limited-capacity attention. *Journal of Experimental Psychology: General, 106*, 226–254.

Nosofsky, R. M. (1986). Attention, similarity, and the identification–categorization relationship. *Journal of Experimental Psychology: General, 115*(1), 39.

Nosofsky, R. M. (1988). Exemplar-based accounts of relations between classification, recognition, and typicality. *Journal of Experimental Psychology: Learning, Memory, and Cognition, 14*, 700–708.

Nosofsky, R. M. (2011). The generalized context model: An exemplar model of classification. In E. M. Pothos & A. Wills (Eds.), *Formal Approaches in Categorization* (pp. 18–39). New York, NY: Cambridge University Press.

Oakhill, J., Garnham, A., & Reynolds, D. (2005). Immediate activation of stereotypical gender information. *Memory & Cognition, 33*, 972–983.

Oberle, C. D., McBeath, M. K., Madigan, S. C., & Sugar, T. G. (2005). The Galileo bias: A naïve conceptual belief that influences people's perceptions and performance in a ball-dropping task. *Journal of Experimental Psychology: Learning, Memory and Cognition, 31*, 643–653.

Olafson, K. M., & Ferraro, F. R. (2001). Effects of emotional state on lexical decision performance. *Brain and Cognition, 45*, 15–20.

Pansky, A., & Koriat, A. (2004). The basic-level convergence effect in memory distortions. *Psychological Science, 15*, 52–59.

Pecher, D., Zeelenberg, R., & Barsalou, L. W. (2003). Verifying different-modality properties for concepts produces switching costs. *Psychological Science, 14*, 119–124.

Posner, M. I., & Keele, S. W. (1968). On the genesis of abstract ideas. *Journal of Experimental Psychology, 77*, 353–363.

Posner, M. I., & Keele, S. W. (1970). Retention of abstract ideas. *Journal of Experimental Psychology, 83*, 304–308.

Prado, J., van der Henst, J-B., & Noveck, I. A. (2008). Spatial associations in relational reasoning: Evidence for a SNARC-like effect. *Quarterly Journal of Experimental Psychology, 61*, 1143–1150.

Pulvermüller, F., Lutzenberger, W., & Preissl, H. (1999). Nouns and verbs in the intact brain: Evidence from event-related potentials and high-frequency cortical responses. *Cerebral Cortex, 9*, 497–506.

Reder, L. M., & Kusbit, G. W. (1991). Locus of the Moses Illusion: Imperfect encoding, retrieval or match? *Journal of Memory and Language, 30*, 385–406.

Rehder, B., & Ross, B. H. (2001). Abstract coherent categories. *Journal of Experimental Psychology: Learning, Memory, and Cognition, 27*, 1261–1275.

Rips, L. J., Shoben, E. J., & Smith, E. E. (1973). Semantic distance and the verification of semantic relations. *Journal of Verbal Learning and Verbal Behavior, 12*, 1–20.

Roediger, H. L., & Crowder, R. G. (1976). A serial position effect in recall of United States presidents. *Bulletin of Psychonomic Society, 8*, 275–278.

Rohrer, D. (2003). The natural appearance of unnatural incline speed. *Memory & Cognition, 31*, 816–826.

Rosch, E. (1975). Cognitive representations of semantic categories. *Journal of Experimental Psychology: General, 104*, 192–233.

Rosch, E., & Mervis, C. B. (1975). Family resemblances: Studies in the internal structure of categories. *Cognitive Psychology, 7*, 573–605.

Rosch, E., Mervis, C. B., Gray, W. D., Johnson, D. M., & Boyes-Braem, P. (1976). Basic objects in natural categories. *Cognitive Psychology, 8*, 382–439.

Rouder, J. N., & Ratcliff, R. (2006). Comparing exemplar- and rule-based theories of categorization. *Current Directions in Psychological Science, 15*, 9–13.

Sachs, J. S. (1967). Recognition memory for syntactic and semantic aspects of connected discourse. *Perception & Psychophysics, 2*, 437–442.

Sachs, J. S. (1974). Memory in reading and listening to discourse. *Memory & Cognition, 2*, 95–100.

Santens, S., & Gevers, W. (2008). The SNARC effect does not imply a mental number line. *Cognition, 108*, 263–270.

Sereno, S. C., O'Donnell, P. J., & Sereno, M. E. (2009). Size matters: Bigger is faster. *Quarterly journal of Experimental Psychology, 62*, 1115–1122.

Shafto, M., & MacKay, D. G. (2000). The Moses, mega-Moses, and Armstrong illusions: Integrating language comprehension and semantic memory. *Psychological Science, 11*(5), 372–378.

Shaki, S., & Fischer, M. H. (2008). Reading space into numbers: A cross-linguistic comparison of the SNARC effect. *Cognition, 108*, 590–599.

Shoben, E. J., Čech, C. G., Schwanenflugel, P. J., & Sailor, K. M. (1989). Serial position effects in comparative judgments. *Journal of Experimental Psychology: Human Perception and Performance, 15*, 273–286.

Shtulman, A., & Valcarcel, J. (2012). Scientific knowledge suppresses but does not supplant earlier intuitions. *Cognition, 124*(2), 209–215.

Solomon, K. O., & Barsalou, L. W. (2004). Perceptual simulation in property verification. *Memory & Cognition, 32*, 244–259.

Summers, W. V., Horton, D. L., & Diehl, V. A. (1985). Contextual knowledge during encoding influences sentence recognition. *Journal of Experimental Psychology: Learning, Memory, and Cognition, 11*, 771–779.

Thompson-Schill, S. L., Kurtz, K. J., & Gabrieli, J. D. E. (1998). Effects of semantic and associative relatedness on automatic priming. *Journal of Memory and Language, 38*, 440–458.

Tversky, B., & Hemenway, K. (1984). Objects, parts, and categories. *Journal of Experimental Psychology: General, 113*(2), 169–193.

Weine, E. R., & Kim, N. S. (2019). Systematic distortions in clinicians' memories for client cases: Increasing causal coherence. *Journal of Experimental Psychology: Learning, Memory, and Cognition, 45*(2), 196–212.

Winer, G. A., Cottrell, J E., Gregg, V., Fournier, J. S., & Bica, L. A. (2002). Fundamentally misunderstanding visual perception: Adults' belief in visual emissions. *American Psychologist, 57*, 417–424.

Winkielman, P., Halberstadt, J., Fazendeiro, T., & Catty, S. (2006). Prototypes are attractive because they are easy on the mind. *Psychological Science, 17*, 799–806.

Yee, E., & Thompson-Schill, S. L. (2016). Putting concepts into context. *Psychonomic Bulletin & Review, 23*(4), 1015–1027.

Zechmeister, E. B., & Nyberg, S. E. (1982). *Human Memory: An Introduction to Research and Theory.* Bekmont, CA: Brooks/Cole Publishing.

PART 3

Special Topics in Memory

CHAPTER 10

Forms of Amnesia

An important issue in memory is not how much people remember but how much they forget. Here we consider forgetting on a pathologically grand scale. **Amnesia** is the catastrophic loss of memories or memory abilities beyond what is expected with normal forgetting, along with otherwise normal intelligence and attention (O'Connor et al., 1995). There are various types of amnesia (Kopelman, 2002). While they vary in their scope and content, they all cripple memory in systematic ways, damaging some memories and leaving others more intact.

Most amnesias are a result of organic brain damage. We begin our coverage by going over two of the more common types of **organic amnesia**, namely retrograde and anterograde amnesia, which are losses of memories from either prior to or after a traumatic brain injury event. We also discuss the transitory loss of memory abilities with transient global amnesia. After that we consider the loss of specific memory abilities, as with semantic amnesia, aphasia, and other conditions. Finally, we cover cases in which there is loss of short-term, rather than long-term, memory function. While most amnesias are organic, some may be a result of a psychological trauma, called psychogenic amnesias. In such cases, the loss of memory may be due to mental trauma and not a problem with the underlying neurophysiology, per se.

RETROGRADE AMNESIA

Retrograde amnesia is a loss of long-term memories prior to a traumatic incident, backward in time. In contrast, anterograde amnesia is a loss of the ability to store new long-term memories, forward in time. Although we consider them separately, it is rare to find a pure case of one or the other—typically both are present to some degree. Some traumas result in more retrograde than anterograde amnesia, whereas others are the opposite. The conditions described here are situations in which one type of amnesia is dominant.

Retrograde amnesia is a loss of long-term memories that were previously accessible (Kapur, 1999). Typically, the personal past is lost. Retrograde amnesia is the sort that people in soap operas tend to get. Usually, in those scenarios, people get hit on the head, and then they cannot remember who they are, where they are, whether they are married, and so on. In real life, things are more complex, and retrograde amnesia has specific defining characteristics.

There are several things that can cause retrograde amnesia, and each involves trauma to the brain that disrupts the **consolidation** (see Chapter 2) of long-term memories (McGaugh, 1966; but see Riccio et al., 2003). Consolidation is a process that makes memories more and more permanent. The easiest memories to disrupt are those that are less consolidated. In severe cases, more stable memories might be disrupted. This may occur either when there has been a disruption to the parts of the brain where the information is held or to the neural mechanisms that are used to retrieve and reconstruct that knowledge.

What can bring about retrograde amnesia? Severe blows to the head are a common cause (and consistent with accounts provided by the entertainment industry). This physical trauma can affect the brain in several ways depending on the nature of the injury, including its location and intensity. Another cause is a cardiovascular incident, such as a stroke. During a stroke there is a disruption of oxygen and nutrients to parts of the brain. If the disruption is brief, many cells will recover, and the memory loss is temporary. However, with longer periods of time, permanent cell damage and cell death occur. With cell death, the patterns of neural information are disrupted, and there is a permanent memory loss. Therefore, stroke victims may need to relearn how to speak and walk.

Ribot's Gradient

One characteristic of retrograde amnesia is a graded loss of memory in which more recent memories are more easily disrupted. In contrast, older memories are more firmly established and difficult to disrupt. This graded pattern of memory loss and retention is **Ribot's gradient** (Ribot, 1882),[1] and it reflects the consolidation of memories in the nervous system. Memory loss is greater as the age of the memory approaches the time of the incident. Basically, the older a memory is, the more consolidated it is, and the less susceptible it is to disruption (Brown, 2002). Figure 10.1 is an illustration of Ribot's gradient for retrograde amnesia for famous faces. There is some regularity in how memories are recovered following brain injury that causes retrograde amnesia, although there is also some variation among individuals (Roberts et al., 2015).

At first glance, Ribot's gradient seems to be the opposite of Ebbinghaus' retention curve. As a reminder, with the Ebbinghaus curve, the older a memory is, the more likely it is forgotten. In contrast, with Ribot's gradient, the older the memory is, the more likely that it has been consolidated, and so it is harder to disrupt and be forgotten. So, which of them is correct? Well, they both are. The Ebbinghaus curve is correct because, over time, more and more information is forgotten. However, keep in mind that most of the forgetting occurs early on, soon after learning. After that, the amount of forgetting tapers off considerably. Moreover, memories are subject to Jost's Law, which is the idea that the rate of

---

1 Like Ebbinghaus' (1885) book, Ribot's (1882) book makes interesting reading, not only for the insights into consolidation and amnesia, but also how he struggles to bring together and interpret concepts and ideas that are taken as a matter of course today. The book is interesting not only for what he got right, but also for what he got wrong.

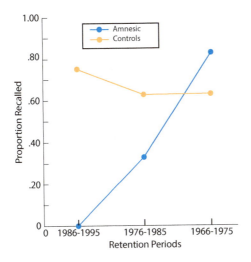

FIGURE 10.1 *Illustration of Ribot's Gradient for a Patient and Controls for Memory for Famous Faces*

Source: Created from data reported in Markowitsch, H. J., Weber-Luxemburger, G., Ewald, K., Kessler, J., & Heiss, W. D. (1997). Patients with heart attacks are not valid models for medial temporal lobe amnesia: A neuropsychological and FDG-PET study with consequences for memory research. *European Journal of Neurology, 4*(2), 178–184

Retrograde amnesia is fairly common. In any situation in which there is a possibility of head trauma, such as that when concussions occur, there is a possibility for retrograde amnesia. Some of you may have had retrograde amnesia, even if in a limited form. A common cause of retrograde amnesia is contact sports, such as with American football.

A study of football players, concussions, and retrograde amnesia was done by Lynch and Yarnell (1973; Yarnell & Lynch, 1973). They lurked on the sidelines during University of Colorado football games. When players were injured, they were tested after they came off the field of play. Neurologically, the players were assessed briefly using funduscopy (using an ophthalmoscope to look into a person's eye), pupil reaction, and extra-ocular-muscle function. These neurological exams revealed nothing remarkable.

For memory testing, six players were identified as having suffered "mild" concussions. Twelve additional players were tested as controls. Eight of these were tested when they came off the field following plays in which they were injured, but not due to head trauma (e.g., torn ligaments). The remaining players were tested after coming off the field after a substitution, but not after an injury.

All the players were tested immediately (within 30 seconds) after coming off the field, as well as three to five minutes later. Memory was assessed by asking the player to state his name, say what position he played and for which team, who his opponents were, and to describe the play that happened.

All the players, both the concussed and the controls, remembered the play that had just occurred when they were questioned within 30 seconds of coming off the field. However, three to five minutes later, or longer, players who had suffered a concussion

STUDY IN DEPTH

could no longer remember the play that led to their injury. They had retrograde amnesia for those events.

This suggests that effects of retrograde amnesia may take time to establish themselves and be observed. Thus, the retrograde amnesia was not immediate. There was a delay between the time of the injury and the onset of the amnesia. It may be that the knowledge of the prior play was still in the players' working memory, but that it could not be consolidated in the hippocampus as part of long-term memory as a result of the head trauma.

forgetting slows down. The reason for this is that more and more memories have been well-consolidated, consistent with Ribot's gradient, making them less likely to be forgotten. Thus, you can see that both Ebbinghaus's forgetting curve and Ribot's gradient contribute to the later likelihood that a memory is available for retrieval.

Much of what is lost in retrograde amnesia are autobiographical memories—memories that refer to events of one's own life, as well as personal semantic information, such as addresses and jobs, and public events, such as news stories. Again, the more recent the memories are, the more likely they are to be lost. Nondeclarative memories are largely preserved, as well as semantic knowledge, although people may not be aware of acquiring this knowledge and may even deny having it.

When there has not been permanent brain damage, the recovery of memories follows a regular pattern, namely Ribot's gradient. Because older memories are more

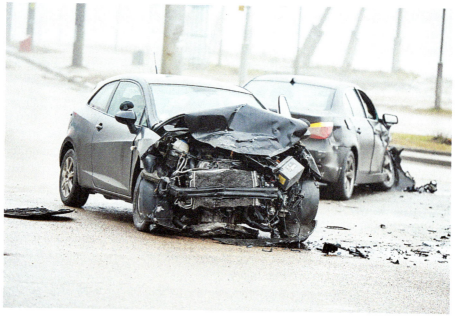

PHOTO 10.1 *Retrograde amnesia can occur if there is a blow to the head, as would occur with a concussion in an automobile collision*

Source: Dmitry Kalinovsky/Shutterstock.com

stable, they are the first to return. As time goes on, more memories are recovered. It is not unusual for many memories to be recovered at or close to their level prior to the incident. However, there is also a time just prior to the trauma for which memories are never recovered. These memories were permanently destroyed because the disruption hits them while they are in a very fragile state.

I had an experience with retrograde amnesia. When I was 21, I worked as a bartender. One night, while driving home after work, I stopped at a red light on Franklin Avenue and was waiting to turn left onto my street, Belle Avenue. There was a car behind me, and behind that car was a police cruiser. When the light turned green, I started to make the left turn, and the cruiser broadsided my car, pushing the driver's side door into the middle of the car (it turned out the officer had just gotten a call and had sped off to answer it with no flashing lights or siren—as reported by the witness in the car behind me). I was taken by ambulance to the hospital half a block away. When I woke up in intensive care the next morning, I had no memory of the accident. And even though it was July, I thought it was April. Over the next few days, my memories gradually returned, but even today, I have no memory of the day of the accident or the accident itself (thank goodness).

Case Studies of Retrograde Amnesia

Not all cases of retrograde amnesia follow the same pattern. What we have seen up to now is a typical pattern, but it can appear in other ways. Stracciari et al. (1994) describe two young men who had closed head injuries resulting in a temporally limited retrograde amnesia. They had trouble remembering what had happened to them during the past year. This amnesia was limited to autobiographical memories but not semantic and public memories (such as current events). Thus, not all information was lost for the amnesic period. However, even important personal information was lost. For example, one of them forgot that he had been dating a woman for six months prior to the accident. This memory loss was profound enough that her name was unfamiliar to him—and he had her name tattooed on his forearm!

Although memories often return during recovery, in more severe cases they do not. One such case is that of P. S., who suffered profound anterograde amnesia as well (McCarthy & Hodges, 1995). As a result of a stroke when he was 67, P. S. sustained damage to his thalamus. The result was retrograde amnesia for all his adult life, except for the period when he was in the British Navy during World War II. Because of his added problem with anterograde amnesia, he believed himself to still be in this time. He interpreted and placed any knowledge within the framework of those war years. For example, while his autobiographical memory was severely compromised, he did have good memory for famous faces of the decades following World War II, and he could place them in the correct temporal sequence. However, when asked to date this information, he would place it in the early to mid-1940s. He did, however, have reasonably good memory for that time. When asked to describe his hometown, he could be very specific, but his description was of the town as it appeared in the 1940s. Here, the thalamus is not the storehouse of memories. Instead, it is a connection between different sources of information that would place memories in time and in P. S.'s life. When this connection was severed, P. S. became trapped in time.[2]

Electroconvulsive Therapy/Shock

Retrograde amnesia can also occur when a powerful electrical current is passed through the brain. In some cases, this is done as part of a therapeutic treatment. This is **Electroconvulsive Therapy**, or **ECT**. For ECT, electrodes are placed on the head. The patient is strapped securely to a table, and a series of electrical pulses are passed through the brain. Unless anticonvulsant drugs are administered, these shocks can make the whole body convulse violently, possibly leading to injury. Basically, the ECT treatment induces a grand mal seizure. This process is repeated 6 to 12 times over a 3- to 5-week period (Cahill & Frith, 1995). It is more often used with depressed patients after there has been little to no response to any other treatments and the patient is in a precarious state. ECT continues to be used and is effective at getting patients to a state where more conventional therapies can be used.

Apart from alleviating depressive symptoms, ECT also induces amnesia. Initially, after ECT, there is a period of anterograde amnesia in which people have trouble learning new things (Cahill & Frith, 1995). More prominent is the retrograde amnesia (Cahill & Frith, 1995; Squire & Cohen, 1979), although some of the memories do eventually return. People undergoing treatment lose memories from the recent past, including memories of the ECT session itself (which is a good thing). The amount of memory loss varies, but it can be as long as one or two years prior to ECT (Squire et al., 1975) (see Figure 10.2). This memory loss is for both

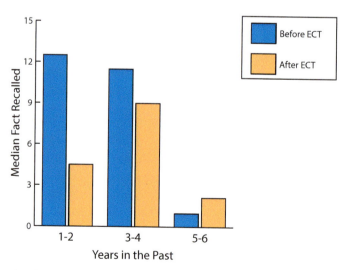

FIGURE 10.2 *Graded Effects of Retrograde Amnesia*

Source: adapted from Squire, L. R., & Cohen, N. (1979). Memory and amnesia: Resistance to disruption develops for years after learning. *Behavioral and Neural Biology, 25*, 115–125

---

2 For another case study of retrograde amnesia, see Hunkin (1997) who describes a person who lost all memories before the age of 19.

autobiographical memories (a more episodic memory loss) and for community-shared public memories (a more semantic memory loss); however, implicit memory seems unaffected (Vakil et al., 2000).[3]

When used to study memory, and not as a treatment, this procedure is called **Electroconvulsive Shock**, or **ECS**. It is used on laboratory animals, such as rats. ECS provides a systematic assessment of retrograde amnesia. When ECS is given to rats shortly after a fear experience, such as receiving a painful shock, retrograde amnesia occurs, and there is no subsequent fear of that situation (Duncan, 1949; Madsen & McGaugh, 1961). In another study by Chorover and Schiller (1965), rats were placed on a platform. If the rats stepped down, they received a shock, so they learned to not step down. Wires that delivered an ECS were attached to the rats' ears, and the amount of time between when rats stepped off the platform and the delivery of the ECS was varied. As can be seen in Figure 10.3, in a study by Duncan (1949), the shorter the delay between the shock and the ECS, the less likely that rats learned to avoid stepping down, because the ECS had disrupted their memories. However, if there was a lengthy period between stepping down and the ECS, this information was stored in the rats' brains and thus was more permanent, stable, and resistant to the disruption by the ECS.

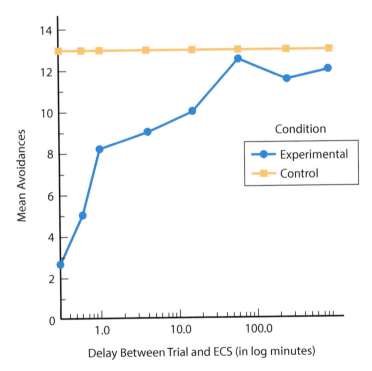

FIGURE 10.3 *Retrograde Amnesia Following Electroconvulsive Shock*

Source: adapted from Duncan, C. P. (1949). The retroactive effect of electroshock on learning. *Journal of Comparative Physiological Psychology, 42,* 32–44

3 For an account of Benjamin Franklin's work on electricity resulting in accidental amnesia and relief from depression when he and his friends were playing around with electricity, see Finger and Zaroub (2006).

Stop and Review

The loss of memories prior to an incident is retrograde amnesia, often involving a disruption of memory consolidation. This loss of memories follows Ribot's gradient, with newer memories being more susceptible to disruption than older memories. Over time, many of the memories initially lost are recovered, although those near the trauma may be gone forever. Retrograde amnesia can be induced using electrical shocks. When this is done therapeutically, it is electroconvulsive therapy, or ECT, whereas when it is done to study memory, it is electroconvulsive shock, or ECS.

ANTEROGRADE AMNESIA

Whereas retrograde amnesia is the loss of memories prior to an incident, **anterograde amnesia** is the inability to store new memories after an incident. This is a more devastating condition. With anterograde amnesia, people lose the ability to fully benefit from their experiences, and they become, in some sense, frozen in time. People with severe anterograde amnesia need to be given the same information repeatedly because they have great difficulty retaining it. Here, we first look at anterograde amnesia in terms of which part of the brain is damaged, namely, either the medial temporal lobes and the hippocampus, or the diencephalon. After this, we consider issues of anterograde amnesia more generally (see Aggleton, 2008, and Aggleton & Brown, 1999, for a suggestion that the same memory processes are disrupted in both cases).

H. M.: Medial Temporal Lobe and Hippocampus

The medial temporal lobes (BA 21) are adjacent to an important memory structure: the hippocampus. Damage to these areas of the brain as a result of surgical intervention, infection, stroke, or anoxia (lack of oxygen to the brain) can result in anterograde amnesia. Perhaps the most famous amnesic was Henry Molaison (February 26, 1926–December 2, 2008), better known as H. M. (Scoville & Milner, 1957). On August 23, 1953, at the age of 27, H. M. had brain surgery to relieve severe epilepsy. He was having several petit mal seizures each day (up to 12 in a two-hour period) and weekly grand mal seizures, often resulting in injury. He was unable to work or lead a normal life. The surgeons removed much of his hippocampus and adjoining cortex on both sides. Brain damage included other structures, such as portions of the amygdala and temporal cortex (Corkin et al., 1997). The parts of the hippocampus that did remain showed evidence of atrophy. In terms of his epilepsy, the operation was a success. The rate and severity of his seizures greatly diminished, although they were still present. Also, his intelligence stayed the same (if not improved), and his personality was unchanged. However, there was an unexpected side effect. H. M. had severe and dense anterograde amnesia. He was not able to learn new things.

Although H. M. had difficulty storing new memories, he had above normal intelligence. He had some retrograde amnesia for the time prior to the operation, but most of his memories were intact (Scoville & Milner, 1957). He had difficulty in daily life because he could not remember much beyond the span of his short-term memory. He often commented that he felt as if he had just awakened from a dream. It was not unusual for him to do a jigsaw puzzle many times or to read the same magazine over and over and not have any memory of having read it before. He enjoyed watching televised news but remembered nothing from it.

While H. M. had severe amnesia, not all his memories were disrupted. He had a good short-term memory (Wickelgren, 1968), and his language abilities were largely intact (Skotko et al., 2005). He could acquire new declarative memories with difficulty if the information was salient and was repeatedly presented over a long period of time. For example, he remembered his father's death after he had been absent from home for about a month (Milner et al., 1968). He also showed evidence of implicit memory, such as perceptual identification (Milner et al., 1968), and procedural memory for motor tasks, such as mirror tracing or pursuit rotor tasks (Corkin, 1968). H. M. was not the only person with severe anterograde amnesia. Other ways of acquiring this condition include loss of oxygen to the brain, brain tumors, neurological disorders such as epilepsy, or viral attacks such as herpes simplex encephalitis.

Diencephalic Anterograde Amnesia

The diencephalon is a collection of brain structures, including the thalamus, hypothalamus, and mammillary bodies. Damage to this area can also cause anterograde amnesia. This is commonly a symptom of **Korsakoff's syndrome**, which occurs in chronic and severe alcoholics. They have damage in many brain areas, including the dorsomedial thalamic nuclei, the mammillary bodies, and the frontal lobe. This extensive brain damage is due to a deficiency in thiamine (vitamin B1) as a result of alcoholism rather than an effect of the alcohol itself. It is also possible for the diencephalon to be damaged in other ways, such as through a stroke.

The diencephalon is associated with frontal lobe processing and the coordination and control of thought. People with anterograde amnesia from damage to these areas, may confabulate (see Chapter 13). This kind of anterograde amnesia may result in a decline in the ability to coordinate information in memory, making it difficult to recover the memory in an effective way. This decreased coordination of information also makes it difficult to retrieve old memories.

Anterograde Amnesia More Generally

The part of memory most affected in anterograde amnesia is conscious, declarative memory, including episodic/autobiographical, as well as semantic knowledge (but see Kitchner et al., 1998). If you were to have a conversation with an anterograde amnesic, he or she might seem more or less normal, maybe a little off. However, if you were to get up, leave, and return ten minutes later, he or she would not recognize you and may claim to have never met you before.

Anterograde amnesics do not show distinctiveness and novelty effects, such as the von Restorff effect (Kishiyama et al., 2004). Due to deficits in long-term memory encoding, they do not have the memories needed to keep track of context. Because distinctiveness is defined by the context in which information is found (e.g., elephant is distinctive in a list of vehicles but not in a list of zoo animals), no von Restorff effect is seen. Relatedly, because these people have less awareness of past encounters, they are less likely to use definite articles when referring to objects (e.g., "the chair") and are more likely to use indefinite articles (e.g., "a chair") (Duff et al., 2011). With standard language use, definite articles refer to things that have been mentioned or encountered before. A shift in language use could reflect changes in the availability of information in memory.

As noted in Chapter 7, episodic memory not only involves memory for past events, but also imagining future events. This is mental time travel. Because mental time travel into the past and the future involve similar neurological processes, people with anterograde amnesia also have trouble imagining the future (Hassabis et al., 2007; Rasmussen & Berntsen, 2014). Thus, anterograde amnesia truly traps people in time. The ability to make decisions may be impaired in anterograde amnesics. This is because they have difficulty tracking how events have unfolded in the past and not because decision making strategies, per se, are impaired (Rosenbaum et al., 2016).

Not all memory functions are seriously affected with anterograde amnesia. For example, short-term memory is largely intact (Baddeley & Warrington, 1970), but people forget things faster (Warrington & Weiskrantz, 1968). Thus, amnesics comprehend events as they happen, but these experiences slip away quickly. Note also that, as with H. M., nondeclarative memory is relatively intact. Anterograde amnesics can learn new procedural tasks, although they may lack conscious awareness of doing so (Brooks & Baddeley, 1976). An example of an anterograde amnesic learning on a mirror tracing task is shown in Figure 10.4.

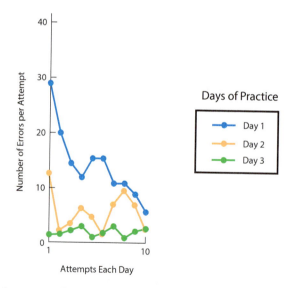

FIGURE 10.4 *Performance of an Anterograde Amnesic on a Mirror Tracing Task, Illustrating Preserved Implicit Memory*

Source: adapted from Blakemore, C. (1977). *Mechanics of the Mind*. Cambridge, UK: Cambridge University Press

Another well-known case of anterograde amnesia is Clive Wearing, a British classical musician who suffered from herpes simplex encephalitis in 1985 (Wilson et al., 1995). Despite his profound anterograde amnesia, his musical abilities remained largely intact, allowing him to play or conduct as he had done before, with degradations noticed only by expert musicians (Wilson & Wearing, 1995).

The preservation of nondeclarative memories also applies to implicit, linguistic tasks (Schacter, 1987), such as the syntactic, semantic, and episodic priming of words (Ferreira et al., 2008; Graf & Schacter, 1985; Graf et al., 1985). However, such priming is likely to be preserved when it depends on perceptual, rather than semantic, characteristics (Rajaram & Coslett, 2000). Amnesics perform similarly to normal people on word fragment, word stem, and perceptual identification tasks (Graf et al., 1984; Warrington & Weiskrantz, 1970). For example, amnesics spend less time viewing pictures that are repeated. That said, if something in a picture has been altered (e.g., the relationship among elements is changed), normal people spend more time looking in the region where the change occurred, whereas amnesics do not (Ryan et al., 2000).

It is important to keep in mind that no memory test is process pure. There is always an influence of multiple memory components. The combined influence of explicit and implicit memory on a direct memory task in amnesics is seen with recall and recognition. Recall requires effort to generate information, whereas recognition requires only that people, at a minimum, believe that the information is old. A feeling of familiarity does not require conscious recollection, but only unconscious, implicit influences. Thus, anterograde amnesics have more difficulty with recall than recognition. In some cases, they may even show no recognition deficit in the face of a clear recall deficit (Hirst et al., 1986; 1988).

Other Case Studies of Anterograde Amnesia

Is it possible for people to have anterograde amnesia for some types of information but not others? One case is that of A. B., who, as a result of a hematoma, had damage to the left posterolateral frontal lobe (BA 4) and adjacent anterior parietal lobe (BA 1, 2, & 3). A. B. could not retain word or sentence lists in short-term memory. However, he could recall complex stories he read or heard. Thus, A. B. had anterograde amnesia for words and unrelated sentences but had more normal memory for complex, interrelated, and meaningful prose (Romani & Martin, 1999). In other words, A. B. had poor memory at the surface form and textbase levels but good memory at the mental model level (see Chapter 7).

Another amnesic with selective problems is T. R. (Sirigu & Grafman, 1996). He suffered cerebral anoxia after heart failure and then had amnesia consistent with damage to the hippocampus. Like many anterograde amnesics, T. R. had difficulty with new episodic memories. However, it was only for certain types of information. He remembered events, but only in terms of what happened and where they happened. He was amnesic for the identities of the people involved and for when the events happened. Thus, there is selective loss for some episodic information, but not for others.

Living with Anterograde Amnesia

As you can imagine, anterograde amnesia impairs the ability to function normally. People with anterograde amnesia may leave kitchen appliances on, fires burning, water running, and so on. They have a tendency to overeat because they consume multiple meals, not remembering that they had just eaten (Higgs et al., 2008). Is there anything that can be done to help these people? Well, it depends on how severe the amnesia is. Some people have relatively mild amnesia, which allows for some independence, whereas others are profoundly affected. Some amnesics are described here for whom treatment has been attempted.

One of these was a special education teacher, Sheila Moakes (Kapur & Moakes, 1995). She became amnesic after an attack of herpes simplex encephalitis, at the age of 32. This damaged parts of her temporal lobe and hippocampus, leaving her with some retrograde amnesia and profound anterograde amnesia. Although she could no longer work as a regular teacher, tracking students across the school year, she was able to tutor students on a lesson-by-lesson basis. She could also do many household tasks but only by keeping to a strict schedule (otherwise she did not do some things and did others repeatedly), and she could do light grocery shopping if she had a list and did not have to go to a new store. She could still drive well, with her only problem being that she could become lost if she ventured too far from home. She did watch television but avoided shows with a plot that must be remembered. She also did not read much for the same reason. Some parts of her life continued to deteriorate. She became distant to her son and lost many of her old friends and was not been able to make new ones. She also lost the motivation to learn new tasks because she knew the enormous effort that would be involved.

If amnesia is milder, people may be aware of the problem and develop strategies to compensate for the loss, such as the case of J. C. (Wilson & Hughes, 1997). He was a former law student, who became amnesic after an attack of herpes simplex encephalitis. Because of some spared memory and his high intelligence and motivation, he was able to overcome this disability to some degree. Although he had to quit law school, he was able to train to become a professional furniture refinisher. Still, it took him 20 trips to learn where to get off the bus for refinishing school. He also went on to start his own business. To keep his life in order, he developed a system using a watch with multiple alarms and a color-coded system for keeping notes about events in his life. If he went to a new restaurant with friends, he needed to write down that he went and what he ate, because he would not remember. He also needed to leave himself constant reminders, such as "clean contact lenses" or "check the oven." His life critically depended on sticky notes.

J. C. showed remarkable adaptation due in large part to the amount of support he gets from family and friends. However, not all anterograde amnesics are so fortunate. For example, Mr. S. became amnesic in his seventies as the result of a stroke (Squires et al., 1997). Although he used a notebook for reminders in the beginning, a lack of reinforcement from his wife and friends, as well as his own lack of motivation, made him soon stop. There was no improvement for Mr. S.

Mixture of Retrograde and Anterograde Amnesia

As noted earlier, it is rare to have only retrograde or anterograde amnesia. Here is a case of severe trauma in which both were present and a description of how they changed over time (as reported in Barbizet, 1970). An overview of the situation is given in Figure 10.5. Initial testing occurred five months after the trauma in which there was both retrograde and anterograde amnesia. For the retrograde amnesia, there was an inability to remember events from two years prior to the accident and only partial memories for the time before that. For the anterograde amnesia, there was an inability to remember much of what happened after coming out of a coma and trouble storing new memories.

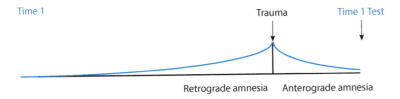

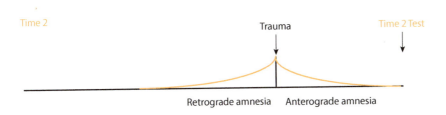

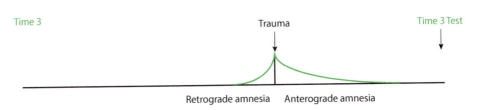

FIGURE 10.5 *Illustration of Brain Damage Resulting in Both Retrograde and Anterograde Amnesias*

Source: adapted from Barbizet, J. (1970). *Human Memory and Its Pathology*. San Francisco, CA: Freeman

As time progressed, things improved. The retrograde amnesia severity eased. By eight months after the trauma, there was dense amnesia for only one year, with partial amnesia for four years prior to that, and most other memories had returned to normal. Ten months later, most of the retrograde amnesia had lifted, leaving only dense amnesia for the two weeks prior to the trauma, never to be recovered. Anterograde amnesia improved as well. By eight months after the trauma, some new information was being stored in long-term memory, and by 18 months memory had returned to normal. It is only for the 3.5-month period after emerging from the coma that there are no memories. Presumably, during this time information was not stored effectively, and so, was never remembered.

Stop and Review

The loss of the ability to store new memories after a trauma is anterograde amnesia. This is caused by damage to either the medial temporal lobes and hippocampus, or to the diencephalon. An example of the first type is the case of H. M., who had his hippocampus surgically removed. Examples of the second are Korsakoff's syndrome patients. People with anterograde amnesia have difficulty learning new information beyond what is held in short-term memory. Most of this loss is for declarative information. They also have trouble imagining future events. Other types of memory are more preserved, such as short-term and nondeclarative memory. People with anterograde amnesia find it difficult to carry on with their lives, although some limited success is possible. It is important to note that while retrograde and anterograde are treated separately here, it is rare to find cases of one, but not the other to some degree.

TRANSIENT GLOBAL AMNESIA

The types of amnesia that we have been discussing are the consequence of a clear traumatic injury, with no ambiguity about what brought it about, and the amnesia lasts for a substantial time. However, there is a type of amnesia that can occur where the cause is organic, but the duration is brief. This is **transient global amnesia**, or **TGA**. The amnesia is transient because it only lasts for a short period of time and does not endure. The amnesia is global, with both retrograde and anterograde components covering almost all memories from a given period. Thus, this is an unusual and hard to study disorder.

TGA episodes are short-lived, lasting only a few hours (typically 3–8). A distribution of TGA durations is shown in Figure 10.6. Thus, TGA is not a permanent change, but a temporary memory state. That said, there is some evidence that deficits may linger for several days (Kessler et al., 2001). The fleeting nature of TGA makes it hard to study. Although the concept of TGA has been around since Ribot (1882) and was originally labelled by Fisher and Adams (1964), it has been difficult to study until recently. Often, by the time an expert is notified, the amnesia has begun to clear. Additionally, many incidents surely go unreported. For example, if people have the beginning of a TGA in the evening, they might go to sleep, and, by morning, most of the symptoms have begun to clear.

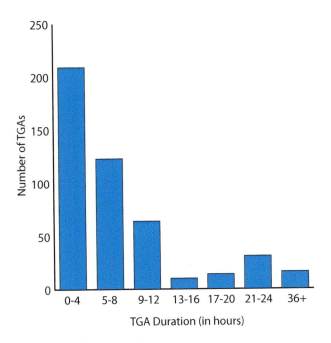

FIGURE 10.6 *Duration of a Transient Global Amnesia*

Source: adapted from Brown, A. S. (1998). Transient global amnesia. *Psychonomic Bulletin & Review, 5,* 401–427

During a TGA attack, people have no memories of the recent past, anywhere from a few hours to several decades, although in most cases the memory loss is for a few months. This range of memory loss is shown in Figure 10.7. As can be seen, the amnesia does not cover all of one's life, but, following Ribot's gradient, with only the weaker, less consolidated memories being prone to disruption. This amnesia can be very dense in terms of the memories that are lost. For example, one man was surprised to see that some fingers on his left hand were missing, having been lost in a farm machinery accident four months before. This suggests that even very traumatic and emotional memories can be disrupted during a TGA.

Often during a TGA episode, people are confused and repeatedly ask the same questions. This is because of an anterograde amnesia component that keeps them from remembering that they had already asked the question and gotten an answer. Although working memory appears fine, episodic knowledge is not retained or recovered. Semantic and procedural knowledge seem unaffected. Some affected people are aware of their memory problems, but many only have a general awareness that something is not right, and may even be unaware of memory problems. They simply know that something is off. People often exhibit signs of anxiety and depression during the TGA state (Hainselin et al., 2012).

Part of what makes TGA so mysterious is that there is no clear indicator of its cause. People seem fine but then are suddenly experiencing a dense memory loss. As illustrated in Figure 10.8, TGAs often occur between the ages of 50 and 70, and typically only occur once in a lifetime. It has been suggested that TGAs are brought

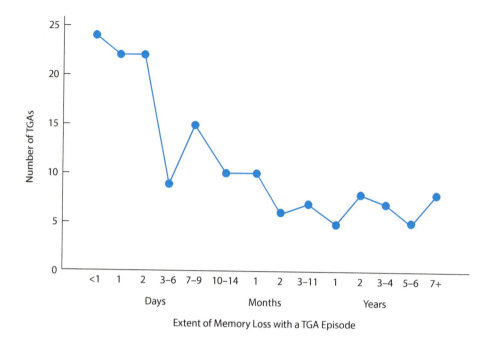

FIGURE 10.7 *Degree of Retrograde Amnesia during a Transient Global Amnesia Episode*

Source: adapted from Brown, A. S. (1998). Transient global amnesia. *Psychonomic Bulletin & Review, 5,* 401–427

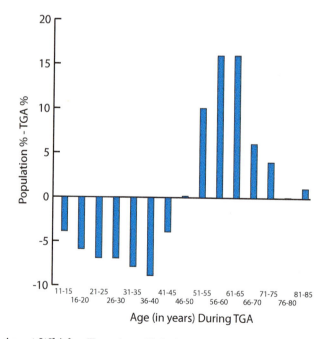

FIGURE 10.8 *Age at Which a Transient Global Amnesia Episode Is Experienced*

Source: adapted from Brown, A. S. (1998). Transient global amnesia. *Psychonomic Bulletin & Review, 5,* 401–427

about by an emotional or physical stress or exertion, such as having an argument, playing an exciting card game, having sex (the most popular way to get it), driving, taking a hot shower, or having a coughing spell.

TGAs may be a result of an ischemia (temporary disruptions of blood flow) in the brain. The parts of the brain that are most often implicated are the temporal lobes, hippocampus, and thalamus (Brown, 1998; Goldenberg, 1995.) There is even some evidence that area CA1 of the hippocampus may be affected (Bartsch & Deuschl, 2010).

Stop and Review

The temporary and extensive loss of memories is transient global amnesia, or TGA. The duration of a TGA episode is typically short, generally lasting less than 24 hours. Despite the limited duration, the amount of memory loss can be extensive, and follows Ribot's gradient. People are often in a confused, anxious, and depressed state during a TGA, and may not be fully aware of their memory problems. TGAs follow periods of stress or excitement and involve a disruption of blood flow.

LOSS OF MEMORY OF SPECIFIC KNOWLEDGE OR SKILLS

The distinction between autobiographical and semantic memories is observed with certain types of amnesia. For example, it is possible for people to have trouble with semantic memory but not autobiographical memory. Yasuda et al. (1997) describe a patient, M. N., who sustained damage from a tumor to her right hemisphere where the frontal and temporal lobes meet. She was able to give accurate accounts of her autobiographical memories, such as where she had gone to school, the places she had worked, and the various illnesses she had. However, she had difficulty identifying and remembering public events, recalling only 20% of those that most people could recall at a 100% level. She also had problems with historical figures and monuments. This problem with semantic memory leads us to a condition called semantic amnesia.

Semantic Amnesia

Semantic amnesia is a deficit in the ability to retrieve semantic knowledge (for a review, see McCarthy & Warrington, 2016). This is a result of damage to the temporal lobes, particularly in the anterolateral portions (BA 38) and more likely with damage to the left hemisphere (Hodges et al. 1992; Snowden et al., 1989). This is rare in the absence of other neurological syndromes, such as Alzheimer's disease. This is because so many sources of damage tend to also affect other areas. Moreover, this part of the brain is well supported, with this part of the temporal lobe being maintained by two major arteries. This makes it less likely to be damaged by a stroke.

People with semantic amnesia have difficulty retrieving word meanings, even for common words, despite otherwise normal language. For example, people with semantic amnesia may not be able to remember what a cat or a robin is or whether a mouse has a beak or a long, skinny tail (Funnell, 1995). This loss is called **anomia** and can be very specific. Patient G. R. had difficulty with famous names but not the names of friends or historical or literary figures (Lucchelli et al., 1997). G. R.'s memory for facts about people was intact, such as knowing their line of work and any distinguishing achievements or physical features. The trouble was in remembering the names of celebrities. For a first-hand account of the experience of anomia, see Ashcraft (1993).

What can distinguish semantic amnesia and anomia from aphasia is that people also have difficulty with semantic judgments that do not require language (Bozeat et al., 2000). People have difficulty not only with the names of objects, but also how they are used. This is **apraxia**. They may try to use objects incorrectly, such as trying to use a match as a pencil. Because of this, these people need to be monitored to avoid harming themselves. That said, they may be able to use some objects appropriately in cases where the use is clear and constrained (Hodges et al., 2000)—for example, using a pair of scissors with a piece of paper. There are only a limited number of ways that the scissors lend themselves to being used, and some people with apraxia perform normally.

Semantic amnesia can be restricted to particular types of information. Patient A. B. R. had semantic amnesia after a period of anoxia during open heart surgery. A. B. R. had trouble identifying pictures (but not names) of famous people (e.g., Queen Elizabeth and Napoleon) and landmarks (e.g., the White House and the Parthenon). The remaining memories were relatively intact (Kartsounis & Shallice, 1996). Another distinction that may be affected is between abstract and concrete ideas. In normal people, concrete ideas (such as sock, pencil, dog, etc.) are easier to remember than abstract ones (such as truth, love, redemption). However, patient D. M. could identify abstract but not concrete words (Breedin et al., 1994). A similar isolation in semantic amnesia can occur for knowledge of natural kinds versus artifacts.

Before leaving semantic amnesia, think about what is going on in episodic memory a little more. As a reminder, with semantic amnesia, despite problems in semantic memory, even complex forms of episodic memory, such as autobiographical memory, appear to be preserved (Simons et al., 2002). These autobiographical memories can be used to guide semantic dementia patients to derive semantic-like knowledge. Memories of experiences can help them derive some semantic understanding, even though semantic memory itself is compromised (Graham et al., 1997). For example, one person could remember the names of people she played golf with frequently by using autobiographical memories, but she could not remember the names of people she had played with in the distant past or the names of famous golfers. Although there is some preserved episodic memory, it is incomplete. This is an odd reversal of Ribot's gradient with semantic amnesia, particularly for semantic aspects of those events, such as people's names (Piolino et al., 2003).

Aphasia, Amusia, and Prospagnosia

Semantic amnesias that are exclusive to specific types of knowledge are treated as separate conditions. In some cases, people may lose the ability to use language, called **aphasia**. Because language is usually located in the left hemisphere of the brain, this is typically a result of damage to that area. There are two general kinds of aphasia. One is **Broca's aphasia**, which occurs when there is damage to caudal portions of the frontal lobe and adjoining portions of the temporal lobe (BAs 44 & 45). This is near the motor cortex of the frontal lobe. In this condition, people have difficulty producing language, but language comprehension is better preserved. Another is **Wernicke's aphasia**, which occurs with damage to the posterior temporal lobe and the adjoining portions of the parietal lobe (BA 22). Here, people have difficulty comprehending language, but language production is better preserved. This decline can get to the point where they have difficulty monitoring their own language. As a result, they produce utterances that are grammatically correct but semantically anomalous. A condition that is related to aphasia is **amusia**. People with this deficit have trouble either comprehending or producing music.

Another specific memory loss is **prosopagnosia**, or a failure to recognize faces. This can occur after damage to the fusiform gyrus (BA 37). People with this condition remember different people but are unable to recognize their faces, even when they

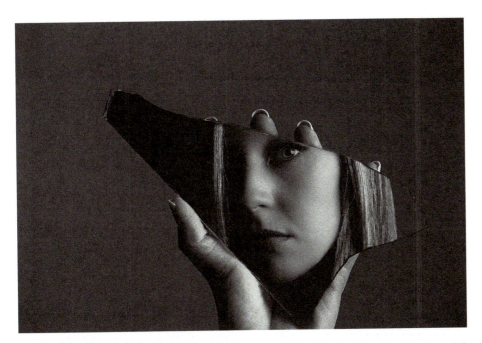

PHOTO 10.2 *Some types of amnesia target only specific memory functions. People with prosopagnosia have trouble recognizing faces. They may not even recognize their own faces in a mirror*

Source: Alta Oosthuizen/Shutterstock.com

know people well. Patients may not even be able to recognize their own faces. These people use other cues to identify people, such as their voice. Different types of memories use different parts of the brain. Memory retrieval is not a discrete process. Instead, people may be able to remember some information but not all of it.

Short-Term Memory Amnesia

Most amnesias affect long-term memory, with preserved short-term memory. However, there are cases where short-term memory is damaged, and long-term memory is less affected (Belleville et al., 2003). One example is K. F. who had a serial position curve recency effect of only one item (normal people have recency effects of five or six) (Shallice & Warrington, 1970). However, long-term memory was relatively intact. Also, there is P. V. (Vallar & Baddeley, 1984; Vallar & Papagno, 1995), who had difficulty remembering spoken words over the short term but had normal memory for visually presented lists and good long-term retention. This led P. V. to have problems "understanding" short sequences that required short-term memory, such as phone numbers or the prices of goods. She also had trouble doing mental calculations.

Many verbal short-term memory amnesias involved damage to the left parietal lobe (Vallar & Papagno, 1995)—in particular, the supramarginal gyrus (BA 40). In some cases, premotor areas of the frontal lobe are also implicated (e.g., Broca's area). This disrupts working memory rehearsal and can spill over to influence more complex thinking, such as sentence comprehension. People with verbal short-term memory amnesia would have difficulty understanding sentences like "Touch the small green square and the large black circle," or "The cat that the dog chased was white." Comprehending these sentences requires keeping track of the words and the order in which they were heard. They are less able to guess the intended message if some words are forgotten. People with short-term memory amnesia must use other sources of information. For example, patient I. R. could not use phonological information to help her remember but could use semantic information from long-term memory (Belleville et al., 2003).

Not all short-term memory amnesias are verbal processing deficits. Some, following damage to the right parietal/occipital lobe, result in visuo-spatial memory problems (Vallar & Papagno, 1995), such as having difficulty counting the number of dots on a computer screen, identifying unfamiliar faces, doing mental rotation, or learning the way around an unfamiliar house.

Stop and Review

It is possible to have selective deficits that target memory for some types of information but leave others relatively intact. With semantic amnesia, people have difficulty retrieving semantic information about the world, which makes it difficult to understand what is going on. However, episodic and autobiographical memories are more preserved. Memory loss can also target specific abilities, such as loss of language skill with aphasia, loss of music skills with amusia, loss of object name knowledge with anomia, and loss of the ability to recognize faces with prosopagnosia. Whereas most amnesias strike long-term memory, it is also possible to have primarily short-term memory damaged.

PSYCHOGENIC AMNESIA

The amnesias that we have seen so far arise from clear physical brain damage. There are other amnesias that may arise from psychological trauma. That is, people may be so psychologically disturbed by something that it causes catastrophic forgetting. These are **psychogenic amnesias** because they are brought about by psychological rather than neurological mechanisms, although in some cases there may be neurological damage that is not detected, making the amnesia only appear to be psychogenic (Kopelman et al., 1994; Markowitsch, 2003). Here, the memory loss is associated with a traumatic event, such as the loss of a beloved parent. The knowledge lost is usually episodic or autobiographical in nature. Semantic and procedural memories remain intact. The memory loss may be a way of coping. If the oppressive knowledge is not consciously remembered, then it will no longer be stressful and anxiety provoking.

A concern with reports of psychogenic amnesia is that some or all these people may be malingering and faking their conditions. In fact, with careful memory tests, some people have been found to be simulating at least some of their symptoms (Kopelman et al., 1994). This may be done because they are trying to avoid prosecution or some other negative outcome. That said, there is also evidence that people who do not claim to remember their crimes may actually be amnestic (Pyszora et al., 2003). Even faking or simulating can influence memory, causing people to have trouble remembering when they need to (Christianson & Bylin, 1999). This is like directed forgetting, although it is possible to eventually recover these memories (Mangiulli et al., 2019). Putting aside the malingerers, let us look at some ideas for what psychogenic amnesia might be, and how it might manifest itself in terms of impaired memory performance.

Repression

One of the best-known forms of psychogenic amnesia is **repression**, a concept associated with Freud and his followers. The idea here is that there are experiences people have that are traumatic or threatening to the point of potentially damaging the ability to function adequately. These can be any number of traumas, including sexual abuse, violence, or even inappropriate sexual desires or feelings. To protect us from these damaging memories, a part of the mind actively represses them to keep them from entering consciousness. Thus, repression is a defense mechanism.

The empirical support for repression is scarce. By its very nature, repression is difficult to study. First, one must recover repressed memories, but a problem is not knowing how accurate such memories are. As we saw in Chapter 13, it is easy for false memories to be generated, and there is no clear way, apart from independent evidence, to distinguish real recovered memories from false ones (Loftus, 1993). An intense debate in memory research was whether recovered repressed memories are real. Some people argued that there is no such thing as repression. All recovered repressed memories are either false memories or not really repressed in the first place. There are two lines of argument for this view. One is that many of the methods used to recover repressed memories are like those that would be used to create false memories. Another point is that the typical outcome for highly traumatic experiences is that people remember them vividly and have difficulty forgetting them, even when they want to, as with people who have PTSD. This is the opposite of repression.

Dissociative Amnesia

Another psychogenic amnesia is **dissociative amnesia** in which people are unable to remember segments of their lives (Kihlstrom & Schacter, 1995). Typically, the forgotten knowledge is either traumatic itself or is associated with a traumatic event. For example, suppose you were the driver of a car in an accident that resulted in someone's death. If this pathologically troubled you, you might acquire dissociative amnesia in which you do not remember the events of that day. What makes this distinct from repression is that people are aware of the memory loss and are troubled by it, whereas this is not the case with repression.

There are three ways for dissociative amnesia to manifest itself (Nemiah, 1979). The first is as a **systematized amnesia**, where people are amnesic for information related to a traumatic event, regardless of when or where it occurred. Second is **localized amnesia**, in which people have trouble remembering events within a block of time, such as a period of hours or weeks. Finally, with **generalized amnesia**, nearly all a person's life is forgotten. These different ways that dissociative amnesia manifests itself illustrate the psychological influence of its origins. This selectivity or breadth of coverage is almost never seen with organic amnesia.

Dissociative Fugue

A more profound psychogenic amnesia is a **dissociative fugue**, in which memory is disrupted to the point that people forget fundamental aspects of their identity, such as who they are, where they live, and what they do for a living (Kihlstrom & Schacter, 1995). There are different fugue states, depending on the nature and extent of the loss (Fisher, 1945; Fisher & Joseph, 1949). First, there may be a change in both identity and location (where the person lives)—this is **fugue and flight**. Second, there may be a loss of memories, but the core identity is intact—this is **memory fugue**. Finally, there may be a reversion to an earlier state of life, with an inability to remember events after that period—this is **regression fugue**. Again, this memory loss is psychological and is not seen with organic damage.

Although conscious awareness of previous memories is rendered inaccessible in the fugue state, if this is like other amnesias, we would expect implicit memory to be unaffected. This has been difficult to test, especially because the fugue state is so rare. However, there is some anecdotal evidence consistent with it. An illustration of preserved implicit memory of a fugal amnesic is a case of a woman who was found wandering around but could provide no information about herself. She was asked to dial a random telephone number. This number turned out to be her mother's (Lyon, 1985).

What is more fascinating is that when people come out of the fugue state, even if it had been going on for years, not only do memories from the original identity return, but memories from the fugue identity are forgotten. This return to the original identity can be slow or fast. Thus, even when there has been a recovery of the original identity, there is still an amnesia associated with this condition.

Dissociative Identity Disorder

A final psychogenic amnesia is involved in **dissociative identity disorder,**[4] in which people act as if they have many separate identities, each with its own autobiographical history. In some cases, these alternative identities are aware of the others. Often one identity has no conscious memories of what another identity learned while he or she was dominant. In dissociative identity disorder, there may be asymmetrical amnesia (Kihlstrom & Schacter, 1995). That is, one identity may remember information that was learned when a second identity was dominant but not vice versa. This resembles a dissociative fugue, where a shift from one identity to another results in amnesic forgetting of information learned while involved with a previous identity.

Still, this amnesia does not apply to all memories. Like organic amnesia, implicit memories may be intact with an otherwise amnesic loss across identities, as with procedural memory learning (Kihlstrom & Schacter, 1995) or priming (Huntjens et al., 2002). These implicit priming effects spread across identities more for tasks that influence perceptual processing, such as picture fragment completion, than for tasks that rely more on conceptual knowledge, such as word stem completion, which can show amnesia across identities (Eich et al., 1997).

Stop and Review

People may, possibly, be amnesic from psychological trauma. Psychogenic amnesias include repression, dissociative amnesia, dissociative fugue, and dissociative identity disorder. Repression involves the mind keeping psychologically threatening information from entering consciousness. The evidence for this condition is weak. Dissociative amnesia is like repression except that people are aware of the memory loss and are bothered by it. Dissociative fugue is a state in which people lose autobiographical memories for an entire prior identity. Memories for the prior identity may return, but with amnesia for the replacement experiences. Finally, dissociative identity disorder involves people having multiple identities, with a frequent symptom being amnesia from one identity to another. This is often asymmetrical and is confined to explicit memory, and less so, if at all, to implicit memory.

4 Formerly Multiple Personality Disorder.

PUTTING IT ALL TOGETHER

Amnesia is the catastrophic loss of memories—a pathological forgetting. The various types of amnesia reinforce the idea that memory is not one thing. It is a made up of different parts and components that typically work together in a harmonious way. Amnesia can be oriented toward the past or the future, as with the distinction between retrograde and anterograde amnesia, each being brought about by different types of brain damage. Amnesia can be shorter in duration, as with some retrograde amnesias and transient global amnesia, or permanently alter people's lives, as with anterograde amnesia. Amnesia can come about from organic or psychologic trauma. The suggested psychogenic amnesias are repression, dissociative amnesia, fugue states, and the memory loss that accompanies dissociative identity disorder.

Much of what we know about memory and the principles that it operates under comes from studies of people with amnesia. The loss of memories can follow Ribot's gradient, highlighting the fact that your memories go through a process of consolidation. The distinction between short- and long-term memories is reinforced by the finding that people can have either short- or long-term memory amnesias. Moreover, short-term memory amnesia may target either verbal or visuo-spatial information. The distinction between declarative and nondeclarative memories is highlighted by the loss of declarative memories in amnesics, with largely preserved nondeclarative memories. Also, highlighting the idea that different kinds of information in memory are processed differently, amnesias can target specific kinds of information. For example, with semantic amnesia, people lose the ability to process certain types of world knowledge. There can also be a loss of language-specific, musical, or face identification memories.

STUDY QUESTIONS

1. How is amnesia different from normal forgetting?
2. How does retrograde amnesia occur? What are some of its defining characteristics? How does this relate to Ribot's gradient?
3. What do electroconvulsive shocks do to memory? How extensive can the damage be?
4. What is anterograde amnesia? Damage to which brain structures produces this condition?
5. What types of memories are damaged in anterograde amnesia? What types of memories are preserved? What is the general prognosis for people with this condition?
6. What is transient global amnesia? How extensive is the loss? How long does it last? Who does this happen to?
7. What are the specific kinds of memory loss that can be targeted by amnesias?
8. What sorts of memory losses occur with short-term memory amnesias? How are these different losses associated with different parts of the brain?

9. What is psychogenic amnesia? What is repression? What is dissociative amnesia? What is a psychogenic fugue? What memory losses can occur in dissociative identity disorder?

KEY TERMS

- amnesia
- amusia
- anomia
- anterograde amnesia
- aphasia
- apraxia
- Broca's aphasia
- consolidation
- dissociative amnesia
- dissociative fugue
- dissociative identity disorder
- Electroconvulsive Shock (ECS)
- Electroconvulsive Therapy (ECT)
- fugue and flight
- generalized amnesia
- Korsakoff's syndrome
- localized amnesia
- memory fugue
- organic amnesia
- prosopagnosia
- psychogenic amnesia
- regression fugue
- repression
- retrograde amnesia
- Ribot's gradient
- semantic amnesia
- systematized amnesia
- transient global amnesia (TGA)
- Wernicke's aphasia

EXPLORE MORE

Here are some additional readings that can allow you to further explore issues of amnesia.

Baddeley, A. D., Kopelman, M. D., & Wilson, B. A. (Eds.). (2003). *The Handbook of Memory Disorders*. Chichester, UK: John Wiley & Sons.

Campbell, R. E., & Conway, M. A. (1995). *Broken Memories: Case Studies in Memory Impairment*. Oxford: Blackwell Publishing.

Corkin, S. (2013). *Permanent Present Tense: The Unforgettable Life of the Amnesic Patient, HM* (Vol. 1000). New York: Basic books.

Parkin, A. J. (1997). *Memory and Amnesia: An Introduction*. New York: Psychology Press.

Ribot, T. A. (1882). *Diseases of Memory: An Essay in the Positive Psychology*. London: Kegan Paul, Trench, & Co.

REFERENCES

Aggleton, J. P. (2008). Understanding anterograde amnesia: Disconnections and hidden lesions. *Quarterly Journal of Experimental Psychology, 61*, 1441–1471.

Aggleton, J. P., & Brown, M. W. (1999). Episodic memory, amnesia and the hippocampal-anterior thalamic axis. *Behavioral and Brain Sciences, 22*, 425–489.

Ashcraft, M. H. (1993). A personal case history of transient anomia. *Brain and Language, 44*, 47–57.

Baddeley, A. D., & Warrington, E. K. (1970). Amnesia and the distinction between long- and short-term memory. *Journal of Verbal Learning and Verbal Behavior, 9*, 176–189.

Barbizet, J. (1970). *Human Memory and Its Pathology*. San Francisco, CA: Freeman.

Bartsch, T., & Deuschl, G. (2010). Transient global amnesia: Functional anatomy and clinical implications. *Lancet Neurology, 9(2)*:205e221.

Belleville, S., Caza, N., & Peretz, I. (2003). A neuropsychology argument for a processing view of memory. *Journal of Memory and Language, 48*, 686–703.

Bozeat, S., Lambon Ralph, M. A., Patterson, K., Garrard, P., & Hodges, J. R. (2000). Non-verbal semantic impairment in semantic dementia. *Neuropsychologia, 38*, 1207–1215.

Breedin, S. D., Saffran, E. M., & Coslett, H. B. (1994). Reversal of the concreteness effect in a patient with semantic dementia. *Cognitive Neuropsychology, 11*, 617–660.

Brooks, D. N., & Baddeley, A. D. (1976). What can amnesic patients learn? *Neuropsychologia, 14*, 111–122.

Brown, A. S. (1998). Transient global amnesia. *Psychonomic Bulletin & Review, 5*, 401–427.

Brown, A. S. (2002). Consolidation theory and retrograde amnesia in humans. *Psychonomic Bulletin & Review, 9*, 403–425.

Cahill, C., & Frith, C. (1995). Memory following electroconvulsive therapy. In A. D. Baddeley, B. A. Wilson, & F. N. Watts (Eds.), *Handbook of Memory Disorders* (pp. 319–335). New York: Wiley.

Chorover, S. L., & Schiller, P. H. (1965). Short-term retrograde amnesia in rats. *Journal of Comparative and Physiological Psychology, 59*, 73–78.

Christianson, S. Å., & Bylin, S. (1999). Does simulating amnesia mediate genuine forgetting for a crime event? *Applied Cognitive Psychology, 13(6)*, 495–511.

Corkin, S. (1968). Acquisition of motor skill after bilateral medial temporal-lobe excision. *Neuropsychologia, 6*, 255–265.

Corkin, S., Amaral, D. G., González, R. G., Johnson, K. A., & Hyman, B. T. (1997). H. M.'s medial temporal lobe lesions: Findings from magnetic resonance imaging. *Journal of Neuroscience, 17*, 3964–3979.

Duff, M. C., Gupta, R., Hengst, J. A., Tranel, D., & Cohen, N. J. (2011). The use of definite references signals declarative memory: Evidence from patients with hippocampal amnesia. *Psychological Science, 22(5)*, 666–673.

Duncan, C. P. (1949). The retroactive effect of electroshock on learning. *Journal of Comparative Physiological Psychology, 42*, 32–44.

Ebbinghaus, H. (1885). *Memory: A Contribution to Experimental Psychology* (H. A. Ruger & C. E. Bussenius, Trans.). New York: Teachers College, Columbia University.

Eich, E., Macaulay, D., Loewenstein, R. J., & Dihle, P. H. (1997). Memory, amnesia, and dissociative identity disorder. *Psychological Science*, 417–422.

Ferreira, V. S., Bock, J. K., Wilson, M. P., & Cohen, N. J. (2008). Memory for syntax despite amnesia. *Psychological Science, 19*, 940–946.

Finger, S., & Zaroub, F. (2006). Benjamin Franklin and shock-induced amnesia. *American Psychologist, 61*, 240–248.

Fisher, C. (1945). Amnesic states in war neuroses: The psychogenesis of fugues. *Psychoanalytic Quarterly, 14*, 437–468.

Fisher, C., & Joseph, E. D. (1945). Fugue with awareness of loss of personal identity. *Psychoanalytic Quarterly, 18*, 480–493.

Fisher, C. M., & Adams, R. D. (1964). Transient global amnesia. *Acta Neurologica Scandinavica. Supplementum, 40*, SUPPL–9.1–83.

Funnell, E. (1995). Objects and properties: A study of the breakdown of semantic memory. *Memory, 3(3–4)*, 497–518.

Goldenberg, G. (1995). Aphasic patients' knowledge about the visual appearance of objects. *Aphasiology, 9*, 50–56.

Graf. P., & Schacter, D. L. (1985). Implicit and explicit memory for new associations in normal and amnesic subjects. *Journal of Experimental Psychology: Learning, Memory, and Cognition, 11*, 501–518.

Graf, P., Shimamura, A. P., & Squire, L. R. (1985). Priming across modalities and priming across category levels: Extending the domain of preserved function in amnesia. *Journal of Experimental Psychology: Learning, Memory, and Cognition, 11*, 386–396.

Graf, P., Squire, L. R., & Mandler, G. (1984). The information that amnesic patients do not forget. *Journal of Experimental Psychology: Learning, Memory, and Cognition, 10*, 164–178.

Graham, K. S., Ralph, M. A. L., & Hodges, J. R. (1997). Determining the impact of autobiographical experience on "Meaning": New insights from investigating sport-related vocabulary and knowledge in two cases with semantic dementia. *Cognitive Neuropsychology*, *14*, 801–837.

Hainselin, M., Quinette, P., Desgranges, B., Martinaud, O., de La Sayette, V., Hannequin, D., Viader, F., & Eustache, F. (2012). Awareness of disease state without explicit knowledge of memory failure in transient global amnesia. *Cortex*, *48*(8), 1079–1084.

Hassabis, D., Kumaran, D., Vann, S. D., & Maguire, E. A. (2007). Patients with hippocampal amnesia cannot imagine new experiences. *Proceedings of the National Academy of Sciences*, *104*(5), 1726–1731.

Higgs, S., Williamson, A. C., Rotshtein, P., & Humphreys, G. W. (2008). Sensory-specific satiety is intact in amnesics who eat multiple meals. *Psychological Science*, *19*, 623–628.

Hirst, W., Johnson, M. K., Kim, J. K., Phelps, E. A., Risse, G., & Volpe, B. T. (1986). Recognition and recall in amnesics. *Journal of Experimental Psychology: Learning, Memory, and Cognition*, *12*, 445–451.

Hirst, W., Johnson, M. K., Phelps, E. A., & Volpe, B. T. (1988). More on recognition and recall in amnesics. *Journal of Experimental Psychology: Learning, Memory, and Cognition*, *14*, 758–762.

Hodges, J. R., Bozeat, S., Lambdon Ralph, M. A., Patterson, K., & Spatt, J. (2000). The role of conceptual knowledge in object use: Evidence from semantic dementia. *Brain*, *123*, 1913–1925.

Hodges, J. R., Patterson, K., Oxbury, S., & Funnell, E. (1992). Semantic dementia: Progressive fluent aphasia with temporal lobe atrophy. *Brain*, *115*, 1783–1806.

Hunkin, N. M. (1997). Focal retrograde amnesia: Implications for the organisation of memory. In A. J. Parkin (Ed.), *Case Studies in the Neuropsychology of Memory* (pp. 63–82). Hove, England: Psychology Press.

Huntjens, R. J. C., Postma, A., Hamaker, E. L., Woertman, L., van der Hart, O., & Peters, M. (2002). Perceptual and conceptual priming in patients with dissociative identity disorder. *Memory & Cognition*, *30*, 1033–1043.

Kapur, N. (1999). Syndromes of retrograde amnesia: A conceptual and empirical synthesis. *Psychological Bulletin*, *125*, 800–825.

Kapur, N., & Moakes, D. (1995). Living with amnesia. In R. E. Campbell & M. A. Conway (Eds.), *Broken Memories: Case Studies in Memory Impairment* (pp. 1–7). Malden, MA: Blackwell.

Kartsounis, L. D., & Shallice, T. (1996). Modality specific semantic knowledge loss for unique items. *Cortex*, *32*, 109–119.

Kessler, J., Markowitsch, H. J., Rudolf, J., & Heiss, W.-D. (2001). Continuing cognitive impairment after isolated transient global amnesia. *International Journal of Neuroscience*, *106*(3–4), 159–168.

Kihlstrom, J. F., & Schacter, D. L. (1995). Functional disorders of autobiographical memory. In A. D. Baddeley, B. A. Wilson, & F. N. Watts (Eds.), *Handbook of Memory Disorders* (pp. 337–364). New York: Wiley.

Kishiyama, M. M., Yonelinas, A. P., & Lazzara, M. M. (2004). The von Restorff effect in amnesia: The contribution of the hippocampal system to novelty-related memory enhancements. *Journal of Cognitive Neuroscience*, *16*, 15–23.

Kitchner, E. G., Hodges, J. R., & McCarthy, R. (1998). Acquisition of post-morbid vocabulary and semantic facts in the absence of episodic memory. *Brain*, *121*, 1313–1327.

Kopelman, M. D. (2002). Disorders of memory. *Brain*, *125*(10), 2152–2190.

Kopelman, M. D., Christensen, H., Puffett, A., & Stanhope, N. (1994). The great escape: A neuropsychological study of psychogenic amnesia. *Neuropsychologia*, *32*(6), 675–691.

Kopelman, M. D., Green, R. E. A., Guinan, E. M., Lewis, P. D. R., & Stanhope, N. (1994). The case of the amnesic intelligence officer. *Psychological Medicine*, *24*(04), 1037–1045.

Loftus, E. F. (1993). The reality of repressed memories. *American Psychologist*, *48*(5), 518.

Lucchelli, F., Muggia, S., & Spinnler, H. (1997). Selective proper name anomia: A case involving only contemporary celebrities. *Cognitive Neuropsychology*, *14*, 881–900.

Lynch, S., & Yarnell, P. R. (1973). Retrograde amnesia: Delayed forgetting after concussion. *American Journal of Psychology, 86*, 643–645.

Lyon, L. S. (1985). Facilitating telephone number recall in a case of psychogenic amnesia. *Journal of Behavior Therapy and Experimental Psychiatry, 16*, 147–149.

Madsen, M. C., & McGaugh, J. L. (1961). The effect of ECS on one-trial avoidance learning. *Journal of Comparative and Physiological Psychology, 54*, 522–523.

Mangiulli, I., Lanciano, T., Van Oorsouw, K., Jelicic, M., & Curci, A. (2019). Do reminders of the crime reverse the memory-undermining effect of simulating amnesia? *Memory & Cognition, 47*(7), 1375–1385.

Markowitsch, H. J. (2003). Psychogenic amnesia. *Neuroimage, 20*, S132–S138.

Markowitsch, H. J., Weber-Luxemburger, G., Ewald, K., Kessler, J., & Heiss, W.-D. (1997). Patients with heart attacks are not valid models for medial temporal lobe amnesia. A neuropsychological and FDG-PET study with consequences for memory research. *European Journal of Neurology, 4*(2), 178–184.

McCarthy, R. A., & Hodges, J. R. (1995). Trapped in time: Profound autobiographical memory loss following a thalamic stroke. In R. Campbell & R. A. Conway (Eds.), *Broken Memories: Case Studies in Memory Impairment*. Cambridge, MA: Blackwell.

McCarthy, R. A., & Warrington, E. K. (2016). Past, present, and prospects: Reflections 40 years on from the selective impairment of semantic memory (Warrington, 1975). *Quarterly Journal of Experimental Psychology, 69*(10), 1941–1968.

McGaugh, J. L. (1966). Time-dependent processes in memory storage. *Science, 153*, 1351–1358.

Milner, B., Corkin, S., & Teuber, H.-L. (1968). Further analysis of the hippocampal amnesic syndrome: 14-year follow-up study of H. M. *Neuropsychologia, 6*, 215–234.

Nemiah, J. C. (1979). Dissociative amnesia: A clinical and theoretical reconsideration. In J. F. Kihlstrom and F. J. Evans (Eds.), *Functional Disorders of Memory* (pp. 303–323). Hillsdale, NJ: Erlbaum.

O'Connor, M., Verfaellie, M., & Cermak, L. S. (1995). Clinical differentiation of amnesic subtypes. In A. D. Baddeley, B. A. Wilson, & F. N. Watts (Eds.), *Handbook of Memory Disorders* (pp. 53–80). New York: Wiley.

Piolino, P., Belliard, S., Desgranges, B., Perron, M., & Eustache, F. (2003). Autobiographical memory and autonoetic consciousness in a case of semantic dementia. *Cognitive Neuropsychology, 20*, 619–639.

Pyszora, N. M., Barker, A. F., & Kopelman, M. D. (2003). Amnesia for criminal offences: A study of life sentence prisoners. *The Journal of Forensic Psychiatry, 14*(3), 475–490.

Rajaram, S., & Coslett, H. B. (2000). Conceptual associative learning in amnesia: A case study. *Journal of Memory and Language, 43*, 291–315.

Rasmussen, K. W., & Berntsen, D. (2014). Autobiographical memory and episodic future thinking after moderate to severe traumatic brain injury. *Journal of Neuropsychology, 8*(1), 34–52.

Ribot, T. A. (1882). *Diseases of Memory: An Essay in the Positive Psychology*. London: Kegan Paul, Trench, & Co.

Riccio, D. C., Millin, P. M., & Gisquet-Verrier, P. (2003). Retrograde amnesia: Forgetting back. *Current Directions in Psychological Science, 12*, 41–44.

Roberts, C. M., Spitz, G., & Ponsford, J. L. (2015). Retrospective analysis of the recovery of orientation and memory during posttraumatic amnesia. *Neuropsychology, 29*(4), 522–529.

Romani, C., & Martin, R. (1999). A deficit in the short-term retention of lexical-semantic information: Forgetting words but remembering a story. *Journal of Experimental Psychology: General, 128*, 56–77.

Rosenbaum, R. S., Kwan, D., Floden, D., Levine, B., Stuss, D. T., & Craver, C. F. (2016). No evidence of risk-taking or impulsive behaviour in a person with episodic amnesia: Implications for the role of the hippocampus in future-regarding decision-making. *Quarterly Journal of Experimental Psychology, 69*(8), 1606–1618.

Ryan, J. D., Althoff, R. R., Whitlow, S., & Cohen, N. J. (2000). Amnesia is a deficit in relational memory. *Psychological Science, 11*, 454–460.

Schacter, D. L. (1987). Memory, amnesia, and frontal lobe dysfunction. *Psychobiology, 15*(1), 21–36.

Scoville, W. B., & Milner, B. (1957). Loss of recent memory after bilateral hippocampal lesions. *Journal of Neurology, Neurosurgery, and Psychiatry, 20*, 11–21.

Shallice, T., & Warrington, E. K. (1970). Independent functioning of verbal memory stores: A neuropsychological study. *Quarterly Journal of Experimental Psychology, 22,* 261–273.

Simons, J. S., Graham, K. S., & Hodges, J. R. (2002). Perceptual and semantic contributions to episodic memory: Evidence from semantic dementia and Alzheimer's disease. *Journal of Memory and Language, 47,* 197–213.

Sirigu, A., & Grafman, J. (1996). Selective impairments within episodic memories. *Cortex, 32,* 83–95.

Skotko, B. G., Andrews, E., & Einstein, G. (2005). Language and the medial temporal lobe: Evidence from H.M.'s spontaneous discourse. *Journal of Memory and Language, 53,* 397–415.

Snowden, J. S., Goulding, P. J., & Neary, D. (1989). Semantic dementia: A form of circumscribed cerebral atrophy. *Behavioral Neurology, 2,* 167–182.

Squire, L. R., & Cohen, N. (1979). Memory and amnesia: Resistance to disruption develops for years after learning. *Behavioral and Neural Biology, 25,* 115–125.

Squire, L. R., Slater, P. C., & Chace, P. M. (1975). Retrograde amnesia: Temporal gradient in very long term memory following electroconvulsive therapy. *Science, 187,* 77–79.

Squires, E. J., Hunkin, N. M., & Parkin, A. J. (1997). Take note: Using errorless learning to promote memory notebook training. In A. J. Parkin (Ed.), *Case Studies in the Neuropsychology of Memory* (pp. 191–203). Hove, England: Psychology Press.

Stracciari, A., Ghidoni, E., Guarino, M., Poletti, M., & Pazzaglia, P. (1994). Post-traumatic retrograde amnesia with selective impairment of autobiographical memory. *Cortex, 30,* 459–468.

Vakil, E., Grunhaus, L., Nagar, I., Ben-Chaim, E., Dolberg, O. T., Dannon, P. N., Schreiber, S. (2000). The effect of electroconvulsive therapy (ECT) on implicit memory: Skill learning and perceptual priming in patients with major depression. *Neuropsychologia, 38,* 1405–1414.

Vallar, G., & Baddeley, A. D. (1984). Fractionation of working memory: Neuropsychological evidence for a phonological short-term store. *Journal of Verbal Learning and Verbal Behavior, 23,* 151–161.

Vallar, G., & Papagno, C. (1995). Neuropsychological impairments of short-term memory. In A. D. Baddeley, B. A. Wilson, & F. N. Watts (Eds.), *Handbook of Memory Disorders* (pp. 135–165). New York: Wiley.

Warrington, E. K., & Weiskrantz, L. (1968). A study of learning and retention in amnesic patients. *Neuropsychologia, 6,* 283–291.

Warrington, E. K., & Weiskrantz, L. (1970). Amnestic syndrome: Consolidation or retrieval? *Nature, 228,* 628–630.

Wickelgren, W. A. (1968). Sparing of short-term memory in an amnesic patient: Implications for strength theory of memory. *Neuropsychologia, 6,* 235–244.

Wilson, B. A., Baddeley, A. D., & Kapur, N. (1995). Dense amnesia in a professional musician following herpes simplex virus encephalitis. *Journal of Clinical and Experimental Neuropsychology, 17*(5), 668–681.

Wilson, B. A., & Hughes, E. (1997). Coping with amnesia: The natural history of a compensatory memory system. In A. J. Parkin (Ed.), *Case Studies in the Neuropsychology of Memory* (pp. 179–190). Hove, UK: Psychology Press.

Wilson, B. A., & Wearing, D. (1995). Prisoner of consciousness: A state of just awakening following herpes simplex encephalitis. In R. Campbell & M. A. Conway (Eds.), *Broken Memories: Case Studies in Memory Impairment.* Cambridge, MA: Blackwell.

Yarnell, P. R., & Lynch, S. (1973). The "ding": Amnestic states in football trauma. *Neurology, 23*(2), 196–197.

Yasuda, K., Watanabe, O., & Ono, Y. (1997). Dissociation between semantic and autobiographical memory: A case report. *Cortex, 33,* 623–638.

CHAPTER 11

Memory for Space and Time

Space and time. For physicists, this is the fabric of reality. Psychologically, these are the primary dimensions for orienting ourselves in our world. Space and time provide a framework for the events that we experience and remember. Spatial information is where things are located and how they are oriented with respect to one another. This is important when we navigate, locate objects, estimate distances, and so on. In this chapter we look at how memory for space corresponds to physical layouts and what distorts our memory. In general, space is a relatively static dimension. We can move from one place to another and back again with ease. In contrast, temporal information is for when things happened, with respect to the present, other events in the past, and even to a standard time scale, such as a calendar. Unlike spatial location, our place in time is always, inexorably, being pushed forward. We cannot go back.

This chapter addresses memory for space (where things are) and time (when things happened). Starting with spatial memory, we cover issues relating to memory psychophysics or how memory for space corresponds to actual, measured space. This is followed by a consideration of the properties of mental maps and how they are created. Then we address memory for time, such as how temporal information is stored in and retrieved. Several theories are considered for how we remember when things happened.

MEMORY FOR SPACE

There have been many studies of spatial memory. In fact, the study of spatial memory in research with rats helped bring an end to radical behaviorist views in psychology (Tolman, 1948). One appeal of spatial knowledge is that we can explicitly measure distances, areas, curvatures, and so on, and then directly compare these measurements to memory of these spatial properties.

Neurologically we can see the specialization and complexity of spatial memory. For example, single cell recordings of the hippocampus and related areas have shown that these areas are important for knowing spatial locations (Burgess, 2002; Kunz et al. 2019; Muller et al., 1987; Shapiro et al., 1997). This includes specialized neurons such as place cells (O'Keefe, & Dostrovsky, 1971), grid cells (Hafting et al., 2005), and boundary cells (Lever et al., 2009), as described in Chapter 2. Moreover, fMRI studies with humans show evidence of a region, the parahippocampal place area (BA 36), that is critical for understanding the spatial structure (Epstein & Kanwisher, 1998) and that disrupts spatial learning if damaged (Epstein et al., 2001).

Moreover, spatial memory is tied up in many of phenomena that affect memory more generally. For example, people better remember the spatial location of pictures when they are emotionally arousing (Mather & Nesmith, 2008). This part of the chapter discusses spatial memory by covering memory psychophysics, memory for information learned from maps, and how our interaction with the world influences spatial memory.

Memory Psychophysics

How well do our memories for space correspond to actual space? The part of psychology that deals with how our experience of the world corresponds to physical properties is **psychophysics**. Many psychophysicists study issues of sensation and perception and have established some "laws" of psychophysical relations. One is **Steven's Law** of psychological magnitude (Stevens & Galantner, 1957). For this law, the relation between actual and perceived magnitudes is a power function that is captured by the formula $\Psi = k\Phi^n$. Here, Ψ corresponds to psychological magnitude. This is related to the actual physical magnitude, Φ, raised to a power, n, and modified by a constant, k.

These same principles can be used to study memory (Algom, 1992). Memory psychophysics has been applied to a number of domains, including memory for size, area, loudness, and labor pains (Algom & Lubel, 1994; Algom et al., 1985; Chew & Richardson, 1980; Kerst & Howard, 1978, 1983; Moyer et al., 1977). Here, we consider memory psychophysics for spatial properties, such as distance and area.

The relation between actual and perceived spatial distance is good. The exponent in Steven's Law is close to 1, which means that our perceptual experience is a near perfect. As for our memory of space, such as distance, the relation is still good, but there are distortions (Wiest & Bell, 1985). This distortion is less when the space was originally viewed all at once compared to when it was inferred from memory from separate experiences (e.g., estimating distances between buildings that are separated by others, so the actual distance cannot be viewed directly). Memory is also compressed when experienced in a virtual environment (e.g., Ziemer et al., 2009). However, this can be mitigated if people can navigate through the virtual space (Waller & Richardson, 2008).

One theory of memory psychophysics of space is of the fuzzy trace variety. This is **Category Adjustment Theory** (Huttenlocher et al., 1991). For this view, performance is a combination of both fine- and coarse-grained memories (Sampaio & Wang, 2017). Objects in space are located within regions that serve as categories or schemas. Thus, people remember the object itself as well as the category to which it belongs. For example, if you are trying to remember where a certain city is located in the country, you may have a fine-grained memory of its actual location on a map, as well as a coarse-grained categorical memory of which state it is in. Memory for space is always a combination of these two influences.

These two sources of spatial knowledge vary in their relative contribution at any given occasion. The more influence that fine-grained memories have during retrieval, the weaker the influence of the coarse-grained memories (Sampaio & Wang, 2008) and vice versa (Kemp, 1988). When a space has clear and obvious boundaries, the coarse-grained categorical information can have an immediate influence; however, when the regions are more subtle, such as a college campus, the influence of such regions on spatial memory can be delayed until knowledge and familiarity builds up (Uttal et al., 2010).

TRY IT OUT

This Try it Out section explores memory for distances using psychophysics. For this task, first set up 12–36 displays of objects at different distances (although you can use area, angles, or something else if you want). One way to do this is to have pairs of small pictures of objects on pieces of paper. Another is to have a variety of objects at different distances from your participants.

Have people estimate those distances. If you have objects on pieces of paper, have people estimate the distances between them in either inches or centimeters. If you use real objects, have people estimate the distances from where they are standing, in feet or meters, to the objects. It does not matter how accurate people are in terms of what they think a foot or a meter is, so long as they are consistent with themselves.

You should have 12 or more participants. Collect this data under two conditions. In one have the people estimate the distances from *perception*—that is, as they are looking at the distance. In the other condition have people estimate the distances from *memory*—that is, have them look at the objects, then either remove the objects or have them turn away, and then have them estimate the distance. The objects for the perception and memory conditions should be different.

After you have collected the data, plot the estimates against the actual distances. For each person, derive an estimate of the slope for the function that best fits those points for each condition. What you should find is that the slope of the function will be smaller in the memory condition than the perception condition, illustrating some compression in spatial memory.

Stop and Review

Memory for space is good. This assessment can be done using psychophysical principles, such as Stevens' Law. There does appear to be some compression of spatial distances in memory. Overall, consistent with the category-adjustment model, spatial memory is a combination of fine-grained, metric memories along with coarse-grained, categorical memories.

Mental Maps

Of course, memory for space is more complex than just remembering distances. You create complex mental representations to guide your travels around the house, through town, and across the country. This section looks at how mental maps are represented and used in memory. First, we consider **spatial theories** that assume that mental maps are structured using some sort of spatial information. This quality of spatial theories makes them straightforward to understand. The simplest version is a mental map that corresponds directly to the space it represents. This is a **metric view**. However, there have been few serious metric theories because mental maps are almost always distorted in some way.

A major influence on mental maps is areas or regions. Space is not uniform. The world is divided into continents, continents are (often) divided into countries, countries are divided into states or provinces, and so on. There are many ways that we chop up space. Locations are often assigned to superordinate locations or regions. The **hierarchical view** (Stevens & Coupe, 1978) is that mental maps are organized the same way. Figure 11.1 gives an example of a hierarchical representation of cities in Colorado and Ohio. This spatial hierarchy reflects the organization of smaller areas into larger ones and can lead people to make errors. When people estimate the direction between two locations, these estimates may be in error if the actual direction differs from the relation between the hierarchical regions. An example is shown in Figure 11.2. People often mistakenly report that San Diego, CA, is west of Reno, NV, because California is generally west of Nevada. However, Reno is actually farther west than San Diego. Thus, the direction of the superordinate regions influences spatial memory. This is not only found for very large spatial structures such as cities and states, but also for smaller environments such as neighborhoods, with people making more directional errors across neighborhoods than within (Han & Becker, 2014).

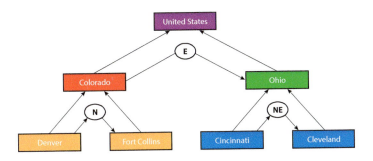

FIGURE 11.1 *Hierarchical Representation of Space*

Source: adapted from Stevens, A., & Coupe, P. (1978). Distortions in judged spatial relations. *Cognitive Psychology, 10*, 422–437

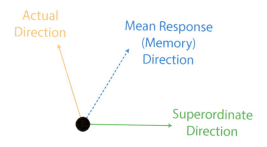

San Diego (California)
to
Reno (Nevada)

FIGURE 11.2 *Distortion of Direction Judgments as Influenced by Superordinate Regions*

Source: created from data reported in: Stevens, A., & Coupe, P. (1978). Distortions in judged spatial relations. *Cognitive Psychology, 10,* 422–437

A mental map based strictly on spatial regions would be categorical. That is, all the locations within a region could be more or less the same, but this is not the case. A theory of mental maps that uses a combination of metric and region information is a **partially hierarchical view** (McNamara, 1986). Some good evidence for this comes from spatial priming studies in which people first memorize a map that was divided into regions. Within each region were a set of locations, such as cities or objects (see Figure 11.3). After memorization, people were given a primed recognition test. That is, a series of location names were given, and the task was to indicate whether those names were on the map. Priming was assessed using response times to the target item as a function of the spatial proximity of the prime item. In general, mental map locations prime one another (McNamara, 1986). An example of such priming is shown in Figure 11.4. There is more priming (people are faster) for close locations (e.g., Fairview and Avon in Figure 11.3) than for far locations (e.g., Casper and Needles). Moreover, regions mediate the amount of priming. For example, keeping Euclidean distance the same, there is less priming across regions (e.g., Bordmann and Stapleton) than within a region (e.g., Fairview and Avon).

As a real-world example, some Germans overestimate distances between cities in the former East and West Germany, even though the country is now united (Carbon & Leder, 2005). Moreover, the more negative their opinion of reunification (i.e., the more salient the East–West differences were in their minds), the greater the overestimation.[1] Thus, this partially hierarchical influence is seen even when the region divisions are subjective rather than objective (McNamara et al., 1989). This increased perceived distance is also observed in virtual environments when the space is perpetually experienced as either a single large space or divided into regions

1 See Maddox et al. (2008) for a related account involving social relations.

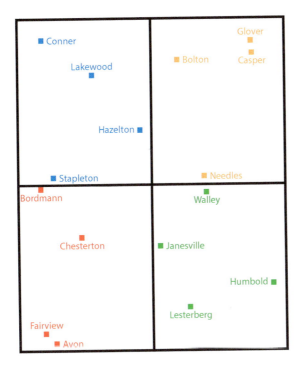

FIGURE 11.3 *Map Used in Spatial Priming Studies*

Source: adapted from McNamara, T. P. (1986). Mental representations of spatial relations. *Cognitive Psychology*, *18*, 87–121

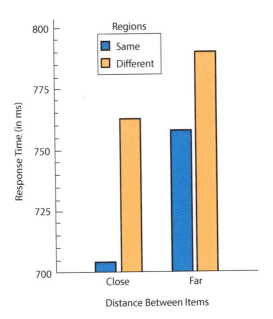

FIGURE 11.4 *Response Times to Probes as a Function of Route Distance*

Source: created from data reported in McNamara, T. P. (1986). Mental representations of spatial relations. *Cognitive Psychology*, *18*, 87–121

by walls coming partially out from the sides (forming a wide doorway from one "region" to the next). The more perceived boundaries there were between a person and a target location, the greater the reported distance (Sturz & Bodily, 2016).

The influence of spatial borders applies not only to spatial memory but also to thinking and decision making about spaces. In a study by Mishra and Mishra (2010), students at the University of Utah were asked to make decisions about which of two locations they would prefer to purchase a vacation home. This could be either in the state of Oregon or the state of Washington. Some students were told that an earthquake had occurred 200 miles from both potential vacation sites. For half of the students, the earthquake was centered in Oregon, and for the others it was centered in Washington. What was found was that students showed a preference for the vacation home in the state that did not have the earthquake centered in it, even though the distance to the earthquake center was the same, and earthquakes do not care about political borders.

Also consistent with a partially hierarchical view is knowledge of geographical position of cities (Friedman & Brown, 2000), which is often clustered based on political/climatic regions. As shown in Figure 11.5, when University of Alberta students were asked to estimate the latitude of North American cities, four categories emerged. These were Canada, the northern United States, the southern United States, and Mexico (with Miami floating in between the United States and Mexico). This occurs even when people are given supporting information, such as map outline (Friedman, 2009). A similar result was observed for students from Southwest Texas State University (Friedman et al., 2002) and Universidad Autónoma de Tamaulipas in Mexico (Friedman et al., 2005). Thus, where people live is less important to how they mentally divide up the world. Figure 11.5 also shows a similar categorical grouping for European cities. Such biases are not observed if maps of imaginary places are used (Newcombe & Chiang, 2007).

Other spatial characteristics can influence mental maps. One is the number of intervening locations on a **route** between two locations. The more locations on a route, the longer the estimated distance (Thorndyke, 1981). This increased crowding causes that part of the mental map to "expand" to accommodate all the places. In one study people memorized a map like the one in Figure 11.6. In this map there are varying numbers of intervening locations between two cities. When memory was tested by having people estimate the distances between pairs of cities, the more intervening cities there were, the greater the distance estimates (see Figure 11.7).

Route distance can also influence memory (McNamara et al., 1984). Given the same Euclidean distance, priming is reduced if there is a long circuitous route between two locations compared to if there is a short and direct one. In one study, students memorized maps like the one in Figure 11.8. The primed recognition test that followed had conditions in which map locations were close in both Euclidean and route distance (e.g., Emmet and Davis), far in both Euclidean and route distance (e.g., Anderson and Berthold), or close in Euclidean distance but far in route distance (e.g., Mantee and Foster). As can be seen in Figure 11.9, if the two locations were far along the route, even if they were spatially close, they were retrieved as if they were spatially far apart.

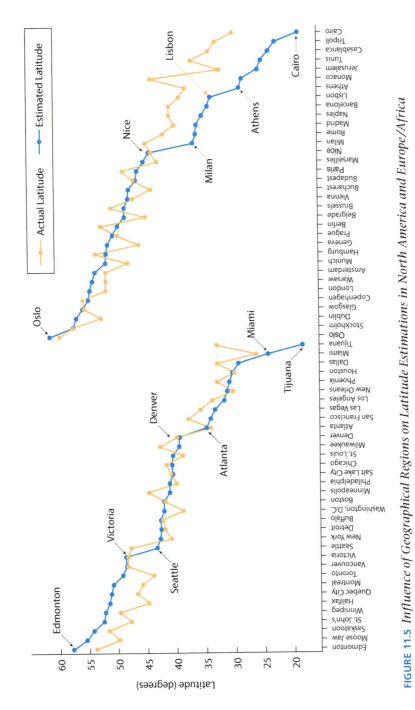

FIGURE 11.5 *Influence of Geographical Regions on Latitude Estimations in North America and Europe/Africa*

Source: Friedman, A., & Brown, N. R. (2000). Reasoning about geography. *Journal of Experimental Psychology: General, 129*, 193–219.

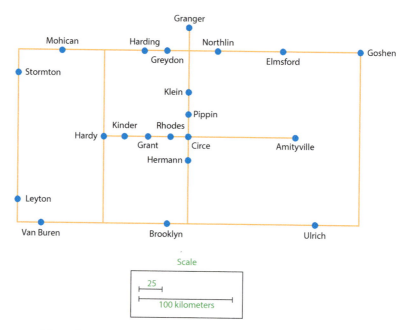

FIGURE 11.6 *Map of Fictitious Area that Varies the Number of Intervening Locations between Cities but Keeps the Distance Relatively Constant*

Source: adapted from Thorndyke, P. W. (1981). Distance estimation from cognitive maps. *Cognitive Psychology, 13,* 526–550

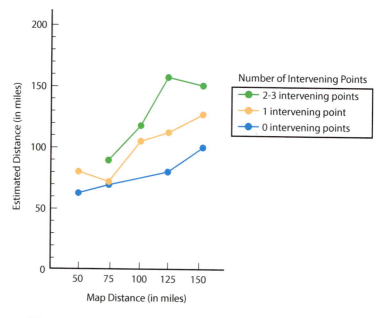

FIGURE 11.7 *Distance Estimate Results as a Function of the Number of Intervening Cities*

Source: adapted from Thorndyke, P. W. (1981). Distance estimation from cognitive maps. *Cognitive Psychology, 13,* 526–550

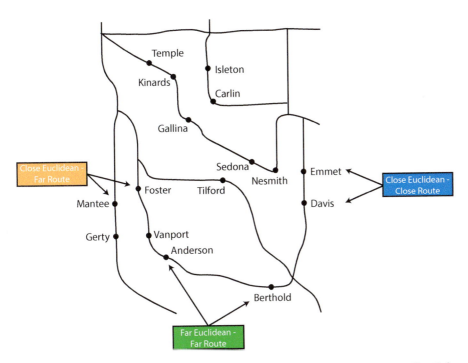

FIGURE 11.8 *Map Used to Study the Effects of Spatial and Route Distance on Spatial Memory*

Source: McNamara, T. P., Ratcliff, R., & McKoon, G. (1984). The mental representation of knowledge acquired from maps. *Journal of Experimental Psychology: Learning, Memory, and Cognition, 10,* 723–732.

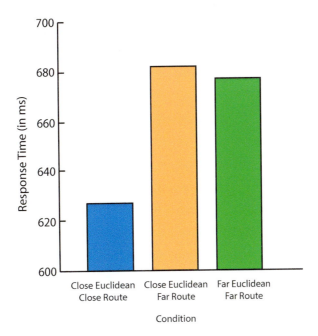

FIGURE 11.9 *Spatial Priming as Affected by Both Euclidean and Route Distance*

Source: created from data reported in McNamara, T. P., Ratcliff, R., & McKoon, G. (1984). The mental representation of knowledge acquired from maps. *Journal of Experimental Psychology: Learning, Memory, and Cognition, 10,* 723–732.

Mental maps are also affected by the temporal order or sequence in which map items are learned. For **temporal theories**, places can be either close or far in temporal proximity in much the same way that they can be close or far in spatial proximity. Typically, spatial and temporal proximity are confounded during learning. Locations that are close in space are also experienced close in time. However, these two dimensions can be dissociated. For example, imagine you learn the map in Figure 11.10 in the order indicated by the arrows (beginning with Gallina). Although you can derive spatial qualities (such as direction and distance) from your mental map, evidence from priming measures suggests that temporal, and not spatial, structure is the primary basis for the mental map (Clayton & Habibi, 1991; Curiel & Radvansky, 1998).

This influence of temporal order for mental maps varies. **Hybrid theories** assume a contribution of both spatial and temporal information. For example, in a study by Curiel and Radvansky (1998), during memorization people either named indicated locations (focusing on identity information) or pointed to named locations (focusing on spatial information). As shown in Table 11.1, there was more temporal priming when people named the location, but more spatial priming when they pointed to the location. Thus, how people learn maps can have a dramatic influence. Spatial and temporal information can work together to influence mental map structure (McNamara et al., 1992). Learning map locations that are close together in both time and space provides the greatest benefit to memory.

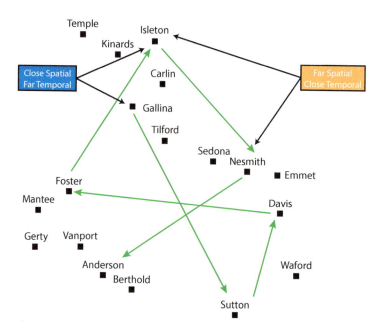

FIGURE 11.10 *Fictitious Map Illustrating the Deconfounding of Spatial and Temporal Proximity with a Partial Temporal Order Indicated by the Arrows*

Source: adapted from Clayton, K., & Habibi, A. (1991). Contributions of temporal contiguity to the spatial priming effect. *Journal of Experimental Psychology: Learning, Memory, & Cognition, 17,* 263–271

TABLE 11.1 *Differences in Spatial and Temporal Priming: Whether People Name Map Locations During Learning in Response to Location Cues or Point to Map Locations in Response to Name Cues*

Condition	Naming	Pointing
Spatial		
Close	690	681
Far	714	730
Priming	24	49
Temporal		
Close	669	721
Far	709	718
Priming	40	−3

Source: Curiel, J. M., & Radvansky, G. A. (1998). Mental organization of maps. *Journal of Experimental Psychology: Learning, Memory, and Cognition, 24*(1), 202–214

Improve Your Memory

Your memory for a space is not like a mental image that can be treated like you are viewing a picture. Instead, it is divided into regions, and these regions affect your use of your mental maps. When learning a new space, it is best not to strive against this bias. This is just how our memories work. To learn a space faster, so that you can use it and navigate in it more effectively, look for a way of dividing a large space into smaller regions. Then, try to learn the locations of individual things within each region. This is another example of chunking in memory.

Mental maps are also influenced by **semantic relationships**. The degree to which different locations are meaningfully similar can accentuate priming, particularly if they are already near one another (McNamara & LeSueur, 1989). For example, people's memory of their college campus shows that their mental maps are also semantically influenced. In priming studies, buildings prime each other more if they serve the same function (i.e., dorms, administration buildings, sports facilities, etc.).

Knowledge can also have spatial influences. As with memory psychophysics, some spatial remembering is a mixture of fine- and coarse-grained information. When given maps in the real world, there may be parts that do not quite line up. For example, on a city map, the streets may not be at 90-degree angles to one another, or the orientation of a town may not square with the standard compass points. Tversky (1981) has shown that when these deviations are present, memories are distorted to smooth out the irregularities. For example, streets are remembered as intersecting at something more closely approximating 90 degrees. As an example of another lining-up distortion, many North Americans assume that South America is more directly south of North America than it is. It is actually more to the east. The western shore of South America is around the same longitude as the eastern shore of North America. People's memories reflect a combination of fine-grained information on the map and more coarse-grained, schematic knowledge about general orientations, causing people to make predictable errors.

The structure of mental maps influences more than just memory for space. It can also influence other types of thinking. Imagine if you memorized a map, such as the map of the research center in Figure 11.11, and then read stories about events

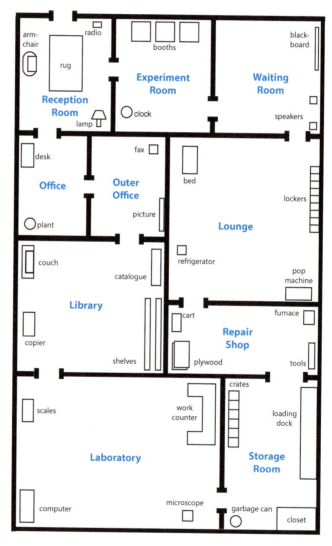

FIGURE 11.11 *Map of the Research Center*

Source: Rinck, M., Hähnel, A., & Becker, G. (2001). Using temporal information to construct, update, and retrieve situation models of narratives. *Journal of Experimental Psychology: Learning, Memory, and Cognition, 27*, 67–80.

that occurred in that area (Morrow et al., 1987). While reading, you would use your mental maps, and these would influence comprehension. If a story character is described as thinking about an object in the building, the time it takes to read that sentence varies as a function of the distance between the character's current location and the object being thought about (Rinck & Bower, 1995). For example, if the story character is in the Repair Shop it will be easier to think of the pop machine (which is only one room away) than the clock, which is three rooms away. In general, the greater the distance, the longer it takes to read. This is the **spatial gradient of availability**. The mental map captures spatial characteristics, and this spills over into comprehension.

Spatial Frameworks

We spend our time in various spaces and regions that are defined in particular ways—a kitchen, a mall, a highway, and so on. These spatial regions are **spatial frameworks**, and how we interact with them affects our memories for them.

When we learn about a location, especially a large one that we cannot see all at once, such as a mall or a town, we may derive our understanding from a map. We study the physical map to create our mental map. One consequence of this is that the orientation of the physical map becomes ingrained into our mental map. Thus, when we need to estimate directions when facing a direction other than the original map orientation, we are slower to respond and may make mistakes (Evans & Pezdek, 1980; He et al., 2018; Waller et al., 2002).[2] It is as if the mental map is viewed as a mental image. The greater the deviation from the orientation in which the map was learned, the more likely that there will be a direction error. An example of this would be viewing a map of an unfamiliar mall that you are in and the orientation of the map does not match the orientation that you are facing when you look at it. If you do not do the requisite mental rotation, then you might head off in the wrong direction.

For example, in Figure 11.12 people who have their mental maps aligned with the current orientation (A) are less likely to make errors than people who have their mental maps misaligned (B). This **orientation effect** is seen in Figure 11.13. This extends to memory for observed spatial layouts (not just maps) that are either static or dynamic (like a soccer game) (Garsoffky et al., 2002). It can also occur when a space is viewed from multiple **perspectives**. Each perspective is stored as an orientation-specific viewpoint (McNamara et al., 2003). However, it is not observed when people actively participate in the situation but only when it is viewed passively, such as by watching a film (Waller et al., 2004).

In general, not surprisingly, spatial memory is better when people actively experience a space (move around in it) rather than passively experience it (watch a video or read a map) (Chrastil & Warren, 2013). If people learn an area, such as a college campus, through experience rather than a map, there is no single orientation (Evans & Pezdek, 1980). Natural exploration exposes you to a wide variety of perspectives, and the experience of different perspectives by actually moving through space is critically important (Holmes et al., 2018). Thus, the

---

2 See Avraamides et al. (2013) for an extension of this to narrative memory.

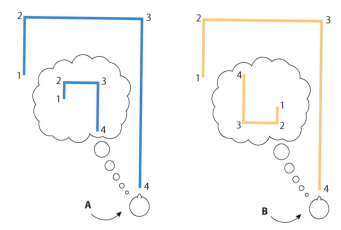

FIGURE 11.12 *Direction Judgment When the Memorized Map Is Aligned or Misaligned with the Current Orientation*

Source: Levine, M., Jankovic, I. N., & Palij, M. (1982). Principles of spatial problem solving. *Journal of Experimental Psychology: General, 111*, 157–175

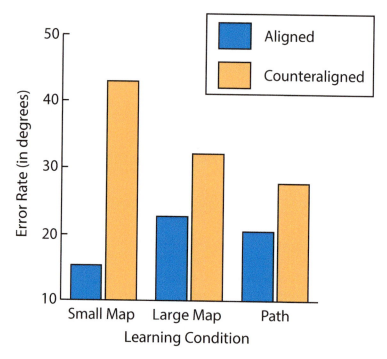

FIGURE 11.13 *Direction Judgment Errors When a Memorized Space Is Aligned or Misaligned with the Current Orientation. This Data Reflects Spaces Memorized Using Small and Large Maps, as Well as by Travelling a Path in an Actual Space*

Source: created from data reported in Levine, M., Jankovic, I. N., & Palij, M. (1982). Principles of spatial problem solving. *Journal of Experimental Psychology: General, 111*, 157–175

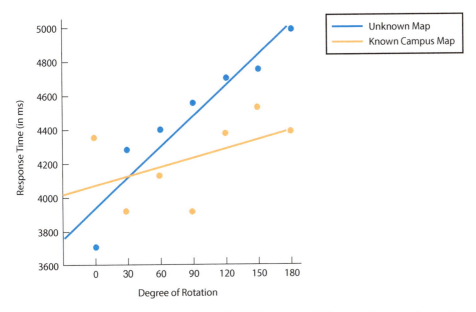

FIGURE 11.14 *Mental Rotation Effects for Unknown and Known Campus Layouts. Mental Rotation Effects Only Observed for the Unknown (Map) Campus Condition*

Source: *created from data reported in* Evans, G. W., & Pezdek, K. (1980). Cognitive mapping: Knowledge of real-world distance and location information. *Journal of Experimental Psychology: Human Learning and Memory, 6,* 13–24.

mental map does not have a preferred viewing orientation. Figure 11.14 shows data from a study in which students made direction judgments for their own campus or for a map of an unfamiliar campus. An orientation effect was only observed for the unfamiliar campus.

Perspective can have other influences. People often overestimate distances to locations near their current location and underestimate those far away. This is shown in a study by Holyoak and Mah (1982). In this study, students at the University of Michigan estimated the relative east–west locations of cities in the United States. Importantly, they made these judgments by imagining they were standing on the West Coast looking eastward, from the East Coast looking westward, or to simply make estimates (keep in mind that they were in Ann Arbor, Michigan). The results, shown in Figure 11.15, reveal that estimates were biased by the perspective taken. People who imagined themselves on the Pacific Coast reported the western cities being farther apart and the eastern cities being closer together, whereas the opposite was true for those who imagined they were standing on the Atlantic Coast. People who were simply asked to estimate locations imposed a Midwesterner's bias by spreading out the distance among cities in the middle of the United States.

Mental maps are often created from experience with an environment or from reading a map. However, sometimes we create mental maps from language—for

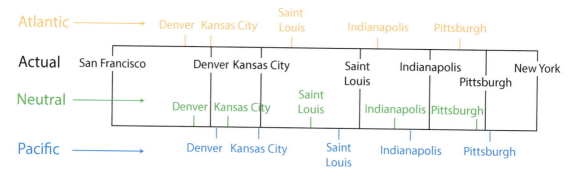

FIGURE 11.15 *Effects of Relative City Locating Depending on the Point of View Taken at Retrieval. The cities tested here were San Francisco, Salt Lake, Denver, Kansas City, Indianapolis, Pittsburgh, and New York*

Source: adapted from Holyoak, K. J., & Mah, W. A. (1982). Cognitive reference points in judgments of symbolic magnitude. *Cognitive Psychology, 14*, 328–352.

example, giving oral directions (e.g., "Go east on Cleveland until you get to Swanson. Turn north. Then turn right at the third stop sign."). Often people navigate with this type of information. How the information is given may not have a major effect on the mental maps in memory (Taylor & Tversky, 1992), although performance tends to be better when people learn from actual maps (Fields & Shelton, 2006).

Landmarks, Route, and Survey Perspectives

Spatial memory plays a vital role in navigation. How do we get from one place to the next? In this section we consider three types of information that can influence navigation. These are landmarks, route, and survey knowledge.

The first type of information that can influence spatial memory and navigation is **landmarks**, which are salient locations in an environment. These can include prominent buildings, bridges, statues, natural features like lakes, and so on. Landmarks are important to spatial memory and mental maps because memories for space are distorted by them. Landmarks help define spatial regions. They may be more effective at helping us develop mental maps than other characteristics, such as boundaries (Zhou & Mou, 2016).

People distort their memory for nonlandmark locations toward the landmarks (Sadalla et al., 1980). For example, a prominent building on a college campus, such as a library, may serve as a landmark and define a region of campus (i.e., what buildings are near it). Conversely, other buildings, such as a dorm, would not be landmarks, and so do not define a region of campus. This influence is mediated by how landmarks are thought about (Bugmann et al., 2007), such as whether people think about how important the landmarks are (larger influences) or how often they are visited (smaller influence). For instance, a tower on a college campus may serve as a notable landmark, but hardly anyone ever actually goes up in it. Landmark influences are observed even when spatial memories are learned verbally, as through a narrative (Ferguson & Hegarty, 1994).

The influence of landmarks on mental maps can be explained using Category Adjustment Theory (Newcombe et al., 1999), which we saw in the section on memory psychophysics. For this theory, people store information about landmarks as categorical information as well as fine-grained information about the locations themselves. Memory then reflects a combination of these, which often results in nonlandmark locations being mentally shifted closer to the landmarks.

A second influence of mental maps is a **route perspective**, which is the view people have when they navigate an environment. In a mental map, route information contains knowledge about which direction to turn (e.g., left or right), how long to travel along a given path, the presence of landmarks, and so on. It typically does not contain environmentally based cues, such as which direction is north, although it can if it is particularly salient (e.g., in the direction of the mountains). In general, route-based processing in spatial memory is supported more by areas in the parietal lobe and the caudate nucleus of the basal ganglia (Burgess, 2002; 2006).

When choosing a route from one place to the next, we can be influenced by several things. When we are traveling to a single destination, there is a bias to select routes that place smaller demands on memory, such as having fewer turns (Bailenson et al., 2000), deviating less from a straight-line (Hochmair & Karlsson, 2005), involving right turns (Scharine & McBeath, 2002), and getting us to the border of the current region quickest (Hochmair et al., 2008). When choosing a route with multiple destinations, we show evidence of the hierarchical structure, preferring routes that either start from outer to inner locations (MacGregor & Ormerod, 1996), that go from one regional cluster to the next (Graham et al., 2000), or that are more in the direction of a final destination (Fu et al., 2015).

The alternative to a route perspective is a **survey perspective**, in which the spatial layout is presented as if it were viewed from high overhead, such as from a helicopter. This is the perspective we have when viewing a map. Compared to route-based knowledge, survey-based knowledge processing is supported more by processing in the hippocampus (Burgess, 2006).

If people verify pictures of the area (walking perspectives or overhead views), memory is better for the perspective in which the information was originally learned (Shelton & McNamara, 2004). Overall, people who are better at remembering orientations, as with the spatial span task (see Chapter 5), do better with route learning, whereas people who are better at perspective tasks, such as mental rotation (also see Chapter 5), do better at survey learning (Fields & Shelton, 2006). This suggests that how information represented in a mental map is influenced by how that information was learned in the first place.

The different types of information that are available in a mental map not only contribute in different ways to spatial thinking and memory but also have different forgetting rates (Ishikawa, 2013). Specifically, survey knowledge (such as route choice, direction judgment, and configuration memory) appears to be retained well, whereas landmark and topological (e.g., what is uphill and downhill) knowledge are forgotten relatively quickly.

People vary in the degree to which they can use mental maps and perspectives (e.g., Rossano et al., 1995). Figure 11.16 divides people into two categories. One is relatively unaffected by how much their mental maps are rotated, whereas the other is susceptible to error (e.g., some people need to rotate a road map to their current driving orientation). People who are better at mental rotation (see Chapter 5) are better at processing survey view information (such as that acquired from maps). Maps sometimes require people to mentally rotate what was acquired from them to match the current directional heading. People who spend more time thinking spatially, such as architecture majors or geologists, do better than others, overall (Campos & Campos-Juanatey, 2019; Holden et al., 2016).

It is clear that there are individual differences in how we use spatial information to create mental maps. Weisberg and Newcombe (2018) identified three types of people. The most efficient and flexible people are *integrators*. They can deftly create, store, and integrate mental map information from their navigation experiences. In the middle are *nonintegrators*. They form mental maps from navigation experiences but have difficulty reconciling multiple experiences. Finally, there are *imprecise navigators*, who have difficulty forming mental maps from their navigation experiences.

These people differ in several ways. For example, integrators do better with mental rotation than nonintegrators, who do better than imprecise navigators. Moreover, integrators and nonintegrators tend to score higher than imprecise navigators on working memory tests. Note that the groups do not differ in general intelligence. Finally, integrators tend to use both survey- and route-based navigation, whereas nonintegrators use route-based navigation, and imprecise navigators struggle in general.

Stop and Review

People create memories of space called mental maps. These mental maps are not metric representations but are influenced and distorted by a range of factors. They are partially hierarchal due to the influence of map regions. They are also influenced by routes, landmarks, semantic relations, and how maps were originally learned. Our use of mental maps is often influenced by and oriented around spatial frameworks, which may reflect the perspective taken during encoding or retrieval. These perspective effects can show a preferred orientation of the mental map, especially for areas that are less familiar. Neurophysiological evidence supports the idea that there are multiple types of knowledge that come together in the creation and use of mental maps.

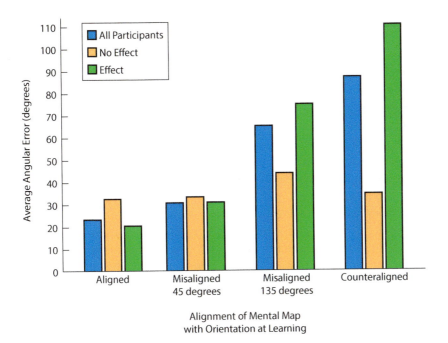

FIGURE 11.16 *Performance of Good and Poorly Misaligned Map Populations*

Source: adapted from Rossano, M. J., Warren, D. H., & Kenan, A. (1995). Orientation specificity: How general is it? *American Journal of Psychology, 108,* 359–380

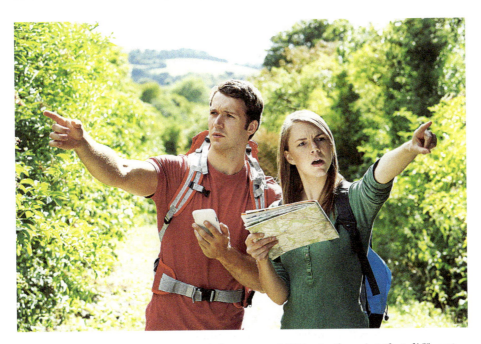

PHOTO 11.1 *People vary in their spatial memory abilities to the point that different people can think that a specific location is in completely different directions*

Source: SpeedKingz/Shutterstock.com

MEMORY FOR TIME

The other physical property we deal with here is time. How do people remember *when* things happened? Like space, memory for time is not perfectly related to the actual flow of time. Instead, there are systematic distortions that vary with respect to the type of temporal information people are trying to remember. There are three ways that people use memory for time (Friedman, 1993). The first is **temporal distance**, which is how long ago in the past an event occurred. The second is **temporal location**, which is knowledge of when an event took place, such as knowing a date. Finally, there is **relative time**, which is knowledge of the relative order of two or more events, such as knowing which came first.

Friedman uses the analogy of an archeologist to explain these three aspects of temporal memory. Temporal distance is like radiocarbon dating used to determine the age of an artifact. Temporal location is like looking at an artifact's characteristics to determine from what time it belongs, perhaps by comparing it to similar artifacts. Finally, relative time is used to place an artifact before or after others, perhaps based on the primitiveness or sophistication of one artifact relative to the others.

Phenomena

Using these three ways of thinking about time, there are a number of phenomena that need to be explained. The first phenomenon is the **memory age effect**. People have difficulty placing events in time. It is not unusual to misremember events as having occurred several years before or after when they actually happened. This distortion of temporal memories, like most memories, is more likely to happen with older memories. That is, the further back in time an event was, the more likely it is that a mistake will be made in remembering when it happened.

Forgetting of information in older memories is not that surprising. That said, as with other memories, there are **serial position curves** in the accuracy with which temporal information is retrieved (Toglia & Kimble, 1976). There is a **primacy effect** with better memory for the time of the first event of a certain type. For example, it is usually easy to remember when you got your first speeding ticket, but harder to remember when subsequent tickets were earned. There is also a **recency effect**, with superior memory for the time of more recent events.

The ability to locate events in time improves as memory for content gets better. An illustration of this **accuracy effect** is a study in which people heard either the melodies or titles of songs that were popular from 2 to 56 years before. Although people could locate songs in time better than chance when they did not consciously remember them (25% accuracy), temporal memory was better if either the melody or the title was recognized (38% accuracy), and was best if they could also remember the lyrics (60% accuracy) (Bartlett & Snelus, 1980). Essentially, the more information that was remembered, the more accurately people knew when the song was popular.

Another temporal memory phenomenon is the **scale effect**, which reflects the fact that memory for when an event occurred may be accurate at one scale of time but distorted at another. For example, people may correctly remember that an event occurred on a Monday but misremember the week it occurred. The scale effect is described in detail in the Study In Depth box.

Memories for when events occurred can also be distorted by a process known as **forward telescoping**. This occurs when an event is placed more recently than when it actually occurred (Bradburn et al., 1987; Thompson et al., 1988). For example, you might think something happened two years ago when it actually happened three years ago. In general, the easier it is to remember or think about an event the more recent it seems (Mrkva et al., 2018).

A related phenomenon is **backward telescoping**. This is when recent events are placed further back in time than they actually occurred. Backward telescoping is largely confined to recent memories (Rubin & Baddeley, 1989). That is, very recent events can seem like they occurred longer ago than they actually did. For example, in the evening, it may seem that the morning's events did not even happen that day.

Telescoping effects reflect uncertainty in memory for time and may be a form of regression to the mean (Rubin & Baddeley, 1989). Forward and backward telescoping can be assessed using memory psychophysics—that is, by looking at which component of the memory processes is affected. Consistent with the presence of both types of telescoping, psychophysical functions using Stevens's Law show slopes that are less than 1 and y-intercepts that are greater than 0 (Ferguson

---

STUDY IN DEPTH

This section describes a study by Thompson et al. (1993) that explored the scale effect in memory for time. This is an interesting study because it uses a diary method, which is uncommon in most research on memory. In this study 33 students from Kansas State University and 30 students from Ohio State University were recruited. The task was for students to first record in diaries the events that they experienced during a semester at college. Each day they recorded one unique experience for that day (so, buying a new sweater at the bookstore would count, but buying a pop out of a machine would not), they could not be too embarrassing (after all, they had to give their diaries to the experimenters), and they had to have short, succinct descriptions. At the end of each week, the students handed in a weekly diary.

At the end of the term the researchers then tested students' memories for the events of that semester. They read aloud individual events from the student's own diaries. The student was to provide the date for when the event happened. To help the students, they were given a blank calendar (with no holidays or other such markers) of the months covered by the term.

What the researchers then did was plot the dates provided in terms of the deviations between the date that the student provided from memory and the actual date. This data,

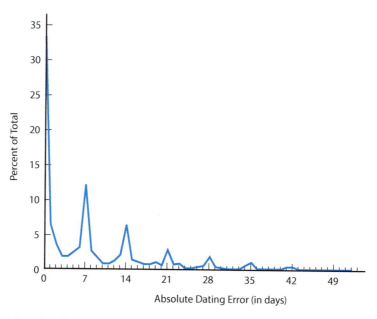

FIGURE 11.17 *Results Showing a Scale Effect in Temporal Estimation*

Source: Thompson, C. P., Skowronski, J. J., & Betz, A. L. (1993). The use of partial temporal information in dating personal events. *Memory & Cognition, 21*(3), 352–360

and the scale effect that it reveals, is shown in Figure 11.17. Notice that there are peaks at regular intervals (every seven days). Thus, as memory for the time of an event became distorted in terms of what week it occurred, there was some memory for the correct day. For example, a student might remember that an event occurred on a Thursday but be wrong about which week.

& Martin, 1983). This means that there is a shift in memory for temporal events away from the extremes and more toward an average amount of time. Looking at memory for events, both in the news and in personal events, for events less than 100 days ago, memory is quite accurate. However, for events between 100 and 1,000 days ago, there is backwards telescoping, whereas for events older than 1,000 days, there is forward telescoping, with older events showing more distortion (Janssen et al., 2006).

Memory is good for the **order information** of a sequence of events. That is, which event came first, second, and so on. Consequently, people can locate events in time by considering event order. Anderson and Conway (1993) found that people better recalled a sequence of life events if they were recalled in a forward order, although a backward order was efficient as well. Recall attempts based on the relative importance of details of an event were difficult. Whitten and Leonard (1981) found that students recall their precollege teachers best when they try to

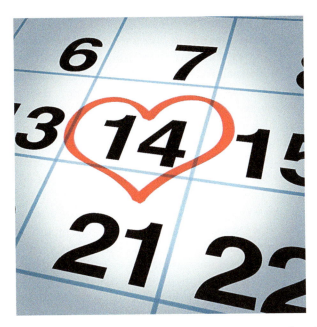

PHOTO 11.2 *We find it hard to locate events of our lives in time, unless there is some well-known date associated with the event, such as a holiday like Valentine's Day. Even then, we might get the day right, but the year wrong*

Source: Lightspring/Shutterstock.com

remember them in a backward order, worse in a forward order, and worst of all in a random order. Thus, in some way, temporal information is encoded as a part of memory.

Processing Factors

Several accounts of temporal memory have been suggested. Following Friedman (1993), here are some of the more prominent ones. These explanations can be broadly classified as being based on distance-based, location-based, and relative time factors. Note that these factors both help determine when events in the past occurred, as well as figuring out when things will happen in the future (Ben Malek et al., 2017).

Distance-based factors involve time estimates based on how far in the past an original event is from the present, perhaps using the strength of the memory (Brown et al., 1985). The longer it has been since a trace was accessed, the weaker it will be. In contrast, stronger traces are often more recent events. Thus, memory strength can be used to determine its age. This can explain the memory age, recency, and relative ordering effects, as well as why events that have been thought about frequently are remembered as being closer to the present. These memories gain strength each time they are retrieved (Brown et al., 1985).

Also, people can use context (Glenberg et al., 1980) because context is constantly in flux. Two events close in time are likely to have similar contexts, but events that are far apart in time have more distinct contexts. These contexts can be either external or internal. For this view, the greater the difference between the current context and the one associated with the memory, the older that trace is assumed to be. Your present situation is generally more like what it was last week, compared to a year ago, or ten years ago.

It should be noted that, overall, distance-based factors have difficulty with the primacy and accuracy effects and forward or backward telescoping. There is little evaluation of the nature of the content of the memory, only its age.

Location-based factors involve locating a memory in time based on its content. The simplest way this could happen is if you store a tag with the memory for the event. That time tag would convey the hour, day, month, year, or whatever was relevant. All you would need to do is read off this information. For example, I know that I officially started my current job on August 23, 1993. This is directly stored in my memory. Although, it has been suggested that time tags may be associated with a biological clock (Tzeng, 1976), most memories do not have such detailed information.

Another way for people to locate a memory is to make inferences using knowledge in the trace. We figure out the time of an event using information we know, as well as similar events whose time is known. For example, I remember an event that happened on May 1, 1983. I remember seeing some people in old convertibles driving through Cleveland's near west side, shouting and waving signs. This was in the late afternoon and I was on my way home from school. I know it was May 1 because these people were members of the local Communist party, and there was also a brief segment about them on the news that night. They were shouting about how there should be a revolt of the workers and that communism should replace the current political system (it did not happen). I know it was May 1 because this is an important date for Communists, and I know it was 1983 because I was coming home from high school, which would have made it 1980, 1981, 1982, or 1983. I also remember discussing this with a girl I was dating at the time, and I did not date her until my senior year, so it must have been 1983. Thus, using my knowledge of the event, along with the circumstances of my life at the time, I can infer the date.

Location-based factors account for the memory age effect due to a loss of either a time tag or context information. As for serial position curves, primacy effects are attributed to both a superior memory for the event itself and any temporal information associated with it. This is helped by the fact that the early occurrence of events of a type makes them temporally distinct. Thus, this makes them better remembered. Scale effects are accounted for by the loss of a time tag, an error at one level of contextual control but not another. For example, remembering an event that occurred at church could be easily reconstructed to be one that occurred on a Sunday, which is likely to be accurate, but the memory is vague enough that the year cannot be reconstructed. Telescoping effects are explained as reconstructive processes by assuming that memories are distorted based on the amount of content recovered. Relative ordering effects can be accounted for by time tags and reconstruction processes, although not as well. Finally, accuracy effects are easily accounted for in that the more that is retained in a memory, the more accurate the time tag or the more reliable the information used for reconstruction.

For **relative time factors**, temporal order information is stored directly in memory. Information about other events and their temporal relation to one another is stored along with the memory of the event itself. This could happen by the associative chaining of memories (Lewandowsky & Murdock, 1989), along with stored associations of prior occurrences of events of the same type. To locate an event in time, one assesses how it is linked with other related events. Did it occur before or after these other events? Thus, by determining where the event is in a sequence, one can figure out its temporal location.

Another way to encode and recover when events happened is to use associations created from prior remindings. Every time an event occurs, the related and similar events are activated in memory (Hintzman et al., 1975). These reminded events then get associated with the memory for the current event. Thus, the more recently an event has occurred, the more events that are associated with it. Of course, the first event of that type has no additional associated memories. Thus, we can locate events in time, at least relatively, by using information about other events that were linked with it during the reminding process. This would explain why it is easier to correctly order events that are similar compared to those that are different.

These views directly account for relative order effects. The storage of order is what these views are all about. Moreover, they can explain other things, such as the memory age effect in that older memories are more likely to have lost the needed associations. They can also explain serial position effects. Older memories have fewer associations, so they are easier to locate in an order. Conversely, a recency effect occurs because newer memories have had the least amount of forgetting and more associations. Forward telescoping is explained as a loss of associations, making the memory seem not so old.

While we may use relative time information, it does not appear to be a major player. In a study by Friedman (2007), people were given pairs of events, such as movies or class announcements, and were asked to judge whether the temporal order of the two was correct. These events were either related or not (such as having the same major actor). If they were related, then people should make relative time associations. However, the results revealed no such process, suggesting that people do not necessarily draw these temporal associations as they experience events.

Category Adjustment Theory

Using an approach similar to understanding spatial memory, Huttenlocher et al. (1990) applied the **category adjustment theory** to temporal memory. Again, this model assumes that memories are stored at two levels: a fine-grained and a coarse-grained level. The coarse-grained level includes large categories of time, such as 7, 10, 14, 21, 30, and 60 days. Estimates of when events happened reflect a combination of detailed and categorical information. The temporal categories place limits on which events could have occurred (such as knowing that a lecture must have happened sometime between the beginning and the end of a semester), as well as a basis for rounding estimates when there is uncertainty at the fine-grained level.

This fuzzy trace approach accounts for memory age and accuracy effects because the forgetting at the fine-grained level is more likely to occur as memories get older. Serial position effects are also explained because those positions are categorically well defined. Recency effects are due to a relatively small amount of forgetting, and primacy effects reflect memories that are more likely to occur at a temporal border and so can be easily located within that category. The use of coarse-grained information explains scale effects because the different temporal scales often correspond to categorical values. Finally, both forward and backward telescoping can be explained as tendencies to use categorical prototypes when fine-grained information is forgotten.

There are other factors that can influence how people locate memories in time. For example, how the information is reported, such as whether it is an absolute or relative time format (Janssen et al., 2006), such as "on Monday" versus "after the fair". People prefer absolute time formats (exact dates) for more recent events and relative time formats for more remote events, consistent with the idea that more recent events are likely to have more details. Moreover, people prefer absolute time formats for personal events compared to news events, consistent with the idea that personal events are more likely to be well encoded and have sufficient details available for absolute dating.

Temporal Duration

Most of the discussion here has been on memory for *temporal location*; that is, when things happened. Another temporal memory characteristic is memory for *temporal duration*; that is, how long an event lasted. Memory for events shows **temporal compression**. That is, when we estimate how long an event lasted, there is a tendency to misremember it taking less time than it did (Conway, 2008). In part, this allows us to review experiences faster than they actually unfolded. This is even observed in event replays in the hippocampus (Skaggs et al., 1996). Also, the more a span of time is divided into sub-events, the less the temporal compression (Jeunehomme et al., 2018; Zakay et al., 1983). That is, for a long stretch of time when not much happened, our memory of how long it took is shorter compared to the same amount of time when lots of things happened. This is a temporal analog to the spatial finding discussed earlier. Temporal compression is greater for future thinking (we often underestimate how long something will take) (Aksentijevic & Treider, 2016). This has been called the *temporal doppler effect* (Caruso et al., 2013).

Another phenomenon is the **return trip effect**. This is the finding that memory for the time it takes to go to someplace seems longer than the time that it takes to return, although the distances are equal. One influence on this has to do with any ambiguity in the trip. For example, when characteristics of the outbound trip are more ambiguous (e.g., going to a new town) than the return trip (e.g., home), then the return trip effect is greater compared to when the two destinations are both less ambiguous (e.g. school and home) (Maglio & Kwok, 2016).

Stop and Review

Memory for time is worse than memory for space. In addition to memory errors due to age and serial position, temporal memory shows scale, telescoping, and compression effects. Despite these errors, people are often able to remember the sequence or order in which events occurred, even if they cannot place them properly in time. Various factors have been suggested as influencing temporal memory. These include distance factors based on the age of the memory, location-based processes based on knowing when the information occurred in time, and relative time-based factors that derive estimates of time based on memory for the order of events. These multiple processes are reflected in mixture models, such as the Category Adjustment Theory, that consider several mental processes acting on memory for time. Finally, memory for temporal duration can be influenced by several factors, such as how many events occurred during a period of time, and how much ambiguity or certainty there is in a future event.

PUTTING IT ALL TOGETHER

This chapter looked at memory for space and time. Your memory for spatial information is fairly good. When distortions occur, they are systematic to the point of obeying psychophysical laws. This often involves a mixture of detailed metric information along with general information about spatial regions, as captured by the category adjustment model. The mental maps in memory can be influenced by spatial regions and the temporal order in which you learned information, as well as by routes and semantic knowledge. They are also modified by the spatial frameworks derived from the perspective you take, although these influences decline with experience. Also important is the presence of landmarks, which can be helpful guides in learning a new space. Finally, people vary in the effectiveness with which they use these different kinds of maps.

Memory for time is less reliable. You can make a number of judgments about temporal memory including judgments of temporal distance (how long ago did an event happen?), temporal location (when did the event happen?), and relative time (which event happened before the other?). Memory for when events occurred is influenced by how old the memories are, as well as by serial position curve. Temporal memory also exhibits a scale effect. You may be accurate at one level of detail but incorrect at another. Memory for time can be distorted forward or backward in time, as with telescoping effects. Finally, you are fairly good at remembering the order in which events occurred, provided that the events are similar in some way.

Several factors can influence memory for when events occurred. Distance-based factors include knowledge of the age of the memory itself, as well as changes in context. Location-based factors involve information in memory itself, including the explicit encoding of temporal information, as well as inferences drawn from memory contents. Finally, relative position factors involve knowing the sequence of events to help determine when a given event may have happened. Overall, like spatial memories, temporal memories are likely a mixture of factors, and this can also be captured by the Category Adjustment Theory.

STUDY QUESTIONS

1. How can psychophysical principles be applied to memory?
2. To what degree and how are memories for space distorted with respect to perceiving a space? Why?
3. What is Category Adjustment Theory and how does it apply to memory for space?
4. What are some of the major factors about a space that can influence the organization of a mental map?
5. What are the different ways of experiencing or learning the information that will go into a mental map, and how do they influence the final nature of that mental map?
6. How good is our memory for time?
7. What are some of the characteristics of memory that affect the ability to remember when something happened?
8. In what ways does memory for time get distorted?
9. What are the major processing factors that account for people's ability to remember when things happened?
10. How does the Category Adjustment Theory account for the variations in our ability to locate memories in time?

KEY TERMS

- accuracy effect
- backward telescoping
- Category Adjustment Theory
- distance-based factors
- forward telescoping
- hierarchical view
- hybrid theories
- landmarks
- location-based factors
- memory age effect
- metric view
- order information
- orientation effect
- partially hierarchical view
- perspectives
- primacy effect
- psychophysics
- recency effect
- relative time
- relative time factors
- return trip effect

- route
- route perspective
- scale effect
- semantic relationships
- serial position curves

- spatial frameworks
- spatial gradient of availability
- spatial theories
- Steven's Law

- survey perspective
- temporal compression
- temporal distance
- temporal location
- temporal theories

EXPLORE MORE

Here are some additional readings to for you to further explore issues having to do with memory for space and time.

Evans, G. W., & Pezdek, K. (1980). Cognitive mapping: Knowledge of real-world distance and location information. *Journal of Experimental Psychology: Human Learning and Memory, 6*, 13–24.

Holyoak, K. J., & Mah, W. A. (1982). Cognitive reference points in judgments of symbolic magnitude. *Cognitive Psychology, 14*, 328–352.

Huttenlocher, J., Hedges, L. V., & Duncan, S. (1991). Categories and particulars: Prototype effects in estimating spatial location. *Psychological Review, 98*, 352–376.

McNamara, T. P. (1986). Mental representations of spatial relations. *Cognitive Psychology, 18*, 87–121.

Thompson, C. P., Skowronski, J. J., Larsen, S. F., & Betz, A. L. (1996). *Autobiographical Memory: Remembering What and Remembering When*. Mahwah, New Jersey: Erlbaum.

Wiest, W. M., & Bell, B. (1985). Stevens's exponent for psychophysical scaling of perceived, remembered, and inferred distance. *Psychological Bulletin, 98*, 457–470.

REFERENCES

Aksentijevic, A., & Treider, J. M. G. (2016). It's all in the past: Deconstructing the temporal Doppler effect. *Cognition, 155*, 135–145.

Algom, D. (1992). Memory psychophysics: An examination of its perceptual and cognitive prospects. In D. Algom (Ed.), *Psychophysical Approaches to Cognition* (pp. 441–513). New York: North Holland.

Algom, D., & Lubel, S. (1994). Psychophysics in the field: Perception and memory for labor pain. *Perception & Psychophysics, 55*, 133–141.

Algom, D., Wolf, Y., & Bergman, B. (1985). Integration of stimulus dimensions in perception and memory: Composition rules and psychophysical relations. *Journal of Experimental Psychology: General, 114*, 451–471.

Anderson, S. J., & Conway, M. A. (1993). Investigating the structure of autobiographical memories. *Journal of Experimental Psychology: Learning, Memory, and Cognition, 19,* 1178–1196.

Avraamides, M. N., Galati, A., Pazzaglia, F., Meneghetti, C., & Denis, M. (2013). Encoding and updating spatial information presented in narratives. *Quarterly Journal of Experimental Psychology, 66*(4), 642–670.

Bailenson, J. N., Shum, M. S., & Uttal, D. H. (2000). The initial segment strategy: A heuristic for route selection. *Memory & Cognition, 28*(2), 306–318.

Bartlett, J. C., & Snelus, P. (1980). Lifespan memory for popular songs. *American Journal of Psychology, 93,* 551–560.

Ben Malek, H., Berna, F., & D'Argembeau, A. (2017). Reconstructing the times of past and future personal events. *Memory, 25*(10), 1402–1411.

Bradburn, N. M., Rips, L. J., & Shevell, S. K. (1987). Answering autobiographical questions: The impact of memory and inference on surveys. *Science, 236,* 157–161.

Brown, N. R., Rips, L. J., & Shevell, S. K. (1985). The subjective dates of natural events in very-long-term memory. *Cognitive Psychology, 17,* 139–177.

Bugmann, D., Coventry, K. R., & Newstead, S. E. (2007). Contextual cues and the retrieval of information from cognitive maps. *Memory & Cognition, 35,* 381–392.

Burgess, N. (2002). The hippocampus, space, and viewpoints in episodic memory. *Quarterly Journal of Experimental Psychology, 55A,* 1057–1080.

Burgess, N. (2006). Spatial memory: How egocentric and allocentric combine. *Trends in Cognitive Sciences, 10*(12), 551–557.

Campos, A., & Campos-Juanatey, D. (2019). Gender differences in the rotation of city maps. *American Journal of Psychology, 132*(3), 303–514.

Carbon, C., & Leder, H. (2005). The wall inside the brain: Overestimation of distances crossing the former Iron Curtain. *Psychonomic Bulletin & Review, 12,* 746–750.

Caruso, E. M., Van Boven, L., Chin, M., & Ward, A. (2013). The temporal Doppler effect: When the future feels closer than the past. *Psychological Science, 24*(4), 530–536.

Chew, E. I., & Richardson, J. T. E. (1980). The relationship between perceptual and memorial psychophysics. *Memory & Cognition, 16,* 25–26.

Chrastil, E. R., & Warren, W. H. (2013). Active and passive spatial learning in human navigation: Acquisition of survey knowledge. *Journal of Experimental Psychology: Learning, Memory, and Cognition, 39*(5), 1520–1537.

Clayton, K., & Habibi, A. (1991). Contribution of temporal contiguity to the spatial priming effect. *Journal of Experimental Psychology: Learning, Memory, & Cognition, 17,* 263–271.

Conway, M. A. (2008). Exploring episodic memory. In E. Dere, A. Easton, L. Nadel, & J. P. Huston (Eds.), *Handbook of Episodic Memory* (Vol. 18, pp. 19–29). Amsterdam, The Netherlands: Elsevier.

Curiel, J. M., & Radvansky, G. A. (1998). Mental organization in maps. *Journal of Experimental Psychology: Learning, Memory, & Cognition, 24,* 202–214.

Epstein, R., DeYoe, E. A., Press, D. Z., Rosen, A. C., & Kanwisher, N. (2001). Neuropsychological evidence for a topographical learning mechanism in parahippocampal cortex. *Cognitive Neuropsychology, 18,* 481–508.

Epstein, R., & Kanwisher, N. (1998). A cortical representation of the local visual environment. *Nature, 392,* 598–601.

Evans, G. W., & Pezdek, K. (1980). Cognitive mapping: Knowledge of real-world distance and location information. *Journal of Experimental Psychology: Human Learning and Memory, 6,* 13–24.

Ferguson, E. L., & Hegarty, M. (1994). Properties of cognitive maps constructed from texts. *Memory & Cognition, 22,* 455–473.

Ferguson, R. P., & Martin, P. (1983). Long-term temporal estimation in humans. *Perception & Psychophysics, 33,* 585–592.

Fields, A. W., & Shelton, A. L. (2006). Individual skill differences and large-scale environmental learning. *Journal of Experimental Psychology: Learning, Memory, and Cognition, 32,* 506–515.

Friedman, A. (2009). The role of categories and spatial cuing in global-scale location estimates. *Journal of Experimental Psychology: Learning, Memory, and Cognition, 35,* 94–112.

Friedman, A., & Brown, N. R. (2000). Reasoning about geography. *Journal of Experimental Psychology: General, 129*, 193–219.

Friedman, A., Kerkman, D. D., & Brown, N. R. (2002). Spatial location judgments: A cross-national comparison of estimation bias in subjective North American geography. *Psychonomic Bulletin & Review, 9*, 615–623.

Friedman, A., Kerkman, D. D., Brown, N. R., Stea, D., & Cappello, H. M. (2005). Cross-cultural similarities and differences in North Americans' geographic location judgments. *Psychonomic Bulletin & Review, 12*, 1054–1060.

Friedman, W. J. (1993). Memory for the time of past events. *Psychological Bulletin, 113*, 44–66.

Friedman, W. J. (2007). The role of reminding in long-term memory for temporal order. *Memory & Cognition, 35*, 66–72.

Fu, E., Bravo, M., & Roskos, B. (2015). Single-destination navigation in a multiple-destination environment: A new "later-destination attractor" bias in route choice. *Memory & Cognition, 43*(7), 1043–1055.

Garsoffky, B., Schwan, S., & Hesse, F. W. (2002). Viewpoint dependency in the recognition of dynamic scenes. *Journal of Experimental Psychology: Learning, Memory, and Cognition, 28*, 1035–1050.

Glenberg, A. M., Bradley, M. M., Stevenson, J. A., Kraus, T. A., Tkachuk, M. J., Gretz, A. L., Fish, J. H., & Turpin, B. M. (1980). A two-process account of long-term serial position effects. *Journal of Experimental Psychology: Human Learning and Memory, 6*, 355–369.

Graham, S. M., Joshi, A., & Pizlo, Z. (2000). The traveling salesman problem: A hierarchical model. *Memory & Cognition, 28*(7), 1191–1204.

Hafting, T., Fyhn, M., Molden, S., Moser, M. B., & Moser, E. I. (2005). Microstructure of a spatial map in the entorhinal cortex. *Nature, 436*(7052), 801–806.

Han, X., & Becker, S. (2014). One spatial map or many? Spatial coding of connected environments. *Journal of Experimental Psychology: Learning, Memory, and Cognition, 40*(2), 511–531.

He, Q., McNamara, T. P., & Kelly, J. W. (2018). Reference frames in spatial updating when body-based cues are absent. *Memory & Cognition, 46*(1), 32–42.

Hintzman, D. L., Summers, J. J., & Block, R. A. (1975). Spacing judgments as an index of study-phase retrieval. *Journal of Experimental Psychology: Human Learning and Memory, 1*, 31–40.

Hochmair, H. H., Büchner, S. J., & Hölscher, C. (2008). Impact of regionalization and detour on ad-hoc path choice. *Spatial Cognition & Computation, 8*(3), 167–192.

Hochmair, H. H., & Karlsson, V. (2005). Investigation of preference between the least-angle strategy and the initial segment strategy for route selection in unknown environments. In C. Freksa, M. Knauff, B. Krieg-Bruckner, B. Nebel, & T. Barkowsky (Eds.), *Spatial Cognition IV* (pp. 79–97). Berlin, Germany: Springer.

Holden, M. P., Newcombe, N. S., Resnick, I., & Shipley, T. F. (2016). Seeing like a geologist: Bayesian use of expert categories in location memory. *Cognitive Science, 40*(2), 440–454.

Holmes, C. A., Newcombe, N. S., & Shipley, T. F. (2018). Move to learn: Integrating spatial information from multiple viewpoints. *Cognition, 178*, 7–25.

Holyoak, K. J., & Mah, W. A. (1982). Cognitive reference points in judgments of symbolic magnitude. *Cognitive Psychology, 14*, 328–352.

Huttenlocher, J., Hedges, L. V., & Bradburn, N. M. (1990). Reports of elapsed time: Bounding and rounding processes in estimation. *Journal of Experimental Psychology: Learning, Memory, and Cognition, 16*, 196–213.

Huttenlocher, J., Hedges, L. V., & Duncan, S. (1991). Categories and particulars: Prototype effects in estimating spatial locations. *Psychological Review, 98*, 352–376.

Ishikawa, T. (2013). Retention of memory for large-scale spaces. *Memory, 21*(7), 807–817.

Janssen, S. M. J., Chessa, A. G., & Murre, J. M. J. (2006). Memory for time: How people date events. *Memory & Cognition, 34*, 138–147.

Jeunehomme, O., Folville, A., Stawarczyk, D., Van der Linden, M., & D'Argembeau, A. (2018). Temporal compression in episodic memory for real-life events. *Memory, 26*(6), 759–770.

Kemp, S. (1988). Memorial psychophysics for visual area: The effect of retention interval. *Memory & Cognition, 16*, 431–436.

Kerst, S. M., & Howard, J. H. (1978). Memory psychophysics for visual area and length. *Memory & Cognition, 6*(3), 327–335.

Kerst, S. M., & Howard, J. H. (1983). Mental processes in magnitude estimation of length and loudness. *Bulletin of the Psychonomic Society, 21*, 141–144.

Kunz, L., Maidenbaum, S., Chen, D., Wang, L., Jacobs, J., & Axmacher, N. (2019). Mesoscopic neural representations in spatial navigation. *Trends in Cognitive Sciences, 23*(7), 615–630.

Lever, C., Burton, S., Jeewajee, A., O'Keefe, J., & Burgess, N. (2009). Boundary vector cells in the subiculum of the hippocampal formation. *The Journal of Neuroscience, 29*(31), 9771–9777.

Levine, M., Jankovic, I. N., & Palij, M. (1982). Principles of spatial problem solving. *Journal of Experimental Psychology: General, 111*, 157–175.

Lewandowsky, S., & Murdock Jr, B. B. (1989). Memory for serial order. *Psychological Review, 96*(1), 25–57.

MacGregor, J. N., & Ormerod, T. (1996). Human performance on the traveling salesman problem. *Perception & Psychophysics, 58*(4), 527–539.

Maddox, K. B., Rapp, D. N., Brion, S., & Taylor, H. A. (2008). Social influences on spatial memory. *Memory & Cognition, 36*, 479–494.

Maglio, S. J., & Kwok, C. Y. N. (2016). Anticipated ambiguity prolongs the present: Evidence of a return trip effect. *Journal of Experimental Psychology: General, 145*(11), 1415–1419.

Mather, M., & Nesmith, K. (2008). Arousal-enhanced location memory for pictures. *Journal of Memory and Language, 58*, 449–464.

McNamara, T. P. (1986). Mental representations of spatial relations. *Cognitive Psychology, 18*, 87–121.

McNamara, T. P., Altarriba, J., Bendele, M., Johnson, S. C., & Clayton, K. N. (1989). Constraints on priming in spatial memory: Naturally learned versus experimentally learned environments. *Memory & Cognition, 17*, 444–453.

McNamara, T. P., Halpin, J. A., & Hardy, J. K. (1992). Spatial and temporal contributions to the structure of spatial memory. *Journal of Experimental Psychology: Learning, Memory, and Cognition, 18*, 555–564.

McNamara, T. P., Hardy, J. K., & Hirtle, S. C. (1989). Subjective hierarchies in spatial memory. *Journal of Experimental Psychology: Learning, Memory, and Cognition, 15*, 211–227.

McNamara, T. P., & LeSueur, L. L. (1989). Mental representations of spatial and nonspatial relations. *Quarterly Journal of Experimental Psychology, 41A*, 215–233.

McNamara, T. P., Ratcliff, R., & McKoon, G. (1984). The mental representation of knowledge acquired from maps. *Journal of Experimental Psychology: Learning, Memory, and Cognition, 10*, 723–732.

McNamara, T. P., Rump, B., & Werner, S. (2003). Egocentric and geocentric frames of reference in memory for large-scale space. *Psychonomic Bulletin & Review, 10*, 589–595.

Mishra, A., & Mishra, H. (2010). Border bias: The belief that state borders can protect against disasters. *Psychological Science, 21*(11), 1582–1586.

Morrow, D. G., Greenspan, S. L., & Bower, G. H. (1987). Accessibility and situation models in narrative comprehension. *Journal of Memory and Language, 26*, 165–187.

Moyer, R. S., Bradley, D. R., Sorensen, M. H., Whiting, J. C., & Mansfield, D. P. (1977). Psychophysical functions for perceived and remembered size. *Science, 200*, 330–332.

Mrkva, K., Travers, M., & Van Boven, L. (2018). Simulation fluency reduces feelings of psychological distance. *Journal of Experimental Psychology: General, 147*(3), 354–276.

Muller, R. U., Kubie, J. L., & Ranck, J. B. (1987). Spatial firing patterns of hippocampal complex-spike cells in a fixed environment. *The Journal of Neuroscience, 7*, 1935–1950.

Newcombe, N. S., & Chiang, N. C. R. (2007). Learning geographical information from hypothetical maps. *Memory & Cognition, 35*, 895–909.

Newcombe, N., Huttenlocher, J., Sandberg, E., Lie, E., & Johnson, S. (1999). What do misestimations and asymmetries in spatial judgement indicate about spatial representation? *Journal of Experimental Psychology: Learning, Memory, and Cognition, 25*(4), 986.

O'Keefe, J., & Dostrovsky, J. (1971). The hippocampus as a spatial map: Preliminary evidence from unit activity in the freely-moving rat. *Brain Research, 34*(1), 171–175.

Rinck, M., & Bower, G. H. (1995). Anaphora resolution and the focus of attention in situation models. *Journal of Memory and Language, 34*, 110–131.

Rossano, M. J., Warren, D. H., & Kenan, A. (1995). Orientation specificity: How general is it? *American Journal of Psychology, 108*, 359–380.

Rubin, D. C., & Baddeley, A. D. (1989). Telescoping is not time compression: A model of the dating of autobiographical events. *Memory and Cognition, 17*, 653–661.

Sadalla, E. K., Burroughs, W. J., & Staplin, L. J. (1980). Reference points in spatial cognition. *Journal of Experimental Psychology: Human Learning and Memory, 5*, 516–528.

Sampaio, C., & Wang, R. F. (2008). Category-based errors and the accessibility of unbiased spatial memories: A retrieval model. *Journal of Experimental Psychology: Learning, Memory, and Cognition, 35*, 1331–1337.

Sampaio, C., & Wang, R. F. (2017). The cause of category-based distortions in spatial memory: A distribution analysis. *Journal of Experimental Psychology: Learning, Memory, and Cognition, 43*(12), 1988–1992. Scharine, A. A., & McBeath, M. K. (2002). Right-handers and Americans favor turning to the right. *Human Factors, 44*, 248–256.

Shapiro, M. L., Tanila, H., & Eichenbaum, H. (1997). Cues that hippocampal place cells encode: Dynamic and hierarchical representation of local and distal stimuli. *Hippocampus, 7*, 624–642.

Shelton, A. L., & McNamara, T. P. (2004). Orientation and perspective dominance in route and survey learning. *Journal of Experimental Psychology: Learning, Memory, and Cognition, 30*, 158–170.

Skaggs, W. E., McNaughton, B. L., Wilson, M. A., & Barnes, C. A. (1996). Theta phase precession in hippocampal neuronal populations and the compression of temporal sequences. *Hippocampus, 6*(2), 149–172.

Stevens, A., & Coupe, P. (1978). Distortions in judged spatial relations. *Cognitive Psychology, 10*, 422–437.

Stevens, S. S., & Galantner, E. H. (1957). Ratio scales and category scales for a dozen perceptual continua. *Journal of Experimental Psychology, 54*, 377–411.

Sturz, B. R., & Bodily, K. D. (2016). Detecting the perception of illusory spatial boundaries: Evidence from distance judgments. *Cognition, 146*, 371–376.

Taylor, H. A., & Tversky, B. (1992). Spatial mental models derived from survey and route descriptions. *Journal of Memory and Language, 31*, 261–292.

Thompson, C. P., Skowronski, J. J., & Betz, A. L. (1993). The use of partial temporal information in dating personal events. *Memory & Cognition, 21*(3), 352–360.

Thompson, C. P., Skowronski, J. J., & Lee, D. J. (1988). Telescoping in dating naturally occurring events. *Memory & Cognition, 16*, 461–468.

Thorndyke, P. W. (1981). Distance estimation from cognitive maps. *Cognitive Psychology, 13*, 526–550.

Toglia, M. P., & Kimble, G. A. (1976). Recall and use of serial position information. *Journal of Experimental Psychology: Human Learning and Memory, 2*, 431–445.

Tolman, E. C. (1948). Cognitive maps in rats and men. *Psychological Review, 55*, 189–208.

Tversky, B. (1981). Distortions in memory for maps. *Cognitive Psychology, 13*, 417–433.

Tzeng, O. J. L. (1976). A precedence effect in the processing of verbal information. *American Journal of Psychology, 89*, 577–599.

Uttal, D. H., Friedman, A., Hand, L. L., & Warren, C. (2010). Learning fine-grained and category information in navigable real-world space. *Memory & Cognition, 38*(8), 1026–1040.

Waller, D., Loomis, J. M., & Haun, D. B. M. (2004). Body-based senses enhance knowledge of directions in large-scale environments. *Psychonomic Bulletin & Review, 11*, 157–163.

Waller, D., Montello, D. R., Richardson, A. E., & Hegarty, M. (2002). Orientation specificity and spatial updating of memories for layouts. *Journal of Experimental Psychology: Learning, Memory, and Cognition, 28*, 1051–1063.

Waller, D., & Richardson, A. R. (2008). Correcting distance estimates by interacting with immersive virtual environments: Effects of task and available sensory information. *Journal of Experimental Psychology: Applied, 14*(1), 61–72.

Weisberg, S. M., & Newcombe, N. S. (2018). Cognitive maps: Some people make them, some people struggle. *Current Directions in Psychological Science, 27*(4), 220–226.

Whitten, W. B., & Leonard, J. M. (1981). Directed search through autobiographical memory. *Memory & Cognition, 9*, 566–579.

Wiest, W. M., & Bell, B. (1985). Stevens's exponent for psychophysical scaling of perceived, remembered, and inferred distance. *Psychological Bulletin, 98*, 457–470.

Zakay, D., Nitzan, D., & Glicksohn, J. (1983). The influence of task difficulty and external tempo on subjective time estimation. *Perception & Psychophysics, 34*(5), 451–456.

Zhou, R., & Mou, W. (2016). Superior cognitive mapping through single landmark-related learning than through boundary-related learning. *Journal of Experimental Psychology: Learning, Memory, and Cognition, 42*(8), 1316–1323.

Ziemer, C. J., Plumert, J. M., Cremer, J. F., & Kearney, J. K. (2009). Estimating distance in real and virtual environments: Does order make a difference? *Attention, Perception, & Psychophysics, 71*(5), 1095–1106.

CHAPTER 12

Autobiographical Memory

Some of our memories involve what most of us would consider to be central to who we are as individuals. These are the memories that help form our identities and give structure to our lives. Knowledge of a person's memory is a very intimate thing. When we meet new people, an important part of getting to know one another is an exchange of memories, often by providing excerpts from our life story. Our memory for our life story is **autobiographical memory**. Autobiographical memory covers events, situations, and other knowledge about yourself that spans your entire life. That said, we also have **vicarious autobiographical memories** from the stories we hear, which are like the memories we create for ourselves (Panattoni & Thomsen, 2018).

This chapter covers general characteristics of autobiographical memories, some methods for studying them, and the various levels of detail in them. We consider how autobiographical memory has a narrative character. It can provide us with different perspectives, which depend on general world knowledge, and can vary across cultures. An important part of autobiographical memory is superior memory for emotional periods of our lives, and the occurrence of involuntary memories. We look at superior memory for surprising events that can give rise to what are known as flashbulb memories. We look at the reminiscence bump for central portions of our lives. Finally, we consider collective memories for large groups of people.

CHARACTERISTICS OF AUTOBIOGRAPHICAL MEMORIES

In this section we examine what autobiographical memories are. This includes their relationship to episodic and semantic memories, their nature, and the ease with which they are retrieved.

Episodic or Semantic?

Because autobiographical memories are about a person's own life, are they a kind of episodic memory? In a way, yes. However, they are much more than that.

Autobiographical memories are more constructive and integrative, often spanning multiple events. In contrast, episodic memories are confined to a single event.

In addition, autobiographical memories contain generic information about you. This can include things such as your address, phone number, job, and so on. Much of your life story involves stable, semantic-like information. Still, autobiographical memories differ from semantic memories, per se, in that they are about ourselves. Moreover, not only does autobiographical memory have semantic aspects, but semantic memory is influenced by autobiographical memory. For example, semantic knowledge of famous people is more accessible if they are autobiographically significant, such as a personal hero (Westmacott & Moscovitch, 2003).

Varieties of Information

Autobiographical memories are about events in our lives and how they are interrelated. This may involve integrating events separated by long periods of time. They are amalgams of all kinds of information, including knowledge of sensory experiences (what things looked, sounded, smelled like, etc.), where things happened, how people acted, what they said, and what emotions were felt (Rubin, 2006). Moreover, autobiographical memories contain interpretive inferences about how one event relates to others and what it means to us.

During retrieval, people typically report general information followed by specific details (Anderson & Conway, 1997). For example, something like

> "I remember when I was in high school back in Cleveland Ohio. I had this Latin teacher. He used to constantly terrorize our class. It was horrible. I remember one day he gave a hard exam. To make sure we did not cheat, he put a chair up on his desk at the front of the class. He then sat on the chair, staring at us all, making us more nervous and tense than we already were."

It is less common for people to start with the details and work out to general information. This suggests that autobiographical memories are organized around general themes. Within these generalized chunks are the details of our lives.

TRY IT OUT

Autobiographical memory has a strong temporal order bias. People prefer remembering events from the beginning to end, rather than the reverse, or even remembering details based on importance. This can be shown by asking people to recall ten details from a set of 12 events.

What you need are a set of 12 life events that most people will have already had. Here is a list that you can use, although you can think of your own:

"going to a birthday party," "getting an important message," "visiting relatives," "going on a shopping trip," "playing a game," "getting a job," "moving to a new home," "learning to drive," "coming home from school," "taking a trip," "meeting a new friend," and "attending a sporting event."

For this study, you need at least 12 participants, although more is better. Read the life event titles to people, one at a time. Have your participants write ten details down on a sheet of paper for each of the 12 events. Next, have the participants recall the details of four of these events in a forward order (from the beginning to the end), four in a backwards order (from the end to the beginning), and recall the details for four events in an importance order, starting with the most important detail and then proceeding to the least important. You should also time how long people take to do each list using a stopwatch. If you can, mix up which events get assigned to which condition for each person, as well as the order of the conditions.

When you are done, average the times for each person for each condition and then average the times across your participants within each condition. What you should find is that people recall more details and/or are fastest when the information was recalled in a forward order compared to a backwards order or based on importance, thereby illustrating the sequential nature of autobiographical memories.

This organizational structure suggests that autobiographical memories are complex. They contain information at a variety of levels of detail and span broad periods of time. This complexity influences retrieval time. It takes longer to retrieve an autobiographical memory (2 to 15 seconds) than a typical episodic or semantic memory (1 or 2 seconds) (Anderson & Conway, 1997). This slower processing time reflects a need to access more information and to sort through and locate specific memories.

There may be gender differences in autobiographical memory. There is a tendency for women to report more episodic elements than men, to have more detailed and evaluative reports, and to have more repetitions (Wang, 2013) They are also more likely to express emotion and report narratives with more connections and elaborations (Grysman et al., 2016). In comparison, men tend to retain more factual information (Schulkind et al., 2012b). That said, whatever is encoded into autobiographical memory is forgotten at similar rates for men and woman (Wang, 2013).

Methods of Autobiographical Memory Study

Autobiographical memory is uniquely personal, and the events occurred long before people step into the laboratory. While many standard methods of assessing memory can be adapted to study autobiographical memory, there are some techniques that are more unique to it. One is the **Galton–Crovitz cue word method**. This was created by Francis Galton (1822–1911) and brought into modern use by Crovitz and Schiffman (1974). This method involves giving people a series of words (such as "tree") and asking them to report the first memory that comes to mind. This technique is used to assess the distribution of memories over a lifetime. This is particularly relevant when we discuss the reminiscence bump.

A problem with autobiographical memory is that the researchers often do not know what people actually experienced. A way to get around this is by using **diary studies** in which participants keep daily records of life events. This allows the experimenter to better test memory accuracy. Because diary studies are long and labor intensive, they are not common. Some diary studies involve only a single person over many years (Linton, 1975; Wagenaar, 1986; White, 2002). Others have several people record information for weeks or months. For example, the assessment of the scale effect in temporal memory (see Chapter 11) involved a diary method. Diary studies can reveal interesting aspects of memory. For example, Linton's (1982) diary study revealed a forgetting curve that was linear, as seen in Figure 12.1, unlike what Ebbinghaus observed.

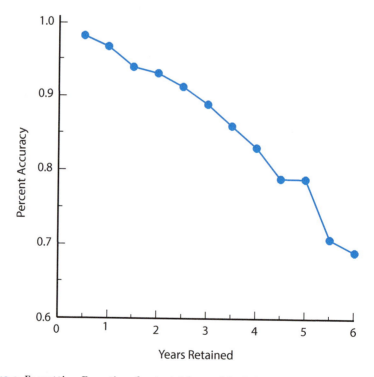

FIGURE 12.1 *Forgetting Function for Autobiographical Memories Recorded in a Diary*

Source: created from data reported in Linton, M. (1982). Transformations of memory in everyday life. In U. Neisser (Ed.), *Memory Observed: Remembering in Natural Contexts.* San Francisco, CA: Freeman

Improve Your Memory

How can you improve your ability to retrieve your autobiographical memories? Well, one way would be to keep a diary. The act of recording daily events improves later memory for them (Szőllősi et al., 2015). The recording process serves to help you rehearse the event, making it more memorable later. Moreover, thinking about your daily events also causes you to draw inferences about how things may be related to each other within the same day or to other events from your own life, thereby weaving your daily events into your life narrative and improving your memory for them.

Functions of Autobiographical Memory

What role does autobiographical memory play? Harris et al. (2014) identified four functions of autobiographical memory. First, it has a **reflective function** in which autobiographical memory is positive self-focused attention aimed at understanding or defining who you are. It provides goals and directions to your life. An example of this is thinking that you should become a physician because you want to help people and you also want to make a good living. Second, autobiographical memory has a **social function** in which it is more positive and other-focused to serve interpersonal and conversational functions. For example, thinking about your life in order to share it in a conversation with someone you have just starting dating, and you want them to get to know you.

Third, autobiographical memory has a **ruminative function** in which memory is self-focused and directed at perceived losses and threats. Examples of this would be thinking about people you know who have died or relationships that have been lost. This is the least used autobiographical memory function. Finally, autobiographical memory has a **generative function** aimed at having a positive impact on the world and creating a legacy. This helps you draw on prior experiences to teach others, develop a sense of achievement, and connection with people from the past. Overall, the uses of these functions decline as one grows older except for generativity, which increases. Note that these functions are also influenced by vicarious experiences of people that we are close to (Lind & Thomsen, 2018).

Stop and Review

Autobiographical memory is made of components of episodic and semantic memories. Autobiographical memories contain information about both individual events and stable characteristics of a person. They are woven out of basic knowledge about the events in our lives along with the inferences and interpretations of those events. These memories are complex and constructive, requiring more time to bring them to mind. Our autobiographical memories play several roles to give structure to our understanding of our lives. These functions include reflecting on past events, interacting with others, ruminating on our past losses, and thinking generatively about the qualities of our lives and how we will be of benefit to those in the future.

LEVELS OF AUTOBIOGRAPHICAL MEMORY

Autobiographical memory is hard to describe because it is made up of different types of information. One way to parse it is by the length of time covered (Conway, 1996). Using this approach, there are three levels that can be identified: (1) the *event level*, which refers to individual events; (2) *general events*, which refer to extended sequences or repeated series of events, often sharing a common component; and (3) *lifetime periods*, which are broad, theme-based portions of a person's life.

An example of these levels is shown in Figure 12.2 (Conway, 1996). At the top are two lifetime periods, which overlap. These are the education and work

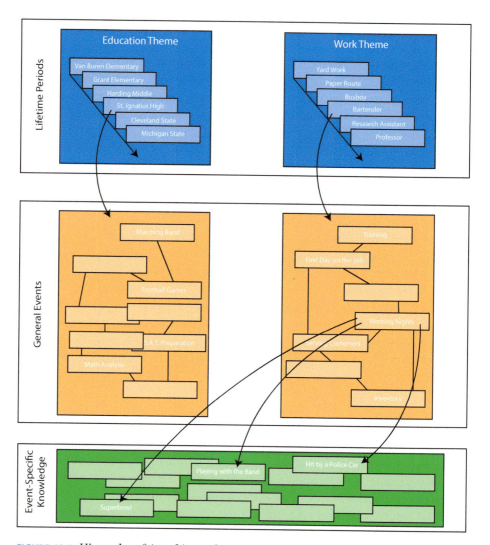

FIGURE 12.2 *Hierarchy of Autobiographical Memories*

Source: adapted from Conway, M. A. (1996). Autobiographical memory. In E. L. Bjork & R. A. Bjork (Eds.) *Memory*. San Diego, CA: Academic Press

themes. Within each of these are several components that make up that theme. Each component is associated with a collection of general events. For example, in the work theme, "working as a bartender" is associated with several general events, such as "first day on the job," "working nights," and "inventory." Each general event is also associated with memories of specific episodes at the lowest level of the hierarchy. Note this division of autobiographical memories also applies to episodic future thinking (D'Argembeau & Demblon, 2012).

Event-Specific Memories

Event-specific memories most closely correspond to episodic memories. These are memories for specific time periods that involve a common activity occurring at a particular place. For example, the Latin teacher sitting on his chair while perched on his desk is an event memory. Event memories contain perceptual and contextual details about what things looked or sounded like, as well as details about time and space. Finally, event memories can contain internal context information, such as emotional reactions, or physiological states.

While most event-specific memories are lost over time, others endure and become important. This is the opposite of many memory processes that move toward making information more semantic and schematic. For an event-specific memory to be retained as a single event, it needs to have some special quality. Pillemer (2001) outlined four ways this can happen. First, they can be memories of initial events that have many goal-relevant memories that follow them—for example, a memory of a childhood experience of going to the hospital for an injury sets a person on the path toward becoming a doctor. Second, they can be memories of turning points when a person's life plan is redirected—for example, being confined to a wheelchair after a car accident. Third, they can be memories of anchoring events that become a basis for a major belief system—for example, having a religious experience. Finally, they can be memories of anomalous events that can guide future behavior—for example, remembering an embarrassing incident at work when you got caught goofing off when the temptation arises to do that again. These qualities of event-specific memories can make them easier to remember and harder to forget.

General Event Memories

At an intermediate level of autobiographical memory are **general events**. One type of general event is a sequence of events that forms a larger episode. For example, the first day on the job is a general event made of the various specific events of that day, such as getting a tour of the building, being assigned a desk, receiving literature on company policies and benefits, and so on. The extension of an event across time and space leads us to unify several smaller events into one memory (Burt et al., 2003).

The other type of general event is a repeating event. For example, your memory for a class taken last year is a general event. The different class sessions are not a sequence of events because they were separated by large periods of time. Still, the repeated event quality of the class was used to organize experiences into a general event of being in the class.

The creation of general event memories requires integrative and interpretive thinking. Integration is needed because different events must be brought together into a common memory. This is clear for recurring situations, such as taking a class. Interpretation is also needed because people must understand how the sub-events go together. For example, in a general event memory of the class, memory for receiving a grade on an exam must be related in some coherent way to the memory for taking the exam and its relation to studying before that.

Lifetime Period Memories

At the highest level are **lifetime periods**. These are long stretches of time that are organized along a common theme, such as "early childhood," "education," or "career." Lifetime periods give us a sense of structure about the progression and development of life in the service of goals or preferences. When we recall autobiographical memories, if they go beyond a single general event, we are likely to confine retrieval to a given theme (Barsalou, 1988). For example, when recalling information about work experiences, we are unlikely to recall information about various relationships we were involved in, unless those relationships overlapped with our work experiences (such as dating a coworker). That said, there may be distinguishing qualities to lifetime periods, even if they share a theme. For example, memories of high school tend to be more socially oriented and positive than memories of middle school (Barzykowski et al., 2019).

Evidence for the Hierarchy

The autobiographical memory hierarchy is more of a heuristic than a hard and fast categorization. There are cases where it is unclear at what level a given memory belongs. For example, is a memory of meeting one's roommate for the first time a single event or a general event of a sequence of events that happened in quick succession? Also, information may be divided into subcomponents at the different levels. A general event may be broken down into other general events. A memory for taking a class may be broken down into different parts of the semester. Thus, there is a recursive quality in which smaller and smaller parts can be nested into a larger description (Barsalou, 1988). An example of this decomposition is shown in Figure 12.3.

We typically have different aspects of our lives going on concurrently. Various extended life events overlap. Thus, there are several ways that autobiographical memories relate to one another (Barsalou, 1988). For example, Figure 12.4 shows events from different lifespan periods overlapping in time. Life does not start and stop depending on our goals and preferences.

Despite the fuzzy nature of the division of autobiographical memory, there is evidence to support this hierarchy, to some degree. For example, lifetime period reports are more likely to be elicited when we are cued to recall an autobiographical

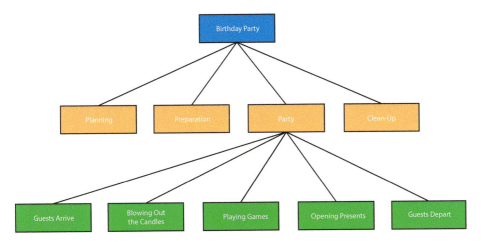

FIGURE 12.3 *The Recursive Process of Breaking Down an Autobiographical Memory into Smaller and Smaller Parts—in This Case, a Memory of a Trip*

Source: adapted from Barsalou, L. W. (1988). The contents and organization of autobiographical memories. In U. Neisser & E. Winograd (Eds.) *Remembering Reconsidered: Ecological and Traditional Approaches to the Study of Memory.* New York: Cambridge University Press

memory in response to a cue word (e.g., tell me a memory of your life based on the word "lock") or a social instruction (e.g., imagine you are describing the event to a friend). In comparison, event-specific reports are more likely to be elicited when there is no specific target audience or after hearing a narrative centered on a lifetime theme (e.g., a description of someone running for high school class president) (Schulkind et al., 2012a). Thus, there is flexibility in how we draw information out of autobiographical memory. Also, over time, the lower we go in the hierarchy, the more likely information is forgotten, with abstract relations in autobiographical memory being retained longer (Mace et al., 2013).

This hierarchy has some neurological support. People with dense amnesia can recall lifetime periods and general events but not specific episodes. One patient, S. S., became amnesic after a case of herpes simplex encephalitis when he was about 40 years old (Cermak & O'Connor, 1983; McCarthy & Warrington, 1992). The virus damaged part of his left hemisphere. Although he had high intelligence, he had severe memory problems. He could not remember specific events from his life but could recount general aspects of his experiences, such as his job. Thus, although he had trouble remembering at the event level, he could remember at the general and lifetime period levels.

A similar case is K. C., who suffered damage to the frontal-parietal region of his left hemisphere and the parietal-occipital region (BAs 7 & 39) of his right hemisphere as the result of a motorcycle accident at the age of 30 (Tulving et al., 1988). He could not remember any life events. For example, he could not remember the circumstances of his brother's tragic drowning ten years before. However, he did remember semantic knowledge of his job, which he had recently begun, and even personally relevant information, such as the floor plan of his childhood

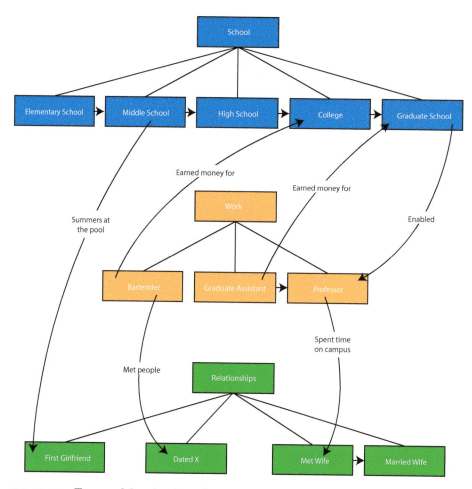

FIGURE 12.4 *Temporal Overlapping of Various Lifetime Periods with Different Themes Based on Common, Shared Specific and General Events*

Source: adapted from Barsalou, L. W. (1988). The contents and organization of autobiographical memories. In U. Neisser & E. Winograd (Eds.) *Remembering Reconsidered: Ecological and Traditional Approaches to the Study of Memory*. New York: Cambridge University Press

home (although he could not say which room was his), the names of his school classmates, and places where he had vacationed. This distinction between what is and what is not remembered supports the idea that autobiographical memory for events is separate from memory of general knowledge.

In contrast, K. S., who had a right anterior temporal lobectomy to control her epileptic seizures, could recall specific life events but not general knowledge about the people involved (Ellis et al., 1989). She also had trouble with the names of famous people and product brands (e.g., Margaret Thatcher or Coca Cola). Thus, in a sense, she had the ability to store memories at the event-specific level but not general events.

Another person with autobiographical memory trouble was P.S., a man in his late 60s with bilateral damage to his thalamus. He had profound anterograde amnesia as well as extensive retrograde amnesia for autobiographical memories, but not semantic, non-personal information (Hodges & McCarthy, 1993). For instance, he could not recall any details of his wedding. He also knew that he had three sons but could not provide any details about their births. He also did not recognize photos of family events. However, he could recognize famous faces and place them in chronological order for when they were famous, but could not remember public events (e.g., the Watergate scandal). Thus, P.S. was unable to remember autobiographical events and the people involved in them.

Stop and Review

Autobiographical memory can be divided into three levels. At the event-specific level are individual events, which is closest to episodic memory. At the general event level are extended and repeated events. Finally, the lifetime period level spans broad, thematically related parts of our lives. This hierarchy is supported by studies of the effectiveness with which people retrieve memories, as well as evidence from brain damaged patients with selective deficits.

AUTOBIOGRAPHICAL MEMORY AS LIFE NARRATIVE

Autobiographical memories are **life narrative** memories (McAdams, 2001). This follows a general human tendency to organize our experiences into stories (Bruner, 1991). People often access information in autobiographical memory using elements found in narratives, such as people, places, activities, and other thematic information (Barsalou, 1988; Conway, 1990). In general, autobiographical memories can be elicited by any event feature that is stored with the event, sometimes involuntarily (Berntsen, 1996).

While autobiographical memories can be triggered by a wide range of cues, such as how things look and sound (Willander et al., 2015), music (Belfi et al., 2016) and olfactory cues (smells) are special. Odors are particularly effective at helping us remember events (Chu & Downes, 2002; de Bruijn & Bender, 2018). They are more likely to elicit memories that we rarely think about (Rubin et al., 1984) and elicit feelings of nostalgia (Reid et al., 2015). Also, odors are more likely to elicit memories from the first decade of life than are words or pictures (Willander & Larsson, 2006). The autobiographical memories elicited by odors tend to be more emotional (Herz, 2004). This may be because the olfactory nerves are strongly connected to the amygdala, which is important for emotion processing. Because smells are more connected to emotional experience, they are more likely to be remembered.

When people are probed for autobiographical memories, they may retrieve them in clusters of other events that occurred at a similar time (Brown & Schopflocher,

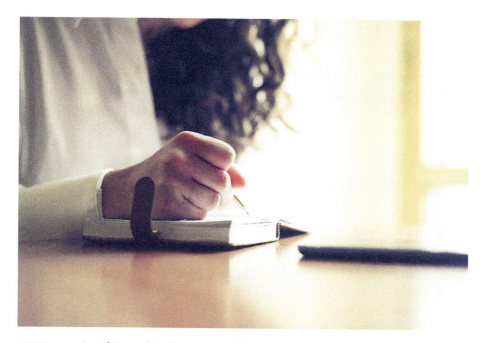

PHOTO 12.1 *Autobiographical memory is like a life narrative. It is the story of ourselves that we tell ourselves and others. It can be improved if one keeps a diary of the events experienced from day to day*

Source: Eugenio Marongiu/Shutterstock.com

1998b), as is expected if they are part of a story. Moreover, people are most often reminded of events that are causally related (either as a cause or an effect) and are reminded of events that share the same person, place, or activity (Brown & Schopflocher, 1998a).

To give autobiographical memories a narrative style, people may draw on semantic memory. As is discussed in Chapter 9, people have scripts for common events. They structure autobiographical memories, giving them a temporal order. We better *recall* life events in a forward order. Although we are faster at *recognizing* important event details (Anderson & Conway, 1993). For example, if you remember a trip to a restaurant, you are more likely to replay it back in your mind in a forward order, as it was experienced. However, if you are thinking of one or two important details, such as a marriage proposal, you would retrieve it quickly without the need to start at the beginning. More generally, our more important autobiographical memories are more likely to be further from the present, both in terms of past and future events, with future events being viewed as being more central than past events. Also, more central life story events are likely to be more emotionally positive (Rubin et al., 2019a).

Narrative structure is important for accurate memory. In a study by Burt et al. (1998), people took photos during their daily lives. Later, they were shown the pictures with the task of putting them in the correct temporal order. Performance was terrible. People were correct only 9% of the time, although they did better if less than a week had passed, in which case they were correct 35% of the time. This low performance is likely because snapshots are just random bits that do not create well-defined narratives, and so are harder to correctly structure and order.

Perspectives in Autobiographical Memory

When you think about events from your life, there may be an accompanying mental visual image (Rubin et al., 2019b). In fact, people who are better able to form mental images are better able to remember autobiographical events (Vannucci et al., 2016). These mental images can vary in their perspective. Sometimes we experience a memory from our original point of view. These are called **field memories** because they capture the original field of view. At other times, we view an event from outside of ourselves and may even see ourselves in it. These are called **observer memories** (Nigro & Neisser, 1983), although some people claim to rarely or never have them (Radvansky & Svob, 2019). The very fact that many of us have observer memories emphasizes the constructive nature of autobiographical memory. Note that there is also a bias for episodic future thoughts to be more from an observer than a field perspective, perhaps because the events have not yet occurred (McDermott et al., 2016).

Three factors that influence how a memory is experienced are shown in Table 12.1. One is the age of the memory. In general, older memories are more likely to be observer memories. A second is emotionality. Generally, the more emotional the memory, the more likely it is experienced as a field memory (Siedlecki, 2015). For example, you are more likely to remember an emotionally intense event, such as getting a marriage proposal, from the perspective that it was experienced. Finally, there is self-awareness in a situation. Generally, the more self-aware we are, the more likely we are trying to understand our role in the larger event, and this tends to lead to more observer memories. For example, an observer memory is more likely to be generated when we remember giving a speech.

TABLE 12.1 *Dimensions and Criteria for Field and Observer Memories*

Dimension	Field Memory	Observer Memory
Age of memory	Newer	Older
Emotionality	More emotional	Less emotional
Self-awareness	Less self-aware	More self-aware

Source: created from description provided in Nigro, G., & Neisser, U. (1983). Point of view in personal memories. *Cognitive Psychology*, 15, 467–482

Schema-Copy-Plus-Tag Model

People use schemas and scripts to help reconstruct incomplete autobiographical memories. The older autobiographical memories are, the more schema-consistent reports are likely to be (Eldridge et al., 1994). However, if you think about your life, it does not feel like you have a memory full of generic, stereotypical events. Instead, you better remember the parts that are unusual. Memory is schematic, but things that are schema-inconsistent are more memorable.

What is the solution to this apparent paradox? Our memories have both schematic and unique aspects of an event. For the **schema-copy-plus-tag model** (Graesser & Nakamura, 1982), when you experience a new event, you first activate the appropriate schema, which is the basis for your event memory. It helps reduce the need to actively think about every little detail. You can simply assume that most details are about the same as they usually are.

In addition, you have "tags" with a memory to denote the important details that were inconsistent with the schema, thereby making memory of that event unique. For example, if you go to a restaurant and the manager tells you that you do not have to pay, this is going to be represented by a tag. Because autobiographical information is focused on the self, people are more likely to show a greater benefit for tagged information when the event memory involves themselves or another familiar person (Colcombe & Wyer, 2002).

Representing autobiographical knowledge this way has two consequences. First, because trivial details are less likely to be directly represented, it is difficult for us to distinguish between schema-consistent parts that were present and those that were not. Second, because the tag is part of the memory, it is easy for us to remember what was odd about an event. This has some unfortunate consequences for education. Students' memories for what happened during class are often better for unusual things that happened, such as spilling coffee or jokes that were told, as compared to the content of the lectures (Kintsch & Bates, 1977).

Cultural Differences

Our autobiographical memories depend on the narratives and stories we are familiar with. Narrative and story forms, as well as life scripts, vary across cultures (Hatiboğlu & Habermas, 2016). Thus, there are cultural differences in autobiographical memories. For example, indigenous Australians have autobiographical memory reports that have more context and detail than non-indigenous Australians (Nile & Van Bergen, 2015). Also, compared to Americans, Japanese people tend to be focused less on the individual and more on the collective (including self-continuity, social-bonding, and behavior-directing aspects of memories of personal events) (Maki et al., 2015). That said, some aspects of autobiographical memory are stable across cultures. For example, across cultures, positive events are more likely to play a central role in defining who we are and are the more important parts of our life stories (Zaragoza et al., 2015).

Stop and Review

Autobiographical memory is a life narrative, paralleling the structure of actual stories. This constructive nature is seen in the distinction between field and observer perspectives of autobiographical memory. Although autobiographical memory construction and retrieval can be guided by schemas in semantic memory, we use tags to help remember the odd, unusual, unexpected, and important aspects of an event. Thus, we have better memory for the unusual details of events rather than the anticipated, common aspects. Finally, because of its narrative structure, people from different cultures with different narrative styles organize and structure their autobiographical memories differently.

EMOTION AND AUTOBIOGRAPHICAL MEMORY

A central aspect of experience is the emotions we feel during events, as well as our emotional reactions when we remember. Like most memories, autobiographical memory has a forgetting curve. People better remember more recent events than older ones (Whitten & Leonard, 1981). However, emotions add complexity. First, the more emotional an event, the more likely it will be remembered (Nadel & Jacobs, 1998). Moreover, consistent with the **Pollyanna principle**, also called the **positivity bias**, over time there is a tendency to remember pleasant events better than unpleasant ones (Wagenaar, 1986) which are forgotten faster (Holmes, 1970; Meltzer, 1930). That is, memory for the good comes to be stronger than the bad (Sedikides & Skowronski, 2020). Moreover, the emotional intensity of negative events is tempered more so than positive events (Cason, 1932; Skowronski et al., 2014; Walker et al., 2003). This is the **fading affect bias**. One last thing to note is that emotional memories are more likely to be accompanied by mental imagery. For example, people make more eye-movements when remembering emotional autobiographical memories (El Haj et al., 2017) and have difficulty if they keep their eyes still (Lenoble et al., 2019).

Although there is a bias to remember more positive life events, there are circumstances when we clearly remember negative events, such as those involving anger, shame, and depression. These negative autobiographical memories differ from positive ones. We tend to focus more on central details and less on peripheral details (Berntsen, 2002), leading to better detailed memory for things in the focus of attention (Kensinger, 2007). This is likely brought on by increased activity in the amygdala during negative events.

The increased focus on central details in an emotional autobiographical memory, at the expense of peripheral details, is called **tunnel memory** (Safer et al., 1998). For example, if you saw an automobile accident, you are likely to better remember aspects about the accident (what colors were the cars) and more poorly remember surrounding details (how many people were in the area). This is because your attention had tunneled in on the central aspects of the emotional event. Tunnel memories also alter other memory phenomena. For example, they

STUDY IN DEPTH

An illustration of the positivity bias in autobiographical memory is a study by Breslin and Safer (2011). This study assessed memories of the major league baseball World Series for 2003 (which was won by the New York Yankees) and 2004 (which was won by the Boston Red Sox). In 2008 they tested 1,563 major league baseball fans. These people were either fans of the Yankees or the Red Socks and lived in Boston, Massachusetts, Cincinnati, Ohio, New York, New York, or Washington, D.C. Of these people, 277 had attended a game in 2008 in one of these cities. Also, 1,286 of them regularly read online Yankees or Red Sox reports during the time that they were questioned. These people were contacted via on-line websites and given a souvenir pen in return for answering a few baseball related questions.

Prior to answering questions about the 2003 and 2004 games, people were reminded of who had won those two years. During testing, people were asked to recall and recognize specific details of those two series. These included questions such as the score of the final game of each series, the winning and losing pitchers' names, the location of the game, and whether the games required extra innings. People were also asked to assess their own memories.

The results are shown in Figure 12.5. People had better memory for events that happened during the World Series when their favorite team won (which resulted in higher levels of positive emotion). That is, there was a positivity bias for people to better remember events for which they had more positive memories.

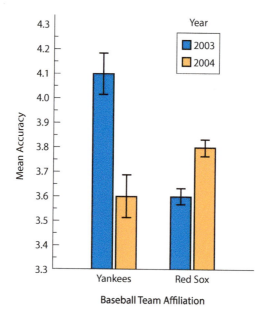

FIGURE 12.5 *Memory for Information about World Series Games for New York Yankees and Boston Red Sox Fans Illustrating the Positivity Bias*

Source: adapted from Breslin, C. W., & Safer, M. A. (2011). Effects of event valence on long-term memory for two baseball championship games. *Psychological Science, 22*(11), 1408–1412

are less likely to exhibit boundary extension (see Chapter 5). Tunnel memories are more common for negative events, perhaps because these central details are more critical in a negative event (e.g., an automobile accident). Positive events are less likely to hinge on a single critical detail (e.g., falling in love). Despite the differences between positive and negative memories, overall, memory is driven more by the intensity of the emotion than by whether it is positive or negative (Talarico et al., 2004).

Some pathologies can influence autobiographical memory. For example, people with depression may have **overgeneral memories** (Williams et al., 2007) in which they recall events with fewer details. There are several reasons for this. First, autobiographical memories are more schema-dependent based on personal concerns and other self-oriented emotional thoughts. Second, autobiographical ideas trigger rumination that further emphasizes personal concerns and emotional thoughts of one's self. Working memory resources are also drained by these interfering thoughts. Finally, overgeneral memories allow a person to avoid thinking about emotionally negative details (Hallford et al., 2018).

Involuntary Memories

While autobiographical memory retrieval may require some time and effort, there are times when autobiographical memories are consciously retrieved spontaneously and involuntarily (Berntsen, 1996; 2001; 2009).[1] An example of an **involuntary memory** might be while you are walking to class in the rain and stepping into a puddle. This spontaneously brings to mind the time you were walking home from school in kindergarten and saw a puddle on the sidewalk with the sky reflected in it. It looked like the puddle had depth and was a window into another world. Involuntary memories occur regularly (Berntsen & Rubin, 2008), at least two to five times a day. They are a basic mode of memory (Berntsen, 2010; Ebbinghaus, 1885) and are likely associated with processing of the default mode network.

Involuntary memories are more likely to be triggered by unique aspects of experience that serve as diagnostic memory cues (Berntsen et al., 2013), and if multiple involuntary memories trigger or cue one another, they often share conceptual characteristics (e.g., the same person) and are from the same lifetime period (Mace & Unlu, 2019). Involuntary memories also tend to be more emotional than voluntary memories and more often are about positive rather than negative events (Berntsen, 1996; 2001).

Involuntary memories not only occur for past events, but also for episodic future thinking. Such spontaneous future-oriented thoughts tend to be more positive than involuntary memories of the past (Berntsen & Jacobsen, 2008). These spontaneously generated future thoughts also tend to be less event specific, and be more on the level of general events (e.g., I should take an advanced chemistry course next semester) or lifetime periods (e.g., I wonder what kind of job I will get after graduation) (Anderson & Dewhurst, 2009).

---

1 See Kvavilashvili and Mandler (2004) for a similar idea for semantic memories, and Jakubowski et al. (2015) for spontaneously having songs pop into our heads.

Stop and Review

Autobiographical memory is affected by emotion, both in terms of mood dependent memory, as well as a positivity bias to remember positive events longer than negative events, consistent with the Pollyanna principle. When people do remember negative events, there is a tendency to have tunnel memories that focus on the more central event details. Finally, memories can come to mind unbidden, as with involuntary memories. Although most of these are emotionally positive, in some cases, they are negative.

FLASHBULB MEMORIES

So far, our discussion of autobiographical memory has focused on more mundane aspects of life. However, we also have memories for surprising and important events. These memories are vivid, have a great deal of detail, and are more resistant to forgetting. Highly detailed memories for surprising events are called **flashbulb memories** (Brown & Kulik, 1977; Hirst & Phelps, 2016) because it is as if the mind had taken a picture of the surprising events as they were occurring.

As examples of flashbulb memories, many people who were around at the time remember where they were and how they heard about the assassination of President Kennedy. A generation later, people can tell you detailed information about hearing about the explosion of the space shuttle *Challenger*. People are also likely to have flashbulb memories for the news of Princess Diana's death (Hornstein et al., 2003) or the terrorist attacks on September 11, 2001 (Schmidt, 2004; Tekcan et al., 2003). Such memories are better if they were personally experienced rather than just heard about (Pillemer, 2009). Note that while most research on flashbulb memories tends to focus on negative events (which tend to make the news broadcasts), they can also happen for positive events (such as finding out that one is going to have a baby). These tend to be much more personal and have a greater impact on our lives (Kraha & Boals, 2014).

A striking feature of flashbulb memories is that they contain detailed information for not only the event itself but also for the context in which it was learned. It is not unusual for people to remember who told them about an event, what the weather conditions were, whom they were with, where they were, what they were wearing, and so on. This contextual information is not directly relevant to what was learned. Still, it seems to be stored at a high level of detail.

Flashbulb Memories Are Special

The original explanation for flashbulb memories was that there is a special memory process, called the "Now Print!" mechanism, somewhere in the neural coding of the memory (Brown & Kulik, 1977). This mechanism is triggered when something of great importance occurs. By storing so many details, it allows people to later

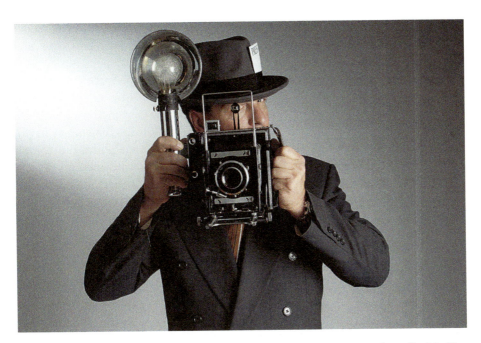

PHOTO 12.2 *When surprising and emotional events happen, we may form flashbulb memories that are highly detailed and longer lasting than our typical event memories. Flashbulb memories are so named because it is as if the brain took a picture of what was happening at the time, although this idea later turned out to be somewhat flawed*

Source: James Steidl/ Shutterstock.com

sort out and identify the important components. This is especially critical for rare events. Thus, it would have some survival value. For example, people are more likely to remember their locations and from whom people heard the news when they encounter surprising events (McKay & Ahmetzanov, 2005), although, interestingly, memory for the emotions experienced at the time are not well remembered (Hirst et al., 2009). That said, other work has failed to support this strong position that flashbulb memories are accurate and unchanging. This is discussed next.

Flashbulb Memories Are Not So Special

It has been suggested that flashbulb memories are just normal memories for important events. They are normal because they can contain errors, be distorted, and be forgotten over time (McCloskey et al., 1988; Schmolck et al., 2000; Talarico & Rubin, 2003). They can also include misinformation from hearing other people's stories of the event (Niedźwieńska, 2003). Flashbulb memories involve people creating autobiographical memory stories for themselves. These accounts then remain relatively stable over long periods of time (Kvavilashvili et al., 2009), although flashbulb memory events experienced as a child may fade over time (Weems et al., 2014).

With flashbulb memories, there is some forgetting, people's accounts change, and incorrect information can creep in. For example, a person might remember that she was having lunch with a friend that she typically has lunch with when she heard the news of an event. However, in truth, the person she remembers having lunch with was somewhere else that day. Thus, flashbulb memories can contain inaccurate information that may be based on schematic reconstructions of what typically happens. Flashbulb memories also may reflect a belief in the accuracy of the memories that emerges from the emotional reaction to the event, rather than the actual accuracy. The stronger the emotional reaction, the more a memory is believed (Talarico & Rubin, 2003). A clear example of how wrong a flashbulb memory can be is seen in the following excerpt from memory researcher Ulric Neisser (1982).

> For many years I have remembered how I heard the news of the Japanese attack on Pearl Harbor, which occurred on the day before my thirteenth birthday. I recall sitting in the living room of our house—we only lived in that house for one year, but I remember it well—listening to a baseball game on the radio. The game was interrupted by an announcement of the attack, and I rushed upstairs to tell my mother. This memory has been so clear for so long that I never confronted its inherent absurdity until last year: no one broadcasts baseball games in December! (It can't have been a football game either: professional football barely existed in 1941, and the college season ended by Thanksgiving.)
>
> (p. 45)

The consensus now is that while flashbulb memories are prone to error, overall they are more detailed, accurate and long-lasting than normal event memories.

Criteria for Flashbulb Memories

Flashbulb memories differ from normal memories, even if they are not perfect. They are better records of the autobiographical experience of a surprising event, but the memory itself may be more normal (Tekcan et al., 2003). What we remember better is our reaction more so than the news itself. Flashbulb memories do have distinguishing qualities, at least phenomenologically (i.e., what they feel like when people remembering them). Moreover, fMRI recordings suggest that during flashbulb memory retrieval there is more right hippocampus and amygdala activity (Metternich et al., 2020).

Under what circumstances are flashbulb memories more likely to be formed? An outline of the more important criteria was provided by Finkenhauer et al. (1998), shown in Figure 12.6. It is one of the best accounts of flashbulb memories

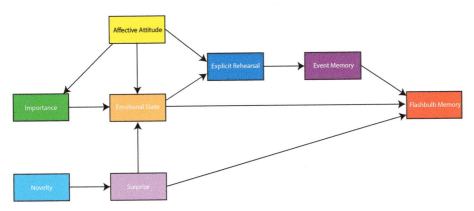

FIGURE 12.6 *Outline of Major Factors in the Creation of Flashbulb Memories*

Source: adapted from Finkenhauer, C., Luminet, O., Gisle, L., El-ahmadi, A., van der Linden, M., & Philipott, P. (1998). Flashbulb memories and the underlying mechanisms of their formation: Toward an emotional-integrative model. *Memory & Cognition, 26,* 516–531

(Luminet, 2009). The first criterion is that the event should be novel. That is, it should be a rare and, most likely, new occurrence. For example, seeing the World Trade Center towers being attacked was a new event, but hearing about a murder on the evening news, sadly, is not. This novelty can lead to a feeling of surprise. This uniqueness and unexpectedness helps it stand out in memory and therefore it is less likely to be influenced by interference. Also, because the event is surprising, people dedicate more effort trying to make sense of the event and its consequences. This makes the flashbulb memory more complex and detailed as well as more enduring.

Flashbulb memory creation requires that the event be important and have consequences for those witnessing or hearing about it. It is critical to remember information that had an impact on our lives, but not to remember more trivial information. For example, the events of September 11, 2001, were important and consequential, but a penny found in a parking lot is not.

The degree to which the events are surprising and important affects emotional reactions. The more intense the reactions, the more likely a flashbulb memory will be formed. Emotionally intense events raise arousal levels, which can aid memory (Bradley et al., 1992). Some flashbulb memories are formed from extremely positive events, such as the flashbulb memories that some Germans formed when the Berlin Wall came down (Bohn & Berntsen, 2007). That said, these positive flashbulb memories tend to be less accurate than the negative ones. Overall, emotions can lead to more attention to an event, more elaborative processing, and more remindings occurring as subsequent consequences are encountered. This all facilitates the retention of a flashbulb memory.

Emotional reactions can override the lack of novelty and surprise for expected events, even if they are repeated, but are emotionally intense. For example, a survey of gay men in the New York City area found that although there were repeated experiences of loved ones dying of AIDS, and the death was expected with the progression of the disease, the emotional intensity of each experience was sufficient to create lasting memories of hearing of the death (Mahmood et al., 2004). Thus, emotional reaction plays a pivotal role in flashbulb memory formation.

Another factor that influences flashbulb memory formation is affective attitude. These are our opinions and beliefs prior to an event that can provide the basis for later elaborative processing. If we lack the requisite knowledge to understand the event, a flashbulb memory is less likely to occur. For example, if a popular sports figure suddenly retires, people who are not fans of that sport consider that news insignificant and do not form a flashbulb memory. In contrast, those who are avid fans may form a flashbulb memory. Curci et al. (2015) found that Italians were more likely to form a flashbulb memory of the unexpected retirement of Pope Benedict XVI if they were practicing Catholics than if they were not, with other normal event memories being similar across the groups.

Finally, people rehearse a flashbulb memory event by discussing it with others. When these events occur, people spend more time thinking about them and how they heard about them, including discussing with others how they heard about the events and their reactions to them. If the event is public, the news media devotes more coverage to it (Koppel et al., 2013). This dwelling on and sharing of the information affects memory. The memory traces are reinforced and strengthened, decreasing the likelihood of forgetting as a form of overlearning.

Stop and Review

Memories of surprising and emotionally engaging events can lead to flashbulb memories that are resistant to forgetting. Originally, flashbulb memories were thought to be highly detailed, accurate, and durable. However, subsequent work has shown that they are prone to distortions and forgetting. Currently, flashbulb memories are viewed as being special but not perfect. The creation of flashbulb memories requires several factors to be in place to occur, which is why they are so rare. These factors include elements of surprise, personal involvement and emotion, and rehearsal.

REMINISCENCE BUMP

Like most memories, autobiographical memories show a forgetting curve. People remember recent events better than older ones (Whitten & Leonard, 1981). Oddly, this forgetting curve extends to events that happened prior to birth (Rubin, 1998; Koppel & Rubin, 2016), which likely reflects interest in historical events that led up to the current situation (Brown, 1990). A major deviation to the forgetting curve considered here is very good memory for life experiences around the age of 20 (between 15 and 25), called the **reminiscence bump**. This interesting

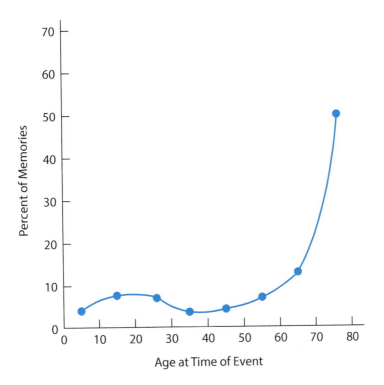

FIGURE 12.7 *The Reminiscence Bump*

Source: an averaging of data reported in Rubin, D. C., Rahhal, T. A., & Poon, L. W. (1998). Things learned in early adulthood are remembered best. *Memory & Cognition, 26,* 3–19

characteristic of autobiographical memory is easier to observe as a person ages. In reminiscence bump studies, the Galton–Crovitz method is often used. For this technique people are given lists of words—such as "bird," "chair," "apple." They are asked to recall the first memory from their lives that comes to mind. Most of these are from the recent past. The further back in time one goes, the fewer memories there are—a forgetting curve. However, there is a bump in the curve around the age of 20, with people recalling more information from this time than would be expected (see Rubin et al., 1998). This reminiscence bump is shown in Figure 12.7.

This phenomenon even influences the life periods from which we derive the topics of our dreams (Grenier et al., 2005) and for information that is not strictly autobiographical, such as memories for famous sports figures (Janssen et al., 2012; but see Koppel & Berntsen, 2016), although it is more likely to be observed for events that are important to a person (Tekcan et al., 2017). Reminiscence bumps for strictly non-autobiographical information may occur as a function of what we were exposed to. There are several explanations for the reminiscence bump. These are covered next.

Cognitive Mechanisms

One explanation for the reminiscence bump is oriented around basic cognitive processes: serial position effects for first experiences of a type (e.g., your first kiss). The reminiscence bump likely occurs around age 20 because this is a time when there is a great deal of change and a number of experiences occur for the first time, such as one's first kiss, first car, first apartment, first job, and so on. Because there are so many firsts, these memories are easier to recall. Thus, the reminiscence bump is partially due to so many primacy effects occurring in close proximity to each other.

A theory of autobiographical memory that is consistent with this is **Transition Theory** (Brown et al., 2016; Svob & Brown, 2012). When there are large changes in a person's life, such as the loss of a one's parents as a child, or moving to a new country, these serve as transitions. These transitions are landmarks for organizing how we think about and remember our lives. These transitions also affect the reminiscence bump in that people who move to a new place show a reminiscence bump for that time (Enz et al., 2016). The later they moved, the later the reminiscence bump. Moving to a new country with a new language provides a lot of novel first experiences (Schrauf & Rubin, 1998). More generally, older adults may divide their life into chapters marked by a series of beginnings and endings (Steiner et al., 2014). These beginnings and endings are more likely to be associated with more new experiences compared to times within a chapter. Around 20 years of age, more people are beginning and ending life chapters than at other ages.

Neurological Changes

Another explanation for the reminiscence bump is neurological. Around the age of 20 is when people are at their neurological peak, when their nervous system is neither maturing nor declining. Thus, we are at our best capacity to encode and store memories. Thus, memory should be more efficient. Prior to this, people have difficulty encoding long-term memories. After this, we begin to see declines in some memory functions, which become more prominent as we age.

Identity Formation

Another explanation for the reminiscence bump is that around the age of 20 people are making a number of decisions about who they are with regard to preferences, ideologies, vocation, and so on (Rathbone et al., 2008). Although we make decisions throughout our lives, there are more of these personally important experiences at this time. These then shape our future choices and our actions and choices become associated with them. As a result, this increased interconnectivity for memories from this time makes them more accessible.

Cultural Schemas

A final explanation for the reminiscence bump is that we have **cultural schemas** or **life scripts** for the important periods and major transition points of our lives (Berntsen & Rubin, 2004). In Western culture this would be things like graduating from school, getting married, buying a house, having a child, and so on. We organize our autobiographical memories using these schemas. When retrieving information, we use these schemas as a guide, thereby producing the reminiscence bump. In a study by Rubin and Berntsen (2003), college students estimated the likelihood that a typical 70-year-old would remember various life events. These estimates were close to the actual pattern shown by older adults. Similarly, Bohn and Berntsen (2011) show that children exhibit a reminiscence bump for their future (projected) lives. This is seen for both cultural life scripted and nonscripted events in Figure 12.8.

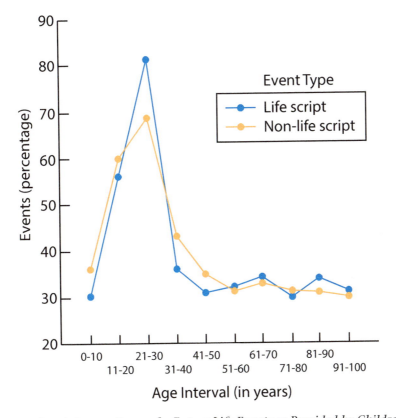

FIGURE 12.8 *Reminiscence Bumps for Future Life Events as Provided by Children. These Occur for Events that Both Do and Do Not Belong to a Culture's Life Script*

Source: an averaging of data reported in: Bohn, A., & Berntsen, D. (2011). The reminiscence bump reconsidered: Children's prospective life stories show a bump in young adulthood. *Psychological Science*, 22(2), 197–202

These data suggest that cultural expectations guide autobiographical memory. We remember more from certain parts of our lives because our culture says that they are more important.

Because most of the events in cultural life schemas are positive (e.g., going to college, getting, married, having a baby, etc.), this contributes to a bias for remembering more positive life events as time goes on (Berntsen & Rubin, 2002). Not surprisingly, this cultural life script account applies to events that are (largely) positive and expected (e.g., getting a first job), but not to surprising and negative events (which are unplanned). Surprising events are often set apart and do not show a reminiscence bump (Dickson et al., 2011).

Another source of support for life scripts is a study by Copeland et al. (2009; see also Koppel & Berntsen, 2014) in which people read a novel (*The Stone Diaries*, by Carol Shields). This book describes a person's entire life. When readers were tested for memory of the novel, a reminiscence bump was found, even though this was a story about someone else's life. Retrieval was guided by a cultural schema and not by first events, neurological development, or development of one's self-identity, all of which are impossible in this case.

Stop and Review

The reminiscence bump is better memory for life events around the age of 20 than would be expected by a normal forgetting curve. There are several factors that play into this. The cognitive factors involve unique and initial experiences. The biological factors involve people being at their neurological peak. The identity formation factors involve the development of one's self-identity. Finally, cultural schemas dictate how life is supposed to progress, and this influences what we remember from our lives.

WE'RE ALL IN THIS TOGETHER

Autobiographical memories are our memories for our life stories. However, we are not islands. We live in families, communities, and nations. These relations affect us. Here we consider group memories. We discuss these in terms of collective memories, living in history, and the cultural transmissions of memories from one generation to the next.

Collective Memory

Collective memories are shared by people in a group, such as a family, a community, or a nation (Hirst et al., 2018; Roediger & Abel, 2015). Collective memories are often for critical events, such as a terrorist attack, as well as more general semantic information about the group, such as its historical founding. This helps define the group's identity (Manier & Hirst, 2008). Collective memories can include wars, national leaders, or even sporting events (Bavassi et al., 2019; Roediger & DeSoto, 2014; Zaromb et al., 2014).

Collective memories show some of the same patterns seen with individual memories. For example, they show forgetting curves, serial position, and von Restorff effects (Roediger & DeSoto, 2014). As an example of a forgetting curve, a study by Fanta et al. (2019) was a historical review of living conditions after major floods. This survey indicated that, in terms of where people chose to live, people abide by memories of a horrific flood experience, but this dies out after a couple of generations.

When people hear public voices (e.g., politicians and journalists), information that they repeat results is retrieval practice that makes the information better remembered. That said, there is also retrieval induced forgetting for related information that is not mentioned (Yamashiro & Hirst, 2020). Collective experiences can be transition events in autobiographical memory, even if they do not directly impact a person (Gu et al., 2017). These may be flashbulb memories of public events. There are even collective future thinking phenomena. As one example, people generally have a more positive attitude of their nation's future than its past (Topcu & Hirst, 2019).

Living in History

Sometimes we live through momentous events that cause a great deal of upheaval, such as wars. This produces many transitions in the lives of those of us who experience those events and leads to better memory for those times, which is the **living-in-history effect** (Brown et al., 2009). This effect is more prominent for negative than positive events. For example, Bohn and Habermas (2016) found that older Germans showed a larger living-in-history effect for negative events, such as World War II, than for positive events, such as the fall of the Berlin Wall. Moreover, living-in-history effects may depend on who experiences them. For example, former East Germans who experienced the fall of the Berlin Wall are more likely to show a living-in-history effect than are former West Germans (Camia et al., 2019). Such traumatic events can lead to a reminiscence bump known as an *upheaval bump* (Brown et al., 2016).

Inter-Generational Memory Transmission

Our memories are also influenced by our parent's memories of their experiences through the stories that they tell us and how often they tell them (Svob & Brown, 2012). This influence is larger when the experiences that the parents went through were traumatic, such as directly encountering warfare (Svob et al., 2016). The intergenerational transmission of memories occurs through the stories that older generations tell younger generations. In can also occur formally, such as the creation of public moments of individuals and events.

More prosaically, Krumhansl and Zupnick (2013) found that when students at Cornell University were probed for memories of popular songs from various decades, there were reminiscence bumps for when people were around the age of 20, as well as another bump for when their parents were around the age of 20. The first bump is a normal reminiscence bump, and the second is due to repeatedly hearing their parents' music.

Stop and Review

Memories are held by groups of people. Collective memories come from shared experiences and discussions. They show many properties of individual memories. Sometimes collective memories are a result of living through historical upheavals, perhaps resulting in flashbulb memories. At other times, they are transmitted across generations through stories and monuments.

PUTTING IT ALL TOGETHER

Your life story is your autobiographical memory. We construct this story into a coherent narrative to tell ourselves and other people. Sometimes this story is recorded in a diary or autobiography, but more often, it is only in our heads and our conversations. Sometimes it is something you are deliberately trying to understand and convey, and other times, parts of the story involuntarily pop into our heads.

Your autobiographical memory is reconstructive and interpretive. It is made up of facts and inferences. Some of these are the general facts of your life, and some are the episodes and scenes from your experiences, the specific events, and general extended and repeated events. Parts of the story are also the general themes that run throughout, such as education, careers, personal relationships, and so on.

You do not assemble an autobiographical story for your own amusement, but to give purpose and meaning to your life. These are the reflective, social, ruminative, and generative functions. The life story you create varies with what you are trying to do at the moment. You can shift your perspective from the one you had at the time or to those of other people This reconstruction and these perspectives can be guided by current knowledge and biases, as well as a more stable understanding of the world from your scripts, schemas, and culture. These schemas can direct what parts of your life you favor and remember better than others. Part of the reason you will remember your late teens and early twenties better is because this is a time of your life when many things are changing and happening for the first time. Moreover, our culture tells us that it is where we should place our emphasis, and we remember more from that time than would otherwise be the case.

That said, autobiographical life stories do not always follow the expected path but take twists and turns in response to the unexpected and unusual events. Sometimes they are so surprising, emotional, and consequential that they seem to have been burned into your memory, as with flashbulb memories. It is an interesting story. Things happen. You react. Some things are good for you, and some of them are bad. While life has pain and suffering, it also has happiness and joy, fear and anger, love and hate. These emotions are a critical part of who you are, how you use autobiographical memory, and they make the story more engaging. Overall, as your autobiographical memory and story develops, the older material takes on a more positive spin. Your life gets better.

Finally, autobiographical memory is shaped by the groups that you belong to, including your family, schools, towns, nations, and so on. These collective memories provide aspects of your identity. They occur through collective experiences, perhaps by living through important moments in history, or by stories that younger generations hear from older generations.

STUDY QUESTIONS

1. In what ways are autobiographical memories like episodic memories? Like semantic memories?
2. How quickly can people retrieve autobiographical information? How does this compare to information learned in the lab? What does this tell us about autobiographical memories?
3. What are some special ways for assessing the autobiographical memories?
4. What are some of the major functions for autobiographical memory in mental life?
5. What are the three levels of autobiographical memory? What are their characteristics?
6. What sort of neurological evidence supports the idea that there are different levels of autobiographical memories?
7. In what ways is autobiographical memory like a story or narrative? How does this affect how autobiographical memories are remembered?
8. What are the two types of perspectives that that occur in an autobiographical memory? What sorts of factors influence which of these two occur?
9. What is better remembered from autobiographical memories, the schema consistent or inconsistent details? What theory accounts for this and how?
10. What role does emotion play in the creation and maintenance of autobiographical memories?
11. What are flashbulb memories? What causes them? How much are they like or unlike regular memories?
12. What is the reminiscence bump? Why does it occur?
13. How do collective memories contribute to our self-identities? Where does this collective knowledge come from?

KEY TERMS

- autobiographical memory
- collective memories
- cultural schemas
- diary studies
- event-specific memories
- fading affect bias
- field memories
- flashbulb memories
- Galton-Crovitz cue word method
- general events

- generative function
- involuntary memory
- life narrative
- life scripts
- lifetime periods
- living-in-history effect
- observer memories
- overgeneral memories
- Pollyanna principle
- positivity bias
- reflective function

- reminiscence bump
- ruminative function
- schema-copy-plus-tag model
- social function
- Transition Theory
- tunnel memory
- vicarious autobiographical memories

EXPLORE MORE

Here are some additional readings that so that you can more deeply explore topics in autobiographical memory.

Berntsen, D. (2009). *Involuntary Autobiographical Memories: An Introduction to the Unbidden Past.* Cambridge, UK: Cambridge University Press.

Bruner, J. (1991). The narrative construction of reality. *Critical Inquiry, 18,* 1–21.

Conway, M. A. (1996). Autobiographical memory. In E. L. Bjork & R. A. Bjork (Eds.), *Memory.* San Diego: Academic Press.

Fivush, R., & Haden, C. A. (Eds.). (2003). *Autobiographical Memory and the Construction of a Narrative Self: Developmental and Cultural Perspectives.* New York: Psychology Press.

Luminet, O., & Curci, A. (Eds.). (2008). *Flashbulb Memories: New Issues and New Perspectives.* New York: Psychology Press.

Radvansky, G. A., & Zacks, J. M. (2014). *Event Cognition.* Oxford: Oxford University Press.

REFERENCES

Anderson, R. J., & Dewhurst, S. A. (2009). Remembering the past and imagining the future: Differences in event specificity of spontaneously generated thought. *Memory, 17*(4), 367–373.

Anderson, S. J., & Conway, M. A. (1993). Investigating the structure of autobiographical memories. *Journal of Experimental Psychology: Learning, Memory, and Cognition, 19*(5), 1178–1196.

Anderson, S. J., & Conway, M. A. (1997). Representations of autobiographical memories. In M. A. Conway (Ed.), *Cognitive Models of Memory.* Cambridge, MA: MIT Press.

Barsalou, L. W. (1988). The contents and organization of autobiographical memories. In U. Neisser & E. Winograd (Eds.) *Remembering Reconsidered: Ecological and Traditional Approaches to the Study of Memory.* New York: Cambridge University Press.

Barzykowski, K., Riess, M., Hajdas, S., & Niedźwieńska, A. (2019). School in our memory: Do we remember our time in middle and high school differently? *Journal of Cognitive Psychology, 31*(4), 438–452.

Bavassi, L., Kaczer, L., & Fernández, R. S. (2019). Maradona in our minds: The FIFA World Cup as a way to address collective memory properties. *Memory & Cognition, 48*(8), 469–480.

Belfi, A. M., Karlan, B., & Tranel, D. (2016). Music evokes vivid autobiographical memories. *Memory, 24*(7), 979–989.

Berntsen, D. (1996). Involuntary autobiographical memories. *Applied Cognitive Psychology, 10,* 435–454.

Berntsen, D. (2001). Involuntary memories of emotional events: Do memories of traumas and extremely happy events differ? *Applied Cognitive Psychology, 15,* S135–S158.

Berntsen, D. (2002). Tunnel memories for autobiographical events: Central details are remembered more frequently from shocking than from happy experiences. *Memory & Cognition, 30*(7), 1010–1020.

Berntsen, D. (2009). *Involuntary Autobiographical Memories: An Introduction to the Unbidden Past.* Cambridge, UK: Cambridge University Press.

Berntsen, D. (2010). The unbidden past: Involuntary autobiographical memories as a basic mode of remembering. *Current Directions in Psychological Science, 19*(3), 138–142.

Berntsen, D., & Jacobsen, A. S. (2008). Involuntary (spontaneous) mental time travel into the past and future. *Consciousness and Cognition, 17*(4), 1093–1104.

Berntsen, D., & Rubin, D. C. (2002). Emotionally charged autobiographical memories across the life span: The recall of happy, sad, traumatic, and involuntary memories. *Psychology and Aging, 17,* 636–652.

Berntsen, D., & Rubin, D. C. (2004). Cultural life scripts structure recall from autobiographical memory. *Memory & Cognition, 32,* 427–442.

Berntsen, D., & Rubin, D. C. (2008). The reappearance hypothesis revisited: Recurrent involuntary memories after traumatic events and in everyday life. *Memory & Cognition, 36,* 449–460.

Berntsen, D., Staugaard, S. R., & Sørensen, L. M. T. (2013). Why am I remembering this now? Predicting the occurrence of involuntary (spontaneous) episodic memories. *Journal of Experimental Psychology: General, 142*(2), 426–444.

Bohn, A., & Berntsen, D. (2007). Pleasantness bias in flashbulb memories: Positive and negative flashbulb memories of the fall of the Berlin Wall among East and West Germans. *Memory & Cognition, 35,* 565–577.

Bohn, A., & Berntsen, D. (2011). The reminiscence bump reconsidered: Children's prospective life stories show a bump in young adulthood. *Psychological Science, 22*(2), 197–202.

Bohn, A., & Habermas, T. (2016). Living in history and living by the cultural life script: How older Germans date their autobiographical memories. *Memory, 24*(4), 482–495.

Bradley, M. M., Greenwald, M. K., Petry, M. C., & Lang, P. J. (1992). Remembering pictures: Pleasure and arousal in memory. *Journal of Experimental Psychology: Learning, Memory, and Cognition, 18,* 379–390.

Breslin, C. W., & Safer, M. A. (2011). Effects of event valence on long-term memory for two baseball championship games. *Psychological Science, 22*(11), 1408–1412.

Brown, N. R. (1990). Organization of public events in long-term memory. *Journal of Experimental Psychology: General, 119,* 297–314.

Brown, N. R., Lee, P. J., Krslak, M., Conrad, F. G., Hansen, T. G. B., Havelka, J., & Reddon, J. R. (2009). Living in history: How war, terrorism, and natural disaster affect the organization of autobiographical memory. *Psychological Science, 20*(4), 399–405.

Brown, N. R., & Schopflocher, D. (1998a). Event clusters: An organization of personal events in autobiographical memory. *Psychological Science, 9,* 470–475.

Brown, N. R., & Schopflocher, D. (1998b). Event cueing, event clusters, and the temporal distribution of autobiographical memories. *Applied Cognitive Psychology, 12,* 305–319.

Brown, N. R., Schweickart, O., & Svob, C. (2016). The effect of collective transitions on the organization and contents of autobiographical memory: A Transition Theory perspective. *American Journal of Psychology, 129*(3), 259–282.

Brown, R., & Kulik, J. (1977). Flashbulb memories. *Cognition, 5,* 73–99.

Bruner, J. (1991). The narrative construction of reality. *Critical Inquiry, 18,* 1–21.

Burt, C. D. B., Kemp, S., & Conway, M. A. (2003). Themes, events, and episodes in autobiographical memory. *Memory & Cognition, 31,* 317–325.

Burt, C. D. B., Watt, S. C., Mitchell, D. A., & Conway, M. A. (1998). Retrieving the sequence of autobiographical event components. *Applied Cognitive Psychology, 12,* 321–338.

Camia, C., Menzel, C., & Bohn, A. (2019). A positive Living-in-History effect: The case of the fall of the Berlin Wall. *Memory, 27*(10), 1381–1389.

Cason, H. (1932). The learning and retention of pleasant and unpleasant activities. *Archives of Psychology, 134,* 1–96.

Cermak, L. S., & O'Connor, M. (1983). The anterograde and retrograde retrieval ability of a patient with amnesia due to encephalitis. *Neuropsychologia, 21,* 213–234.

Chu, S., & Downes, J. J. (2002). Proust nose best: Odors are better cues of autobiographical memory. *Memory & Cognition, 30,* 511–518.

Colcombe, S. J., & Wyer, R. S. (2002). The role of prototypes in the mental representation of temporally related events. *Cognitive Psychology, 44,* 67–103.

Conway, M. A. (1990). Associations between autobiographical memories and concepts. *Journal of Experimental Psychology: Learning, Memory, and Cognition, 16,* 799–812.

Conway, M. A. (1996). Autobiographical memory. In E. L. Bjork & R. A. Bjork (Eds.), *Memory.* San Diego, CA: Academic Press.

Copeland, D. E., Radvansky, G. A., & Goodwin, K. A. (2009). A novel study: Forgetting curves and the reminiscence bump. *Memory, 17,* 323–336.

Crovitz, H. F., & Schiffman, H. (1974). Frequency of episodic memories as a function of their age. *Bulletin of the Psychonomic Society, 4*(5), 517–518.

Curci, A., Lanciano, T., Maddalena, C., Mastandrea, S., & Sartori, G. (2015). Flashbulb memories of the Pope's resignation: Explicit and implicit measures across differing religious groups. *Memory, 23*(4), 529–544.

D'Argembeau, A., & Demblon, J. (2012). On the representational systems underlying prospection: Evidence from the event-cueing paradigm. *Cognition, 125*(2), 160–167.

de Bruijn, M. J., & Bender, M. (2018). Olfactory cues are more effective than visual cues in experimentally triggering autobiographical memories. *Memory, 26*(4), 547–558.

Dickson, R. A., Pillemer, D. B., & Bruehl, E. C. (2011). The reminiscence bump for salient personal memories: Is a cultural life script required? *Memory & Cognition, 39*(6), 977–991.

Ebbinghaus, H. (1885). *Memory: A Contribution to Experimental Psychology* (H. A. Ruger & C. E. Bussenius, Trans.). New York: Teachers College, Columbia University.

Eldridge, M. A., Barnard, P. J., & Bekerian, D. A. (1994). Autobiographical memory and daily schemas at work. *Memory, 2,* 51–74.

El Haj, M., Nandrino, J. L., Antoine, P., Boucart, M., & Lenoble, Q. (2017). Eye movement during retrieval of emotional autobiographical memories. *Acta Psychologica, 174,* 54–58.

Ellis, A. W., Young, A. W., & Critchley, E. M. R. (1989). Loss of memory for people following temporal lobe damage. *Brain, 112,* 1469–1483.

Enz, K. F., Pillemer, D. B., & Johnson, K. M. (2016). The relocation bump: Memories of middle adulthood are organized around residential moves. *Journal of Experimental Psychology: General, 145*(8), 935–940.

Fanta, V., Šálek, M., & Sklenicka, P. (2019). How long do floods throughout the millennium remain in the collective memory? *Nature Communications, 10*(1), 1–9.

Finkenhauer, C., Luminet, O., Gisle, L., El-Ahmadi, A., van der Linden, M., & Philippot, P. (1998). Flashbulb memories and the underlying mechanisms of their formation: Toward an emotional–integrative model. *Memory & Cognition*, *26*, 516–531.

Graesser, A. C., & Nakamura, G. V. (1982). The impact of a schema on comprehension and memory. *The Psychology of Learning and Motivation*, *16*, 59–109.

Grenier, J., Cappeliez, P., St-Onge, M., Vachon, J., Vinette, S., Roussy, F., Mercier, P., Lortie-Lussier, M., & de Koninck, J. (2005). Temporal references in dreams and autobiographical memory. *Memory & Cognition*, *33*, 280–288.

Grysman, A., Fivush, R., Merrill, N. A., & Graci, M. (2016). The influence of gender and gender typicality on autobiographical memory across event types and age groups. *Memory & Cognition*, *44*(6), 856–868.

Gu, X., Tse, C. S., & Brown, N. R. (2017). The effects of collective and personal transitions on the organization and contents of autobiographical memory in older Chinese adults. *Memory & Cognition*, *45*(8), 1335–1349.

Hallford, D. J., Austin, D. W., Raes, F., & Takano, K. (2018). A test of the functional avoidance hypothesis in the development of overgeneral autobiographical memory. *Memory & Cognition*, *46*(6), 895–908.

Harris, C. B., Rasmussen, A. S., & Berntsen, D. (2014). The functions of autobiographical memory: An integrative approach. *Memory*, *22*(5), 559–581.

Hatiboğlu, N., & Habermas, T. (2016). The normativity of life scripts and its relation with life story events across cultures and subcultures. *Memory*, *24*(10), 1369–1381.

Herz, R. S. (2004). A naturalistic analysis of autobiographical memories triggered by olfactory, visual, and auditory stimuli. *Chemical Senses*, *29*, 217–224.

Hirst, W., & Phelps, E. A. (2016). Flashbulb memories. *Current Directions in Psychological Science*, *25*(1), 36–41.

Hirst, W., Phelps, E. A., Buckner, R. L., Budson, A. E., Cuc, A., Gabrieli, J. D. E., Johnson, M. K., Lustig, C., Lyle, K. B., Mather, M., Meksin, R., Mitchell, K. J., Ochsner, K. N., Schacter, D. L., Simons, J. S., & Vaidya, C. J. (2009). Long-term memory for the terrorist attack of September 11: Flashbulb memories, event memories, and the factors that influence their retention. *Journal of Experimental Psychology: General*, *138*, 161–176.

Hirst, W., Yamashiro, J. K., & Coman, A. (2018). Collective memory from a psychological perspective. *Trends in Cognitive Sciences*, *22*(5), 438–451.

Hodges, J. R., & McCarthy, R. A. (1993). Autobiographical amnesia resulting from bilateral paramedian thalamic infarction: A case study in cognitive neurobiology. *Brain*, *116*, 921–940.

Holmes, D. S. (1970). Differential change in affective intensity and the forgetting of unpleasant personal experiences. *Journal of Personality and Social Psychology*, *15*, 234–239.

Hornstein, S. L., Brown, A. S., & Mulligan, N. W. (2003). Long-term flashbulb memory for learning of Princess Diana's death. *Memory*, *11*, 293–306.

Jakubowski, K., Farrugia, N., Halpern, A. R., Sankarpandi, S. K., & Stewart, L. (2015). The speed of our mental soundtracks: Tracking the tempo of involuntary musical imagery in everyday life. *Memory & Cognition*, *43*(8), 1229–1242.

Janssen, S. M. J., Rubin, D. C., & Conway, M. A. (2012). The reminiscence bump in the temporal distribution of the best football players of all time: Pelé, Cruijff or Maradona? *Quarterly Journal of Experimental Psychology*, *65*(1), 165–178.

Kensinger, E. A. (2007). Negative emotion enhances memory accuracy: Behavioral and neuroimaging evidence. *Current Directions in Psychological Science*, *16*, 213–218.

Kintsch, W., & Bates, E. (1977). Recognition memory for statements from a classroom lecture. *Journal of Experimental Psychology: Human Learning and Memory*, *3*, 150–159.

Koppel, J., & Berntsen, D. (2014). The cultural life script as cognitive schema: How the life script shapes memory for fictional life stories. *Memory*, *22*(8), 949–971.

Koppel, J., & Berntsen, D. (2016). The reminiscence bump in autobiographical memory and for public events: A comparison across different cueing methods. *Memory*, *24*(1), 44–62.

Koppel, J., Brown, A. D., Stone, C. B., Coman, A., & Hirst, W. (2013). Remembering President Barack Obama's inauguration and the landing of US Airways Flight 1549: A comparison of the predictors of autobiographical and event memory. *Memory*, *21*(7), 798–806.

Koppel, J., & Rubin, D. C. (2016). Recent advances in understanding the reminiscence bump: The importance of cues in guiding recall from autobiographical memory. *Current Directions in Psychological Science, 25*(2), 135–140.

Kraha, A., & Boals, A. (2014). Why so negative? Positive flashbulb memories for a personal event. *Memory, 22*(4), 442–449.

Krumhansl, C. L., & Zupnick, J. A. (2013). Cascading reminiscence bumps in popular music. *Psychological Science, 24*(10), 2057–2068.

Kvavilashvili, L., & Mandler, G. (2004). Out of one's mind: A study of involuntary semantic memories. *Cognitive Psychology, 48*, 47–94.

Kvavilashvili, L., Mirani, J., Schlagman, S., Foley, K., & Kornbrot, D. E. (2009). Consistency of flashbulb memories of September 11 over long delays: Implications for consolidation and wrong time slice hypotheses. *Journal of Memory and Language, 61*(4), 556–572.

Lenoble, Q., Janssen, S. M. J., & El Haj, M. (2019). Don't stare, unless you don't want to remember: Maintaining fixation compromises autobiographical memory retrieval. *Memory, 27*(2), 231–238.

Lind, M., & Thomsen, D. K. (2018). Functions of personal and vicarious life stories: Identity and empathy. *Memory, 26*(5), 672–682.

Linton M. (1975). Memory for real-world events. In D. A. Norman & D. E. Rumelhart (Eds.) *Explorations in Cognition*, San Francisco, CA: Freeman.

Linton, M. (1982). Transformations of memory in everyday life. In U. Neisser (Ed.), *Memory Observed: Remembering in Natural Contexts*. San Francisco, CA: Freeman.

Luminet, O. (2009). Models for the formation of flashbulb memories. In O. Luminet & A. Curci (Eds.), *Flashbulb Memories: New Issues and New Perspectives* (pp. 51–76). New York: Psychology Press.

Mace, J. H., Clevinger, A. M., & Bernas, R. S. (2013). Involuntary memory chains: What do they tell us about autobiographical memory organisation? *Memory, 21*(3), 324–335.

Mace, J. H., & Unlu, M. (2019). The role of lifetime periods in the organisation of episodic memories. *Memory, 27*(8), 1167–1174.

Mahmood, D., Manier, D., & Hirst, W. (2004). Memory for how one learned of multiple deaths from AIDS: Repeated exposure and distinctiveness. *Memory & Cognition, 32*, 125–134.

Maki, Y., Kawasaki, Y., Demiray, B., & Janssen, S. M. J. (2015). Autobiographical memory functions in young Japanese men and women. *Memory, 23*(1), 11–24.

Manier, D., & Hirst, W. (2008). A cognitive taxonomy of collective memories. *Cultural memory Studies: An International and Interdisciplinary Handbook*, 253–262.

McAdams, D. P. (2001). The psychology of life stories. *Journal of General Psychology, 5*, 100–122.

McCarthy, R. A., & Warrington, E. K. (1992). Actors but not scripts: The dissociation of people and events in retrograde amnesia. *Neuropsychologia, 30*, 633–644.

McCloskey, M. Wible, C. G., & Cohen, N. J. (1988). Is there a special flashbulb-memory mechanism? *Journal of Experimental Psychology: General, 117*, 171–181.

McDermott, K. B., Wooldridge, C. L., Rice, H. J., Berg, J. J., & Szpunar, K. K. (2016). Visual perspective in remembering and episodic future thought. *Quarterly Journal of Experimental Psychology, 69*(2), 243–253.

McKay, D. G., & Ahmetzanov, M. V. (2005). Emotion, memory, and attention in the taboo Stroop paradigm: An experimental analogue of flashbulb memories. *Psychological Science, 16*, 25–32.

Meltzer, H. (1930). Individual differences in forgetting pleasant and unpleasant experiences. *Journal of Educational Psychology, 21*, 399–409.

Metternich, B., Spanhel, K., Schoendube, A., Ofer, I., Geiger, M. J., Schulze-Bonhage, A., Mast, H., & Wagner, K. (2020). Flashbulb memory recall in healthy adults–a functional magnetic resonance imaging study. *Memory, 28*(4), 461–472.

Nadel, L., & Jacobs, W. J. (1998). Traumatic memory is special. *Current Directions in Psychological Science, 7*(5), 154–157.

Niedźwieńska, A. (2003). Misleading postevent information and flashbulb memories. *Memory, 11*(6), 549–558.

Neisser, U. (1982). Snapshots or benchmarks? In U. Neisser (Ed.), *Memory Observed: Remembering in Natural Contexts* (pp. 43–48). San Francisco, CA: Freeman.

Nigro, G., & Neisser, U. (1983). Point of view in personal memories. *Cognitive Psychology, 15,* 467–482.

Nile, E., & Van Bergen, P. (2015). Not all semantics: Similarities and differences in reminiscing function and content between Indigenous and non-Indigenous Australians. *Memory, 23*(1), 83–98.

Panattoni, K., & Thomsen, D. K. (2018). My partner's stories: Relationships between personal and vicarious life stories within romantic couples. *Memory, 26*(10), 1416–1429.

Pillemer, D. B. (2001). Momentous events and the life story. *Journal of General Psychology, 5,* 123–134.

Pillemer, D. B. (2009). "Hearing the news" versus "being there": Comparing flashbulb memories and recall of first hand experiences. In O. Luminet & A. Curci (Eds.), *Flashbulb Memories: New Issues and New Perspectives* (pp. 125–140). New York: Psychology Press.

Radvansky, G. A., & Svob, C. (2019). Observer memories may not be for everyone. *Memory, 27*(5), 647–659.

Rathbone, C. J., Moulin, C. J. A., & Conway, M. A. (2008). Self-centered memories: The reminiscence bump and the self. *Memory & Cognition, 36,* 1403–1414.

Reid, C. A., Green, J. D., Wildschut, T., & Sedikides, C. (2015). Scent-evoked nostalgia. *Memory, 23*(2), 157–166.

Roediger, H. L., & Abel, M. (2015). Collective memory: a new arena of cognitive study. *Trends in Cognitive Sciences, 19*(7), 359–361.

Roediger, H. L., & DeSoto, K. A. (2014). Forgetting the presidents. *Science, 346*(6213), 1106–1109

Rubin, D. C. (1998). Knowledge and judgments about events that occurred prior to birth: The measurement of the persistence of information. *Psychonomic Bulletin & Review, 5,* 397–400.

Rubin, D. C. (2006). The basic-systems model of episodic memory. *Perspectives on Psychological Science, 1,* 277–311.

Rubin, D. C., & Berntsen, D. (2003). Life scripts help to maintain autobiographical memories of highly positive, but not highly negative, events. *Memory & Cognition, 31,* 1–14.

Rubin, D. C., Berntsen, D., Deffler, S. A., & Brodar, K. (2019a). Self-narrative focus in autobiographical events: The effect of time, emotion, and individual differences. *Memory & Cognition, 47*(1), 63–75.

Rubin, D. C., Deffler, S. A., & Umanath, S. (2019b). Scenes enable a sense of reliving: Implications for autobiographical memory. *Cognition, 183,* 44–56.

Rubin, D. C., Groth, E., & Goldsmith, D. J. (1984). Olfactory cuing of autobiographical memory. *American Journal of Psychology, 97,* 493–507.

Rubin, D. C., Rahhal, T. A., & Poon, L. W. (1998). Things learned in early adulthood are remembered best. *Memory & Cognition, 26,* 3–19.

Safer, M. A., Christianson, S. Å., Autry, M. W., & Österlund, K. (1998). Tunnel memory for traumatic events. *Applied Cognitive Psychology, 12,* 99–117.

Schmidt, S. R. (2004). Autobiographical memories for the September 11th attacks: Reconstructive errors and emotional impairment of memory. *Memory & Cognition, 32,* 443–454.

Schmolck, H., Buffalo, E. A., & Squire, L. R. (2000). Memory distortions over time: Recollections of the O. J. Simpson trial verdict after 15 and 32 months. *Psychological Science, 11,* 39–45.

Schrauf, R. W., & Rubin, D. C. (1998). Bilingual autobiographical memory in older adult immigrants: A test of cognitive explanations of the reminiscence bump and the linguistic encoding of memories. *Journal of Memory and Language, 39,* 437–457.

Schulkind, M., Rahhal, T. A., Klein, M. R., & Lacher, S. R. (2012a). The specificity and organisation of autobiographical memories. *Memory, 20*(8), 923–934.

Schulkind, M., Schoppel, K., & Scheiderer, E. (2012b). Gender differences in autobiographical narratives: He shoots and scores; she evaluates and interprets. *Memory & Cognition, 40*(6), 958–965.

Sedikides, C., & Skowronski, J. J. (2020). In human memory, good can be stronger than bad. *Current Directions in Psychological Science, 29*(1), 86–91.

Siedlecki, K. L. (2015). Visual perspective in autobiographical memories: Reliability, consistency, and relationship to objective memory performance. *Memory, 23*(2), 306–316.

Skowronski, J. J., Walker, W. R., Henderson, D. X., & Bond, G. D. (2014). The fading affect bias: Its history, its implications, and its future. *Advances in Experimental Social Psychology, 49*, 163–218.

Steiner, K. L., Pillemer, D. B., Thomsen, D. K., & Minigan, A. P. (2014). The reminiscence bump in older adults' life story transitions. *Memory, 22*(8), 1002–1009.

Svob, C., & Brown, N. R. (2012). Intergenerational transmission of the reminiscence bump and biographical conflict knowledge. *Psychological Science, 23*(11), 1404–1409.

Svob, C., Brown, N. R., Takšić, V., Katulić, K., & Žauhar, V. (2016). Intergenerational transmission of historical memories and social-distance attitudes in post-war second-generation Croatians. *Memory & Cognition, 44*(6), 846–855.

Szőllősi, Á., Keresztes, A., Conway, M. A., & Racsmány, M. (2015). A diary after dinner: How the time of event recording influences later accessibility of diary events. *Quarterly Journal of Experimental Psychology, 68*(11), 2119–2124.

Talarico, J. M., LaBar, K. S., & Rubin, D. C. (2004). Emotional intensity predicts autobiographical memory experience. *Memory & Cognition, 32*, 1118–1132.

Talarico, J. M., & Rubin, D. C. (2003). Confidence, not consistency, characterizes flashbulb memories. *Psychological Science, 14*, 455–461.

Tekcan, A. İ., Boduroglu, A., Mutlutürk, A., & Erciyes, A. A. (2017). Life-span retrieval of public events: Reminiscence bump for high-impact events, recency for others. *Memory & Cognition, 45*(7), 1095–1112.

Tekcan, A. I., Ece, B., Gülgöz, S., & Er, N. (2003). Autobiographical and event memory for 9/11: Changes across one year. *Applied Cognitive Psychology, 17*, 1057–1066.

Topcu, M. N., & Hirst, W. (2019). Remembering a nation's past to imagine its future: The role of event specificity, phenomenology, valence, and perceived agency. *Journal of Experimental Psychology: Learning, Memory, and Cognition, 46*(3), 563–579.

Tulving, E., Schacter, D. L., McLachlan, D. R., & Moscovitch, M. (1988). Priming of semantic autobiographical knowledge: A case study of retrograde amnesia. *Brain and Cognition, 8*, 3–20.

Vannucci, M., Pelagatti, C., Chiorri, C., & Mazzoni, G. (2016). Visual object imagery and autobiographical memory: Object Imagers are better at remembering their personal past. *Memory, 24*(4), 455–470.

Wagenaar, W. A. (1986). My memory: A study of autobiographical memory over six years. *Cognitive Psychology, 18*, 225–252.

Walker, W. R., Skowronski, J. J., & Thompson, C. P. (2003). Life is pleasant—and memory helps keep it that way! *Review of General Psychology, 7*, 203–210.

Wang, Q. (2013). Gender and emotion in everyday event memory. *Memory, 21*(4), 503–511.

Weems, C. F., Russell, J. D., Banks, D. M., Graham, R. A., Neill, E. L., & Scott, B. G. (2014). Memories of traumatic events in childhood fade after experiencing similar less stressful events: Results from two natural experiments. *Journal of Experimental Psychology: General, 143*(5), 2046–2055.

Westmacott, R., & Moscovitch, M. (2003). The contribution of autobiographical significance to semantic memory. *Memory & Cognition, 31*, 761–774.

White, R. (2002). Memory for events after twenty years. *Applied Cognitive Psychology, 16*(5), 603–612.

Whitten, W. B., & Leonard, J. M. (1981). Directed search through autobiographical memory. *Memory & Cognition, 9*(6), 566–579.

Willander, J., & Larsson, M. (2006). Smell your way back to childhood: Autobiographical odor memory. *Psychonomic Bulletin & Review, 13*, 240–244.

Willander, J., Sikström, S., & Karlsson, K. (2015). Multimodal retrieval of autobiographical memories: Sensory information contributes differently to the recollection of events. *Frontiers in Psychology, 6:* 1681.

Williams, J. M. G., Barnhofer, T., Crane, C., Herman, D., Raes, F., Watkins, E., & Dalgleish, T. (2007). Autobiographical memory specificity and emotional disorder. *Psychological Bulletin, 133*(1), 122–148.

Yamashiro, J. K., & Hirst, W. (2020). Convergence on collective memories: Central speakers and distributed remembering. *Journal of Experimental Psychology: General, 140*(3), 463–481.

Zaragoza Scherman, A., Salgado, S., Shao, Z., & Berntsen, D. (2015). Event centrality of positive and negative autobiographical memories to identity and life story across cultures. *Memory, 23*(8), 1152–1171.

Zaromb, F., Butler, A. C., Agarwal, P. K., & Roediger, H. L. (2014). Collective memories of three wars in United States history in younger and older adults. *Memory & Cognition, 42*(3), 383–399.

CHAPTER 13

Memory and Reality

O ur memory is our contact with the world beyond the present. We make assessments about the nature of reality, how it works, and what has happened in the past, based on what we remember. Most of the time our memories are fairly accurate, and we get along fine. However, other times, what we remember and what happened may differ. For example, if you misremember that you turned off the oven before you left for vacation, when in reality you left it on, you risk burning down your house, or at least a much larger utility bill. What are the circumstances that cause memory and reality to part ways?

In this chapter we discuss several factors related to how memory and reality square up. The first issue is how we keep track of where our memories come from, or source monitoring, which includes unconscious plagiarism, or cryptomnesia, and false fame effects. We also examine the sleeper effect and how this affects our attitudes and opinions. We then move on to cases where we remember things that never happened, called false memories. This includes implanted memories and those recovered under hypnosis. Finally, we look at how the normal use of information in memory can change it, as with verbal overshadowing, the revelation effect, and memory blending.

SOURCE MONITORING

Many of the issues that we have seen so far have been on what a memory is about. While this is important, another critical factor is knowing *where* a memory came from. For example, was a story on the news or from a friend? Was it all just a dream? The ability to keep track of where memories come from is **source monitoring**,[1] and it involves processes over and above those used to assess whether something is old or new (Johnson et al., 1993; 1994). However, as complex as it is, source monitoring does not require conscious awareness of the original source. Accurate source judgments are regularly made using vague and partial information associated with feelings of familiarity (Meissner et al., 2002).

---

1 A related phenomenon is **destination memory**, our ability to remember to whom we have told things (Gopie & MacLeod, 2009). Note also that changing the color of a word or background, or other such manipulation, is a change in item features or context, not a manipulation of source.

Source monitoring requires people to integrate source and content information into a common memory. Later, there is an active search of memory for source information. This involves different parts of the brain. The integration of information involves the hippocampus. In comparison, the search for source information, being a controlled memory process, involves the anterior prefrontal cortex (BA 10) and posterior hippocampal activities (Davachi et al., 2003; Simons et al., 2017), whereas the retrieval of that information emphasizes the temporal lobes (Senkfor & Van Petten, 1998), as well as the parietal lobes when there is conscious recollection (Leynes & Phillips, 2008).

Types of Source Information

Different types of information are used to evaluate the source of a memory. People can make fairly accurate judgments based only on partial or unconscious information (Hicks et al., 2002). One type is **perceptual detail**. This is perceptual information that is encoded into a memory, such as what you were looking at or hearing at the time. Memories for events that were experienced often have more perceptual detail than those created from hearing about an event from someone else or imagining it. For example, we find it easier to discriminate between words we actually said versus words that we only imagined being said. The difference in perceptual experiences in these two cases is pronounced. However, we find it harder to remember words that another person actually said versus "hearing" the words in our minds as if they were spoken by that person (Johnson et al., 1988). This is because they have similar perceptual or pseudoperceptual qualities.

We also use **contextual information** about the situation in which a memory was acquired. For example, if we remember seeing a plane crash while we were at an airport, it is more likely that the event was witnessed. However, if we remember seeing the plane crash while we were sitting in the living room, it is more likely that it was seen on the news. Thus, we can use expectancies based on context to help make source monitoring decisions (Bayen et al., 2000).

Overall, we better remember a source when it is an expected source than if it is from an unexpected source, suggesting that some guessing is involved (Bayen et al., 2000). These expectancy influences are more likely to operate at retrieval than at encoding (Hicks & Cockman, 2003). For example, it is easier to recall that a reminder to call your mother came from your sister than from your professor because the first is more expected, even if the second were true.

A third type of source information is the amount of **semantic detail** and/or **affective information** available. This is how much we were mentally and emotionally involved in events. This can include thoughts that we have (e.g., "Man, Bob must really be stupid to ask if gravity's getting heavier") or emotional reactions (e.g., "I remember feeling really queasy when I saw what the car accident had done to that girl's face"). Such information can help you figure out where a memory came from. Source information is less likely to be bound to emotional memories (Cook et al., 2007), perhaps because in emotional events we tend to focus attention on the central object and less on the context or source. This is less true if source information provides insight into misbehaving people, such as if they are cheaters (Bell et al., 2012), as shown in Figure 13.1.

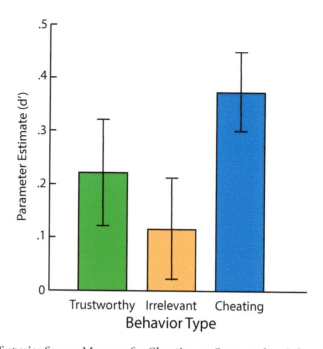

FIGURE 13.1 *Superior Source Memory for Cheating as Compared to Other Behaviors*

Source: adapted from Bell, R., Buchner, A., Erdfelder, E., Giang, T., Schain, C., & Riether, N. (2012). How specific is source memory for faces of cheaters? Evidence for categorical emotional tagging. *Journal of Experimental Psychology: Learning, Memory, and Cognition, 38*(2), 457–472

A final type of source information is **cognitive operations**, the mental processes done when first thinking about information. This includes retrieving information from long-term memory, manipulating it, trying to generate a mental image, and so on. This is more likely to be present in memories of things that were only thought about. When we think about things, we not only remember what we were thinking about, but also the mental activity that we used to generate those ideas. For example, if you were trying to remember something your significant other said in the middle of an argument, you might think was this (1) a real argument or (2) something you imagined he or she said when you could not talk directly to him or her (most people seem to be brilliant at winning these arguments). An imaginary argument would involve more cognitive operations. Source memory may sometimes show a generation effect (see Chapter 3) and be better for information that people generated (because of the stored cognitive operations) compared to something that was simply read (Geghman & Multhaup, 2004).

Types of Source Monitoring

There are three types of source monitoring (Johnson et al., 1993): internal source monitoring, external source monitoring, and reality monitoring. Table 13.1 provides a summary of each to help orient you.

TABLE 13.1 *Types of Source Monitoring and How They Relate to Different Types of Source Information*

Type	Perceptual Detail	Contextual Information	Semantic Detail	Emotional Reactions	Cognitive Operations
Internal	+	+	−	−	−
External	+	+	+	+	−
Reality	+	+	+	+	+

Source: Generated from information reported in Johnson, M. K., Hashtroudi, S., & Lindsay, D. S. (1993). Source monitoring. *Psychological Bulletin*, *114*(1), 3–28.

Internal source monitoring involves distinguishing between actions we either thought about or actually did. People trying to remember if they locked the back door before going on vacation, are engaged in internal source monitoring. Perceptual detail is important here because actions actually done have more perceptual details in memory (e.g., remembering seeing the key turning in the lock), whereas events that were only thought about have fewer. A similar point can be made for context. Semantic detail and emotional reactions are low because these actions were generated by people and so are unlikely to be reacted to. Finally, cognitive operations are high in both because people plan to carry out an action. The question is whether it was actually done.

As an example of internal source monitoring, Foster and Garry (2012) had students at Victoria University of Wellington assemble a toy vehicle by following a plan. During the assembly, the participants did some steps but not others. Those steps not taken were done by an experimenter while the student's eyes were closed. What is interesting is that people were more likely to make internal source monitoring errors when they could see all of the pieces laid out during building than when they only saw the pieces they needed for the current step. The additional perceptual information of consistently seeing the pieces and imaging how they would be assembled increased the possibility of an internal source monitor error.

A second type of source monitoring is **external source monitoring**, in which people distinguish between two external sources. Who told you this, Susan or John? Did you read about this on a website or a supermarket tabloid? Here, perceptual detail is important because different external sources have different perceptual details (e.g., a man's or a woman's voice). Contextual information is also informative. For example, imagine deciding which of two people told you something. If you always see one person in your neighborhood and the other on campus, then knowing where you heard it can help you narrow it down. Semantic detail and emotional reactions can be used similarly. Finally, because the information is coming from outside of us, cognitive operations are low and not very informative. Another factor is whether a source was involved in the described event. For example, you might hear about a train wreck from someone who was on the train or from a news reporter. In general, we more accurately remember sources when we were involved in the event (de Pereyra et al., 2014).

Reality monitoring (Johnson & Raye, 1981) involves distinguishing between memories of events that happened and those that were only imagined. For example, did witnesses to a car accident see broken glass, or did they only hear someone speak of broken glass later? It is more common for people to mistakenly think they saw things that were only imagined than the reverse (Henkel, 2012). Note also that people are also less likely to make reality monitoring errors for emotionally charged information (Kensinger & Schacter, 2006).

Perceptual detail is important for reality monitoring. Real events have more perceptual details than imagined events. Moreover, real event memories have more contextual information than imagined events. Semantic detail and emotional reactions are more developed in memories of real events. Lastly, knowledge about cognitive operations is scarcer for real events than for imagined events. Still, reality monitoring errors do occur. For example, in a study by Intraub and Hoffman (1992), a week after viewing photographs and reading descriptions of scenes, people frequently mistook pictures of scenes that they had only read about as having been seen, but rarely the reverse.

SOURCE MONITORING ERRORS

Source monitoring is pertinent for this chapter because source information grounds our memories in reality. We are reasonably accurate about knowing where our knowledge came from. However, errors can be made. For example, repeated attempts to remember, which can produce reminiscence and hypermnesia, can also increase the likelihood of confusing an imagined event for a real one (Henkel, 2004). This is because the repeated retrievals of imagined information may introduce perception-like qualities to the memory (through the process of imagination) and make a memory seem more like something that actually happened.

When source monitoring errors occur, people's understanding of the world and what actually happened are at odds. As one example, for an error in internal source monitoring, people believe they had done something that was not actually done. As an example, people may believe that they read some fact about a president of the United States in a history book, when in reality, they had watched a historical movie.

Source misattributions can be biased to make ourselves look good. In a study of choice making (Mather et al., 2000), people had to pick between two alternatives—for example, which of two people they would go out with on a blind date. Several characteristics of each person were given. Some were positive (e.g., "always interesting to talk to") and others were negative (e.g., "awkward in social situations such as parties"). Later, people identified which characteristics belonged to each dating prospect. People tended to misremember positive characteristics of the other choice as belonging to the one they picked and, to misremember negative attributes of the person they picked as belonging to the person they rejected. This does not occur when options are assigned rather than chosen (Mather et al., 2003). Thus, our choices can distort our memories. We tend to think of the things we choose as being more positive than they are and the things we do not choose as being more negative than they are.

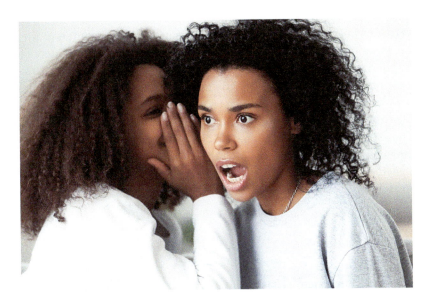

PHOTO 13.1 *Source monitoring is an important part of how we use our memories. We not only need to know the "what" of memory content, but also the "from where." For example, if you know a secret, it would be a god idea to know from whom that secret came in order to avoid embarrassment*

Source: fizkes/shutterstock.com

TRY IT OUT

This Try It Out section is for assessing source monitoring. As a reminder, there are three basic types of source monitoring: internal, external, and reality monitoring. You can do whichever version you find the most interesting.

First, create a list of 40 five- to seven-letter two-syllable nouns. Then, randomly assign these words to two conditions that we will call A and B. Have 12–24 people go through the list, presenting the words in one of the three ways described below. At the end of the list, give people a distractor task to do for five–ten minutes to occupy their time. For example, you could have them solve math problems to help allow some forgetting to occur. At the end of the distractor period, give your participants the entire list of 40 words and have them indicate from which source the word originated. After you collect your data, average the number of correct responses for each source type. What you should find is that people make source monitoring errors.

For *internal source monitoring*, have people read 20 of the words out loud, and have them read 20 of the words silently to themselves. For the memory test, have people indicate whether the words were said or just imagined. Most of the source monitoring errors should be cases where people say that words they only imagined were actually said.

For *external source monitoring* you will need two experimenters (if they are of the same gender, then that is even better). Have the experimenters taking alternating turns reading the words aloud, with one person reading 20 words and the other reading the rest. For the memory test, have participants indicate which words were said by which person.

For *reality monitoring*, as the experimenter, read 20 of the words aloud, and have your participants imagine the other 20 words being said in your voice. For the memory test, have them indicate whether the words were said or just imagined. Most of the source monitoring errors should be people reporting that words they only imagined were actually said.

Cryptomnesia

Knowing where information comes from can have important consequences. For example, it is important to know whether an idea is your own or someone else's. When we present someone else's idea as our own, this is plagiarism, which is bad. However, not all plagiarism is intentional. Some plagiarism is unconscious and unintentional. It occurs when people come up with ideas that they believe are their own but in fact were encountered in the past. This unconscious plagiarism is **cryptomnesia** (Gingerich & Sullivan, 2013). One theory of cryptomnesia is that it is a reality monitoring error. People retain the content information, but after some time has passed, and/or because little attention was paid during encoding, the source memory is weak and has no influence. Memories of plagiarized ideas have similar phenomenological characteristics as accurate memories. Consequently, the feeling of familiarity produced by a plagiarized memory only boosts people's confidence in the idea. (Brédart et al., 2003).

Another way that source monitoring errors produce cryptomnesia is by having people take existing ideas and elaborate or improve on them (Stark & Perfect, 2006). For example, people might try to think of novel uses for an object, like a brick. Then, during an elaboration phase, people try to improve on ideas, both their own and those of other people. After elaborating, there are now memories for cognitive operations associated with each idea, and another person's idea seems more like something people would have thought of themselves, rather than something that was heard from someone else. Cryptomnesia gets worse the more people elaborate on an idea (Stark & Perfect, 2008). This is why people working in groups where everyone is generating ideas and trying to improve on each other's ideas may later lead to people misremembering which ideas were generated by other people, and thus lead to cryptomnesia.

False Fame

A powerful way to manipulate memory is to influence the frequency that something is encountered. Information that is repeatedly encountered is more likely to be remembered, and may be overlearned and chronically available (see Chapter 7). However, different memory components are forgotten at different rates. Information content may be remembered for a long time, but source knowledge may be lost. People may need to reconstruct this missing information perhaps by assessing how familiar a memory seems. A source monitoring error that is familiarity-based is the **false fame effect** (Jacoby et al., 1989a). This is the tendency to think that people are famous, or more famous than they really are, because their names are familiar. With the false fame effect it may be possible to take people who have utterly no fame whatsoever and make them "famous" overnight. This is done using the principle of mere exposure (see Chapter 6).

To study the false fame effect, a researcher might give people a list of names. Some names are of people who were mildly famous. These are names that most students might recognize but could not quite remember who they are. The other names are not famous, such as Sebastian Wiesdorf, Larry Jacoby, or Gabriel Radvansky. The task is to go through the list and pick out who is famous and who is not. Later, people would be given a new list of names consisting of famous people, nonfamous people whose names were seen before, and new nonfamous names. Half of the people would be given this new list immediately after the first, but the other half are given the list on the next day. People who got the second list the next day are twice as likely to call nonfamous people famous simply because they had seen those names earlier but forgotten where they saw them. Thus, those names became famous overnight!

This false fame effect can occur if people are distracted during encoding by another task (such as listening to a series of numbers, waiting for three odd numbers in a row) (Jacoby et al., 1989b). Because a name is familiar, people say that it is famous. The link between memory content and source is disconnected (Steffens et al., 2000). There is an unconscious influence of prior memories (this name was encountered before) on conscious efforts to make a decision (is this name famous?). This is one reason why some people say that there is no such thing as bad publicity. People may remember that they have encountered a name before but not why. The more times a name is seen or heard, the more familiar it is, and the more famous and likable that person seems. (It is not a good idea to overdo it. Eventually people can connect the unflattering information with a name, as with the name Hitler.)

Social Influences and the Sleeper Effect

Memory for source can also be affected by social factors, such as stereotypes. When asked to remember from whom a set of statements came, people may misattribute statements to people based on social stereotypes (Bayen et al., 2000). For example, people are more likely to attribute the statement "I'll come talk to you as soon as I wash up" to a doctor and the statement "I had a deposition yesterday" to a lawyer, even if the opposite was true.

A phenomenon in social psychology that involves source monitoring is the **sleeper effect** (see Kumkale & Albarracín, 2003). This occurs when people hear some propaganda from a source of either high or low credibility. A high credibility

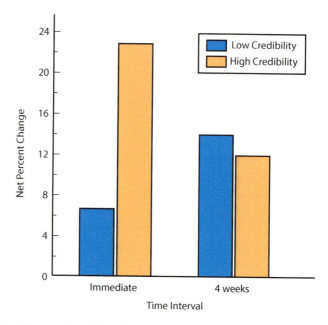

FIGURE 13.2 *An Illustration of the Sleeper Effect*

Source: adapted from Hovland, C. I., & Weiss, W. (1951). The influence of source credibility on communication effectiveness. *Public Opinion Quarterly, 15,* 635–650

source might be scientist, and a low credibility source might be a member of the Ku Klux Klan. If the source has low credibility, then people initially discount it. However, after a few days, weeks, or months, people remember the information but now consider it more credible than before. What previously seemed unreasonable has, with the simple passage of time, become reasonable (Hovland & Weiss, 1951). The sleeper effect is shown in Figure 13.2 which conveys how much attitudes towards ideas changed after hearing opinions from high and low credibility sources, both immediately and after a four-week delay. The sleeper effect occurs when source information in memory becomes disconnected from the content. As a result, people are more willing to accept ideas because they no longer have the source information that would make it suspect (Underwood & Pezdek, 1998).

Several components must be in place to observe a sleeper effect. First, people must pay attention to the message to set up a memory trace of the content. Second, the message source should be discounted after the message was given, preventing people from discounting the message during encoding. Finally, people should evaluate the trustworthiness of the source immediately afterward. This provides time for the source information to be forgotten (Pratkanis et al., 1988).

A related finding is the **wishful thinking bias**, which is a tendency to misremember desirable information as having come from reliable sources and undesirable information as having come from unreliable sources (Gordon et al., 2005). This is especially true for things that have implications for yourself (Barber et al., 2009). For example, if you hear someone say about you, "Boy, she is really smart," you are more likely to misremember this as having been said by a reliable source, such as your professor, as compared to a less reliable source, such as your bus driver, even if the opposite is true. This is even more likely because it was a positive statement about you and not someone else. The opposite is true for negative statements.

Stop and Review

In addition to remembering information content, it is helpful to know where memories came from. This is source monitoring. People use various types of information to make source memory decisions. This can include perceptual details and contextual information in the memory, semantic details and affective responses, as well as any cognitive operations about what they were thinking at the time the memory was created. Source monitoring includes discriminating between multiple external sources, whether one thought something or actually did it (internal), or if some event actually happened or was just thought about (reality). Although we are reasonably accurate at source monitoring, errors can occur, as with unconscious plagiarism (cryptomnesia), false fame, and sleeper effects. In all these cases, we remember the content information but forget from where it originated.

FALSE MEMORIES

An important issue is that people sometimes "remember" things that never happened. These are **false memories**. Sometimes false memories can cause serious problems. A good example of this is erroneous information from eyewitness testimony.

Deese–Roediger–McDermott (DRM) Paradigm

A simple way to create false memories is by using a word list-learning paradigm. This paradigm, regularly used by memory researchers, is commonly known as the **DRM paradigm**, after the first researchers to use it, namely Deese (1959) and Roediger and McDermott (1995). First, people hear a list of words, such as those in Table 13.2. Then, they try to recall those words. Of course, people typically recall only some of the list. The interesting thing is that people often systematically misremember words that were not on the list. For example, for the list in Table 13.2, people often mistakenly say that they heard the word "sleep" even though it was not there (Gallo, 2010). This process of creating false memories can occur in as little as four seconds (Atkins & Reuter-Lorenz, 2008), suggesting that we create false memories as we actively comprehend the world around us.

Over time, DRM false memories stay with us. They may even be more durable than memories of studied words. This can be seen in the data from a study by Thapar and McDermott (2001) shown in Figure 13.3. While the rate of recalling particular words declines in both cases, the rate of change is greater for words that were actually heard. This difference may happen because the critical false word

TABLE 13.2 *Words that May Lead to a False Memory for the Word "Sleep"*

bed	doze
rest	slumber
awake	snore
tired	nap
dream	peace
wake	yawn
snooze	drowsy
blanket	

Source: adapted from Roediger, H. L., & McDermott, K. B. (1995). Creating false memories: Remembering words not presented in lists. *Journal of experimental psychology: Learning, Memory, and Cognition, 21*(4), 803–814

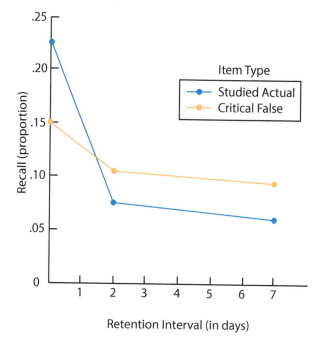

FIGURE 13.3 *Changes in the Rate of Giving False Memories in the DRM Paradigm for Both Actually Studied and Critical False Words*

Source: generated from data reported in Thapar, A., & McDermott, K. (2001). False recall and false recognition induced by presentation of associated words: Effects of retention interval and level of processing. *Memory & Cognition, 29*(3), 424–432

is strongly related to all the other words that were heard. This larger number of semantic associations may lead it to be reported over longer periods of time.

False memories occur more frequently when they are plausible. People are likely to misremember the word "sleep" because all the other words in the list are strongly associated with "sleep" (Cann et al., 2011). These false memories are guided by how many associations in semantic memory there are between the words that were actually seen (the more the better), as well as the general recallability of the actual list words (the fewer the better) (Roediger et al., 2001). A larger number of associations makes it more likely that a false memory word will be primed or unconsciously activated. The less recallable the actual items are, the more likely people will do some guessing or memory reconstruction, making it more likely that a false memory item will be "remembered." These false memories are based on partial information (Heit et al., 2004). For example, people may misremember the source (it was thought about but not heard) or may use more gist than verbatim memories (Brainerd et al., 2001; 2003).

Because memories for pictures are more detailed and less gist oriented, they are less likely to show this effect (Hege & Dodson, 2004). People are also less likely to have DRM false memories if the speaker has a foreign accent which presumably focuses attention more on perceptual qualities, making it less likely that a false memory will be generated (Romero-Rivas et al., 2019).

TRY IT OUT

For an assessment of false memories, you can do a DRM study. First generate lists of 15 words each that have an unmentioned word with which all the others have a strong association. You can use the sleep list shown in Table 13.2 or one of the other three lists provided below. For even more lists you can go to the library and look up Roediger and McDermott's (1995) paper, which has an appendix at the end with several lists of this type.

Once you have your lists of words, read aloud to people each list of 15 words. Read these words one at a time at a rate of about one word per second. When you are done reading, give each of your participants a sheet of paper. For each list have people try to recall as many words as they can remember by writing them down on the paper. This can be done individually or in groups, but you should have at least 24 participants.

After the participants are done recalling, go on to the next list. Once they have gone through all the lists, collect their response sheets. From the response sheets get the proportion of the words that were actually heard that were remembered later. You may also want to keep track of where on the original list the words that were actually remembered came from. Were they from the beginning of the list, the middle, or the end? Also, tabulate the number of false memories that occurred. That is, determine the proportion of the lists that resulted in people reporting a false memory. You might also want to keep track of what part of their recall output the false memory was reported in. Was it near the beginning, in the middle, or near the end? What you should find is that most of these false memories occurred towards the end.

Bread: butter, food, eat, sandwich, rye, jam, milk, flour, jelly, dough, crust, slice, wine, loaf, toast

Needle: thread, pin, eye, sewing, sharp, point, prick, thimble, haystack, thorn, hurt, injection, syringe, cloth, knitting

Soft: hard, light, pillow, plush, loud, cotton, fur, touch, fluffy, feather, furry, downy, kitten, skin, tender

This DRM false memory effect is supported by ERP measures. At encoding when there will be later false memories, the neural ERP signal suggests that during encoding people are paying less attention to the details of the real information (Urbach et al., 2005). Moreover, fMRI recordings have found that false memories are associated with more activity in brain areas used for mental images (see a description of imagery inflation later), particularly the anterior cingulate cortex (BA 24), precuneus (BA 7), and right inferior parietal lobe (BA 40) (Gonsalves et al., 2004).

At retrieval, the P300 component of an ERP signal occurs *about* 300 ms after people are given a memory probe and is associated with recognition. With false memories, the P300 is observed earlier than with true recognition (Miller et al., 2001). Also, there is less gamma band activity during the recall of false memories, particularly in the hippocampus and left temporal lobe (Sederberg et al., 2007). Overall, this suggests that people are making memory decisions faster as if they are being less thorough and using less information.

This creation of false memories is influenced by several factors. When people have DRM false memories, they are often influenced by both associative information (what other words are associated with those that were heard) and gist-based thematic information (in a fuzzy trace way). False memories are more likely to be caused by associative processes immediately after exposure, but over time (such as a week), false memories are more likely to be caused by gist-based thematic processes (Carneiro et al., 2017).

Another mechanism is the operation of inhibition (see Chapter 8) that is involved in directed forgetting (Kimball & Bjork, 2002). When people are asked to forget a set of words that regularly elicits a false memory, then the rate of producing false memories increases. Apparently, the instruction to forget inhibits the memory for that list, thereby making access to memories for the entire list harder. As a result, people have trouble discriminating between what was actually heard and what was not. Thus, more false memories are produced. In other words, trying to forget what was actually heard before makes it harder to distinguish reality from imagination.

False Memories from Integration

Another way people can misremember is when information that was presented at different times is integrated into a single memory. With integration, what were actually several events are misremembered as one. This may involve the schema integration processes discussed in Chapter 9. People may misremember different pieces of information as being part of the same event if they "seem" like they should go together.

One example of integration is a study by Bransford and Franks (1971) in which people heard a list of sentences, shown in Table 13.3. As they were listening, people had to answer questions about the sentences, also shown in the table. (Go ahead and read the sentences and answer the questions now.) Afterward, people identified which sentences they had seen and rated their confidence in their memory. A portion of this recognition test is shown in Table 13.4. Try to identify which sentences you remember seeing and which you do not. Also, rate how confident you are. After you have done this, look back at Table 13.3 to see which sentences were actually there.

The important thing here is that the study and test sentences varied in the number of simple idea units (called propositions) they had, which could be 1, 2, 3, or all 4 propositions. For example, in one sentence "The ants were in the kitchen" is a one-proposition sentence, "The ants in the kitchen ate the jelly" is two, "The ants in the kitchen ate the jelly, which was on the table" is three, and "The ants in

TABLE 13.3 *Sentences Used in the Bransford and Franks (1971) Study*

The ants ate the sweet jelly, which was on the table.	The ants ate what?
The ants in the kitchen ate the jelly, which was on the table.	The ants were where?
The ants in the kitchen ate the jelly.	What was in the kitchen?
The ants ate the sweet jelly.	The jelly was what?
The ants were in the kitchen	What was in the kitchen?
The jelly was on the table.	What was on the table?

Source: adapted from Bransford, J. D., & Franks, J. J. (1971). The abstraction of linguistic ideas. *Cognitive Psychology, 2*, 331–350

TABLE 13.4 *Recognition Test from the Bransford and Franks (1971) Study*

The ants in the kitchen ate the sweet jelly, which was on the table.

The ants in the kitchen ate the sweet jelly.

The ants ate the sweet jelly.

The sweet jelly was on the table.

The ants ate the jelly, which was on the table.

The jelly was sweet.

The ants ate the jelly.

Source: adapted from Bransford, J. D., & Franks, J. J. (1971). The abstraction of linguistic ideas. *Cognitive Psychology, 2*, 331–350

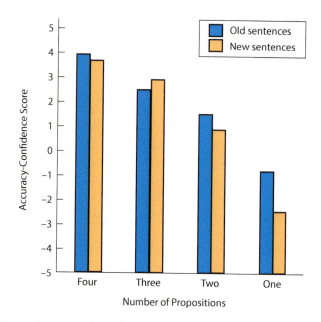

FIGURE 13.4 *Recognition Test Data from the Bransford and Franks (1971) Study. The Accuracy Score Reflects the Combined Influences of People's Selection on Items along with Their Confidence in Having Heard Items Before*

Source: adapted from Bransford, J. D., & Franks, J. J. (1971). The abstraction of linguistic ideas. *Cognitive Psychology, 2*, 331–350

the kitchen ate the sweet jelly, which was on the table" has all four propositions. On the memory test, the more propositions a test sentence had, the more likely people "remembered" it. A sentence with four propositions that was not read was more likely to be "recognized" than a sentence with only one proposition that was actually read. Moreover, confidence ratings showed the same pattern and increased with the number of propositions, as shown in Figure 13.4.

The explanation for this is that when people heard the sentences because there is overlap in content, they are likely to be interpreted as referring to a common situation. This makes information integration easy. This integrated representation is then used to make memory judgments. Items that contain more propositions more closely match the memory trace and so are more likely to be recognized and given higher confidence ratings. People use memories of entire events that they created, not memories for what they actually experienced. While this information integration is a false memory because people never actually saw some information together, this appears to rely on different memory processes than those for DRM false memories because performance on these two tasks are unrelated (Varga et al., 2019).

Stop and Review

The separation of memory and reality is most salient when people have false memories for events that never happened. In the DRM paradigm, people regularly report remembering words that were not actually encountered. This happens because the critical false memory word is strongly associated with the ones that actually occurred. This is supported by both behavioral and neurological data. False memories also come about through our natural impulse to integrate information that is about a common event. As a result, we lose our memories for the individual encounters and misremember what individual pieces were learned apart from the others.

IMPLANTED MEMORIES

In the preceding examples, the false information was never explicitly conveyed. However, it is possible to have false memories implanted in people, intentionally or unintentionally, from some outside source (Loftus, 2004; see Scoboria et al., 2018, for how to evaluate implanted memories). In these cases, information is introduced in a way that leads people to adopt the memory as a real event from their lives.

For example, imagine that I tell you that your mother says that when you were eight years old you got lost in a mall. I then, over a stretch of time, repeatedly ask you if you remember that incident. The repeated attempts to remember would cause you to try to imagine this event, and you start to confuse your imagination with reality. Alternatively, if you hear me say that I remember a story about whales on the news, you might later misremember reading the story on the internet (Meade & Roediger, 2002). This is because you remember something about a whale story, and you know that you read lots of things on the internet. You put these two things together to form a false memory. Finally, if you are told that, as a child, you had an unpleasant experience with a food that you do not eat often (e.g., egg salad), you then avoid that food in the future, as if you had a real taste aversion experience (Bernstein & Loftus, 2009). Here, the imagining of the described event eventually gets treated as a real one, and this alters your behavior.

Note that false memories are not only for visual/verbal information. They also occur for other experiences, such as being misled to believe an instrument (e.g., drums) was heard in a piece of music (Anglada-Tort et al., 2019). Another example is that people may misremember pain they experienced. If they are shown pain ratings and are told that these were the ratings they gave earlier, even when they are not, their memories of pain shift toward the new (false) ratings (Urban et al., 2019). In general, when we off-load memories (by writing them down, putting them into our phones, taking pictures, etc.), if those externalized memories are altered, this also alters the memories in our mind (Risko et al., 2019).

For implanted false memories, again, the likelihood of creating one is a function of how plausible it is (Pezdek et al., 1997). In one study, students were asked to judge how well their own memories corresponded with those of their parents. During this time, the researchers relayed a description of an event that was said to be described by the student's mother but that had never happened. This event was consistent with being raised either Jewish or Catholic. Jewish students were more likely to have a false memory for the Jewish event than the Catholic event, and vice versa, as shown in Figure 13.5. Thus, implanted false memories are

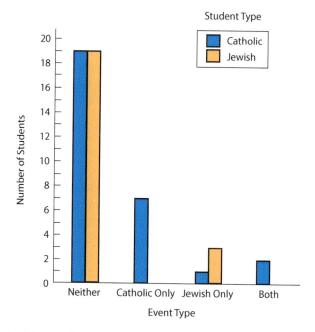

FIGURE 13.5 *False Memory Reports for Implanted Memories Consistent with a Catholic or Jewish Family Event*

Source: generated from data reported in Pezdek, K., Finger, K., & Hodge, D. (1997). Planting false childhood memories: The role of event plausibility. *Psychological Science, 8,* 437–441

more likely for plausible events. That said, it is possible to implant false memories of implausible events. For example, reading articles about demonic possession can make it seem more plausible, leading to a false memory of witnessing demonic possession (Mazzoni et al., 2001).

In some unfortunate cases, people may experience implanted memories from overzealous and substandard therapists looking for repressed memories (Loftus, 1993). The suggestion that these "memories" have been repressed makes it more likely that people will accept them as real. The normal scrutiny of the memory content and source does not seem to take place.

Increasing Implanted Memories

A technique that makes the creation of implanted false memories more likely is imagination, which also increases our confidence in the false memories. This is called **imagination inflation** (Garry & Polaschek, 2000). Imagination makes memory traces richer and gives them pseudoperceptual qualities, making them seem real. Suppose people heard about an event but did not see it. If they also imagined the event, they are more likely to come to believe that it was seen (Henkel et al., 2000). Imagination inflation has a greater influence when people take a first-person perspective (Libby, 2003) or with repeated imaginings (Thomas & Loftus, 2002). Both increase the perceptual "experience" in the memories, making them seem more real. Over time, if imagined false memories are strong enough, people may claim to consciously "remember" doing imagined events, even if they are odd, such as sitting on dice (Thomas & Loftus, 2002).

Given the power of imagination inflation, it is not surprising that actually viewing pictures can also make false memories more likely[2] (Garry & Gerrie, 2005). If people see photos of themselves at the age that an event was supposed to have occurred, they are more likely to create false memories (Lindsay et al., 2004). Viewing old photos gives memory some concrete perceptual information to put into the false memories, along with any additional information that is triggered. Similarly, if people see pictures of places under divided attention, when the encoding of source information is poorer, they may later misremember having been at those places (Brown & Marsh, 2008). This influence of photos on false memories is also seen for news events. People are more likely to change their memories, even when either warned that some of the images may be altered, or the photos were so badly altered so that they were obvious fakes (Nash, 2018). Finally, although it seems unlikely, it is even possible for people to implant false memories into themselves. See the Study In Depth box to read about this.

STUDY IN DEPTH

This section describes a study by Zaragoza et al. (2001). In this study, 98 students at Kent State University first watched an eight-minute excerpt from a live action Disney film about two brothers at camp. This portion of the study provided the event knowledge that would be manipulated later.

After viewing the film segment, the students were asked 12 experimental questions about the movie. Eight of these questions were about incidents or details that actually occurred in the film. The other four were about things that did not occur. For example, a question might be "The chair broke and Delaney fell on the floor. Where was Delaney bleeding?" In fact, the character did not bleed. All the students were verbally asked questions by an experimenter and gave spoken responses, which were recorded.

Thirty students were in a control group that were told to answer as best that they could, but were not forced to generate false information if they did not know the answer, or if they did not believe an event occurred. The remaining 68 students were in the experimental group. They were told to answer the questions the best that they could. Moreover, if there was a question that did not correspond to an event that they remembered from the film, they were supposed to guess and generate an answer. Thus, this group knew that they were creating answers and not remembering that information from the film. In addition, for the experimental group, the researchers also manipulated the feedback that people received for their false memory guesses. For half of these, the students received confirmatory feedback (such as "Yes, that's right"), and for the other half, they received neutral feedback (such as "Okay").

A week later, the students returned and were met by a new experimenter. This person told the students that the prior experimenter had made some mistakes and had asked questions about things that never happened in the film. Thus, if anything, students were biased to be more conservative in their memory reports. During testing, people received 23 questions of the form "When you watched the video, did you see _____?" Some

---

2 Although narratives have an even bigger influence (Garry & Wade, 2005).

of these were about answers that the student provided, and some of these were about answers that another student provided. Some of the questions were about information that they generated false answers to, and the rest were about things that actually happened in the film. Finally, four to six weeks later, the students who were asked to generate false answers were asked to return once more. This time they were asked to write down everything that they could remember from the film.

What is interesting is that students who knowingly confabulated answers in the first part of the study, in the second part accepted 32% of these answers as being the truth, compared to 8% in the control group (which provides an index of guessing). Moreover, if the experimenter had provided supportive, confirmatory feedback for a made-up response, then the rate of accepting self-implanted false memories was higher (38%) than if only neutral feedback had been given (26%). Finally, in the final recall task four to six weeks later, falsely generated knowledge was included in their recalls 27% of the time when the feedback was confirmatory and 13% of the time when the feedback was neutral. Thus, even minimal external support of self-implanted false memories boosts their creation tremendously.

More generally, when people tell lies, this has a lasting impact. Memories are altered to conform to the lies, particularly when lying involves some sort of fabrication of new additional information rather than leaving some things out (Otgaar & Baker, 2018).

Related to imagination inflation is the finding that repeating things can make it seem more real and believable (Dechêne et al., 2010). This is the **illusory truth effect**. People are *more* likely to think that something is true if they have heard it multiple times. This even occurs for highly implausible ideas, such as "A single elephant weighs less than a single ant" (Fazio et al., 2019). Thus, even when the base level of truth is extremely low, the level of acceptance goes up with repetition. This occurs because of the greater familiarity of the information, which makes it easier to process, and therefore makes it feel true.

Although people can falsely remember implanted information, there are some qualities that distinguish true from false memories. True memories are often richer in detail, are more emotional, are more likely to be consciously "recollected," and are more likely to be field memories. In contrast, false memories are more likely to be stereotypical events, to be "known," and to be observer memories (Heaps & Nash, 2001). That said, these are general tendencies and are not defining criteria that can diagnose whether a given memory is real. True and false memories overlap a great deal on all these dimensions. These are only trends that characterize the false memories from true memories. It is like saying men are taller than women. While this is true in general, there is a great deal of overlap between these two distributions. Just as you cannot make firm judgments about the sex of people given their height, you cannot use such qualities of a memory to determine if it is true or false.

The Misinformation Effect

The storage of incorrect and false information in memory not only applies to knowledge about events that one experienced, as is the case with many of the false memories discussed in this chapter, but also can happen for general, semantic knowledge. The **misinformation effect** is the finding that people alter memory reports to conform to incorrect information that was recently encountered and which contradicts their prior semantic knowledge (Rapp, 2016).

As an example of the misinformation effect, when people read fictional stories about real people, they tend to misremember some of the fictional information as being real. The fictional knowledge gets integrated with the real knowledge. Although people are aware that the story contained some fictional information, they also think that they knew some of the fictional information *before* reading the story (Marsh et al., 2003). What is more, if people are warned about this kind of memory distortion, even before they read, they still incorporate the inaccurate information into their semantic memories (Marsh & Fazio, 2006). As another example, although people know correct information ahead of time, such as the fact that the Pacific is the largest ocean, if they are exposed to misinformation, such as reading a story that states that the Atlantic is the largest ocean, people mistakenly use the misinformation to answer general knowledge questions soon after (Fazio et al., 2013).

The misinformation effect is more likely to emerge after people have recently taken a test on the critical information (Chan & LaPaglia, 2013). This may be because the testing reactivates the requisite knowledge, which then is in a malleable state, prone to alteration, consistent with the idea of reconsolidation (see Chapter 2). How well people do this can vary and is related to their susceptibility to DRM false memories (Zhu et al., 2013), suggesting that the same memory retrieval processes that segregate true from false memories are operating in both cases.

False Memories: A Social Contagion

As with source monitoring, false memories can be influenced by social factors. People are more willing to say that they "remember" events that were only imagined if other people claim that they saw them (Reysen, 2007; Roediger et al., 2001) or if they have a conversation with someone about a shared event (Rush & Clark, 2014). This influence of other people's memory reports on your own memory is sometimes called a "social contagion." Just hearing other people relate events may cause us to remember them as if we experienced them.

That said, talking with other people does not always lead to more false memories. For example, with the DRM paradigm, people working in actual groups recall more accurately presented words than people working in nominal groups or alone. However the rate of recalling false memories does not change (Maki et al., 2008). Thus, the proportion of memories that are labeled as false decreases, while the absolute rate of reporting false memories stays the same.

The social influence of implanted false memories is also affected by the people involved. For example, social contagions are less likely if people think that the person that they are hearing false information from has consumed alcohol recently (Thorley & Christiansen, 2018). False memories are more likely for people who are more prone to dissociative experiences (e.g., driving and not remembering what happened the past few miles). Such people have a harder time distinguishing between what was real versus what was imagined or only plausible. Furthermore, false memories are more likely to occur when the people who provide the implanted information have more extroverted personalities. This is particularly strong when the people doing the remembering are more introverted (Porter et al., 2000) or are the first to recall something (Wright & Carlucci, 2011), suggesting some sort of primacy effect in terms of the preference for which information in memory is more accurate.

Emotional Connections

The influence of emotion on false memories is complicated (Bookbinder & Brainerd, 2016). In the DRM paradigm, compared to emotionally neutral items, false memories are more likely if words are emotionally negative, but less likely if they are emotionally positive (Brainerd et al., 2008). The explanation is that negative emotional content encourages us to rely more on gist-based processing, causing us to be more willing to remember something that is consistent with the actual information, producing a false memory. However, positive information encourages more item-specific, verbatim memories, which decreases the likelihood of false memories.

In comparison to the emotional content itself, our emotional mood can also influence the creation of false memories. In the DRM paradigm, relative to people who are in a neutral mood, false memories are more likely for people who are in a positive mood and less likely for those in a negative mood (Storbeck & Clore, 2005), although this may due to emotional intensity rather than negativity (Corson & Verrier, 2007). Positive moods encourage relational processing, which encourages the activation of a common associate concept, whereas negative moods encourage

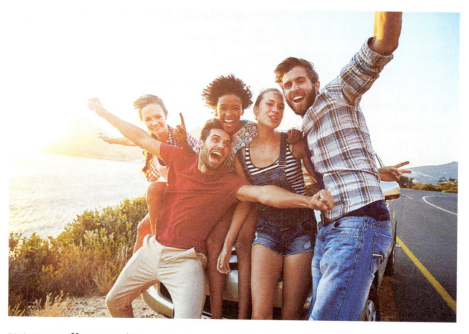

PHOTO 13.2 *Your emotions can influence the likelihood of forming false memories—although people are more likely to form false memories of negative information, people are more likely to form false memories when they are in a positive mood and may hear incorrect information from other people*

Source: monkeybusinessimages/iStock/Thinkstock

MEMORY AND REALITY **443**

item-specific processing, which discourages the activation of what would become the false memory.

Hypnosis and Memory

If you are not familiar with the state of **hypnosis**, it is a real thing. It is an altered state of consciousness in which people are more willing to accept and follow the suggestions of the hypnotist.[3] We vary in the degree to which we can be hypnotized. Some people are not at all susceptible, whereas others are highly susceptible, to the point of being able to experience auditory, visual, or tactile illusions as suggested by the hypnotist.

While there are many interesting topics that can be explored with hypnosis, the issue at hand is how hypnosis influences memory. Does it make memory better, worse, or have no appreciable effect? At first blush, it seems that hypnosis has a beneficial effect on memory. If you put people under hypnosis and ask them to recall things, they report more than if they are not under hypnosis. There are also anecdotal reports about the effectiveness of hypnosis on memory.

One case involves the Chowchilla kidnapping (as reported by Smith, 1983). In 1976, members of the Symbionese Liberation Army (a militant radical sect) kidnapped, at gunpoint, a bus full of schoolchildren and their driver. They were herded into two vans and taken to an old rock quarry where the students and bus driver were placed into a buried chamber. Eventually the driver and students were able to dig themselves out and go to the police. When questioned, the bus driver said that he had tried to memorize the van license plates as they were being loaded into them. However, because he was so agitated while being held at gunpoint, he was unable to recall the plate numbers. At this point, a decision was made to hypnotize him in the hope that this would help him remember. While under hypnosis, the driver called out two license plate numbers. One of these, except for one digit, turned out to be the plate number for one of the vans. This information eventually led to the arrest and conviction of the kidnappers. With reports such as this, it can be seen why some people would view hypnosis as a memory technique with great practical potential.

Perhaps more familiar are cases where people are hypnotized in therapeutic situations. The movie *Communion* provides a striking example of this when a man is hypnotized and recalls his abduction by aliens. More down-to-earth and common are cases where people are hypnotized in therapy sessions to remember aspects of their past that they may have forgotten because they had been traumatized by the event. Often these approaches take the view that memory is like a videotape that accurately records events and can be played back with a high level of accuracy if the proper technique is used. This is incorrect.

There is no doubt that people report more memories under hypnosis, but there are serious problems. For one, there is a larger risk that the memories reported are inaccurate (Scoboria et al., 2002; Smith, 1983). The new accurate information that is reported under hypnosis is no different from the hypermnesia that one would see with repeated recall (see Chapter 3). As a reminder, when people are

---

3 It may be that it is the suggestions, not the hypnotic state itself, that are relevant, Kirsch et al., 2007.

asked to remember something repeatedly, they can often remember things in later attempts that they had forgotten previously. This was demonstrated in a study by Dinges et al. (1992), in which people were given 40 line drawings to look at and memorize. People were then asked repeatedly to report what they had seen either when they were hypnotized or not. A forced recall test (see Chapter 3) was used to recall 40 things. Thus, hypnotized and unhypnotized people reported the same overall amount of information. What was found was that there was no difference in how much was recalled when people were either hypnotized or not. Consistent hypermnesia was observed in all cases. Thus, hypnosis adds little to the ability to remember beyond what is normally seen (for a review, see Mazzoni et al., 2014). That said, one way that false memory implantation has been used in a potentially beneficial way is to implant positive memories in hypnotized people to counter feelings of anxiety (Nourkova & Vasilenko, 2018).

Stop and Review

False memories can be implanted from outside sources, including self-implantation. The likelihood of a false memory being implanted is increased the more retrieval attempts there are and by engaging in mental imagery and imagination of the implanted events. Moreover, implanted false memories can be made for otherwise well-known semantic knowledge of the world (the misinformation effect). The formation of false memories is affected by our emotions. We are more likely to form false memories of negative emotional content, but are more likely to form false memories when we are in a positive mood. False memory implanting unintentionally occurs as part of our interactions with other people when there is a sharing of experiences, particularly when the other people are more extroverted and trusted. False memories also arise through hypnosis, and they are often remembered at a high level of confidence. All of that said, while we can be easily misled in some circumstances, our grip on reality is fairly firm, and we tend not to create false memories wildly.

FALSE MEMORIES THROUGH NORMAL MEMORY USE

Every time we use our memories, we change them in some way. Different things that we do with the knowledge alter our memories' content. In this section we look at examples of normal ways of using memory that can lead to changed memories. These are verbal overshadowing, the revelation effect, and the blending of memories.

Verbal Overshadowing

When we talk about things that we have seen, our memories can be changed by this. This is **verbal overshadowing**. When we describe an event, we create a verbal memory of our description. Because verbal information differs from visual information, our memory for what we said alters our memory for what we saw. This is a fuzzy trace view that suggests that memory is a mixture of various traces. Overall, our more recent verbal memories overshadow our older visual memories.

As an example of this, students at the University of Washington, in a study by Schooler and Engstler-Schooler (1990), watched a video of a bank robbery. Afterward, some people spent five minutes writing a description of the robber's face. Everyone was then shown a set of eight pictures of similar faces and had to pick out which one was the robber. Students who described the robber's face correctly picked it out less often than students who did not write a description. Thus, memory was worsened by talking about the experience. Verbal overshadowing can even occur when naming pictures of objects (e.g., saying "chair" to a picture of a chair) (Lupyan, 2008). It should be noted that verbal overshadowing does not occur if people only read a description— only when they actually generate a description does it occur (Dodson et al., 1997).

Verbal overshadowing of memory for a face can occur even when it was not the face that was described. in a study by Dodson et al. (1997), verbal overshadowing occurred even when people wrote a description of another face. Westerman and Larsen (1997) found verbal overshadowing after people wrote descriptions of a car that was in a scene. Even here, memory for a face was worse. Thus, verbal overshadowing influences the types of information used during retrieval. There is a shift from visual to verbal knowledge. In general, talking about things can sometimes make memory worse. Finally, there is evidence that verbalization may be a form of retrieval induced forgetting in that details that are not talked about will be forgotten, even for emotionally intense events, such as hearing of the September 11, 2001, terrorist attacks (Coman, et al., 2009).

While verbal overshadowing occurs, it is not true that providing verbal descriptions always makes memory worse. In some cases, *verbal facilitation* can occur (e.g., Brown & Lloyd-Jones, 2005; 2006; Lyle & Johnson, 2004). For example, if people are presented a series of faces and provide a description of each one as it occurs (in a control condition, no description is provided), they adopt strategies of encoding faces to memory which can take advantage of these verbal descriptions.

Revelation Effect

When we interact with the world, sometimes information is revealed slowly. At such times we may be trying to figure out what we are dealing with. Because of this revelation process, people are more likely to recognize information as old, for both old and new information. This is the **revelation effect** (Watkins & Peynircioğlu, 1990; see Aßfalg et al., 2017, for a meta-analysis). There are several ways that the revelation effect is studied. For one, a word might be revealed one letter at a time until the person can make a recognition judgment (e.g., M _ _ _ _ _, M _ _ O _ _, M _ _ O _ Y, etc.). The revelation effect occurs only when we think that we are remembering a prior event. It does not occur if we either know that no such episode occurred or if we engage in semantic memory retrieval (Frigo et al., 1999).

The revelation effect appears because people are using memory familiarity (Westerman & Greene, 1996; but see Hicks & Marsh, 1998). As people go through the revelation process, the information feels more familiar (because they have now been thinking about it for some time), so they are more willing to claim it was seen before. This occurs even when people had not heard something before but were subjected to subliminal suggestions that they had (Frigo et al., 1999). ERP recordings of the frontal lobes show that there is greater cortical activity for information that was revealed, consistent with the idea that people are relying on memory familiarity (Azimian-Faridani & Wilding, 2004).

Consistent with this familiarity idea, the revelation effect is more likely when people are less able to consciously recollect the circumstances in which information was learned and need to rely on feelings of familiarity. Thus, having a longer delay between the original presentation and the memory test or presenting the information faster makes it harder for people to encode it in a way that makes conscious recollection possible (Landau, 2001). This feeling of familiarity may even come in the form of general activation by a presumably unrelated prior task, rather than revelation itself, such as doing a working memory span task prior to recognition (Westerman & Greene, 1998) or by solving a problem such as an anagram (Dougal & Schooler, 2007). However, when retrieval emphasizes conscious recollection, the revelation effect may not be observed (Westerman, 2000).

The revelation effect not only applies to simple items, like words, but also to complex events (Bernstein et al., 2002; 2004). If people go through a process of trying to uncover their memories, this very uncovering process can increase the likelihood that a person will falsely claim that a memory is real. Thus, efforts at recovering previously hidden memories by engaging in imagination can lead people to believe in false memories.

The revelation effect is similar to other phenomena, such as the mere exposure (Chapter 6) and false fame effects, in that memory is altered by prior encounters. More false memory reports occur if people are exposed to a brief preview of something, such as a word, face, or scene. This preview makes the thing seem more familiar, and we are more likely to report that we had encountered it earlier (other than the preview) (Brown & Marsh, 2009; Jacoby & Whitehouse, 1989; Titchener, 1928). This may partially explain a déjà vu experience. Sometimes we get an initial glance of something, and then, later, when we look at it more carefully, it seems oddly familiar.

Improve Your Memory

One of the primary concerns about memory for many people is that their memories are accurate. The very term "false" in false memory has a negative connotation. So, what can be done to make our memories more accurate? As you have seen, there are a number of things that can cause memory and reality to become disconnected. In terms of source monitoring, remember that this is a problem-solving process. Cognition is putting many different pieces of information together to figure out the source of a memory. At the time of the event, if remembering the source is going to be important, do what you can to make it salient in memory. For example, if you heard a secret from Elise, try to form a mental image of Elise carrying a briefcase full of secrets. This will make the knowledge more memorable so that you can bring it to mind when needed. Afterward, you will just need to work with whatever knowledge you have. In general, be aware of circumstances when source memory can fail you so that you do not put yourself in an embarrassing situation.

In terms of the false memories that are generated through processes such as those found in the DRM and integration paradigms, keep in mind that this involves a mental process that is normally valuable, namely making inferences. As was noted in Chapter 8, some of the sins of forgetting exist because they are often actually virtues. Just be aware that sometimes you may be mistaken, and that other people may remember accurately. To avoid the implanting of false memories, if an event is important to remember, first, try to avoid talking to other people when it is reasonable to do so. This may preserve the accurate portions of the memory. Alternatively, allowing yourself to imagine events, causing imagination inflation, leads you to say that events might have happened, when they did not. Finally, talking about events can sometimes cause memories to be distorted and lost, as with verbal overshadowing. This is why some people do not like to talk about movies or television shows just after they watched them. Giving them some time will allow them to be consolidated and not be lost through verbal overshadowing.

Memory Blending

A final way that false memories can be created is when information from different memories are blended during retrieval. As a reminder, some aspects of memory retrieval are reproductive. That is, information that was encountered before is directly retrieved from memory in more or less the same form that it was originally encountered and encoded. For example, when you remember the name of the street you grew up on, you are reproducing this information. That said, much of our memory is reconstructive. That is, we have bits and pieces stored in memory, and we reconstruct those memories from other knowledge that we have. This might be done using schemas and scripts (see Chapter 9). As a result of these reconstructive processes, elements from different events may be blended together during retrieval to form a composite memory of an event that never actually happened (Devitt et al., 2016). This is more likely to happen when the original events are similar in some way. For example, if you made multiple trips to visit the Smithsonian museums in Washington D.C., you might combine different trips into a single composite memory.

This kind of memory blending may also happen when you watch other people doing something (Lindner et al., 2010) or when you engage in counterfactual thinking and imagine how the world may have been different (what if you actually had picked up that litter on the way to school and thrown it away instead of just letting it sit there?). Again, people may blend imagined and actual events to form a new memory (Gerlach et al., 2013).

There are several examples of memory blending that have been discussed elsewhere in this book. For instance, the integrative false memories discussed earlier are a form of memory blending. The use of schemas and scripts, as described in

Chapter 9, to fill in the gaps in our memories is another. Also, formal memory models, such as MINERVA 2, described in Chapter 18, incorporate the idea that memory retrieval always involves a blending of memories.

CONFABULATION

Up to now we have been discussing disconnections between memory and reality that might occur in normal individuals. However, certain kinds of brain damage can result in patients reporting things that are clearly not based on reality but are false memories that they generate. These are false memories and not lies because the patient believes them to be true at the time that they are reported. There is no intention to deceive. The creation of false memories because of brain injury is **confabulation**. For example, after his stroke, my grandfather would tell stories of things my father did when he was younger, even though my father never did those things. Those were events that my grandfather had seen in a television show.

Confabulation is a symptom that may occur with damage to the frontal lobes. This can be thought of as damage to the central executive of working memory. Patients report what they believe to be the truth. Even when the confabulations are bizarre, the people are unaware of any problems. For example, a man might claim to have been married for only three years but have two full grown children as a result of that marriage. Another feature of confabulation is that people might see an object in the environment which could trigger a confabulatory report. For example, a patient might see a picture in a room of a tropical beach. This could trigger a report of the time the patient went on a trip to Hawaii, even though that person had never actually been there.

With confabulation people are not able to effectively monitor memory and evaluate the results of their own retrieval. Thus, incorrect information is reported as if it were true. Confabulatory reports are often confined to episodic memory, with a strong metamemory sense of remembering. Semantic memory is largely unaffected (Barba, 1993). So, people are unconsciously inventing information about their lives, while their general understanding of how the world is structured and operates is relatively intact.

Stop and Review

False memories can be created through what would seem to be the normal use of memory. For example, describing a witnessed event can lead to memory distortions, even when the part of the event being described is not what is tested later. Also, the gradual recovery or revelation of information during a memory search can create false memories. The build-up of partial memories leads to greater feelings of familiarity. False memories can also be created through a blending of related memories in a (false) composite memory. Finally, some kinds of brain damage, particularly damage associated with the frontal lobes, can cause affected people to have trouble regulating their memory processes, causing them to confabulate memories of events that never actually happened.

PUTTING IT ALL TOGETHER

Typically, you remember things that happened. However, sometimes you remember things that did not. False memories can come about through how the material was encoded, stored, and retrieved. During encoding, you may use semantic world knowledge to make inferences, and these inferences then get remembered as actual events. This may be what happens in the DRM paradigm. This is more likely for negative content, which may encourage you to form inferences. Alternatively, false memories may be implanted by others (or even self-implanted). This is more likely when retrieval attempts are repeated, you engage in mental imagery, or are encouraged by other people, as with hypnosis. One thing that happens with hypnosis, and other circumstances, is that knowledge may come to consciousness slowly, leading to greater feelings of familiarity. This gradual revelation may lead you to treat false memories as real.

During storage, false memories may be generated by combining information from experiences that you encountered separately. If they refer to a common situation, they are integrated into a single memory. These blended memories may not be distinguished from the individual memories that were used to construct them. Alternatively, talking about an event produces verbal memories that can overshadow an original memory, causing distortions. This overshadowing can even occur for otherwise well-known world knowledge, as with the misinformation effect.

During retrieval, a memory can be in error if you lose source information. When these mistakes occur, you may use knowledge in an inappropriate manner, such as with cryptomnesia, the false fame effect, and the sleeper effect. This is more likely when you are in a good mood and are not being careful in how you retrieve and appraise information from memory. With some kinds of brain damage, you might not be able to regulate the flow and evaluation of information during retrieval. This can cause you to confabulate and believe false memories, even if they are bizarre.

A final point of note. The bulk of this chapter focused on situations in which memory is in error. This does happen. That said, it is also important to keep in mind that much of what we remember is reasonably accurate and reliable (Brewin et al., 2020). If it were not, our ability to function would be greatly compromised. It is also important to note that just because someone exhibits one type of error (e.g., DRM false memory), does not mean that they are susceptible to other types of errors (e.g., misinformation effects or imagination inflation) (Nichols & Loftus, 2019). They are not.

STUDY QUESTIONS

1. What is source monitoring? How is it different from destination memory?
2. What are the different types of information that memory uses to perform source monitoring?
3. What are the different types of source monitoring?

4. Generally speaking, what happens when a source monitoring error occurs? More specifically, what are some of the ways that source monitoring errors produce problems?

5. What are cryptomnesia, the false fame effect, the sleeper effect, and the wishful thinking bias? How are each of these related to the process of source monitoring?

6. How can false memories be created by hearing related sets of information as in the DRM paradigm?

7. How might false memories be created through an integration process?

8. How are false memories implanted? What can be done to influence the probability that a false memory will be created?

9. How might semantic memory be distorted in the misinformation effect?

10. Under what circumstances might false memories become a social contagion?

11. How is the creation of false memories influenced by emotions?

12. What is the best way to describe the effect of hypnosis on attempts to remember?

13. What is the influence on memory of providing a verbal description of a witnessed event?

14. Does slowly revealing information to people make memory more or less accurate? Why?

15. How can memory be disconnected from reality through processes that result in memory blending?

16. What is confabulation, and how does it arise?

KEY TERMS

- affective information
- cognitive operations
- confabulation
- contextual information
- cryptomnesia
- destination memory
- DRM paradigm
- external source monitoring
- false fame effect
- false memories
- hypnosis
- illusory truth effect
- imagination inflation
- internal source monitoring
- misinformation effect
- perceptual detail
- reality monitoring
- revelation effect
- semantic detail
- sleeper effect
- source monitoring
- verbal overshadowing
- wishful thinking bias

EXPLORE MORE

Here are some additional readings that can provide better insight into issues of memory and reality.

Gallo, D. A. (2010). False memories and fantastic beliefs: 15 years of the DRM illusion. *Memory & Cognition, 38*(7), 833–848.

Garry, M., & Polaschek, D. L. L. (2000). Imagination and memory. *Current Directions in Psychological Science, 9*, 6–10.

Johnson, M. K., Hashtroudi, S., & Lindsay, D. S. (1993). Source monitoring. *Psychological Bulletin, 114*, 3–28.

Brainerd, C. J., & Reyna, V. F. (2005). *The Science of False Memory*. Oxford: Oxford University Press.

Roediger, H. L., & McDermott, K. B. (1995). Creating false memories: Remembering words not presented in lists. *Journal of Experimental Psychology: Learning, Memory, and Cognition, 21*, 803–814.

Westerman, D. L. (2000). Recollection-based recognition eliminates the revelation effect in memory. *Memory & Cognition, 28*, 167–175.

REFERENCES

Anglada-Tort, M., Baker, T., & Müllensiefen, D. (2019). False memories in music listening: Exploring the misinformation effect and individual difference factors in auditory memory. *Memory, 27*(5), 612–627.

Atkins, A. S., & Reuter-Lorenz, P. A. (2008). False working memories? Semantic distortion in a mere 4 seconds. *Memory 7 Cognition, 36*, 74–81.

Azimian-Faridani, N., & Wilding, E. L. (2004). An event-related potential study of the revelation effect. *Psychonomic Bulletin & Review, 11*, 926–931.

Aßfalg, A., Bernstein, D. M., & Hockley, W. (2017). The revelation effect: A meta-analytic test of hypotheses. *Psychonomic Bulletin & Review, 24*(6), 1718–1741.

Barba, G. D. (1993). Confabulation: Knowledge and recollective experience. *Cognitive Neuropsychology, 10*, 1–20.

Barber, S. J., Gordon, R., & Franklin, N. (2009). Self-relevance and wishful thinking: Facilitation and distortion in source monitoring. *Memory & Cognition, 37*, 434–446.

Bayen, U. J., Nakamura, G. V., Dupuis, S. E., & Yang, C. L. (2000). The use of schematic knowledge about sources in source monitoring. *Memory & Cognition, 28*, 480–500.

Bell, R., Buchner, A., Erdfelder, E., Giang, T., Schain, C., & Riether, N. (2012). How specific is source memory for faces of cheaters? Evidence for categorical emotional tagging. *Journal of Experimental Psychology: Learning, Memory, and Cognition, 38*(2), 457–472.

Bernstein, D. M., Godfrey, R. D., Davidson, A., & Loftus, E. F. (2004). Conditions affecting the revelation effect for autobiographical memory. *Memory & Cognition, 32*, 455–462.

Bernstein, D. M., & Loftus, E. F. (2009). The consequences of false memories for food preferences and choices. *Perspectives on Psychological Science, 4*, 135–139.

Bernstein, D. M., Whittlesea, B. W. A., & Loftus, E. F. (2002). Increasing confidence in remote autobiographical memory and general knowledge: Extensions of the revelation effect. *Memory & Cognition, 30*, 432–438.

Bookbinder, S. H., & Brainerd, C. J. (2016). Emotion and false memory: The context–content paradox. *Psychological Bulletin, 142*(12), 1315–1351.

Brainerd, C. J., Payne, D. G., Wright, R., & Reyna, V. F. (2003). Phantom recall. *Journal of Memory and Language, 48*, 445–467.

Brainerd, C. J., Stein, L. M., Silveira, R. A., Rohenkohl, G., & Reyna, V. F. (2008). How does negative emotion cause false memories? *Psychological Science, 19*, 919–925.

Brainerd, C. J., Wright, R., Reyna, V. F., & Mojardin, A. H. (2001). Conjoint recognition and phantom recollection. *Journal of Experimental Psychology: Learning, Memory, and Cognition, 27*, 307–327.

Bransford, J. D., & Franks, J. J. (1971). The abstraction of linguistic ideas. *Cognitive Psychology, 2*, 331–350.

Brédart, S., Lampinen, J. M., & Defeldre, A. C. (2003). Phenomenal characteristics of cryptomnesia. *Memory, 11*, 1–11.

Brewin, C. R., Andrews, B., & Mickes, L. (2020). Regaining consensus on the reliability of memory. *Current Directions in Psychological Science, 29*(2), 121–125.

Brown, A. S., & Marsh, E. J. (2008). Evoking false beliefs about autobiographical experience. *Psychonomic Bulletin & Review, 15*, 186–190.

Brown, A. S., & Marsh, E. J. (2009). Creating illusions of past encounter through brief exposure. *Psychological Science, 20*, 534–538.

Brown, C., & Lloyd-Jones, T. J. (2005). Verbal facilitation of face recognition. *Memory & Cognition, 33*, 1442–1456.

Brown, C., & Lloyd-Jones, T. J. (2006). Beneficial effects of verbalization and visual distinctiveness on remembering and knowing faces. *Memory & Cognition, 34*, 277–286.

Cann, D. R., McRae, K., & Katz, A. N. (2011). False recall in the Deese–Roediger–McDermott paradigm: The roles of gist and associative strength. *Quarterly Journal of Experimental Psychology, 64*(8), 1515–1542.

Carneiro, P., Garcia-Marques, L., Lapa, A., & Fernandez, A. (2017). Explaining the persistence of false memories: A proposal based on associative activation and thematic extraction. *Memory, 25*(8), 986–998.

Chan, J. C., & LaPaglia, J. A. (2013). Impairing existing declarative memory in humans by disrupting reconsolidation. *Proceedings of the National Academy of Sciences, 110*(23), 9309–9313.

Coman, A., Manier, D., & Hirst, W. (2009). Forgetting the unforgettable through conversation: Socially shared retrieval-induced forgetting of September 11 memories. *Psychological Science, 20*, 627–633.

Cook, G. I., Hicks, J. L., & Marsh, R. L. (2007). Source monitoring is not always enhanced for valenced material. *Memory & Cognition, 35*, 222–230.

Corson, Y., & Verrier, N. (2007). Emotions and false memories: Valence or arousal? *Psychological Science, 18*, 208–211.

Davachi, L., Mitchell, J. P., & Wagner, A. D. (2003). Multiple routes to memory: Distinct medial temporal lobe processes build item and source memories. *Proceedings of the National Academy of Sciences, 100*(4), 2157–2162.

Dechêne, A., Stahl, C., Hansen, J., & Wänke, M. (2010). The truth about the truth: A meta-analytic review of the truth effect. *Personality and Social Psychology Review, 14*(2), 238–257.

de Pereyra, G., Britt, M. A., Braasch, J. L. G., & Rouet, J. F. (2014). Reader's memory for information sources in simple news stories: Effects of text and task features. *Journal of Cognitive Psychology, 26*(2), 187–204.

Deese, J. (1959). On the prediction of occurrence of particular verbal intrusions in immediate recall. *Journal of Experimental Psychology, 58*, 17–22.

Devitt, A. L., Monk-Fromont, E., Schacter, D. L., & Addis, D. R. (2016). Factors that influence the generation of autobiographical memory conjunction errors. *Memory, 24*(2), 204–222.

Dinges, D. F., Whitehouse, W. G., Orne, E. C., Powell, J. W., Orne, M. T., & Erdelyi, M. H. (1992). Evaluating hypnotic memory enhancement (hypermnesia and reminiscence) using multitrial forced recall. *Journal of Experimental Psychology: Learning, Memory, and Cognition, 18*, 1139–1147.

Dodson, C. S., Johnson, M. K., & Schooler, J. W. (1997). The verbal overshadowing effect: Why descriptions impair face recognition. *Memory & Cognition, 25*, 129–139.

Dougal, S., & Schooler, J. W. (2007). Discovery misattribution: When solving is confused with remembering. *Journal of Experimental Psychology: General, 136*, 577–592.

Fazio, L. K., Barber, S. J., Rajaram, S., Ornstein, P. A., & Marsh, E. J. (2013). Creating illusions of knowledge: Learning errors that contradict prior knowledge. *Journal of Experimental Psychology: General, 142*(1), 1–5.

Fazio, L. K., Rand, D. G., & Pennycook, G. (2019). Repetition increases perceived truth equally for plausible and implausible statements. *Psychonomic Bulletin & Review, 26*(5), 1705–1710.

Foster, J. L., & Garry, M. (2012). Building false memories without suggestions. *American Journal of Psychology, 125*(2), 225–232.

Frigo, L. C., Reas, D. L., & LeCompte, D. C. (1999). Revelation without presentation: Counterfeit study list yields robust revelation effect. *Memory & Cognition, 27*, 339–343.

Gallo, D. A. (2010). False memories and fantastic beliefs: 15 years of the DRM illusion. *Memory & Cognition, 38*(7), 833–848.

Garry, M., & Gerrie, M. P. (2005). When photographs create false memories. *Current Directions in Psychological Science, 14*, 321–325.

Garry, M., & Polaschek, D. L. L. (2000). Imagination and memory. *Current Directions in Psychological Science*, *9*, 6–10.

Garry, M., & Wade, K. A. (2005). Actually, a picture is worth less than 45 words: Narratives produce more false memories than photographs do. *Psychonomic Bulletin & Review*, *12*, 359–366.

Geghman, K. D., & Multhaup, K. S. (2004). How generation affects source memory. *Memory & Cognition*, *32*, 819–823.

Gerlach, K. D., Dornblaser, D. W., & Schacter, D. L. (2014). Adaptive constructive processes and memory accuracy: Consequences of counterfactual simulations in young and older adults. *Memory*, *22*(1), 145–162.

Gingerich, A. C., & Sullivan, M. C. (2013). Claiming hidden memories as one's own: A review of inadvertent plagiarism. *Journal of Cognitive Psychology*, *25*(8), 903–916.

Gonsalves, B., Reber, P. J., Gitelman, D. R., Parrish, T. B., Mesulam, M-M., & Paller, K. A. (2004). Neural evidence that vivid imagining can lead to false remembering. *Psychological Science*, *15*, 655–660.

Gopie, N., & MacLeod, C. M. (2009). Destination memory: Stop me if I've told you this before. *Psychological Science*, *20*(12), 1492–1499.

Gordon, R., Franklin, N., & Beck, J. (2005). Wishful thinking and source monitoring. *Memory & Cognition*, *33*, 418–429.

Heaps, C. M., & Nash, M. (2001). Comparing recollective experience in true and false autobiographical memories. *Journal of Experimental Psychology: Learning, Memory, and Cognition*, *27*, 920–930.

Hege, A. C. G., & Dodson, C. S. (2004). Why distinctiveness information reduces false memories: Evidence for both impoverished relational-encoding and distinctiveness heuristic accounts. *Journal of Experimental Psychology: Learning, Memory, and Cognition*, *30*, 787–795.

Heit, E., Brockdorff, N., & Lamberts, K. (2004). Strategic processes in false recognition memory. *Psychonomic Bulletin & Review*, *11*, 380–386.

Henkel, L. A. (2004). Erroneous memories arising from repeated attempts to remember. *Journal of Memory and Language*, *50*, 26–46.

Henkel, L. A. (2012). Seeing photos makes us read between the lines: The influence of photos on memory for inferences. *Quarterly Journal of Experimental Psychology*, *65*(4), 773–795.

Henkel, L. A., Franklin, N., & Johnson, M. K. (2000). Cross-modal source monitoring confusions between perceived and imagined events. *Journal of Experimental Psychology: Learning, Memory, and Cognition*, *26*, 321–335.

Hicks, J. L., & Cockman, D. W. (2003). The effect of general knowledge on source memory and decision processes. *Journal of Memory and Language*, *48*, 489–501.

Hicks, J. L., & Marsh, R. L. (1998). A decrement-to-familiarity interpretation of the revelation effect from forced-choice tests of recognition memory. *Journal of Experimental Psychology: Learning, Memory, & Cognition*, *24*, 1105–1120.

Hicks, J. L., Marsh, R. L., & Ritschel, L. (2002). The role of recollection and partial information in source monitoring. *Journal of Experimental Psychology: Learning, Memory, & Cognition*, *28*, 503–508.

Hovland, C. I., & Weiss, W. (1951). The influence of source credibility on communication effectiveness. *Public Opinion Quarterly*, *15*, 635–650.

Intraub, H., & Hoffman, J. E. (1992). Reading and visual memory: Remembering scenes that were never seen. *American Journal of Psychology*, *105*, 101–114.

Jacoby, L. L., Kelley, C., Brown, J., & Jasechko, J. (1989a). Becoming famous overnight: Limits on the ability to avoid unconscious influences of the past. *Journal of Personality and Social Psychology*, *56*, 326–338.

Jacoby, L. L., & Whitehouse, K. (1989). An illusion of memory: False recognition influenced by unconscious perception. *Journal of Experimental Psychology: General*, *118*, 126–135.

Jacoby, L. L., Woloshyn, V., & Kelley, C. (1989b). Becoming famous without being recognized: Unconscious influences of memory produced by dividing attention. *Journal of Experimental Psychology: General*, *118*, 115–125.

Johnson, M. K., Foley, M. A., & Leach, K. (1988). The consequences for memory of imagining in another person's voice. *Memory & Cognition*, *16*, 337–342.

Johnson, M. K., Hashtroudi, S., & Lindsay, D. S. (1993). Source monitoring. *Psychological Bulletin*, *114*, 3–28.

Johnson, M. K., Kounios, J., & Reeder, J. A. (1994). Time-course studies of reality monitoring and recognition. *Journal of Experimental Psychology: Learning, Memory, and Cognition, 20*, 1409–1419.

Johnson, M. K., & Raye, C. L. (1981). Reality monitoring. *Psychological Review, 88*, 67–85.

Kensinger, E. A., & Schacter, D. L. (2006). When the Red Sox shocked the Yankees: Comparing negative and positive memories. *Psychonomic Bulletin & Review, 13*, 757–763.

Kimball, D. R., & Bjork, R. A. (2002). Influences of intentional and unintentional forgetting on false memories. *Journal of Experimental Psychology: General, 131*, 116–130.

Kirsch, I., Mazzoni, G., & Montgomery, G. H. (2007). Remembrance of hypnosis past. *American Journal of Clinical Hypnosis, 49*(3), 171–178.

Kumkale, G. T., & Albarracín, D. (2003). The sleeper effect in persuasion: A meta-analytic review. *Psychological Bulletin, 130*, 143–172.

Landau, J. D. (2001). Altering the balance of recollection and familiarity influences the revelation effect. *American Journal of Psychology, 114*, 425–437.

Leynes, P. A., & Phillips, M. C. (2008). Event-related potential (ERP) evidence for varied recollection during source monitoring. *Journal of Experimental Psychology: Learning, Memory, and Cognition, 34*, 741–751.

Libby, L. K. (2003). Imagery perspective and source monitoring in imagination inflation. *Memory & Cognition, 31*, 1072–1081.

Lindner, I., Echterhoff, G., Davidson, P. S. R., & Brand, M. (2010). Observation inflation: Your actions become mine. *Psychological Science, 21*(9), 1291–1299.

Lindsay, D. S., Hagen, L., Read, J. D., Wade, K. A., & Garry, M. (2004). True photographs and false memories. *Psychological Science, 15*, 149–154.

Loftus, E. F. (1993). The reality of repressed memories. *American Psychologist, 48*, 518–537.

Loftus, E. F. (2004). Memories of things unseen. *Current Directions in Psychological Science, 13*, 145–147.

Lupyan, G. (2008). From chair to "chair": A representational shift account of object labeling effects on memory. *Journal of Experimental Psychology: General, 137*, 348–369.

Lyle, K. B., & Johnson, M. K. (2004). Effects of verbalization on lineup face recognition in an interpolated inspection paradigm. *Applied Cognitive Psychology, 18*, 393–403.

Maki, R. H., Weigold, A., & Arellano, A. (2008). False memory for associated word lists in individuals and collaborating groups. *Memory & Cognition, 36*, 598–603.

Marsh, E. J., & Fazio, L. K. (2006). Learning errors from fiction: Difficulties in reducing reliance on fictional stories. *Memory & Cognition, 34*, 1140–1149.

Marsh, E. J., Meade, M. L., & Roediger, H. L. (2003). Learning facts from fiction. *Journal of Memory and Language, 49*, 519–536.

Mather, M., Shafir, E., & Johnson, M. K. (2000). Misremembrance of options past: Source monitoring and choice. *Psychological Science, 11*, 132–138.

Mather, M., Shafir, E., & Johnson, M. K. (2003). Remembering chosen and assigned options. *Memory & Cognition, 31*, 422–433.

Mazzoni, G. A. L., Laurence, J. R., & Heap, M. (2014). Hypnosis and memory: Two hundred years of adventures and still going! *Psychology of Consciousness: Theory, Research, and Practice, 1*(2), 153–167.

Mazzoni, G. A. L., Loftus, E. F., & Kirsch, I. (2001). Changing beliefs about implausible autobiographical events: A little plausibility goes a long way. *Journal of Experimental Psychology: Applied, 7*, 51–59.

Meade, M. L., & Roediger, H. L. (2002). Explorations in the social contagion of memory. *Memory & Cognition, 30*, 995–1009.

Meissner, C. A., Brigham, J. C., & Kelley, C. M. (2002). The influence of retrieval processes in verbal overshadowing. *Memory & Cognition, 29*, 176–186.

Miller, A. R., Baratta, C., Wynveen, C., & Rosenfeld, J. P. (2001). P300 latency, but not amplitude or topography, distinguishes between true and false recognition. *Journal of Experimental Psychology: Learning, Memory, and Cognition, 27*, 354–361.

Nash, R. A. (2018). Changing beliefs about past public events with believable and unbelievable doctored photographs. *Memory, 26*(4), 439–450.

Nichols, R. M., & Loftus, E. F. (2019). Who is susceptible in three false memory tasks? *Memory, 27*(7), 962–984.

Nourkova, V. V., & Vasilenko, D. A. (2018). On the advantage of autobiographical memory pliability: Implantation of positive self-defining memories reduces trait anxiety. *Memory*, 26(7), 869–881.

Otgaar, H., & Baker, A. (2018). When lying changes memory for the truth. *Memory*, 26(1), 2–14.

Pezdek, K., Finger, K., & Hodge, D. (1997). Planting false childhood memories: The role of event plausibility. *Psychological Science*, 8, 437–441.

Porter, S., Birt, A. R., Yuille, J. C., & Lehman, D. R. (2000). Negotiating false memories: Interviewer and rememberer characteristics relate to memory distortion. *Psychological Science*, 11, 507–510.

Pratkanis, A. R., Greenwald, A. G., Leippe, M. R., & Baumgarder, M. H. (1988). In search of reliable persuasion effects: III. The sleeper effect is dead: Long live the sleeper effect. *Journal of Personality and Social Psychology*, 54, 203–218.

Rapp, D. N. (2016). The consequences of reading inaccurate information. *Current Directions in Psychological Science*, 25(4), 281–285.

Reysen, M. B. (2007). The effects of social pressure on false memories. *Memory & Cognition*, 35, 59–65.

Risko, E. F., Kelly, M. O., Patel, P., & Gaspar, C. (2019). Offloading memory leaves us vulnerable to memory manipulation. *Cognition*, 191, 103954.

Roediger, H. L., & McDermott, K. B. (1995). Creating false memories: Remembering words not presented in lists. *Journal of Experimental Psychology: Learning, Memory, and Cognition*, 21, 803–814.

Roediger, H. L., Meade, M. L., & Bergman, E. T. (2001). Social contagion of memory. *Psychonomic Bulletin & Review*, 8, 365–371.

Roediger, H. L., Watson, J. M., McDermott, K. B., & Gallo, D. A. (2001). Factors that determine false recall: A multiple regression analysis. *Psychonomic Bulletin & Review*, 8, 385–407.

Romero-Rivas, C., Thorley, C., Skelton, K., & Costa, A. (2019). Foreign accents reduce false recognition rates in the DRM paradigm. *Journal of Cognitive Psychology*, 31(5–6), 507–521.

Rush, R. A., & Clark, S. E. (2014). Social contagion of correct and incorrect information in memory. *Memory*, 22(8), 937–948.

Schooler, J. W., & Engstler-Schooler, T. Y. (1990). Verbal overshadowing of visual memories: Some things are better left unsaid. *Cognitive Psychology*, 22, 36–71.

Scoboria, A., Mazzoni, G., Kirsch, I., Milling, L. S. (2002). Immediate and persisting effects of misleading questions and hypnosis on memory reports. *Journal of Experimental Psychology: Applied*, 8, 26–32.

Scoboria, A., Otgaar, H., & Mazzoni, G. (2018). Defending and reducing belief in memories: An experimental laboratory analogue. *Memory & Cognition*, 46(5), 770–786.

Sederberg, P. B., Schulze-Bonhage, A., Madsen, J. R., Bromfield, E. B., Litt, B., Brandt, A., & Kahana, M. J. (2007). Gamma oscillations distinguish true from false memories. *Psychological Science*, 18, 927–932.

Senkfor, A. J., & Van Petten, C. (1998). Who said what? An event-related potential investigation of source and item memory. *Journal of Experimental Psychology: Learning, Memory, and Cognition*, 24, 1005–1025.

Simons, J. S., Garrison, J. R., & Johnson, M. K. (2017). Brain mechanisms of reality monitoring. *Trends in Cognitive Sciences*, 21(6), 462–473.

Smith, M. C. (1983). Hypnotic memory enhancement of witnesses: Does it work? *Psychological Bulletin*, 94, 387–407.

Stark. L-J. & Perfect, T. J. (2006). Elaboration inflation: How your ideas become mine. *Applied Cognitive Psychology*, 20, 641–648.

Stark. L-J. & Perfect, T. J. (2008). The effects of repeated idea elaboration on unconscious plagiarism. *Memory & Cognition*, 36, 65–73.

Steffens, M. C., Buchner, A., Martensen, H., & Erdfelder, E. (2000). Further evidence on the similarity of memory processes in the process dissociation procedure and in source monitoring. *Memory & Cognition*, 28(7), 1152–1164.

Storbeck, J., & Clore, G. L. (2005). With sadness comes accuracy; with happiness, false memory: Mood and the false memory effect. *Psychological Science*, 16, 785–791.

Thapar, A., & McDermott, K. B. (2001). False recall and false recognition induced by presentation of associated words: Effects of retention interval and level of processing. *Memory & Cognition*, 29(3), 424–432.

Thomas, A. K., & Loftus, E. F. (2002). Creating bizarre false memories through imagination. *Memory & Cognition, 30,* 423–431.

Thorley, C., & Christiansen, P. (2018). The impact of own and others' alcohol consumption on social contagion following a collaborative memory task. *Memory, 26*(6), 727–740.

Titchener, E.B. (1928). *A Text-Book of Psychology.* New York: Macmillan.

Underwood, J., & Pezdek, K. (1998). Memory suggestibility as an example of the sleeper effect. *Psychonomic Bulletin & Review, 5,* 449–453.

Urbach, T. P., Windmann, S. S., Payne, D. G., & Kutas, M. (2005). Mismaking memories: Neural precursors of memory illusions in electrical brain activity. *Psychological Science, 16,* 19–24.

Urban, E. J., Cochran, K. J., Acevedo, A. M., Cross, M. P., Pressman, S. D., & Loftus, E. F. (2019). Misremembering pain: A memory blindness approach to adding a better end. *Memory & Cognition, 47*(5), 954–967.

Varga, N. L., Gaugler, T., & Talarico, J. (2019). Are mnemonic failures and benefits two sides of the same coin?: Investigating the real-world consequences of individual differences in memory integration. *Memory & Cognition, 47*(3), 496–510.

Watkins, M. J., & Peynircioğlu, Z. F. (1990). The revelation effect: When disguising test items induces recognition. *Journal of Experimental Psychology: Learning, Memory, and Cognition, 16,* 1012–1020.

Westerman, D. L. (2000). Recollection-based recognition eliminates the revelation effect in memory. *Memory & Cognition, 28,* 167–175.

Westerman, D. L., & Greene, R. L. (1996). On the generality of the revelation effect. *Journal of Experimental Psychology Learning, Memory, and Cognition, 22,* 1147–1153.

Westerman, D. L., & Greene, R. L. (1998). The revelation that the revelation effect is not due to revelation. *Journal of Experimental Psychology Learning, Memory, and Cognition, 24,* 377–386.

Westerman, D. L., & Larsen, J. D. (1997). Verbal-overshadowing effect: Evidence for a general shift in processing. *American Journal of Psychology, 110,* 417–428.

Wright, D. B., & Carlucci, M. E. (2011). The response order effect: People believe the first person who remembers an event. *Psychonomic Bulletin & Review, 18*(4), 805–812.

Zaragoza, M. S., Payment, K. E., Ackil, J. K., Drivdahl, S. B., & Beck, M. (2001). Interviewing witnesses: Forced confabulation and confirmatory feedback increase false memories. *Psychological Science, 12,* 473–477.

Zhu, B., Chen, C., Loftus, E. F., Lin, C., & Dong, Q. (2013). The relationship between DRM and misinformation false memories. *Memory & Cognition, 41*(6), 832–838.

CHAPTER 14

Memory and the Law

Memory has practical and important applications. Currently, for most of you, one of the more important applications is the learning of a large set of facts that can be written on an exam or used to develop a term paper. Hopefully, some of what you have learned here can be applied to make those efforts more successful. There are other applications outside of the classroom. A salient one is memory in the legal arena. Arriving at a just and legal outcome may involve people using their memories effectively. If memory is more accurate, then investigators, judges, and juries can come to more appropriate conclusions. However, as we have seen, memory reports may be inaccurate, even though people are doing their best. In a legal setting, memory errors can lead to miscarriages of justice, with guilty individuals not being held accountable or innocent people being punished for things that they did not do.

This chapter looks at five ways that memory can influence legal matters. The first is the accuracy of eyewitness memory. That is, how well does an eyewitness remember what they saw? The second is the confidence eyewitnesses have in their memories. The third is the development of a cognitive interview to gather information in a way to get the most out of a person's memory. The fourth is the use of memory to identify a perpetrator from a lineup. For the fifth, we consider how memory processes influence the effectiveness of juries.

EYEWITNESS TESTIMONY

When an automobile accident occurs or a crime is committed, an important source of evidence is **eyewitness testimony**. Eyewitnesses can provide information that cannot be obtained any other way. Moreover, if it is a serious enough case to warrant a jury trial, eyewitnesses can provide some of the most convincing evidence to jurors. Thus, the accuracy, stability, and scope of eyewitness memories are critically important. It is vital to understand how accurate such accounts are, even in the absence of any desire to mislead on the part of a witness.

We begin by looking at some things that can affect eyewitness memory. For instance, how can the wording of a question influence memory? What influence does misleading information have on memory and why? How does the witness's emotional state at the time of the event affect later memory? Are there other aspects of the event that influence later memory?

Wording Effects

To get information from a witness, questions must be asked. How questions are worded can influence what is remembered. People reconstruct their memories of an event based on the questions they are asked, which serve as memory cues. Take the example of an automobile accident involving two cars.[1] In some studies, people watched a film of a car accident. Note that in the actual film, there was no broken glass. Yet, as part of a set of questions, people were asked if they had seen any broken glass. In this case, the critical question included the verbs "smashed" or "hit" to describe the accident. What was found was that the more severe the verb, the more likely it was that people claimed to have seen broken glass (Loftus & Palmer, 1974). People reported broken glass 16% of the time when they heard "smashed" in the question but only 7% of the time when they heard "hit." People in a control condition said "yes" to the broken glass question only 6% of the time. Thus, the wording of a question can influence eyewitness memory.

This influence of wording even occurs for what might seem to be subtle differences, such as whether a question contained the article "a" or "the." In one study (Loftus & Zanni, 1975), people saw a car accident film. They then wrote a summary of what they saw and answered some questions. One question was either "Did you see *a* broken headlight?" or "Did you see *the* broken headlight?" The difference between the articles "a" and "the" is important because "a" does not presuppose the existence of a broken headlight, whereas "the" does. Half the time the questioned item was present in the film, and half the time it was not. When the item was not in the film (e.g., no broken headlight), people claimed they saw it 7% of the time when "a" was used, but 18% of the time when "the" was used. The error rate more than doubled following a change in a small function word.

Misleading Post-event Information

As you may have guessed, because it is so easy to alter memory reports based on the wording of a question, it is also alarmingly easy to alter memory by giving misleading information afterward, whether intentionally or not. This is called **misleading post-event information**. This misinformation enters memory, and people have difficulty distinguishing it from accurate memories. These memory distortions come from hearing other people describe the event, with memory reports being distorted in the direction of what a person has heard other people say (Wright et al., 2009). The effect of misleading post-event information can be exacerbated by the presence of nonverbal information that supports the incorrect information, such as gestures (Gurney et al., 2014). We first look at how to assess the influence of misleading post-event information and then consider some theories that try to explain how this happens.

---

1 A commonly cited study is by Loftus and Palmer (1974), in which people were asked, "How fast were the cars going when they smashed/collided/bumped/hit/contacted each other?" What was found was that the speed estimates varied by nearly 10 miles per hour, depending on which verb was used. However, this effect has been difficult to replicate (Lipscomb et al., 1985; McAllister et al. 1988; Read et al., 1978; Read & Bruce, 1984).

A standard approach for assessing the influence of misleading post-event information on memory was developed by Loftus et al. (1978). First, people watch an accident or crime on video. For example, people might see an accident in which a driver goes past a yield sign. Then, people are asked questions about the video. A critical question refers to an object that was in the scene, such as "Did another car pass the red convertible when it was stopped at the yield sign?" Because the sign mentioned in the question is in the video, this is the *consistent* condition. In other cases, this question refers to an object that was not in the scene, such as "Did another car pass the red convertible when it was stopped at the stop sign?" Because no stop sign was in the video, this is the *misleading* condition. Finally, in a third *control* condition, the question was a neutral reference to the critical object, such as "Did another car pass the red convertible when it was stopped at the traffic sign?"

After viewing the event and answering a critical question (among others), people make a decision about what they saw—such as choosing between pictures or verbal descriptions. For example, people might make a choice about whether the car had stopped at a stop sign or a yield sign. Although memory is better in the consistent condition (relative to the control condition), performance is worse in the misleading condition. The results of one study are shown in Figure 14.1. This

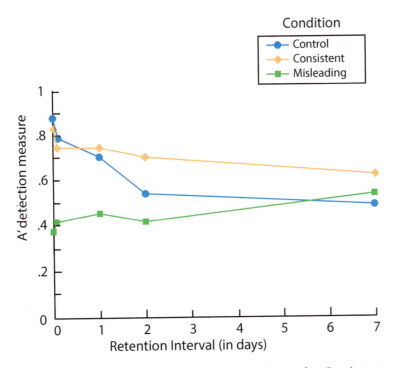

FIGURE 14.1 *Proportion Correct for Selecting the Correct Item after Consistent, Misleading, or Neutral Information over Several Days*

Source: generated from data reported in Loftus, E. F., Miller, D. G., & Burns, H. J. (1978). Semantic integration of verbal information into a visual memory. *Journal of Experimental Psychology: Human Learning and Memory, 4*, 19–31

shows that people incorporated the misleading information into their memory of the event. Moreover, while performance for the correct information declined over time for the control and consistent conditions, for the misleading condition performance stayed relatively low and the same over time.

This misleading post-event information effect is stable. It is more pronounced the longer the delay between witnessing an event and the time the misleading information is encountered (Loftus et al., 1978). It also occurs when the misleading information is presented prior to witnessing the event (Eakin et al., 2003). Because people are trying to understand what they witnessed, misleading information that provides some sort of causal explanation for what happened is more likely to be misremembered (Chrobak & Zaragoza, 2013; Rindal et al., 2017). People can even mislead themselves. Witnesses who give false information (i.e., deliberately lie about what they saw) have a poorer memory when they later try to remember accurately. They retrieve less true information and are more likely to have their lies intrude on their memory (Pickel, 2004). In their minds, their lies have become truths.

TRY IT OUT

A paradigm in research on eyewitness memory is on misleading post-event information. In this paradigm, people witness an event, and then afterward, they are exposed to information that is inconsistent with what was actually observed. To assess this, first, get a video of some extended event. This video can be one that you make or one that you find on the internet. The video can be an automobile accident or a crime, but it does not have to be. All it needs to be is a video that shows something happening. It does not even need to be live action. It could be animated. This video should be a few minutes long and contain enough elements that would allow you to later mislead your viewers.

From this video identify some element about which you will mislead some people. Come up with an alternative that would be plausible in that situation, but which was not actually seen. For example, a road sign could be a stop sign in the video, and you could choose yield sign as the misleading item. Alternatively, if the video is of a crime, the criminal could move a calculator on a desk in the video, and you could use a cell phone as your misleading item. Choose whatever makes sense for the event that you picked.

For this study you will need at least three groups with 20 or more people in each. These groups will be (a) control, (b) consistent, and (c) misled. At the beginning of the study, have all three groups watch the same video. Then, give participants a short distractor task in which they do something unrelated to the task at hand for five minutes. For example, you could have them solve Sudoku puzzles.

After the distractor period, give the participants a series of questions about the video. Twelve to 20 questions should be sufficient. All but one question should be about things that happened, such as "Was the car following a truck when it passed the drugstore?" Overall, half of the questions should elicit a "yes" answer and half a "no" answer. Importantly, among the filler questions, you should have a critical one. For the neutral group, the question should refer to the item in general terms, such as "Did the car turn right at the traffic sign?" For the consistent group, the question should refer to the actual item, such as "Did the car turn right at the stop sign?" Finally, for the misled group, the question should refer to the misleading item, such as "Did the car turn right at the yield sign?" This question should be worded so that the assumption in the question is that the misleading item is true.

After the question period, there should be another distractor period like the earlier one. After that, you should have a final forced-choice recognition test. This test should be about a dozen items. For each item, the question should ask about some detail of the video, and there should be three options to choose from. For example, a question might be "What was the car following when it passed the drugstore: (a) truck, (b) SUV, (c) motorcycle?" The critical item will assess whether people will distort their memories in favor of the misleading post-event information. This critical question should contain answers that are the original item, the misleading item, and a new item. For example, the critical question could be "At what sort of traffic sign did the car turn right: (a) stop sign, (b) yield sign, (c) no parking sign?"

After your participants are done, collect their responses. Total up the number of correct, misled, and other answers for the critical item and see how the rates of these responses varied across the three groups. What you should find is that the rate of reporting the misled items should be greater for the misled group than the other two groups. For interesting variants, you can look at different types of videos, different ways of presenting the misleading information, different retention intervals, or anything else that you think could influence the outcome.

Several explanations have been given for how eyewitness memory reports are altered by misleading post-event information. These theories vary in the fate of the original information, and how the misleading information dominates later responses. The three that are covered here are memory replacement theory, memory coexistence theory, and source monitoring theory. Each has some support, and it is likely that the misleading post-event information effect is driven by multiple causes (Loftus & Hoffman, 1989).

For **memory replacement theory** (Loftus, 1979), misleading information replaces or overwrites the original memory, which is permanently lost or altered. This can be seen when people are given three alternatives on the memory test in which one was the original item (e.g., yield sign), one was the misleading item (e.g., stop sign), and a third was a new item (e.g., no parking sign). After the initial response, people selected their best second-guess. If people initially selected the misleading item, the probability of selecting the correct item as a second guess is at chance. If the original memory was still present, then performance should have been higher. This is consistent with the idea that the original information is absent from memory.

A second view, **blocking theory**, is that the original and misleading information coexist in memory, but the original information is being blocked by the newer information. Because the misleading information is more recent, it has a stronger activation level in memory. Thus, it obscures the original memory, making it hard for a witness to be accurate. It has been shown that if people are asked to recall an event prior to being exposed to misinformation, they are more likely to accept the misinformation (Chan et al., 2009). Recalling the event may make it easier to bind and integrate the misinformation into memory, blocking access to the original memory. This is like the processes of reconsolidation in which memories are altered.

It may even be the case that the original memory is inhibited, similar to what happens with retrieval practice (MacLeod & Saunders, 2005). In a study by Berkerian and Bowers (1983), if the context was adequately reinstated at the time the questions were asked, then the effect of misleading post-event information was reduced or eliminated. This was done by having the questions match the order of the original event rather than a random order. In another study by Christiaansen and Ochalek (1983), people were warned before the memory test that some questions contained misleading information. With this warning, people could disregard some things and perform more like people who were not misled. Thus, they could remove the memory traces containing the misleading information that had blocked access to the original memory and focus only on those traces for the original event. Finally, even when there appears to be no memory for the original event on a direct memory test, like recognition, there is evidence that the information is still present when an indirect memory test is used, such as lexical decision (Dodson & Reisberg, 1991).

A third view, **source monitoring theory**, suggests that there may be a source monitoring problem (see Chapter 13) playing into the misleading post-event information effect. Witnesses who encounter misleading information generally remember where it came from (Zaragoza & Koshmider, 1989). However, errors do occur. These source monitoring errors are more likely for people who are more dissociative thinkers and can more readily disengage from external reality (they also show a lower correspondence between their accuracy and their confidence) (Cann & Katz, 2005).

It should be noted that when people create incorrect descriptions this makes memory even worse (Lane & Zaragoza, 2007), particularly if such self-generated false reports are used to help explain why something *may* have happened (Chrobak & Zaragoza, 2013). People even come to accept as real the memories that were generated as part of a false confession (Porter & Baker, 2015; Shaw & Porter, 2015). This heightened belief in self-implanted memories is because self-generated inaccuracies bring the misinformation, generation, and verbal overshadowing effects together to work against accurate source monitoring. Reflective thinking makes the aspects of memory that distinguish source more obscure, leading to an increase in source monitoring errors. The more thematically similar misleading information is to the witnessed event, the more likely that errors are made.

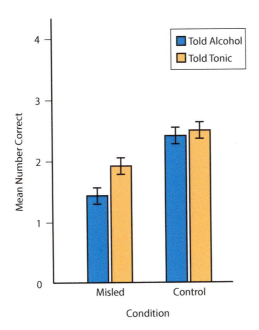

FIGURE 14.2 *Influence of Perceived Alcohol Consumption on Memory Performance*

Source: adapted from Assefi, S. L., & Garry, M. (2003). Absolut memory distortions: Alcohol placebos influence the misinformation effect. *Psychological Science, 14*, 77–80

Just because people encounter misleading information does not mean that memory is altered. It depends on the trustworthiness of the source. For example, misleading information about an accident is more likely to have an effect if people think it came from a bystander than if it came from a driver involved in the wreck (Dodd & Bradshaw, 1980).

Physiological state can also influence eyewitness memory. For example, people who consume alcohol prior to witnessing an event remember less, although what they do remember is just as accurate as people who were sober (Altman et al., 2018; Flowe et al., 2016; Hagsand et al., 2017). In an interesting twist, Assefi and Garry (2003) found that people were more susceptible to misinformation if they thought they had recently consumed alcohol (even though they had not because the experimenters gave them drinks that only tasted like alcohol), as seen in Figure 14.2. Thus, even implicit social demands can influence eyewitness memory. What was more disconcerting was that not only did people who *thought* they had consumed alcohol make more errors, but they were also more confident in their answers.

Witness Collaboration

There has been a great deal of evidence over the years that witnesses can contaminate one another's memories. Moreover, witnesses working together could also suffer from the effects of collaborative inhibition (see Chapter 8). However, there is also evidence emerging that witnesses can help each other remember more. This generally works by first having witnesses recall an event individually and then collaboratively. This way, memory reports can be garnered prior to any possibility of contamination.

Under these circumstances, collaborating witnesses can prune out the errors that they remember individually, without altering the amount of correct information remembered (Vredeveldt et al., 2016). This occurs both when collaborative remembering is done by people who are familiar with one another or not (Vredeveldt et al., 2019). Collaborators who do this often acknowledge other people's statements, as well as repeat, rephrase, and elaborate on what the other person said. All of this can bolster memory when the collaborators are accurate. Moreover, after collaborative remembering, witnesses may become less susceptible to misleading suggestions (Rossi-Arnaud et al., 2019).

Arousal Influences

Events involving eyewitnesses are often not standard and mundane. Instead, they are emotion-arousing situations, such as when someone witnesses a violent car accident or is a victim of a serious crime. How do intense emotions affect eyewitness memory? Do emotions make memory better? Do they make it worse? Well, the picture is somewhat complicated, although there is no doubt that memory is influenced by emotion (see Deffenbacher et al., 2004 for a meta-analysis) or arousal from physical exertion (Hope et al., 2012). This relationship is outlined by Christianson (1992).

One view is that emotion and memory follow the **Yerkes–Dodson law** (Yerkes & Dodson, 1908). According to this view, arousal is a continuum, with memory being an inverted-U-shaped function, as shown in Figure 14.3. At low

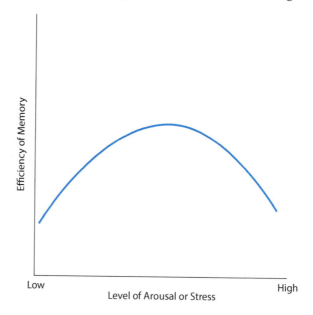

FIGURE 14.3 *The Yerkes-Dodson Law*

levels of arousal, people do not encode information very well. This is like trying to study when you are tired. As arousal increases, performance increases as well, up to a point. There is a level where memory is maximized. Beyond that point, people are over-aroused, and memory worsens. This is like trying to study when you are preparing to go out on a hot date. Thus, people who are bystanders to a violent crime are likely to remember more than the victims. The bystander would be closer to the optimum arousal level, whereas victims could be too highly aroused.

Overall, memory does follow the Yerkes–Dodson law. However, the situation is more complicated than this. The ability to remember details under different levels of arousal depends on the type of details. At high levels of emotion, memory for peripheral details (e.g., the color of a car, someone's clothing, the actions of bystanders, etc.) is worse. However, memory for central details (e.g., what a robber said) is better. This is consistent with the **Easterbrook hypothesis** (Easterbrook, 1959) which says that at higher levels of emotional intensity, people restrict attention to a narrower range of details. Attention is more focused (Kensinger et al., 2007; but see Laney et al., 2005), a process called **cue utilization**. At normal emotion levels, people notice a variety of things in their environment, giving more attention to various details. However, during an emotional event, attention focuses in on the principal parts of that event and less on other details (see also, tunnel memories in Chapter 12). Thus, peripheral details are less well remembered, whereas the central details are better remembered. For example, if you encountered two people in a nonstressful event, you might remember their faces equally well. However, if you met them as part of a stressful event, where one was a bank robber and another was a person in line, the cue utilization that occurs would lead you to pay more attention to, and thus better remember, the robber's face relative to the other customer's face.

Although high levels of emotion can lead to more accurate memory for a narrower range of information, this does not mean that people do not report a wide range of things. Although accurate memory is present for the focal details, people can still fill in memories with what they *expect* to be present based on their schemas and scripts. For example, people who see both emotional and neutral pictures show boundary extension effects (see Chapter 5) of similar magnitudes (Candel et al., 2003). In effect, they are interpreting their memories of the pictures they have viewed using their expectations of what likely extended beyond the boundaries of the images.

A good example of the influence of emotional intensity is the **weapon focus effect**, which is an increase in memory for a weapon (such as a gun, knife, cleaver, etc.) along with a decline in memory for other details (Maass & Köhnken, 1989; see Fawcett et al., 2013 for a meta-analysis). Recordings of eye movements while watching pictures that depict a crime show that people spend more time looking at what a person is holding if it is a weapon than if it is a neutral object (Loftus et al., 1987). This even occurs when a weapon is present but not involved in a violent action (Kramer et al., 1990). The barrel of a gun or the blade of a knife is a point of interest to people, and they spend a lot of time looking at such things. At some

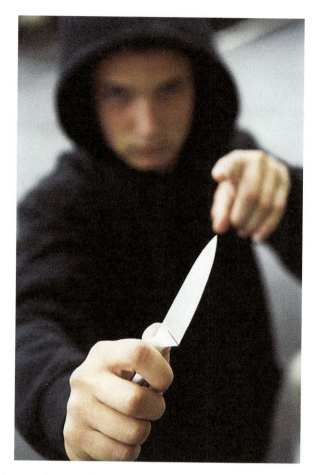

PHOTO 14.1 *Memory for eyewitnessed events can be influenced by the level of arousal experienced. Attention and memory tends to narrow in on central aspects of the event, as with the weapon focus effect*

Source: Monkey Business Images/ Shutterstock.com

level, we want to know whether the weapon will be used against us. This increased attention to a weapon increases memory for it and decreases memory for other aspects of the event, such as a perpetrator's face.

John Dean's Memory

One of the more famous cases of memory in legal proceedings is John Dean's memory for the cover-up of the Watergate break-in during President Nixon's administration leading to the president's resignation. John Dean, a White House advisor, testified before Congress against President Nixon and the other coconspirators about the cover-up in terms of what was going on in the White House. What was remarkable about Dean's testimony was the number of conversations he claimed to remember and the degree of accuracy with which he remembered them. (His initial statement to Congress was 245 pages). His memory was so remarkable that reporters nicknamed him "the human tape recorder."

The interesting thing is that soon after John Dean had given his testimony, real tape recordings emerged that Nixon had secretly made of White House conversations. At that point, it was possible to compare Dean's memory with the recordings and perform a scientific study of memory for conversations that had legal implications. This is just what was done (Neisser, 1981).

In comparing the initial testimony concerning things that were claimed to have been said and the actual conversation on the tapes, John Dean hardly ever got it *exactly* right. Many things that he claimed were said were never actually said at specific meetings. For example, with regard to one White House meeting, Dean claimed that Nixon had asked him to sit down, had asked Halderman (another aid) to keep him posted, and had praised Dean for doing a good job. Also, John Dean claimed that he himself had made statements about not really wanting to take credit for his efforts and that the cover-up would eventually unravel. The tapes revealed that none of these statements were made during the particular meeting in question.

However, a comparison of Dean's statements and the tapes also indicated no attempt to lie on Dean's part. The tapes do corroborate important points in Dean's testimony, such as the fact that the White House was aware of and was involved in the cover-up. Often the distortions in Dean's testimony reflected a schematization of his prior memory. His memory reflected the events in a cleaned-up fashion. Also, Dean misremembers himself as playing a more central role in the conversations than was the case. This self-centered bias is an expected aspect of anyone's memory of any event. This is because our memory of an event includes both the things that objectively occurred and our own subjective thoughts and emotions that would be stored as part of the memory trace. Any act of remembering will involve these components.

Stop and Review

While eyewitness testimony is generally accurate, it can be altered. The way a question is worded can bias how people misremember an event. People also incorporate misleading information into their reports, either because the original memory is altered or replaced, because a misleading memory has blocked access to the original, accurate memory, or because of problems with source memory. Eyewitness memory is affected by a witness's level of arousal. Consistent with the Yerkes–Dodson law, at high levels of arousal, overall memory is worse. This is because attention during encoding is focused on fewer, critical details, consistent with the Easterbrook hypothesis. This is seen in the weapon focus effect. Furthermore, John Dean's memory provides evidence for the idea that an eyewitness may be inaccurate for some of the details but be spot on for the gist of a crime.

EYEWITNESS CONFIDENCE

Is there any way to assess how accurate eyewitness reports are, especially when there are few to no other sources of corroborating evidence? Intuitively it seems that eyewitness confidence should be an indicator of memory accuracy. However, the monitoring of one's own memory is imperfect (see Chapter 15). The same applies to eyewitness accounts. It is possible to have people who are very confident that an innocent person committed a crime. For eyewitness identification, the relation between accuracy and reported confidence is far from perfect. In terms of memory for details, confidence is more reliable for central as compared to peripheral details (Roberts & Higham, 2002). Thus, it is possible to have witnesses who are very confident and still wrong.

Eyewitness confidence is influenced by several factors. One is **post-identification feedback**, which is information about the quality of an eyewitness's report. For example, if positive feedback is given to a witness, such as "Good. You identified the suspect," then the confidence in memory increases, compared to when no feedback is given. This can lead witnesses to embellish claims about the quality of their view of the crime, the clarity of their memory, and the speed with which they remember identifying the person (Wells & Bradfield, 1998; 1999). Of course, there is no way for such a comment to actually improve any of these qualities of memory.

Also, telling somewhat what other witnesses reported increases confidence. For example, after a lineup identification for an offender, if a witness is told that another witness picked the same person, confidence increases. However, if the person hears that another witness picked someone else, confidence decreases (Luus & Wells, 1994). Thus, the relation between accuracy and confidence can be distorted by subsequent information.

Witness confidence is also influenced by how many times questions are asked. The more people are asked about an accident, the more confidence they have in their memories. In general, the passage of time typically makes memories worse, not better. Still, confidence increases with more retellings. This also occurs for misleading post-event information (Shaw & McClure, 1996). This increase in confidence from repeated retellings is unrelated to memory accuracy.

Repeated questioning makes information easier to access and more salient in memory (remember it is impossible to probe a memory without changing it). Increased retrieval fluency may lead people to be more confident in their accuracy (Shaw, 1996; but see Odinot & Wolters, 2006). This is important because judges and juries are often swayed by the confidence a witness has. By the time a witness gets to trial, the same questions have been answered many times, thereby increasing confidence without increasing accuracy. Trying to make people aware of the relationship between their level of confidence and memory accuracy may either have no effect or actually worsen things (Robinson & Johnson, 1998). Finally, eyewitness confidence can be influenced by external motivation to remember accurately. This is illustrated in detail in the Study In Depth box.

To address the issue of how eyewitness confidence and motivation can affect eyewitness accuracy, let us look in detail at a study by Shaw and Kerr (2003). This study assessed the eyewitness memory of 75 students at Lafayette College. An event was identified by the researchers for which the students would be tested later. Specifically, during the third week of the academic term, the students heard a nine-minute presentation from the college counseling center.

Five days later, the students were given a surprise memory test about what they remembered. The test consisted of a randomized list of 12 three-alternative multiple-choice questions about the classroom visitor's appearance and what she talked about. The students were also asked to rate their confidence in their answers to each question. The students could go through the memory test at their own pace.

Critically for this study, for half of the students there was no extra motivation to remember accurately (the control group). However, the other half (the experimental group) were told that they could get a prize if their answers were correct. Specifically, the person with the most correct answers would get $25, and the next highest ten scorers would get a candy bar of their choice. Thus, half of the students were extra motivated to be correct. How did this additional motivation affect memory?

Extra motivation did not alter the accuracy of the memory reports and confidence ratings. People were similarly accurate no matter which group they were in. However, motivation did affect the relationship between accuracy and confidence. For the control group, the correlation between accuracy and confidence was relatively good: $r = .44$. However, for the students with the extra motivation, the correlation was horrible: $r = .05$. By encouraging people to try harder, a great deal of effort is associated with each memory retrieval attempt. Thus, it becomes harder for people to identify what was easy to remember and what was hard. As a result, the usefulness of the confidence ratings drops. This is important because eyewitnesses to accidents and crimes are often motivated to try hard to remember. Such an external motivation may end up backfiring.

Stop and Review

Although eyewitness confidence is often used as an indicator of accuracy, the real relationship between confidence and accuracy is lower than would be desired. Moreover, this relationship is worsened by several factors, including reinforcing feedback, repeated attempts to remember, and external encouragement to try to remember more accurately.

THE COGNITIVE INTERVIEW

Given that eyewitness memory can be error prone, can anything be done to improve these reports? Research has led to information gathering methods to increase accuracy and decrease the impact of misinformation. One of these is the **cognitive**

interview. This technique uses basic memory principles to maximize the amount of correct information and minimize the amount of incorrect information (Fisher et al., 2011; Geiselman et al., 1984; see Memon, et al., 2010 for a meta-analysis). The cognitive interview focuses on five retrieval processes.

The first is to use the principles of encoding specificity and mood dependent learning (see Chapter 7). There should be an attempt to reinstate the external and internal contexts of the event. This can include having people imagine being back at the scene and feeling how they felt at the time. Reinstating the context serves as a retrieval cue, making it more likely that people can access their memories. As a reminder, context is most likely to influence memory retrieval during recall with weaker memory traces—just as in the case of investigator interviews.

Second, because people sometimes retrieve only partial information, as with the tip-of-the-tongue state (see Chapter 9), witnesses are encouraged to report whatever they can, however partial or insignificant it may seem at the time. For example, if a witness cannot remember someone's name but can remember how many syllables it had or what letter it began with, then it should be reported. Information, even in a fragmentary state, can potentially be useful to investigators.

Third, there are often many retrieval pathways to a given memory. When we forget, we may be able to retrieve a memory later if we take a different approach (see Chapters 7 and 8). This can be done by reporting an event in a variety of orders. Starting at different points emphasizes different types of information, and different details are reported. This enhances eyewitness reports.

Fourth, people may report information from different perspectives (see Chapter 9). Altering perspective may make some information more salient and more likely to be reported. Thus, the witness's report is more complete. Alternative perspectives provide alternative retrieval pathways, allowing information to be remembered that might otherwise have been missed.

Finally, interviewers are discouraged from interrupting a witness's report. By disrupting people, the flow of the retrieval plan is disturbed, and more weakly stored information might not be reported. This is like the part-set cuing effect (see Chapter 9), in which providing people with part of a learned set of information can result in the probability of recalling a given item decreasing rather than increasing. In short, interrupting people disrupts their idiosyncratic retrieval plans, thereby worsening memory.

The cognitive interview has been modified to elicit more accurate eyewitness reports. An enhanced cognitive interview places the witness more in control of the retrieval of memories (Fisher & Geiselman, 1992). Moreover, a shortened version has been devised to elicit the needed information in less time (Bensi et al., 2011).

The cognitive interview is an effective eyewitness memory tool. It can boost the reports of accurate information by more than 50% without noticeable changes in the amount of incorrect information (Fisher et al., 1989). The cognitive interview takes more time to administer than a standard interview. However, given the amount of extra work that might be needed without it, the cost is well worth it.

Improve Your Memory

Most of what you remember does not come from witnessing an accident or a crime (thankfully). That said, there are some lessons to be learned and applied to your everyday situations. For example, you can take the techniques that are used for the cognitive interview and apply them to your everyday memories. This can include trying to mentally reinstate the context and emotional state you were in when you experienced an event, not being shy about using whatever partial information you may have available, trying different ways of thinking about the event, and giving yourself some time to let weaker aspects of the memory come to mind. You should also adopt a healthy skepticism of your confidence in your memories. Remember, the accuracy–confidence correlation is generally positive. That said, you can be confident about something and still be wrong. Finally, try to keep the limits of memory in mind when listening to other people describing events that they remember. They may be inaccurate about things, even things that they are confident about. This healthy skepticism can be useful if you ever serve as a juror for a trial.

Stop and Review

Although eyewitness memory is imperfect, by using what we know about memory we can do things that increase accuracy. The cognitive interview does this by considering what is known about the influences of learning context, partial retrieval, hypermnesia, and part-set cuing on memory to avoid situations that deter accurate remembering.

EYEWITNESS IDENTIFICATION

Eyewitnesses may be asked to identify people, particularly the culprits of crimes. An eyewitness must remember reliably and accurately. However, as we have seen, we are prone to forgetting, which can lead us to make errors. For eyewitness identification, this can lead to two undesirable outcomes: (1) failing to identify a perpetrator or (2) misidentifying an innocent person as the perpetrator. In cases of DNA exoneration of previous convictions, erroneous eyewitness identification was the primary cause of the imprisonment of innocent people. Several things can influence a witness's memory of a person involved in a crime. Some of these are beyond the control of the legal system, such as whether a perpetrator was carrying a weapon (which reduces accuracy), how good the lighting was at the time, how far away the perpetrator was from the eyewitness (Lampinen et al., 2014), and how much stress the eyewitness was experiencing at the time (Valentine & Mesout, 2009). However, steps can be taken to increase identification accuracy (Clark & Godfrey, 2009; Wells et al., 2006).

Mugshots

Mugshots are a standard way to help identify perpetrators. Essentially, an eyewitness is shown a series of photographs of people who have been involved in previous crimes. If a witness can identify the perpetrator from this set of faces, investigators can more quickly solve the crime. However, mugshots can also have negative effects on memory. If people are shown a series of mugshots, and the perpetrator is not among them, the eyewitness may sometimes still pick out a person from the series of mugshots. When people do this, the ability to identify the perpetrator later is lower than for people who do not incorrectly identify someone (Gorenstein & Ellsworth, 1980). Essentially, memory for the selected mugshot interferes with, and makes it harder to retrieve, the memory of the face of the perpetrator.

When a perpetrator is not among the mugshots, witnesses may later pick out another person whose mugshot was viewed earlier, even if that person was not identified during that time (Memon, et al., 2002). Witnesses may pick these people because they are familiar, not realizing that the familiarity is due to previously seeing the mugshot rather than seeing the perpetrator. People have better memory for having seen a face before, than remembering *where* they saw that face (Brown et al., 1977). Thus, problems in source monitoring can lead to errors in eyewitness identification.

A process that also focuses on face memory is to have a sketch artist make a drawing of a perpetrator. This is a type of recall memory. Unfortunately, individual drawings created using this method are poorer than one would hope. That said, morphing the drawings from several witnesses can produce a more accurate image (Wells & Hasel, 2007). The poor recall observed here is likely because people do not encode faces as sets of features but in a more holistic fashion.

Unconscious Transference

An important aspect of eyewitness memory that investigators cannot control is **unconscious transference**. This occurs when a person mistakenly identifies an innocent bystander as the perpetrator (Ross et al., 1994). In such cases, people remember seeing the offender and others but then become confused. As a result, an innocent bystander is incorrectly remembered as being the person who committed the crime.

A particularly compelling description of unconscious transference is provided by Baddeley et al. (2015, p. 344). In 1975, Donald Thompson, an Australian psychologist, was accused of raping a woman in her apartment and leaving her unconscious. The day after the rape he was picked up by the police. The woman who had been raped had accused him as being the culprit and identified him out of a police lineup. However, he was clearly innocent of the crime. Why? Well, at the very time the rape was happening he was far away giving a live television interview on the unreliability of eyewitness testimony. Additionally, part of that interview was with a member of the Australian Civil Rights Committee and the Assistant Commissioner of Police. When Thompson explained to the arresting officers that he had these people as witnesses for his alibi, they replied "Yes, and I suppose you've got Jesus Christ and the Queen of England, too!" So, how could such a false accusation from the victim occur as part of this traumatic event? Well, just prior to and during the rape, the woman's television was on and this live broadcast was playing. She accurately remembered Thompson's face as part of the event (it was on the television) but mistakenly remembered how he was involved.

What happens with unconscious transference is that witnesses remember seeing people as bystanders but also as perpetrators. This is a memory blending theory of unconscious transference (Ross et al., 1994). This may occur because witnesses know that each person was involved in the event, but they have trouble remembering the role each one played (Kersten et al., 2013). Thus, an eyewitness may remember that two people were involved, one as the perpetrator and the other as a bystander, but then later confuse the roles. Another view is a source monitoring theory of unconscious transference (Read, 1994). Here, witnesses remember people but fail to remember the situation in which they interacted with them. As a result, witnesses may be more likely to misattribute the source of a memory as a case of remembering the person as the perpetrator.

Lineups

One factor that can affect eyewitness identification is what happens during a lineup. Suspect identification is a recognition process. This can be a live lineup, but more often this is a photo lineup. Witnesses compare their memories with what they see: the faces in a lineup. During identification, people make judgments based not only on how well a given person matches their memory, but also how well the different people in the lineup compare to one another in terms of how much they resemble the offender. This is the **relative judgment principle** (Wells, 1984; but see Fife et al., 2014). According to this principle, witnesses may select someone from a lineup not because this was who they saw, but because, compared to the others, that person most closely resembles the criminal. Thus, **lineup similarity**—the physical resemblances of lineup members—is important. Lineups with fillers who do not resemble a suspect are biased toward the witness choosing a suspect, even if they are not the offender. An example of this was conveyed by Colloff et al. (2016, p. 1227).

> In 1986, a woman viewed a lineup and identified the police suspect, Leonard Callace, as her attacker. She had described the attacker as a White male with reddish-blonde Afro-style hair and a full beard. But Callace—who had a full beard and straight hair—appeared in the lineup with 5 men who had only moustaches. After Callace served 6 years in prison, DNA evidence revealed he was not the attacker.

When lineup fillers fit the basic description given by the witness, people need to use memory more carefully, and their selections are more diagnostic (Wells et al., 1993). With similar fillers, the identification of guilty suspects is roughly the same as when they are dissimilar, but the identification of innocent suspects decreases considerably (Lindsay & Wells, 1980).

Eyewitness identification can also be influenced by the instructions given, such as whether the instructions include a statement that the perpetrator might not be present. This explicitly allows the possibility of the witness not identifying anyone. Without this simple instruction, there is a bias to select *someone*. Thus, innocent people may be identified just because they resemble the perpetrator. In comparison, with this additional instruction, people feel less compelled to pick someone, and the false identification rate drops dramatically (Malpass & Devine, 1981). In general, the rate of false identification drops by about 42 percent when this instruction is included. The rate of not selecting a perpetrator drops by only about 2 percent (Steblay, 1997).

Finally, eyewitness identification is also influenced by how a lineup is presented. The traditional lineup—what you see in movies and television—is a **simultaneous lineup**, where all of the alternatives are shown together, and the witness is asked to select one. Another type is a **sequential lineup**, where the witness sees one person at a time. How well people make decisions under these conditions has been a concern and is not just limited to eyewitness identification (Basu & Savani, 2019). As one example, similar principles seem to operate when trying to decide which product to buy. While there is some evidence that sequential lineups may lead to fewer errors (Lindsay & Wells, 1985; see Steblay et al., 2011, for a meta-analysis), more recent work suggests that simultaneous lineups may be better (Clark et al., 2014). These types of lineups allow people to make better recognition decisions because alternatives can be more easily compared.

Sequential lineups also are prone to shifts in an eyewitness's response criteria (bias) as they progress through the lineup. Witnesses are more likely to adopt a stricter (more conservative) criterion for people seen earlier, and a looser (more liberal) criterion for people seen later. Thus, this may introduce a bias in the ability to identify a perpetrator (Meisters et al., 2018).

Stop and Review

As with other memories, the act of using a memory can change it. Having seen a face before in mugshots can mistakenly lead people to think that it was the face of the perpetrator. Also, an eyewitness may make an unconscious transference error and misremember a bystander as the perpetrator. Additionally, the type of lineup used can influence memory. Finally, lineup accuracy is increased if people are explicitly reminded that they can say "not present" if the person is not there.

JURIES

The influence of memory in legal arenas affects areas other than eyewitnesses. Another important setting is juries. Jury trials, while fairly efficient, are not as crisp and clean as one would hope. Here we look at two ways that memory can influence jury decisions apart from other cognitive factors (Salerno & Diamond, 2010). These are the order in which information is encountered and the ability to disregard inappropriate information.[2]

---

2 For a compelling description of jurors' understanding of memory principles during a murder trial, see Brainerd (2013).

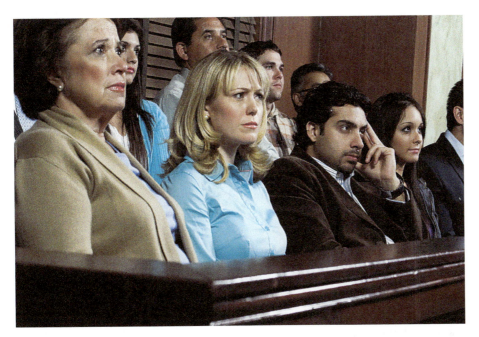

PHOTO 14.2 *It is important to understand how memory works when considering how people make decisions on a jury. Each juror is prone to the same memory distortions*

Source: sirtravelalot/Shutterstock.com

Information Order

When jurors hear evidence, they try to mentally construct an understanding of the event as a coherent story, much like what happens with autobiographical memory (see Chapter 12). Only in this case the memory is for other people's experiences (Pennington & Hastie, 1986; 1988). Juror memories are affected by the order in which they learn information, just like other settings. This order influences the decisions rendered later. There are two ways to assess how information order affects jury decisions. The first is a step-by-step process in which people render preliminary decisions after each piece of information is given. Under these circumstances, people show a recency effect (Pennington & Hastie, 1992). That is, decisions are more influenced by what was learned most recently. The most recent information is most available in memory, so people are more likely to rely on it.

The other way to assess the influence of information order is to have people make decisions after all the information is given. Here, one of two things can happen. If people are given background information, such as a motive for a killing, then decisions show a recency effect. However, if they are not given background information, but are given only reports from various witnesses, then people show a primacy effect (Kersholt & Jackson, 1998). This happens because background information provides a starting point, and people are more willing to adjust their opinions based on new information. However, without this background information, people try to make a coherent story with the information they have. Thus, they need to keep more information of their own creation active in working memory and are more reluctant to alter their prior understanding of the events, which would require more mental effort.

Jurors may hear contradictory testimony, sometimes from the same witness. How is memory affected by these inconsistencies? Are jurors more affected by the initial statement or the later, contradictory statement? As it turns out, they are affected by both. For inconsistent testimony from a given witness, jurors remember and note both statements and tend to place less emphasis on such testimony when making their decisions (Berman & Cutler, 1996).

Inadmissible Evidence

A problem that can arise before a jury trial (as with pretrial publicity) or during the trial itself, is when jury members are exposed to inadmissible evidence. If this happens, a judge has a couple of choices. One is to declare a mistrial and the other is to instruct the jurors to disregard or ignore the inadmissible evidence. Clearly, the second alternative is preferable if the jury can be trusted to do so because it makes the process quicker.

The instruction to disregard evidence is essentially directed forgetting (see Chapter 8). The question here is how well does the instruction to forget work in a real-world setting? When memory for inadmissible evidence is tested for, jurors' memories for the inadmissible evidence are poorer than for admissible evidence. Thus, there is some success in forgetting. However, when looking at assessments of a defendant's attributes (e.g., friendly, dishonest, etc.) and decisions to convict or acquit, there continues to be an influence of the inadmissible evidence. The presence of damaging inadmissible evidence biases jurors toward a guilty verdict, whereas supporting inadmissible evidence biases jurors toward a not guilty verdict (Golding & Hauselt, 1994; Thompson et al., 1981). Generally, people continue to use information they were supposed to disregard to make attributions about a person (Wyer & Unverzagt, 1985). This is because the memories for inadmissible information may have been suppressed, and people have difficulty accessing the source in long-term memory (Bjork & Bjork, 2003). Thus, jurors may remember the information but not where it came from. As a result, they forget that they are supposed to forget it. This is a form of the sleeper effect.

This influence of the to-be-forgotten information on decision making is also affected by jurors' opinions about the source or nature of the information. Directed forgetting is less efficient, and the opinions are more biased when the jurors believe that information is accurate and relevant to the defendant, such as when the information is described as confidential but inadvertently presented. However, directed forgetting is more efficient and opinions less biased when the jurors believe that the information is inaccurate and irrelevant to the defendant (Golding et al., 1990). For example, forgetting is more efficient if the information referred to another person in a different case. Alternatively, if the jurors are suspicious of the source of the inadmissible evidence, it does not affect their decision making (Fein et al., 1997). For example, if people are exposed to pretrial publicity that is damaging to the defendant, and then later learn that this information was leaked by a source trying to unfairly discredit the defendant, then jurors successfully forget it.

There are clear influences of inadmissible evidence on the decisions of individual jurors. While this may be troubling, the influences of this ineffective forgetting can be mediated or softened during the deliberation process where the jurors discuss the case with each other and come to a consensus about the verdict (London & Nunez, 2000). The collective memory efforts of the jury dampen the implicit influences of to-be-forgotten and inappropriate information. The information is weakened and cannot compete with the stronger, explicit, knowledge that is being openly discussed during deliberation.

As a final point, not all inadmissible evidence comes from external sources. Sometimes it comes from the jurors themselves. When people think about events, they may think about how things might have been different. This is **counterfactual thinking**. When people engage in counterfactual thinking, they are likely to focus on behaviors that are outside of a person's normal routine. Jurors are more likely to award a victim a larger compensation if the defendant did something out of the ordinary because it is easier to imagine that person doing something different. However, if the victim did something outside of his or her normal routine, then the juries tended to award a smaller compensation. It is as if they are, in part, unconsciously blaming the victim. Moreover, the smaller the size of people's working memory spans, the less likely they are to suppress these irrelevant thoughts when making decisions (Goldinger et al., 2003).

Stop and Review

Memory is important for juries. Their decisions are influenced by the order in which information is heard. The also vary in their effectiveness at suppressing, or forgetting, inadmissible evidence. Even when they try to conform to instructions, the decisions juries reach can be biased in the direction of the inappropriate information due to unconscious processes. That said, the collective deliberation process can mitigate some distorting effects of memory.

PUTTING IT ALL TOGETHER

Memory has practical value that is important for our society to be well-functioning and fair. This is seen clearly in the legal arena. Problems can arise when we lose knowledge of the source of a memory or our reports of events become distorted. This may happen when we are asked questions with biased wording; when we encounter misinformation; when we become confused about who a perpetrator was and who were just bystanders, or faces in a set of mugshots or a lineup. Please note that while eyewitness memory can be distorted, overall, much of what eyewitnesses remember is accurate, especially prior to encountering potential sources of contamination (Wixted et al., 2018).

Other aspects of memory bring about fair and just outcomes. While our emotions can limit the overall scope of our knowledge, they are also a focusing lens to better remember more critical, central details. This is the distinction between the Yerkes–Dodson law and the Easterbrook hypothesis. Furthermore, while confidence in our memories is not ideal, it does have some merits, so long as we guard against situations that can throw confidence and accuracy out of whack. This includes comments and feedback that are given later, as well as the number of times a memory is reported. The study of human memory and legal issues are brought together with the cognitive interview to provide society with guidelines to increase to the effectiveness of the pursuit of justice.

Finally, memory also has an important influence on juror decision making. Under some circumstances, the testimony that we hear most recently has a greater influence, a kind of recency effect, whereas under other circumstances, there is a preference to base decisions on the earlier information. As jurors, we also may find it hard to forget information that was deemed inadmissible, especially when it may seem relevant. That said, the jury deliberation process, in which we work together, can mitigate and correct some of these biases and errors.

STUDY QUESTIONS

1. How can an eyewitness's memory be altered by what they hear after witnessing an event?
2. What are some likely effects of misleading post-event information?
3. What are some of the theoretical explanations for the misleading post-event information effect?
4. How does an eyewitness's arousal level at the time of an event affect memory? What theory best captures this?
5. How does the presence of a weapon during a crime affect memory?
6. What do the findings about John Dean's testimony tell us about eyewitness memory?
7. What is the relationship between eyewitness confidence and accuracy? How can this be altered, and with what outcome?
8. How does the cognitive interview work to produce more accurate memory reports?
9. How is eyewitness identification affected by the use of mugshots? By different types of lineups? By things that are said by an investigator?
10. How is eyewitness identification affected by the presence of bystanders, in terms of unconscious transference?
11. How does the order in which jurors hear things affect their memories?
12. What happens in the memories of jurors when they are instructed to disregard inadmissible evidence? How does this influence their decision making?

KEY TERMS

- blocking theory
- cognitive interview
- counterfactual thinking
- cue utilization
- Easterbrook hypothesis
- eyewitness testimony

- memory replacement theory
- misleading post-event information
- post-identification feedback
- relative judgment principle

- sequential lineup
- simultaneous lineup
- source monitoring theory
- unconscious transference
- weapon focus effect
- Yerkes–Dodson law

EXPLORE MORE

Here are some additional readings that you can use to further explore some of the ideas about how memory can impact legal issues.

Brainerd, C. J. (2013). Murder must memorise. *Memory*, *21*(5), 547–555.

Christianson, S. Å. (1992). Emotional stress and eyewitness memory: A critical review. *Psychological Bulletin*, *112*, 284–309.

Fawcett, J. M., Russell, E. J., Peace, K. A., & Christie, J. (2013). Of guns and geese: A meta-analytic review of the "weapon focus" literature. *Psychology, Crime & Law*, *19*(1), 35–66.

Fisher, R. P., & Geiselman, R. E. (1992). *Memory Enhancing Techniques for Investigative Interviewing: The Cognitive Interview*. Springfield, IL: Charles C. Thomas.

Lampinen, J. M., Neuschatz, J. S., & Cling, A. D. (2012). *The Psychology of Eyewitness Identification*. New York: Taylor & Francis.

Neisser, U. (1981). John Dean's memory: A case study. *Cognition*, *9*, 1–22.

REFERENCES

Altman, C. M., Schreiber Compo, N., McQuiston, D., Hagsand, A. V., & Cervera, J. (2018). Witnesses' memory for events and faces under elevated levels of intoxication. *Memory*, *26*(7), 946–959.

Assefi, S. L., & Garry, M. (2003). Absolute memory distortions: Alcohol placebos influence the misinformation effect. *Psychological Science*, *14*, 77–80.

Baddeley, A. D., Eysenck, M. W., & Anderson, M. C. (2015). *Memory*. New York: Psychology Press.

Basu, S., & Savani, K. (2019). Choosing among options presented sequentially or simultaneously. *Current Directions in Psychological Science*, *28*(1), 97–101.

Bensi, L., Nori, R., Gambetti, E., & Giusberti, F. (2011). The enhanced cognitive interview: A study on the efficacy of shortened variants and single techniques. *Journal of Cognitive Psychology*, *23*(3), 311–321.

Berkerian, D. A., & Bowers, J. M. (1983). Eyewitness testimony: Were we misled? *Journal of Experimental Psychology: Learning, Memory, and Cognition*, *9*, 139–145.

Berman, G. L., & Cutler, B. L. (1996). Effects of inconsistencies in eyewitness testimony on mock-juror decision making. *Journal of Applied Psychology*, *81*, 170–177.

Bjork, E. L., & Bjork, R. A. (2003). Intentional forgetting can increase, not decrease, residual influences of to-be-forgotten information. *Journal of Experimental Psychology: Learning, Memory, and Cognition, 29,* 524–531.

Brainerd, C. J. (2013). Murder must memorise. *Memory, 21*(5), 547–555.

Brown, E., Deffenbacher, K., & Sturgill, W. (1977). Memory for faces and the circumstances of encounter. *Journal of Applied Psychology, 62,* 311–318.

Candel, I., Merckelbach, H., & Zandbergen, M. (2003). Boundary distortions for neutral and emotional pictures. *Psychonomic Bulletin & Review, 10,* 691–695.

Cann, D. R., & Katz, A. N. (2005). Habitual acceptance of misinformation: Examination of individual differences and source attributions. *Memory & Cognition, 33,* 405–417.

Chan, J. C. K., Thomas, A. K., & Bulevich, J. B. (2009). Recalling a witnessed event increases eyewitness suggestibility: The reversed testing effect. *Psychological Science, 20,* 66–73.

Christiaansen, R. E., & Ochalek, K. (1983). Editing misleading information from memory: Evidence for the coexistence of original and postevent information. *Memory & Cognition, 11,* 467–475.

Christianson, S. Å. (1992). Emotional stress and eyewitness memory: A critical review. *Psychological Bulletin, 112,* 284–309.

Chrobak, Q. M., & Zaragoza, M. S. (2013). When forced fabrications become truth: Causal explanations and false memory development. *Journal of Experimental Psychology: General, 142*(3), 827–844.

Clark, S. E., & Godfrey, R. D. (2009). Eyewitness identification evidence and innocence risk. *Psychonomic Bulletin & Review, 16,* 22–42.

Clark, S. E., Moreland, M. B., & Gronlund, S. D. (2014). Evolution of the empirical and theoretical foundations of eyewitness identification reform. *Psychonomic Bulletin & Review, 21*(2), 251–267.

Colloff, M. F., Wade, K. A., & Strange, D. (2016). Unfair lineups make witnesses more likely to confuse innocent and guilty suspects. *Psychological Science, 27*(9), 1227–1239.

Deffenbacher, K. A., Bornstein, B. H., Penrod, S. D., & McGorty, E. K. (2004). A meta-analytic review of the effects of high stress on eyewitness memory. *Law and Human Behavior, 28*(6), 687–706.

Dodd, D. H., & Bradshaw, J. M. (1980). Leading questions and memory: Pragmatic constraints. *Journal of Verbal Learning and Verbal Behavior, 19,* 695–704.

Dodson, C. S., & Riesberg, D. (1991). Indirect testing of eyewitness memory: The (non)effect of misinformation. *Bulletin of the Psychonomic Society, 29,* 333–336.

Eakin, D. K., Schreiber, T. A., & Sergent-Marshall, S. (2003). Misinformation effects in eyewitness memory: The presence and absence of memory impairment as a function of warning and misinformation accessibility. *Journal of Experimental Psychology: Learning, Memory, and Cognition, 29,* 813–825.

Easterbrook, J. A. (1959). The effect of emotion on cue utilization and the organization of behavior. *Psychological Review, 66,* 183–201.

Fawcett, J. M., Russell, E. J., Peace, K. A., & Christie, J. (2013). Of guns and geese: A meta-analytic review of the "weapon focus" literature. *Psychology, Crime & Law, 19*(1), 35–66.

Fein, S., McCloskey, A. L., & Tomlinson, T. M. (1997). Can the jury disregard that information? The use of suspicion to reduce the prejudicial effects of pretrial publicity and inadmissible testimony. *Personality and Social Psychology Bulletin, 23,* 1215–1226.

Fife, D., Perry, C., & Gronlund, S. D. (2014). Revisiting absolute and relative judgments in the WITNESS model. *Psychonomic Bulletin & Review, 21*(2), 479–487.

Fisher, R. P., & Geiselman, R. E. (1992). *Memory Enhancing Techniques for Investigative Interviewing: The Cognitive Interview.* Springfield, IL: Charles C. Thomas.

Fisher, R. P., Geiselman, R. E., & Amador, M. (1989). Field test of the cognitive interview: Enhancing the recollection of actual victims and witnesses of crime. *Journal of Applied Psychology, 74,* 722–727.

Fisher, R. P., Milne, R., & Bull, R. (2011). Interviewing cooperative witnesses. *Current Directions in Psychological Science, 20*(1), 16–19.

Flowe, H. D., Takarangi, M. K. T., Humphries, J. E., & Wright, D. S. (2016). Alcohol and remembering a hypothetical sexual assault: Can people who were under the influence of alcohol during the event provide accurate testimony? *Memory, 24*(8), 1042–1061.

Geiselman, R. E., Fisher, R. P., Firstenberg, L., Hutton, L. A., Sullivan, S. J., Avetissian, I. V., & Prosk, A. L.

(1984). Enhancing of eyewitness memory: An empirical evaluation of the cognitive interview. *Journal of Police Science and Administration, 12,* 74–80.

Golding, J. M., Fowler, S. B., Long, D. L., & Latta, H. (1990). Instructions to disregard potentially useful information: The effects of pragmatics on evaluative judgments and recall. *Journal of Memory and Language, 29,* 212–227.

Golding, J. M., & Hauselt, J. (1994). When instructions to forget become instructions to remember. *Personality and Social Psychology Bulletin, 20,* 178–183.

Goldinger, S. D., Kleider, H. M., Azuma, T., & Beike, D. R. (2003). "Blaming the victim" under memory load. *Psychological Science, 14,* 81–85.

Gorenstein, G. W., & Ellsworth, P. C. (1980). Effect of choosing an incorrect photograph on a later identification by an eyewitness. *Journal of Applied Psychology, 65,* 616–622.

Gurney, D. J., Pine, K. J., & Wiseman, R. (2013). The gestural misinformation effect: Skewing eyewitness testimony through gesture. *American Journal of Psychology, 126*(3), 301–314.

Hagsand, A. V., Roos af Hjelmsäter, E., Granhag, P. A., Fahlke, C., & Söderpalm Gordh, A. (2017). Witnesses stumbling down memory lane: The effects of alcohol intoxication, retention interval, and repeated interviewing. *Memory, 25*(4), 531–543.

Hope, L., Lewinski, W., Dixon, J., Blocksidge, D., & Gabbert, F. (2012). Witnesses in action: The effect of physical exertion on recall and recognition. *Psychological Science, 23*(4), 386–390.

Kensinger, E. A., Garoff-Eaton, R. J., & Schacter, D. L. (2007). Effects of emotion on memory specificity: Memory trade-offs elicited by negative visually arousing stimuli. *Journal of Memory and Language, 56,* 575–591.

Kersten, A. W., Earles, J. L., & Upshaw, C. (2013). False recollection of the role played by an actor in an event. *Memory & Cognition, 41*(8), 1144–1158.

Kerstholt, J. H., & Jackson, J. L. (1998). Judicial decision making: Order of evidence presentation and availability of background information. *Applied Cognitive Psychology, 15,* 445–454.

Kramer, T. H., Buckhout, R., & Eugenio, P. (1990). Weapon focus, arousal, and eyewitness memory. *Law and Human Behavior, 14,* 167–184.

Lampinen, J. M., Erickson, W. B., Moore, K. N., & Hittson, A. (2014). Effects of distance on face recognition: Implications for eyewitness identification. *Psychonomic Bulletin & Review, 21*(6), 1489–1494.

Lane, S. M., & Zaragoza, M. S. (2007). A little elaboration goes a long way: The role of generation in eyewitness suggestibility. *Memory & Cognition, 35,* 1255–1266.

Laney, C., Campbell, H. V., Heuer, F., & Reisberg, D. (2005). Memory for thematically arousing events. *Memory & Cognition, 32,* 1149–1159.

Lindsay, R. C. L., & Wells, G. L. (1980). What price justice? Exploring the relationship of lineup fairness to identification accuracy. *Law and Human Behavior, 4,* 303–313.

Lindsay, R. C. L., & Wells, G. L. (1985). Improving eyewitness identifications from lineups: Simultaneous versus sequential lineup presentation. *Journal of Applied Psychology, 70,* 556–564.

Lipscomb, T. J., Bregman, N. J., & McAllister, H. A. (1985). A developmental inquiry into the effects of postevent information on eyewitness accounts. *The Journal of Genetic Psychology, 146*(4), 551–556.

Loftus, E. F. (1979). The malleability of human memory: Information introduced after we view an incident can transform memory. *American Scientist, 67,* 312–320.

Loftus, E. F., & Hoffman, H. G. (1989). Misinformation and memory: The creation of new memories. *Journal of Experimental Psychology: General, 118(1),* 100–104.

Loftus, E. F., Loftus, G. R., & Messo, J. (1987). Some facts about "weapon focus." *Law and Human Behavior, 11,* 55–62.

Loftus, E. F., Miller, D. G., & Burns, H. J. (1978). Semantic integration of verbal information into a visual memory. *Journal of Experimental Psychology: Human Learning and Memory, 4,* 19–31.

Loftus, E. F., & Palmer, J. C. (1974). Reconstruction of automobile destruction: An example of the interaction between language and memory. *Journal of Verbal Learning and Verbal Behavior, 13,* 585–589.

Loftus, E. F., & Zanni, G. (1975). Eyewitness testimony: The influence of the wording of a question. *Bulletin of the Psychonomic Society, 5,* 86–88.

London, K., & Nunez, N. (2000). The effect of jury deliberations on jurors' propensity to disregard inadmissible evidence. *Journal of Applied Psychology, 85*, 932–939.

Luus, C. A. E., & Wells, G. L. (1994). The malleability of eyewitness confidence: Co-witness and perseverance effects. *Journal of Applied Psychology, 79*, 714–723.

Maass, A., & Köhnken, G. (1989). Eyewitness identification: Simulating the "weapon effect." *Law and Human Behavior, 13*, 397–408.

MacLeod, M. D., & Saunders, J. (2005). The role of inhibitory control in the production of misinformation effects. *Journal of Experimental Psychology: Learning, Memory, and Cognition, 31*, 964–979.

Malpass, R. S., & Devine, P. G. (1981). Eyewitness identification: Lineup instructions and the absence of the offender. *Journal of Applied Psychology, 66*, 482–489.

McAllister, H. A., Bregman, N. J., & Lipscomb, T. J. (1988). Speed estimates by eyewitnesses and earwitnesses: How vulnerable to postevent information? *The Journal of General Psychology, 115*(1), 25–35.

Meisters, J., Diedenhofen, B., & Musch, J. (2018). Eyewitness identification in simultaneous and sequential lineups: An investigation of position effects using receiver operating characteristics. *Memory, 26*(9), 1297–1309.

Memon, A., Hope, L., Bartlett, J., & Bull, R. (2002). Eyewitness recognition errors: The effects of mugshot viewing and choosing in young and old adults. *Memory & Cognition, 30*, 1219–1227.

Memon, A., Meissner, C. A., & Fraser, J. (2010). The cognitive interview: A meta-analytic review and study space analysis of the past 25 years. *Psychology, Public Policy, and Law, 16*(4), 340–372.

Neisser, U. (1981). John Dean's memory: A case study. *Cognition, 9*, 1–22.

Odinot, G., & Wolters, G. (2006). Repeated recall, retention interval and the accuracy–confidence relation in eyewitness memory. *Applied Cognitive Psychology, 20*(7), 973–985.

Pennington, N., & Hastie, R. (1986). Evidence evaluation in complex decision making. *Journal of Personality and Social Psychology, 51*, 242–258.

Pennington, N., & Hastie, R. (1988). Explanation-based decision making: Effects of memory structure on judgment. *Journal of Experimental Psychology: Learning, Memory, and Cognition, 14*, 521–533.

Pennington, N., & Hastie, R. (1992). Explaining the evidence: Tests of the story model for juror decision making. *Journal of Personality and Social Psychology, 62*, 189–206.

Pickel, K. L. (2004). When a lie becomes the truth: The effects of self-generated misinformation on eyewitness memory. *Memory, 12*, 14–26.

Porter, S. B., & Baker, A. T. (2015). CSI (crime scene induction): Creating false memories of committing crime. *Trends in Cognitive Sciences, 19*(12), 716–718.

Read, J. D. (1994). Understanding bystander misidentifications: The role of familiarity and contextual knowledge. In D. F. Ross, J. D. Read, & M. P. Toglia (Eds.), *Adult Eyewitness Testimony: Current Trends and Developments* (pp. 56–79). Cambridge, UK: Cambridge University Press.

Read, J. D., Barnsley, R. H., Ankers, K., & Whishaw, I. Q. (1978). Variations in severity of verbs and eyewitnesses' testimony: An alternative interpretation. *Perceptual and Motor Skills, 46*(3), 795–800.

Read, J. D., & Bruce, D. (1984). On the external validity of questioning effects in eyewitness testimony. *Applied Psychology, 33*(1), 33–49.

Rindal, E. J., Chrobak, Q. M., Zaragoza, M. S., & Weihing, C. A. (2017). Mechanisms of eyewitness suggestibility: Tests of the explanatory role hypothesis. *Psychonomic Bulletin & Review, 24*(5), 1413–1425.

Roberts, W. T., & Higham, P. A. (2002). Selecting accurate statements from the cognitive interview using confidence ratings. *Journal of Experimental Psychology: Applied, 8*, 33–43.

Robinson, M. D., & Johnson, J. T. (1998). How not to enhance the confidence-accuracy relation: The detrimental effects of attention to the identification process. *Law and Human Behavior, 22*, 409–428.

Ross, D. R., Ceci, S. J., Dunning, D., & Toglia, M. P. (1994). Unconscious transference and mistaken identity: When a witness misidentifies a familiar but innocent person. *Journal of Applied Psychology, 79*, 918–930.

Rossi-Arnaud, C., Spataro, P., Bhatia, D., & Cestari, V. (2019). Collaborative remembering reduces suggestibility: A study with the Gudjonsson Suggestibility Scale. *Memory, 27*(5), 603–611.

Salerno, J. M., & Diamond, S. S. (2010). The promise of a cognitive perspective on jury deliberation. *Psychonomic Bulletin & Review, 17*(2), 174–179.

Shaw, J. S. (1996). Increases in eyewitness confidence resulting from postevent questioning. *Journal of Experimental Psychology: Applied, 2*, 126–146.

Shaw, J. S., & Kerr, T. K. (2003). Extra effort during memory retrieval may be associated with increases in eyewitness confidence. *Law and Human Behavior, 27*, 315–329.

Shaw, J. S., & McClure, K. A. (1996). Repeated postevent questioning can lead to elevated levels of eyewitness confidence. *Law and Human Behavior, 20*, 629–653.

Shaw, J. S., & Porter, S. (2015). Constructing rich false memories of committing crime. *Psychological Science, 26*(3), 291–301.

Steblay, N. M. (1997). Social influence in eyewitness recall: A meta-analytic review of lineup instruction effects. *Law and Human Behavior, 21*, 283–297.

Steblay, N. K., Dysart, J. E., & Wells, G. L. (2011). Seventy-two tests of the sequential lineup superiority effect: A meta-analysis and policy discussion. *Psychology, Public Policy, and Law, 17*(1), 99.

Thompson, W. C., Fong, G. T., & Rosenhan, D. L. (1981). Inadmissible evidence and juror verdicts. *Journal of Personality and Social Psychology, 40*, 453–463.

Valentine, T., & Mesout, J. (2009). Eyewitness identification under stress in the London Dungeon. *Applied Cognitive Psychology, 23*(2), 151–161.

Vredeveldt, A., Hildebrandt, A., & Van Koppen, P. J. (2016). Acknowledge, repeat, rephrase, elaborate: Witnesses can help each other remember more. *Memory, 24*(5), 669–682.

Vredeveldt, A., Van Deuren, S., & Van Koppen, P. J. (2019). Remembering with a friend or a stranger: Comparing acquainted and unacquainted pairs in collaborative eyewitness interviews. *Memory, 27*(10), 1390–1403.

Wells, G. L. (1984). The psychology of lineup identification. *Journal of Applied Social Psychology, 14*, 89–103.

Wells, G. L., & Bradfield, A. L. (1998). "Good, you identified the suspect": Feedback to eyewitnesses distorts their reports of the witnessing experience. *Journal of Applied Psychology, 83*, 360–376.

Wells, G. L., & Bradfield, A. L. (1999). Distortion in eyewitnesses' recollections: Can the postidentification-feedback effect be moderated? *Psychological Science, 10*, 138–144.

Wells, G. L., & Hasel, L. E. (2007). Facial composite production by eyewitnesses. *Current Directions in Psychological Science, 16*, 6–10.

Wells, G. L., Memon, A., & Penrod, S. D. (2006). Eyewitness evidence: Improving its probative value. *Psychological Science in the Public Interest, 7*, 45–75.

Wells, G. L., Rydell, S. M., & Seelau, E. P. (1993). The selection of distractors for eyewitness lineups. *Journal of Applied Psychology, 78*, 835–844.

Wixted, J. T., Mickes, L., & Fisher, R. P. (2018). Rethinking the reliability of eyewitness memory. *Perspectives on Psychological Science, 13*(3), 324–335.

Wright, D. B., Memon, A., Skagerberg, E. M., & Gabbert, F. (2009). When eyewitnesses talk. *Current Directions in Psychological Science, 18*, 174–178.

Wyer, R. S., & Unverzagt, W. H. (1985). Effects of instructions to disregard information on its subsequent recall and use in making judgments. *Journal of Personality and Social Psychology, 48*, 533–549.

Yerkes, R. M., & Dodson, J. D. (1908). The relation of strength of stimulus to rapidity of habit-formation. *Journal of Comparative Neurology and Psychology, 18*, 459–482.

Zaragoza, M. S., & Koshmider, J. W. (1989). Misled subjects may know more than their performance implies. *Journal of Experimental Psychology: Learning, Memory, and Cognition, 15*, 246–255.

CHAPTER 15

Metamemory

Much of how our memories affect thinking and behavior occurs out of conscious awareness. Still, we do have some conscious insights into our memories. There are also instances in which we forget, yet have some inkling that we have this knowledge hidden away somewhere. To remember effectively, we need some awareness and control of our own memories. This is **metamemory**—the awareness of our own memories. This refers to both the contents of memory, as well as how to use it.

There are many ways to approach metamemory. First, we examine theories of metamemory, and then we cover some phenomena, including our ability to judge when we have learned something or whether we will later remember things that are currently forgotten. We also look at how we know that we *don't* know something. After this we cover the phenomenology of memory (what it feels like to remember or forget) and how what we know biases what we remember. Finally, we explore how to use what we know about our memories to improve them, including the use of mnemonics and some consideration of people with exceptional memories.

GENERAL PROPERTIES AND THEORIES OF METAMEMORY

Before addressing various aspects of metamemory, we will go over some basic concepts and theories. First, we cover the difference between cues and targets. After that, there is an overview of general theories of how metamemory judgments are made—namely, the cue utilization, accessibility, and competition hypotheses.

Cues and Targets

Memory traces that people make judgments about are **targets,** and the questions or prompts are **cues**. So, if someone were to ask you if you remember your thirteenth birthday, your memory for the birthday would be the target, and the question would be the cue.

Target-based sources are information from the memory trace about which the judgment is made, including information that was retrieved from memory, as well as the ease with which it is recovered. In comparison, cue-based sources are information gleaned from a memory cue, such as a question (Schwartz, 1994). Metamemory judgments are better in proportion to the familiarity of the cue information. Thus, if someone asks you a question about a topic that you are relatively familiar with, you are more inclined to say that you know the answer based on the familiarity of the concepts in the question. Now, let us look at three general theories of metamemory.

Cue Utilization Hypothesis

For the **cue utilization hypothesis** (Reder, 1987) metamemory judgments are based on the familiarity of the information in a cue. The emphasis is on cue-based information. The more familiar the cue contents are, the more likely that we will judge that the knowledge is in memory. Imagine if someone asked you if you know your grandmother's maiden name. If you know a lot about your family, you might recognize this as a familiar topic and say to yourself, "This is something I know." However, if you are unfamiliar with your family's history, you might recognize this as a topic you know little about and say to yourself, "I have no clue."

Accessibility Hypothesis

For the **accessibility hypothesis** (Koriat, 1993), metamemory judgments are inferential. People make inferences about what is in memory based on the information at hand, including partial retrievals. There are two sources of information that can be used. One is the *amount* of information that is activated. The more that is activated, the more likely that the knowledge is in memory. For example, if you cannot think of someone's name, but you know what letter it begins with, how many syllables it has, and so on, then you have a lot of information, and are more likely to judge that the name is in memory.

The other source of information is the *intensity* of the activated memory traces. This includes the ease of access, the vividness of any imagery, how specific the information is, and so on. The stronger the retrieved information, the more likely the knowledge is in memory. For example, if you are asked what your best friend's mother's maiden name is, several names might be activated, but only very weakly. As a result, you would decide that you do not know this. The cue utilization is more apt for metamemory decisions that are made under time pressure, otherwise the accessibility hypotheses is more appropriate (Metcalfe & Finn, 2008b).

Competition Hypothesis

For the **competition hypothesis** (Schreiber, 1998), metamemory judgments are influenced by memory competition during retrieval. Thus, the emphasis is also on target-based sources. Metamemory judgments are greater with less competition. When only a few traces are involved, the search process is targeted and is likely to produce the desired information. In contrast, if many traces are involved, resulting in interference, then it is less likely that the knowledge will be retrieved. The more competition among the traces, the more difficult retrieval will be.

Stop and Review

Metamemory judgments involve a cue and a target. The cue is the question about your memory, and the target is the contents of the memory itself. There are several theories of metamemory. One is that decisions are based on the familiarity of the cues. Another is that judgments are based on a partial memory search. Finally, metamemory judgments may reflect how much interference is experienced during retrieval.

KNOWING WHAT IS KNOWN

So, how well do we know our own memories? This includes assessments of how well information was learned, whether things that have been forgotten are still known, and how we know that we don't know something. The next sections address these issues.

Judgments of Learning

When learning, it is helpful to know how well new materials are stored in long-term memory. Information that is poorly learned should be studied more, and information that is well learned does not need as much further study. Estimates for how well we have learned something are called **judgments of learning**, or **JOLs** (Arbuckle & Cuddy, 1969). Studies of JOLs have shown that we are poor estimators of how much we actually learned. The question is, why?

One theory is the **inability hypothesis**. The idea is that JOLs are poor because we have little conscious awareness of our own mental processes (Nisbett & Wilson, 1977). We lack sufficient insight into ourselves and our memories. So much information is below conscious awareness that we are almost guaranteed to be wrong more often than we are right.

An alternative is the **monitoring-retrieval hypothesis**, which states that JOLs are poor because we are assessing whether we can retrieve information. When JOLs are made soon after the information was encountered, that information is still in working memory. Thus, we think that the information is better learned than it actually is. If some delay or interruption is present, then we could more accurately assess whether the material can be retrieved from long-term memory.

These theories were compared by Nelson and Dunlosky (1991, but see Kimball et al., 2012). They elicited JOLs either immediately or after a delay. If the inability hypothesis is correct, then a delay should not matter. However, if the monitoring-retrieval hypothesis is correct, then after a delay, working memory is cleared out, and people will depend more on long-term memory and judge future performance more accurately. In one study (Dunlosky & Nelson, 1994), people learned a set of words either through rote rehearsal or by forming mental images. As discussed in Chapter 3, memory is better when people use imagery. As shown in Figure 15.1, when people made JOLs immediately after studying, there was little to no distinction made between how well they thought they had learned in the two conditions. However, with a delay, the difference between JOLs was the same as what is revealed by actual memory performance.

These JOL improvements are consistent with Koriat's (1993) accessibility hypothesis. The low correspondence between immediate JOLs and later memory is due to a mismatch between conditions when people study (the information is present) versus at test (the information is absent), making it difficult to predict future memory (Koriat & Bjork, 2006). JOLs are more accurate the closer the conditions at the time the judgments were made to those during memory retrieval. When people can better assess what is in long-term memory, JOL estimates are more accurate.

Koriat (1997) outlined how JOLs are affected by three types of cues that are available to us: extrinsic, intrinsic, and mnemonic. **Extrinsic cues** are aspects of the learning situation, such as massed or distributed practice, or presentation times. We are not attuned to how these influence learning, and JOLs are generally not affected by extrinsic cues.

Intrinsic cues are aspects of the material being learned, such as the perceived ease or fluency of learning. In contrast to extrinsic cues, JOLs are sensitive to

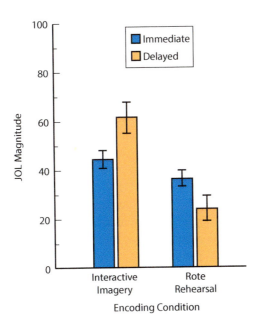

FIGURE 15.1 *Judgments of Learning: Words Were Learned under Imagery or Rote Memorization Instructions, Given either Immediately or after a Delay*

Source: adapted from Dunlosky, J., & Nelson, T. O. (1994). Does the sensitivity of judgments of learning (JOLs) to the effects of various activities depend on when the JOLs occur? *Journal of Memory and Language, 33,* 545–565

intrinsic cues. This is in line with the cue utilization hypothesis. That said, JOLs can be misled by irrelevant characteristics of the materials. For example, people say that information was better learned if it was presented in a larger font or heard at a louder level (Peynircioğlu & Tatz, 2019; Rhodes & Castel, 2008; 2009), perhaps because this makes it seem more important (Luna et al., 2019).

Finally, **mnemonic cues** are memory-based sources of information. These are assessments of how we have done on previous judgments. Over time, with practice, if we continue to make JOLs, we shift from using intrinsic cues to mnemonic cues (Ariel & Dunlosky, 2011). This is in line with the accessibility hypothesis.

Additional information does not always improve JOLs. In some cases, they can worsen. For example, multiple study–test cycles can worsen JOLs over time (Koriat, 2002). Declines in JOLs also occur when there is competition among memory traces. For the fan effect (see Chapter 8), retrieval is harder with more associations with a concept. This also lowers JOLs (McGuire & Maki, 2001). When additional memory traces compete with a desired trace, people judge that they do not know the information, thus JOL estimates worsen. This is in line with the competition hypothesis. Finally, things that are irrelevant can intrude on the JOLs. Alban and Kelley (2013) found that people gave higher JOLs if they were holding a heavier rather than a lighter clipboard while making their judgments. Presumably, the extra effort of holding a heavy clipboard got translated into greater effort spent learning, and so, increased JOLs.

In addition to providing guidance about whether something has been learned, JOLs have other memory benefits. People who give JOLs have better memories compared to those who do not (Rhodes & Tauber, 2011). In a sense, a JOL is a self-imposed testing effect (Akdoğan et al., 2016)[1].

Although JOLs can be inaccurate, we do have some sense of our own learning. JOLs impact the **allocation of study time** (Metcalfe & Finn, 2008a). Ideally, study time should maximize the amount of new knowledge that is learned. Spending all your time on material you already know well is less effective. It may increase overlearning, but it does not help you learn new things.

Although we can allocate study time based on a goal to learn certain things over others (Ariel et al., 2009), in general, we regulate study time based on how easy we think information is to learn. However, this is not always effective. People may choose distributed practice for easy items and massed practice for difficult items, which is ineffective (Son, 2004; but see Benjamin & Bird, 2006). When people first encounter information, they tend to put more effort into learning the harder items, often using massed practice (which gives the illusion of harder studying). Because these items are so difficult, people have trouble learning anything new. They spend more effort on things that are far from being learned. As a result, there is little gain of new knowledge. This is the **labor-in-vain effect** (Nelson & Leonesio, 1988).

However, the picture is not completely dismal. As people gain experience with the new material, study time allocation becomes more effective. People shift to spending more time on material that is just beyond their current ability. This is the **region of proximal learning** (Metcalfe, 2002; 2009). This method is more efficient

---

1 Conversely, testing during learning can also improve judgments of future memory (Barenberg & Dütke, 2019).

because people spend less time on knowledge that is well beyond their ability. Instead, they focus on things that can help them ratchet up to the next level. Moreover, people who study information in the region of proximal learning are less likely to mind wander while studying (Xu & Metcalfe, 2016).

As mentioned in Chapter 7, memory can be boosted if people take a test after studying as compared to simply studying some more. This is the testing effect. Another cause of the testing effect is that, after testing, people are better able to distribute their study time because they now have explicit knowledge of what they do and do not know (Soderstrom & Bjork, 2014). Overall, we have some awareness of our own learning. We do better when we pace our own learning rather than follow along at a set pace (Markant et al., 2014). That said, a major problem is that even when students know what the best study strategies are, and they express an intention to follow them at the beginning of a term, they often do not follow through (Blaisman et al., 2017).

Improve Your Memory

One of the primary reasons that we want to improve our memories is to make it easier for us to learn new things. This is particularly true for things that we learn in school. As is illustrated in this part of the chapter, sometimes we are not very good at knowing when we have learned something well enough. So, what can you do to improve this? Well, first off, as you are studying, write down a list of topics and questions that cover the material that you are studying. After you have read through and studied the material, set it aside and do something else for a while. Then come back to your list and see which of those topics and questions you can retrieve from memory. If you do retrieve them, then it is more likely that you have learned that material. If not, then you can better target your study time later.

Because you are only testing yourself on the material you initially determined to be important, this opens up the possibility that there can still be gaps in your knowledge. This is why you should try to find time to study with your classmates, quiz each other, and find out what you may have missed. Other people remember and think about the material differently from you and interacting with them allows you to more completely learn the material in a shorter amount of time than if you simply work by yourself. As always, be sure to begin with the material that overlaps the most with what you already know and work your way out to the more difficult material. This way you will not waste as much of your study time.

Feeling of Knowing

When you forget things, it does not always feel the same. Sometimes you do not know something, and it seems like you never learned it. Other times, you do not know the answer, but you feel that it is somewhere in memory, and if you heard or saw it, you would be able to identify it. These differences are revealed by **feeling of knowing**, or **FOK**, judgments (Hart, 1965).

To get FOK judgments, people are asked a series of moderately difficult questions, such as, "Who was Richard Nixon's vice president before Gerald Ford?" Some things were never learned, but others were learned but are no longer prominent. After failing to recall an answer, people make an FOK judgment by rating how likely it is that they would identify the answer on a later recognition test. Then, at the end, people are given a recognition test to see how good their FOK judgments were. In general, FOK judgments are reasonably good predictors, although there are some deviations.

For the cue-utilization hypothesis (Reder, 1987), FOK judgments are based on the familiarity of the information in the question or cue. One way to test this is by using the "game show" method (Reder, 1987) in which people are given a question and then either answer it (control condition) or indicate that they know the answer (game show condition). This is like a game show in which the contestants are asked a question and the one who hits the buzzer first gets to answer. This technique reveals that people know whether they have information in memory before they can retrieve it, as shown in Figure 15.2. Moreover, the rate at which people indicate that they know an answer is related to the familiarity of the information in the question, and not necessarily what is in memory (Reder & Ritter, 1992). Similarly, people give higher FOK ratings to things they think they ought to know, rather than what they actually do know (Costermans et al., 1992). In general, FOK involves a controlled assessment of memory and so people with frontal lobe damage are less accurate on FOK tasks (Janowski et al., 1989).

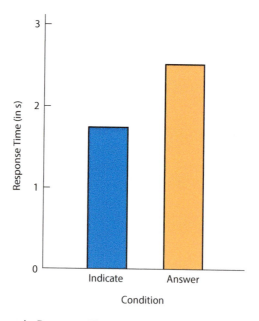

FIGURE 15.2 *Difference in Response Times: People Either Had to Answer a Question (Control) or Indicate that They Knew the Answer (Game Show)*

Source: generated from data reported in Reder, L. M. (1987). Strategy selection in question answering. *Cognitive Psychology, 19,* 90–91

FOK judgments are related to how much partial information is retrieved (Koriat, 1993). Most of this partial information is semantic attributes of what we are trying to remember (Koriat et al., 2003), such as failing to recall a name but knowing that the person was a nineteenth-century composer who lived in Germany. However, metamemory judgments can be tricked. For example, FOK increases when information is revealed slowly rather than presented all at once, showing a revelation effect (see Chapter 13) (Young et al., 2009). With lots of accurate partial information, there is a high correspondence between FOK ratings and future memory. However, if the partial information is incorrect, the correspondence is lower. Thus, the relation between FOK ratings and actual memory is not ideal.

Partial information also predicts whether what is eventually retrieved is "remembered" or is just "known" (Hicks & Marsh, 2002; see the remember-know section later in this chapter). A cue-utilization account applies more to the early stages of the processing, which is related to "known" information. However, an accessibility account applies more to later stages, when familiarity with the cue is high and people get past the initial evaluation stage (Koriat & Levy-Sadot, 2001) and focus more on "remembered" information. Finally, FOK judgments are affected by the number of competitors involved. If people are trying to remember something, FOK ratings are higher if that memory has fewer competitors (Schreiber, 1998), in line with the competition hypothesis.

Tip-of-the-Tongue State

A **tip-of-the-tongue (TOT) state** is when we fail to recall information but feel that we are about to retrieve it. It is on the tip of our tongues (Brown & McNeill, 1966).[2] This is like a FOK judgment. However, FOK judgments test whether we think the information can be remembered, whereas a TOT state indicates that remembering is imminent (Brown, 1991).

There are several characteristics of TOT states that have been identified (Brown, 1991). First, we experience them about once a week on average. Second, there is often some information available. We typically can think of words that are like the one that is needed, either in terms of meaning, sound, or both. Also, we may be aware of the first letter of a word or the number of syllables that the word has (Brown et al., 2013). Third, we often have trouble with proper nouns, such as names. Fourth, we may be aware of the first letter or sound of the word, and perhaps the last one as well, along with the number of syllables. Finally, the occurrence of TOT states is not related to current feelings of stress or anxiety.

One theory of the TOT state is the **incomplete activation view** (Brown & McNeill, 1966). A TOT state occurs when the search range has not been sufficiently narrowed. There are too many possibilities, so we cannot retrieve the desired word. Another theory is a **blocking view** in which TOT states occur when related but inappropriate competitors are activated to a greater degree, and block access to the appropriate information. Because these wrong traces have been retrieved recently, they are more available, and so are more likely to be retrieved again. We keep

2 See Thompson et al. (2005) for an account of a tip-of-the-fingers (TOF) state for deaf signers.

retrieving the wrong memories. This starts a vicious cycle, resulting in the TOT state. After some time, if you stop trying to retrieve the memory, the activation level of the blocking trace(s) goes down, and it becomes easier to access the information you had so much trouble getting at before.

Knowing that You Don't Know

Sometimes we feel like we know something, even if we cannot remember it at the moment. Other times, we know that we just **don't know** something. No matter how long we search, the information will never be remembered. For example, if I asked you "When was the city of Lakewood, Ohio, founded?" "Is *scissel* a word?" or "Does President Obama use an electric toothbrush?" most of you know immediately that you do not know the answer. People make these "don't know" judgments as rapidly as, if not faster than they do about knowledge that is actually in memory (Kolers & Palef, 1976). Why does this occur?

Feeling that we don't know something is different from feeling that we do (Liu et al., 2007).When we are asked about very unfamiliar topics, we rapidly make a judgment based on the information in the question, consistent with the cue-utilization hypothesis (Reder, 1987). For a question with very unfamiliar information, because the memory retrieval process does not get very far, we quickly identify the information as unknown. In general, things that we claim that we don't remember were generally never encountered before. They are accompanied by an absence of any feeling of familiarity, let alone recollection (Coane & Umanath, 2019).

In support of this, in a study by Glucksberg and McCloskey (1981), people first explicitly learned that they did not know certain pieces of information, such as "It is unknown whether John has a pencil" (*explicit don't know*) along with items that were known, such as "John has a shovel" (*true*) and "John does not have a chair" (*false*). After learning, people made "yes," "no," and "don't know" responses to these items, as well as to new items that they would not have known about. People were slower and less accurate in saying that they did not know something if they had previously learned that they did not know it than if they had never studied it (see Figure 15.3). Thus, by having something in memory for the "don't know" facts that were learned, there is now something in memory to access, and so retrieval slows down accordingly. However, when nothing was learned, there is nothing in memory, and so rapid "don't know" responses are made. "Don't know" responses are faster when there is no relevant information in memory, but they are hindered when there is relevant information in memory, even when this is knowledge that the information is not known.

When asked questions about things we do not have in memory, if the information is distinctive, it will not connect with many memory traces. This is a failure to retrieve any information in a very short time. Based on this lack of retrieval, we can judge that the information is not known (Ghetti, 2003). This is consistent with the accessibility hypothesis.

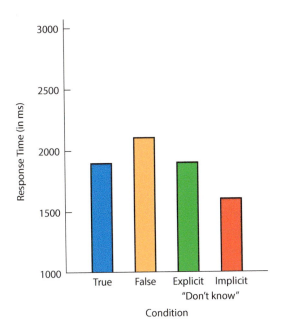

FIGURE 15.3 *Difference in Response Times: Questions were True, False, or Unknown—"Don't Know" Responses Were for Facts that Were Either Learned Earlier as "Don't Know" (Explicit) or Not (Implicit)*

Source: generated from data reported in Glucksberg, S., & McCloskey, M. (1981). Decisions about ignorance: knowing that you don't know. *Journal of Experimental Psychology: Human Learning and Memory, 7,* 311–325

Stop and Review

Judgments of learning are important for effective studying. Unfortunately, the relationship between JOLs and later accuracy is often low. Part of this is because people make JOLs before clearing out working memory. People use their JOLs to manage their study time in inefficient ways and may spend too much effort on material that is too difficult, laboring-in-vain. With more experience, people learn to use what is already known as a springboard for learning new things. When people forget something, they can estimate whether they know it, even if it is not currently available, using feeling-of-knowing judgments. These are based on either partial information or an assessment of the familiarity of a cue. When remembering seems imminent, it is a tip-of-the-tongue, or TOT, state. Finally, when there is no information in memory, people can quickly say that they don't know something.

MEMORY PHENOMENOLOGY

In this section we look at the phenomenology or conscious experience of remembering. We first look at the difference between conscious and unconscious memories as outlined by the remember–know distinction. Then we cover how errors in recollection lead us to misunderstand what things were like in the past, as with the hindsight bias.

Remember versus Know

Up to this point we have been talking about metamemory judgments for information that we either do or do not remember. Now, we consider cases where people rate the quality of what they do remember by making a **remember–know judgment** (Gardiner, 1988). If the remembering experience is accompanied by a conscious recollection of the circumstances in which the information was learned, this is a "remember" experience[3]. In contrast, if people do not consciously recollect, but only have a feeling of familiarity, this is a "know" experience.

A great deal of research has been done on the remember-know distinction (Gardner & Java, 1990; 1991; Gardiner & Parkin, 1990). It appears that "remember" and "know" responses reflect relatively independent qualities of memory (Dudukovic & Knowlton, 2006). Research has shown a double dissociation between these responses. That is, things that affect one type of response do not affect the other, and vice versa. Thus, remembering and knowing capture different qualities of memory.

"Remember," but not "know," responses are affected by elaborative rehearsal, generation effects, frequency of occurrence, divided attention at learning, the retention interval (if less than a day), reading silently or aloud, intentional versus incidental learning, serial position, and external context (Gruppuso et al., 2007). As an example, if you read something aloud, you are more likely to have a "remember" experience than if you read it silently. However, the probability of giving a "know" judgment would be the same, regardless of how you read the text. Also, as mentioned earlier in the text, if you walk through a doorway, this makes memory worse and this affects "remember" responses, but not "know" responses (Seel et al., 2019).

In contrast, "know," but not "remember," responses are affected by the amount of maintenance rehearsal, repetition priming, stimulus modality (e.g., visual or auditory), and suppression of focal attention. For example, if you engage in maintenance rehearsal and repeat a word over and over, this does not alter the degree to which you later recollect it. However, if you did remember it, you would be more likely to say that you "know" that you learned it.

There are cases where "remember" and "know" responses are both affected but in opposite ways. For example, word versus nonword memory, massed versus distributed practice, gradual versus abrupt presentations, and learning in a way that emphasizes similarities or differences (Cook et al., 2006). For example, with massed practice, "remember" responses are less likely and "know" response are more likely. In other cases, "remember" and "know" responses are similarly affected, such as by the retention interval (if more than a day), the amount of unfamiliar information, and long versus short response deadlines (when people must respond by a certain time).

---

3 Rubin et al., 2003, suggest that "remember" responses reflect a belief that an event occurred.

This distinction between "remember" and "know" responses corresponds to different memory qualities. "Remember" responses correspond to knowledge-based, conceptually driven processes, and "know" responses correspond to perceptually based, data-driven processes (Rajaram, 1993). This is supported neurologically. For example, relative to "know" responses, "remember" responses involve greater parietal lobe activity (Curran, 2000), greater EEG activity (Burgess & Ali, 2002) and more hippocampal activity, whereas "know" responses reflect more parahippocampal activity (Meeter et al., 2005).

This distinction between "remember" and "know" responses reveals differences between expert's and novice's memories. The influence of prior knowledge, such as schemas, on retrieval is often observed with recall but less frequently with recognition. Experts almost always recall more than novices, but they may not differ on recognition tests. This is related to the fact that experts are more likely to give "remember" reports, whereas novices are more likely to say that they "know" them. Long and Prat (2002) did a study of students at the University of California, Davis. They had students read stories based on the television series *Star Trek*. Some of the students were experts (people who watch the show a lot), and some were novices (people who saw the show only occasionally). The two groups did similarly on a recognition test. However, the experts were more likely to report that they remembered reading the items, whereas the novices were more likely to say that they knew them. The experts' prior knowledge allowed them to spend more time making inferences and elaborating on the memories they were creating, which made it more likely that they would have an experience of remembering it.

Recognition without Awareness

The difference between "remember" and "know" responses reflects differences in conscious experience, explicit and implicit memory, and direct and indirect memory assessment. Our metamemory abilities are limited. There are many memory processes that occur beyond awareness. This is even true for things that seem like we should have conscious awareness of, but we do not.

A simple form of memory retrieval is recognition. Something is encountered in the environment and we either recognize it as having been encountered before or not. This awareness of "pastness" should seemingly be conscious, even if we cannot explicitly say when or where in the past it happened. However, **recognition without awareness** occurs in which we recognize things that we have seen before, without the conscious awareness that we have done so (Peynircioğlu, 1990). We feel like these recognition judgments are being made at chance.

In one example of recognition without awareness, Voss et al. (2008) showed people a series of kaleidoscope images. Then, they were to select the ones that they had seen earlier from a set of old and new images. Although people felt like they were guessing, performance was well above chance. Thus, they recognized previously seen items, with no conscious awareness of doing so. This unconscious recognition is accompanied by changes in ERP signals 200–400 ms after the presentation of a

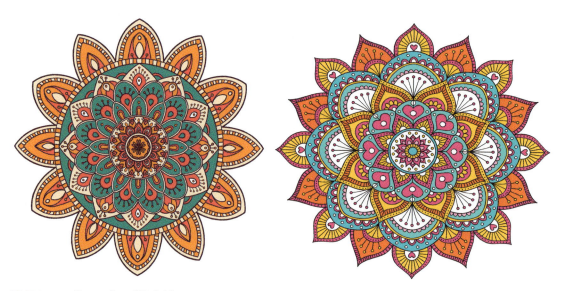

PHOTO 15.1 *Examples of Kaleidoscope Images Similar to the Ones Used to Assess Recognition without Awareness*

Source: (left) Evgenia L/Shutterstock.com; (right) Fairy-N/Shutterstock.com

test image (Voss & Paller, 2006). It is regularly observed with a variety of materials, including line drawings (Cleary et al., 2004), faces (Cleary & Specker, 2007), scenes (Cleary & Reyes, 2009), spoken words (Cleary et al., 2007), songs (Kostic & Cleary, 2009), and odors (Cleary et al., 2010).

Craik et al. (2015) suggested that recognition without awareness has two requirements. First, the knowledge must be encoded into memory. If not, then there can be no recognition because there are no memories. The second requirement is that information about context should be weak or absent. People would then have no feeling that something was experienced in the past.

Hindsight Bias

People tend to think of events as being more deterministic after they happen than they thought they would be before they occurred. This is the **hindsight bias**, and this increased deterministic thought after the fact is called "creeping determinism" (Fischhoff, 1975). For memory, the hindsight bias is seen when people remember their mental state as being different from what it really was. People misremember their memory as being more like their current knowledge state.

As an illustration of this, in a study by Safer et al. (2001) bereaved spouses rated their grief six months after the death and then four and a half years later. At the second rating, people also rated how much grief they felt at the six-month period. Although most people said they felt more grief at the six-month period than currently, their memory was positively related to their current level of grief. Thus, they misremembered their emotional states in hindsight based on their current state.

The hindsight bias pervades many aspects of life. Other examples are memories for predictions of outcomes of the Rodney King civil rights trial (Gilbertson et al., 1994), the Clarence Thomas Supreme Court Justice confirmation vote (Dietrich & Olson, 1993), the probability of a medical diagnosis being correct (Arkes et al., 1981), the results of political elections (Blank et al., 2003), the outcome of sporting events (Leary, 1981), and the inevitability of a work layoff (Mark & Mellor, 1991). This reinforces the idea that memories are in a constant state of flux and what we currently remember is, in part, due to our experiences and current state.

The hindsight bias also applies to romantic relationships. Our memories of our relationships are biased in the direction of our current opinion of the relationship. People who are happy with their relationship remember events more positively than people who are unhappy (McFarland & Ross, 1987). Moreover, even when relationship satisfaction is constant, people misremember the relationship as improving over time (Sprecher, 1999). This leads to an unusual idea that people in satisfactory relationships, even for marriages of over 20 years, are biased to remember the past as being worse than it really was, although they remember the relationship positively overall. This bias is a trick that makes the relationship seem as though it is improving more than it actually is (Karney & Coombs, 2000). Thus, as a result, people have a more positive attitude toward their relationship than if memory were accurate.

The hindsight bias is driven by a need to reconcile one's current view with memory for the past. For example, people show a larger hindsight bias when outcome information is surprising than if it is congruent with what one knows (Ash, 2009). The act of trying to make sense of a surprising outcome leads us to think more about the information, reconciling it with what is already known, thereby leading to the false impression that the information was better known than it actually was. The hindsight bias is not inevitable. For example, it can be reduced or eliminated if people are told ahead of time that they will be asked to remember both original judgments and the knowledge that was acquired later (Van Boekel et al., 2017).

A major variant of the hindsight bias is the **knew-it-all-along effect** (Wood, 1978). In studies of this phenomenon people are asked to evaluate information in some way at Stage 1—for example, judging whether a series of statements are true or false, such as "Lhasa is the capital of Nepal." Then, at Stage 2, people are given feedback about the information encountered at Stage 1, such as learning that Kathmandu is the capital of Nepal. This feedback is likely to be knowledge that the person did not have at Stage 1. Finally, in Stage 3, people indicate their memory for what they knew at Stage 1. Compared to people who got no feedback at Stage 2, metamemory reports of prior knowledge are biased toward the information learned during Stage 2. After Stage 2, people have a hard time remembering what it was like not knowing something, as if they knew it all along.

The knew-it-all-along effect can be reversed if the more recent learning is discredited. For example, if you did not know the capital of Nepal originally, were then told the name, you might show a knew-it-all-along effect. However, if you were then told that the Stage 2 information was wrong, this reverses the bias to say that the information was known all along, and there is a more accurate assessment of what was and was not known (Erdfelder & Bechner, 1998).

In general, it is hard to remember what it was like when we did not know something. College professors are no exception. If you have ever felt that some of your instructors have talked over your head, it may not necessarily be because they were arrogant or uncaring. The problem may have been that, because of the knew-it-all-along effect, they were having trouble remembering what it was like to learn the course material for the first time.

Another illustration of the hindsight bias is memory for remembering and forgetting. How well do we remember whether we had remembered or forgotten something previously? Joslyn et al. (2001) tested people one day and six weeks after learning. At the six-week session, people were asked whether they had remembered or forgotten items at the first session. People were more accurate at remembering their previous successes than their previous forgetting. About half the time people had originally forgotten something, it was later reported that it had been remembered. Thus, there is a metamemory bias to think that we have better memories than we do.

Memory can also be affected by our **beliefs** about memory. Winkielman and Schwartz (2001) told some people that sad events fade faster from memory, whereas others were told that happy events fade faster. People who were told that sad memories are forgotten faster were more likely to rate their childhood as less happy. It is as if people think that if they have forgotten more sad memories, then their childhood must have been less happy than they would have otherwise rated it.

While current knowledge can influence memory of prior knowledge, it is not the case that we have completely lost the original information. If the current knowledge state is discredited, we can disregard it and gain more accurate access to the original knowledge state. In a study by Hasher et al. (1981), Temple University students were first given a set of statements to rate as either true or false. In a second stage, they were told that some of the items were either true or false. Importantly, at the third stage, some of the students were told that the information they were given in the second stage was incorrect. If the second stage information was discreditation, then people accurately remembered their original opinion in the first stage. In contrast, people who received no discrediting showed the standard knew-it-all-along effect. This reinforces the idea that our memories are using multiple sources of knowledge and that what we remember is the degree to which these different memory traces and processes are emphasized.

A similar reduction of the knew-it-all-along effect occurs if people are asked to retrieve only information that was recently learned, rather than what they remember knowing before learning (Begg et al., 1996). Source monitoring helps us assess whether our knowledge is recent. Simply encouraging people to try harder

To better understand how beliefs and the hindsight bias can influence metamemory judgments, let us go over a study by Henkel and Mather (2007). The aim of this study was to assess whether people's beliefs about their choices change their memories for what those choices were. Specifically, people tend to misremember the features of various options that they were given to be more consistent with their own choices.

This study involved testing 80 students at Fairfield University who were asked to read through five scenarios in which they had to pick between two options. These scenarios involved making choices between roommates, summer internships, apartments, used cars, and potential dating partners. The order in which these scenarios were presented was randomized for each participant.

For each scenario, each of two options had both positive and negative features, and people were asked to pick which of these they would prefer. For example, for the used cars scenario there were ten features for each car. Five of the features were positive and five were negative. The positive and negative features were randomly assigned to each choice. The options for two cars are listed below. People read through the descriptions at their own pace.

Car 1	Car 2
Hard to find service outlets	No warranty
Has a dent from a previous accident	Some rust on exterior
Seats are very comfortable	High resale value
Good handling on turns	Has airbags
High mileage on odometer	Needs a few repairs
Makes an unidentified rattling sound	Not much trunk space
Prestigious model	Powerful engine
Air conditioning included	Previous owner took good care of car
Does not do well in bad weather	Not fuel efficient
Stereo included	Has a sun roof

Two days later, people returned and were given a memory test for the features of the options they had seen. For each scenario, these tests were randomly ordered lists of the features of the two choices, along with some additional features that were not seen. People were told to indicate whether each feature belonged to their original choice, the other choice, or was new.

What was found was that people were more likely to misremember the positive features as being for the choice they selected, and the negative features for the choice they selected against. Thus, people have a memory bias to think that things that are consistent with their own beliefs have more positive and fewer negative characteristics than they actually do.

does not help. While asking people to consider alternatives is helpful, asking them to try to remember something, even after it becomes harder to think of alternatives, may increase the hindsight bias. This happens because the additional retrieval attempts make the outcome seem more like it was already known (Sanna & Schwartz, 2004).

Stop and Review

Remembering is accompanied by different conscious experiences. "Remember" responses are associated with conscious recollection, whereas "know" responses are associated with unconscious feelings of familiarity. We are influenced by unconscious processes, even for basic direct memory tasks, such as recognition. This is recognition without awareness. Metamemory awareness sometimes leads people astray, as with the hindsight bias, in which we assess the past in a way that is more consistent with the present. Another example of this is the knew-it-all-along effect. Finally, our assessments of our own memories can influence how we believe or understand our memories to work, even if these beliefs are inaccurate.

MNEMONICS

When we are aware of the limitations of our own learning and memory, we can take steps to address them. One thing we can do is to use metamemory techniques, known as mnemonics. **Mnemonics** are mental or physical devices used to help people remember. In some cases, the mnemonics involve the application of principles of memory that we have already discussed and that we know improve memory, such as the use of mental imagery (Morris et al., 1978). Of course, the use of multiple strategies provides a larger boost to memory (Morris et al., 2005).

There are several ready-made mnemonic devices that can be used to help remember larger sets of information. One example is the **peg-word mnemonic**, in which people use a known sequence of items, or "pegs," on which to "hang" other pieces of information. For example, people might memorize the sequence "One is a bun, two is a shoe, three is a tree, (and so on)." This structure can then be used as a set of pegs for other information. For example, suppose you needed to go to the grocery store to buy onions, milk, and watermelon. You could use the peg word mnemonic by forming a mental image of sliced onions on a bun, a shoe full of milk, and watermelons hanging from a tree. When you get to the store, your sequence of pegs will help you remember the images you formed, and thus help you remember what to buy. Part of the reason the peg-word mnemonic works (as well as the method of loci, described next) is that there is an encouragement to form and use mental images (Wang & Thomas, 2000).

Another common mnemonic is the **method of loci** (Yates, 1966). Here, people first have a set of well-known locations, such as rooms in a house, places along a familiar path, and so on. A more linear path (e.g., a route to work) can be more effective than a set of locations with no clear linear ordering (Massen et al., 2009). People then imagine things at each location. To continue our grocery shopping example, you might mentally place the onions in the living room, cartons of milk at the foot of the stairs, and watermelons in the dining room. Then, to remember, you take a mental tour of your home. The method of loci builds on the fact that the hippocampus is important for spatial information, as well as declarative memories in general. The method of loci is better than other memory techniques, such as imaging survival scenarios, as with adaptive memory (see Chapter 7) (Kroneisen & Makerud, 2017).

A concern might be that, for the method of loci, people would need a new set of locations each time they want to learn something. Otherwise, proactive interference builds up (see Chapter 8) and the effectiveness of a set of locations decreases with each use. While proactive interference does occur, it is not the repeated use of the same spatial locations that produces it, but any overlap in the contents of the material (De Beni & Cornoldi, 1988). Repeated use of the same locations with the method of loci does not create additional proactive interference. There is something about spatial locations that allows them to be used over and over with less interference than is experienced with other types of concepts.

Other mnemonics take advantage of the information itself. A **rhyming mnemonic** takes all the information and forms a rhyme from it. For example, "Thirty days hath September, April, June, and November" is a rhyming mnemonic for the number of days in the months. **Acronyms** are a mnemonic in which the first letters of a phrase are used to help us remember. For example, the word HOMES is an acronym for the names of the five great lakes: Huron, Ontario, Michigan, Erie, and Superior. Finally, **acrostics** are a mnemonic in which the first letters of the items are used as the basis of forming a memorable phrase. For example, the phrase "On old Olympus' towering top, a Finn and German vault and hop" is used to help people remember the names of the twelve cranial nerves in the correct order: olfactory, optic, oculomotor, trochlear, trigemenal, abducens, facial, auditory, glossopharyngal, vagus, accessory, and hypoglossal. Remembering the phrase provides the cues for the appropriate names and sequence.

There are many mnemonics we can use. Sometimes a mnemonic is a simple cue, like tying a string around your finger or switching a wedding ring from one hand to the other, to remember to do something in the future (prospective memory). Other times, the structure of a mnemonic helps us remember the information itself, such as the knuckle mnemonic, which is another way of remembering how many days there are in each month (see Figure 15.4). For all mnemonics, the ability to cue memory is at work, in much the same way as the other sorts of cues we have talked about (see Chapter 7). Anything can be a mnemonic, so long as it is well structured. Mnemonics can even be done using the steps you go through to make a sandwich (Bouffard et al., 2018).

As noted in Chapter 7, information can be represented in memory at different levels. For example, text memory involves three levels of representation: the

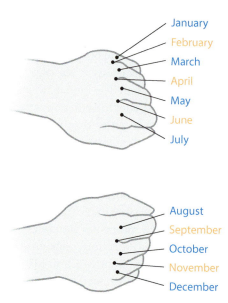

FIGURE 15.4 *The Knuckle Mnemonic*

surface form (verbatim memory), the textbase (memory for the ideas in a text), and the mental model (the situation described by the text). While the surface form and textbase levels are forgotten rapidly, memory at the mental model level is more stable, showing less forgetting (Fisher & Radvansky, 2018). The benefit of event cognition and narrative memory applies not only to memory for stories and situations you have encountered, it can also be turned around. You can use a **story mnemonic** to help you learn information that is not in a story form to begin with. As an example, Bower and Clark (1969) gave two groups of students 12 sets of ten words each to learn in order. One group was told to learn the words and their order as best as possible. This was the *control group*. The other group was told to make up a story starting with the first word and going to the second. This was the *narrative group*. As shown in Figure 15.5, averaged across lists, people who created stories remembered the information much better. Thus, if you are looking for a way to better learn material that you are struggling with, try to make a story out of it.

Stop and Review

People can use metamemory knowledge to help them remember, as with mnemonics. Some mnemonics simply involve an application of memory-based principles. Others are more formal and rely on learning a new structure, as with the peg-word mnemonic. In comparison, other mnemonics use some well-known or readily available structure that can then be used as a guide, as with the method of loci. Other mnemonics use language, as with rhymes, acronyms, and acrostics. Mnemonics use any stable structure, including physical cues, such as a string tied around one's

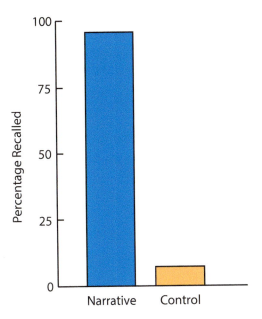

FIGURE 15.5 *Memory for Words as a Function of People Using a Story Mnemonic or Simply Trying to Remember as Effectively as They Can*

Source: generated from data reported in Bower, G. H., & Clark, M. C. (1969). Narrative stories as mediators for serial learning. *Psychonomic Science, 14*(4), 181–182.

TRY IT OUT

An important feature of metamemory is the ability to exert some control over your own learning and memory. For this Try It Out section we look at the use of mnemonics and mental imagery (Neath, 1998). Ideally you should have at least 16 participants in each of two groups.

First, create a list of 40 concrete nouns (things like dog, house, or rope, and not like truth, justice, or hope). Give your participants 20 random pairings of these words. Tell people that they will later need to be able to recall the second word when given the first word. For one group (the control group) simply tell them to memorize the word pairs as efficiently as possible. For the second group (the imagery group) tell them to try to form a mental image in their mind that involves the two objects interacting in some way (they don't need to tell you what the images are). Give people in both groups about five seconds per word pair during the study portion. Alternatively, you could use other mnemonics, such as the method of loci, the story mnemonic, or some other memory device, to see how these affect later memory.

At the end of the study portion, give people the first words of each pair and see if they can recall the second. You can do this by simply providing them a sheet of paper with the first words written in a column and have them write down the other work next to the appropriate first word. Total up and average the number of items remembered in each group. What you should find is that people who use imagery as a mnemonic should remember more of the words than the control group.

finger. Finally, the story mnemonic is an effective way of storing new information in memory.

EXCEPTIONAL MEMORY

Having an awareness of your own memory is helpful. Further improvements can occur as your range of knowledge is broadened. The more you know, the easier it is to remember because it is easier to organize and chunk information. Thus, expertise can cause you to have what would otherwise seem an exceptional memory for certain types of information.

We saw some of this in Chapter 4 with the case of S. F., a runner who extended his digit span to over 80 items (Ericsson et al., 1980; see also Ericsson et al., 2017 for a person with a digit span of 300). Another example is taxi drivers' memories for street names. Their superior memory is due to both the large amount of knowledge they have about streets in their city and the highly organized way that this information is represented. Information is chunked based on routes through the city (how they use this knowledge), rather than spatial proximity, semantic relatedness, or alphabetical order (Kalakoski & Saariluoma, 2001).

Other exceptional memories are cases when people use implicit knowledge. Speakers of tonal languages, such as Mandarin Chinese and Vietnamese, have better memory for musical pitches and are more likely to have perfect pitch than speakers of nontonal languages, such as English (Deutsch, 2002). Because those languages place a greater demand on remembering pitch, this knowledge is then applied, at an unconscious level, to memory for tone pitches in music.

MEMORISTS

People with exceptional memories are called **mnemonists** or **memorists**. We use the term memorist here because they are not necessarily relying on mnemonics (Neisser, 1982). A well-known memorist was Solomon V. Shereshevsky, better known as S., a man who lived in the Soviet Union in the early to mid-twentieth century (Luria, 1968). S. worked as a newspaper reporter in Moscow and had the uncanny ability to accurately remember many details of an event without taking notes. S.

had a short-term memory span of over 70 items, with the additional amazing ability of recalling them in any order requested. He could also recall lists of items years after hearing them only once. It is important to note that S. did not think that his memory was markedly better than anyone else's.

A major contributor to S.'s ability was the fact that he had synesthesia. This is a condition in which sensory qualities from different modalities intrude on one another. For example, different sounds may also be experienced as colors. S.'s synesthesia made his memory traces richer and more detailed, allowing them to endure, be highly structured in memory, and be recalled accurately. While S.'s condition allowed him to remember exceptionally large sets of items, there were some drawbacks. For one, because he was so dependent on sensory and perceptual qualities, he found it difficult to comprehend and think about abstract ideas.

Not all memorists have an unusual neurological condition. There are a number of accounts of memorists and the techniques they use (Gordon et al., 1984; Hunt & Love, 1972; 1983; Wilding & Valentine, 1997). To get an idea of how people become memorists, we look at three in detail, all of whom were in the *Guinness Book of World Records* for reciting pi from memory.

The first is Rajan Mahadevan (Biederman et al., 1992; Thompson et al., 1993; Thompson et al., 1991) who set the record on July 5, 1981, by reciting pi out to 31,811 digits in 3 hours and 49 minutes. His memory ability was first observed at the age of five when his parents hosted a dinner party for 50 people and he memorized, in just a few minutes, the license plate numbers of all of the guests' cars and then reported them back. Rajan has a letter span of 13, a visual digit span of 28, and an auditory digit span of 43. One strategy he used was keeping track of the position of an item in a sequence and then used this sequence to report information back. His exceptional memory was confined to digits and similar information. He sometime extended his memorization approach to other types of information but not always with the same level of success. For example, when given a list of words, he was less likely to use semantic relations. Moreover, his memory for stories and spatial information was in the normal range. Rajan also memorized information from a text or lectures. However, as many professors will tell you, while memorization is important, what is just as important is the ability to apply and use that knowledge.

The second pi memorist is Hideaki Tomoyori who set his record on March 9, 1987, by reciting pi out to 40,000 digits in 13 hours and 6 minutes (Takahashi et al., 2006). Tomoyori had good skills for memorizing long lists of numbers, but his memory for word lists and stories was not exceptional. Tomoyori accomplished his task using a digit-symbol mnemonic in which the Japanese symbols for digits were combined to form words and then images. The digit-symbol mnemonic is like assigning letters to numbers in English, (e.g., 1 = t, d or th; 2 = n; 3 = m; etc.). Thus, his approach was very different from Rajan's. He also had a large, but not far from normal, digit span of ten for auditory digits and eight for visual digits. His word and story memories were not different from everyone else. Thus, Tomoyori achieved his feat not through an innate talent, but through the persistent application of a particular strategy and a lot of effort.

Tomoyori's record was bettered by the pi memorist Chao Lu, who, on November 20, 2005, recalled pi out to 67,890 digits in 24 hours and 4 minutes (Hu et al., 2009). Lu did this by using the phonology, or word sounds, of the various digits to recode the information linguistically, much like Tomoyori, and then developed stories for himself out of this. However, he also developed techniques based on the shapes of the characters for the digits and their meanings. Lu had a normal digit span of about nine digits. Overall, these three memorists accomplished similar tasks using different talents and strategies.

Extreme Memory Abilities

So far, we have discussed memorists who are using either synesthesia or some mental technique, such as the story mnemonic, to help them remember large amounts of information. Recent work suggests that there may be a small set of individuals who have amazingly good memories for events of their lives. These people have **highly superior autobiographical memory**. Studies of this condition started with a single case of a woman with the ability to remember nearly all of the events of her life from around the age of 14 onward (Parker et al., 2006). However, subsequent work has reported other people who also have exceptional memory for their life events (LePort et al., 2017).

People with this condition have remarkable memory for the events of their lives and public events (e.g., a baseball game). They can provide accurate information about the days and dates of those events (e.g., on what day did Jimmy Carter receive his Nobel Prize?). People with highly superior autobiographical memory remember the day of the week an event happened on, as well as what happened during a public or personal (autobiographical) event, at an accuracy level of about 80%, whereas most of the rest of us remember this information at a rate of about 10%. Thus, their event memory is stunningly good.

This storage, encoding, and retrieval of event memories appears to happen without any special effort. It occurs as a matter of course during the unfolding of their lives. They are not using a mnemonic, such as calendar calculation. Other than their highly superior autobiographical memory, their cognitive processing does not differ from controls (LePort et al., 2017). One difference may be that these people are better at mentally stimulating events, which may help them rehearse and consolidate autobiographical memories (Patihis, 2016). They also may be more liberal in their response bias (more willing to say that something was seen before (Frithsen et al., 2019)).

Many people may have this condition and not realize it because their memories for events have always been very good, and they may assume that other people have similar abilities. This superior memory ability is limited to events. It does not extend to memory for typical laboratory tasks, such as learning lists of words or digits.

Neuroimaging of the brains of these people show some potential areas of differences from normal brains (although keep in mind that the number of such people tested is quite small). This has been done using fMRI and diffusion tensor imaging. These analyses suggest that there are neurological differences in the parahippocampal gyrus (BA 36), the inferior and middle temporal gyri and temporal pole (BAs 20, 21 and 38, respectively), the anterior insula, and the uncinate fasciculus (white matter connections among many of these structures). There is also less gray matter in part of the basal ganglia and intraparietal sulcus (Palombo et al., 2018). Thus, their event memory skill may be due to underlying neurological differences and not to how they have trained themselves to use their memories.

Another condition is, in some ways, the opposite of highly superior autobiographical memory. This is **severely deficient autobiographical memory** in which people have severe problems remembering life events, but do not display problems on standard memory and cognition tasks (e.g., Palombo et al., 2015). This condition is less well understood. These people may have smaller hippocampal mass in some areas, as well as be less likely to engage the brain's autobiographical memory networks. Moreover, they seem deficit in visual imagery processing (Palombo et al., 2018), a condition known as *aphantasia*. Thus, they have difficulty forming and storing autobiographical memories of events. The rapid loss of autobiographical memory with this condition is shown in Figure 15.6, compared to normal controls, over ten years of autobiographical memory.

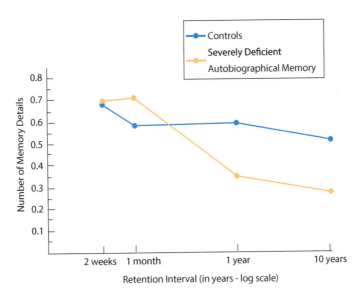

FIGURE 15.6 *Retention of Autobiographical Memories over Ten Years for a Control Group and Severely Deficient Autobiographical Memory*

Source: derived from data reported in Palombo, D. J., Alain, C., Söderlund, H., Khuu, W., & Levine, B. (2015). Severely deficient autobiographical memory (SDAM) in healthy adults: A new mnemonic syndrome. *Neuropsychologia, 72*, 105–118

Eidetic Imagery

Some people think they have photographic memories. This would be the ability to use mental images in a way that resembles perceptually viewing an image. This is called **eidetic imagery** (Gray & Gummerman, 1975). Someone with this ability would have an extraordinary memory for things seen earlier, showing little to no distortion. In general, there is little support for the existence of eidetic imagery. For the most part, people who report having eidetic imagery are instead using other memory skills to a high degree, often restricted to a limited range of knowledge.

Stop and Review

Some people have exceptional memories. In some cases, this comes with expertise and practice with mnemonics. Some memorists have memory skills that seem to defy the imagination but are limited to certain types of information. Other memorists have synesthesia, which they can use to aid memory. People with highly superior autobiographical memory can remember events and dates from nearly all their lives, well beyond the accuracy found with most people. In comparison, people with severely deficient autobiographical memory have great difficulty remembering life events. Finally, despite claims to the contrary, there is little evidence to suggest that photographic memory exists.

PUTTING IT ALL TOGETHER

While most memories and memory processes are unconscious, there is much that is open to consciousness. This is the domain of metamemory, your awareness, monitoring, and control of your own memories. Metamemory is important for knowing what is in memory and how to remember more effectively. In terms of what is in memory, you can estimate whether you have learned something (and you are better at this if you wait for information to move out of working memory) and how to allocate your study time. During studying you may be tempted to spend too much time on difficult items, consistent with the labor-in-vain effect. However, over time, you may drift more towards studying those items just beyond your current state of knowledge, in the region of proximal learning. Part of the problem with assessing the contents of your memory, is that you are sometimes biased by what you know, as with the hindsight bias, and the knew-it-all-along effect.

In terms of how to remember something, it is clear that you use knowledge about both the questions you are asked (the cues), the answers that you know (the targets), and any trouble you have remembering (such as the competition from interference). Remembering and forgetting are associated with different subjective feelings. When something is forgotten, it feels different if you have some knowledge (partial retrieval) versus if you know absolutely nothing. There is also the distinct feeling that retrieval is imminent with the tip-of-the-tongue phenomenon. Moreover, it feels different to "remember" than to "know." The "remember" responses are related to conscious recollection, whereas the "know" responses are related to unconscious retrieval. This unconscious retrieval may even bring about recognition without awareness in which you recognize something without conscious awareness of having encountered it before.

To get at the contents of memories you may use mnemonics that organize the storage and retrieval of material. Most of us are not memorists with highly skilled memories or have conditions, such as synesthesia, or highly superior autobiographical memory. However, if you do, you can exploit these to gain a better command over your memory. None of us have eidetic memories. Still, you can use what knowledge you have to improve how you use your memory.

STUDY QUESTIONS

1. What is metamemory? How does it differ from other kinds of memory?
2. What are the sources of information available to people when making metamemory judgments?
3. What are the major classes of theories of metamemory? How do they suggest that people use the different types of information that are available when making metamemory judgments?
4. How accurate are judgments of learning and how are they made? What can be done to improve judgments of learning?
5. What sort of cues are available to people when they are assessing whether they have learned something? Which are they more or less likely to use?
6. How effective are people at allocating their study time, and why? In what ways are people ineffective? What are more effective ways to allocate study time?
7. What are feeling-of-knowing judgments? When are they given? How accurate are they?
8. What is the difference between feeling-of-knowing judgments and the tip-of-the-tongue state? What are some of the unique characteristics of the tip-of-the-tongue state? Why do they occur?
9. How do people assess that they do not know something?
10. What is the difference between "remember" and "know" responses? What evidence is there that these tap into different memory processes?
11. What is the recognition without awareness phenomenon, and why does it occur?
12. What are the hindsight bias and the knew-it-all-along effects? How can they be avoided?
13. How do people's beliefs about how their memories work influence their ability to make judgments about their own memories?

14. What neurological structures are strongly associated with metamemory performance?

15. How do mnemonics work? What are some examples of mnemonics?

16. What are some of the ways that people can exhibit exceptional memory performance?

KEY TERMS

- accessibility hypothesis
- acronyms
- acrostics
- allocation of study time
- beliefs
- blocking view
- competition hypothesis
- cue utilization hypothesis
- cues
- eidetic imagery
- extrinsic cues
- feeling of knowing (FOK)
- highly superior autobiographical memory

- hindsight bias
- inability hypothesis
- incomplete activation view
- intrinsic cues
- judgments of learning (JOLs)
- knew-it-all-along effect
- labor-in-vain effect
- memorists
- metamemory
- method of loci
- mnemonic cues
- mnemonics
- mnemonists

- monitoring retrieval hypothesis
- peg-word mnemonic
- recognition without awareness
- region of proximal learning
- remember–know judgment
- rhyming mnemonic
- severely deficient autobiographical memory
- story mnemonic
- targets
- tip-of-the-tongue (TOT) state

EXPLORE MORE

Here are some additional readings so that you can further explore issues involving metamemory.

Brown, A. S. (1991). A review of the tip-of-the-tongue experience. *Psychological Bulletin, 109*, 204–223.

Cleary, A. M., & Greene, R. L. (2000). Recognition without identification. *Journal of Experimental Psychology: Learning, Memory, and Cognition, 26*(4), 1063–1069.

Dunlosky, J., & Bjork, R. A. (2013). *Handbook of Metamemory and Memory*. New York: Psychology Press.

Gardiner, J. M., & Java, R. I. (1993). Recognising and remembering. In A. F. Collins, S. E. Gathercole, M. A. Conway, & P. E. Morris (Eds.), *Theories of Memory* (pp. 163–188). Hillsdale, NJ: Erlbaum.

Thompson, C. P., Cowan, T. M., & Frieman, J. (1993). *Memory Search by a Memorist*. Hillsdale, NJ: Erlbaum.

REFERENCES

Akdoğan, E., Izaute, M., Danion, J. M., Vidailhet, P., & Bacon, E. (2016). Is retrieval the key? Metamemory judgment and testing as learning strategies. *Memory, 24*(10), 1390–1395.

Alban, M. W., & Kelley, C. M. (2013). Embodiment meets metamemory: Weight as a cue for metacognitive judgments. *Journal of Experimental Psychology: Learning, Memory, and Cognition, 39*(5), 1628–1634.

Arbuckle, T. Y., & Cuddy, L. L. (1969). Discrimination of item strength at time of presentation. *Journal of Experimental Psychology, 81*, 126–131.

Ariel, R., & Dunlosky, J. (2011). The sensitivity of judgment-of-learning resolution to past test performance, new learning, and forgetting. *Memory & Cognition, 39*(1), 171–184.

Ariel, R., Dunlosky, J., & Bailey, H. (2009). Agenda-based regulation of study-time allocation: When agendas override item-based monitoring. *Journal of Experimental Psychology: General, 138*, 432–447.

Arkes, H. R., Wortmann, R. L., Saville, P. D., & Harkness, A. R. (1981). Hindsight bias among physicians weighing the likelihood of diagnosis. *Journal of Applied Psychology, 66*, 584–588.

Ash, I. K. (2009). Surprise, memory, and retrospective judgment making: Testing cognitive reconstruction theories of the hindsight bias effect. *Journal of Experimental Psychology: Learning, Memory, and Cognition, 35*, 916–933.

Barenberg, J., & Dutke, S. (2019). Testing and metacognition: Retrieval practise effects on metacognitive monitoring in learning from text. *Memory, 27*(3), 269–279.

Begg, I. M., Robertson, R. K., Gruppuso, V., Anas, A., & Needham, D. R. (1996). The illusory-knowledge effect. *Journal of Memory and Language, 35*, 410–433.

Benjamin, A. S., & Bird, R. D. (2006). Metacognitive control of the spacing of study repetitions. *Journal of Memory and Language, 55*, 126–137.

Biederman, I., Cooper, E. E., Fox, P. W., & Mahadevan, R. S. (1992). Unexceptional spatial memory in an exceptional memorist. *Journal of Experimental Psychology: Learning, Memory, and Cognition, 18*, 654–657.

Blaisman, R. N., Dunlosky, J., & Rawson, K. A. (2017). The what, how much, and when of study strategies: Comparing intended versus actual study behavior. *Memory, 25*(6), 784–792.

Blank, H., Fischer, V., & Erdfelder, E. (2003). Hindsight bias in political elections. *Memory, 11*, 491–504.

Bouffard, N., Stokes, J., Kramer, H. J., & Ekstrom, A. D. (2018). Temporal encoding strategies result in boosts to final free recall performance comparable to spatial ones. *Memory & Cognition, 46*(1), 17–31.

Bower, G. H., & Clark, M. C. (1969). Narrative stories as mediators for serial learning. *Psychonomic Science, 14*(4), 181–182.

Brown, A. S. (1991). A review of the tip-of-the-tongue experience. *Psychological Bulletin, 109*, 204–223.

Brown, A. S., Burrows, C. N., & Caderao, K. C. (2013). Partial word knowledge in the absence of recall. *Memory & Cognition, 41*(7), 967–977.

Brown, R., & McNeill, D. (1966). The "tip of the tongue" phenomenon. *Journal of Verbal Learning and Verbal Behavior, 5*, 325–337.

Burgess, A. P., & Ali, L. (2002). Functional connectivity of gamma EEG activity is modulated at low frequency during conscious recollection. *International Journal of Psychophysiology, 46*, 91–100.

Cleary, A. M., Konkel, K. E., Nomi, J. S., & McCabe, D. P. (2010). Odor recognition without identification. *Memory & Cognition, 38*(4), 452–460.

Cleary, A. M., Langley, M. M., & Seiler, K. R. (2004). Recognition without picture identification: Geons as components of the pictorial memory trace. *Psychonomic Bulletin & Review, 11*(5), 903–908.

Cleary, A. M., & Reyes, N. L. (2009). Scene recognition without identification. *Acta Psychologica, 131*(1), 53–62.

Cleary, A. M., & Specker, L. E. (2007). Recognition without face identification. *Memory & Cognition, 35*(7), 1610–1619.

Cleary, A. M., Winfield, M. M., & Kostic, B. (2007). Auditory recognition without identification. *Memory & Cognition, 35*(8), 1869–1877.

Coane, J. H., & Umanath, S. (2019). I don't remember vs. I don't know: Phenomenological states associated with retrieval failures. *Journal of Memory and Language, 107,* 152–168.

Cook, G. I., Marsh, R. L., & Hicks, J. L. (2006). The role of recollection and familiarity in the context variability mirror effect. *Journal of Experimental Psychology: Learning, Memory, and Cognition, 32,* 828–835.

Costermans, J., Lories, G., & Ansay, C. (1992). Confidence level and feeling of knowing in question answering: The weight of inferential processes. *Journal of Experimental Psychology: Learning, Memory, & Cognition, 18,* 142–150.

Craik, F. I. M., Rose, N. S., & Gopie, N. (2015). Recognition without awareness: Encoding and retrieval factors. *Journal of Experimental Psychology: Learning, Memory, and Cognition, 41*(5), 1271.

Curran, T. (2000). Brain potentials of recollection and familiarity. *Memory & Cognition, 28,* 923–938.

De Beni, R., & Cornoldi, C. (1988). Does the repeated use of loci create interference? *Perceptual and Motor Skills, 67,* 415–418.

Deutsch, D. (2002). The puzzle of absolute pitch. *Current Directions in Psychological Science, 11,* 200–204.

Dietrich, D., & Olson, M. (1993). A demonstration of hindsight bias using the Thomas confirmation vote. *Psychological Reports, 72,* 377–378.

Dudukovic, N. M., & Knowlton, B. J. (2006). Remember–know judgments and retrieval of contextual details. *Acta Psychologica, 122,* 160–173.

Dunlosky, J., & Nelson, T. O. (1994). Does the sensitivity of judgments of learning (JOLs) to the effects of various activities depend on when the JOLs occur? *Journal of Memory and Language, 33,* 545–565.

Erdfelder, E., & Buchner, A. (1998). Decomposing the hindsight bias: A multinomial processing tree model for separating recollection and reconstruction in hindsight. *Journal of Experimental Psychology: Learning, Memory, and Cognition, 24,* 387–414.

Ericcson, K. A., Chase, W. G., & Faloon, S. (1980). Acquisition of a memory skill. *Science, 208*(4448), 1181–1182.

Ericsson, K. A., Cheng, X., Pan, Y., Ku, Y., Ge, Y., & Hu, Y. (2017). Memory skills mediating superior memory in a world-class memorist. *Memory, 25*(9), 1294–1302.

Fischhoff, B. (1975). Hindsight is not equal to foresight: The effect of outcome knowledge on judgment under uncertainty. *Journal of Experimental Psychology: Human Perception and Performance, 1*(3), 288.

Fisher, J. S., & Radvansky, G. A. (2018). Patterns of forgetting. *Journal of Memory and Language, 102,* 130–141.

Frithsen, A., Stark, S. M., & Stark, C. E. L. (2019). Response bias, recollection, and familiarity in individuals with Highly Superior Autobiographical Memory (HSAM). *Memory, 27*(6), 739–749.

Gardiner, J. M. (1988). Functional aspects of recollective experience. *Memory & Cognition, 16*(4), 309–313.

Gardiner, J. M., & Java, R. I. (1990). Recollective experience in word and nonword recognition. *Memory & Cognition, 18,* 23–30.

Gardiner, J. M., & Java, R. I. (1991). Forgetting in recognition memory with and without recollective experience. *Memory & Cognition, 19,* 617–623.

Gardiner, J. M., & Parkin, A. J. (1990). Attention and recollective experience in recognition memory. *Memory & Cognition, 18,* 579–583.

Ghetti, S. (2003). Memory for nonoccurrences: The role of metacognition. *Journal of Memory and Language, 48,* 722–739.

Gilbertson, L. J., Dietrich, D., Olson, M., & Guenther, R. K. (1994). A study of hindsight bias: The Rodney King case in retrospect. *Psychological Reports, 74,* 383–386.

Glucksberg, S., & McCloskey, M. (1981). Decisions about ignorance: Knowing that you don't know. *Journal of Experimental Psychology: Human Learning and Memory, 7,* 311–325.

Gordon, P., Valentine, E., & Wilding, J. (1984). One man's memory: A study of a mnemonist. *British Journal of Psychology, 75,* 1–14.

Gray, C. R., & Gummerman, K. (1975). The enigmatic eidetic image: A critical examination of methods, data, and theories. *Psychological Bulletin, 82,* 383–407.

Gruppuso, V., Lindsay, D. S., & Masson, M. E. J. (2007). I'd know that face anywhere! *Psychonomic Bulletin, & Review, 14,* 1085–1089.

Hart, J. T. (1965). Memory and the feeling-of-knowing experience. *Journal of Educational Psychology, 56,* 208–216.

Hasher, L., Attig, M. S., & Alba, J. W. (1981). I knew it all along: Or did I? *Journal of Verbal Learning and Verbal Behavior, 20,* 86–96.

Henkel, L. A., & Mather, M. (2007). Memory attributions for choices: How beliefs shape our memories. *Journal of Memory and Language, 57,* 163–176.

Hicks, J. L., & Marsh, R. L. (2002). On predicting the future states of awareness for recognition of unrecallable items. *Memory & Cognition, 30,* 60–66.

Hu, Y., Ericsson, K. A., Yang, D., & Lu, C. (2009). Superior self-paced memorization of digits in spite of a normal digit span: The structure of a memorist's skill. *Journal of Experimental Psychology: Learning, Memory, and Cognition, 35,* 1426–1442.

Hunt, E., & Love, T. (1972). How good can memory be? In A.W. Meltin, & E. Martin (Eds), *Coding Processes in Human Memory,* pp. 237–260. Washington, D.C.: Winston-Wiley.

Hunt, E., & Love, T. (1983). The second mnemonist. In U. Neisser (Ed), *Memory Observed: Remembering in Natural Context,* pp. 390–398. San Francisco, CA: W.H. Freeman.

Janowsky, J. S., Shimamura, A. P., & Squire, L. R. (1989). Memory and metamemory: Comparisons between patients with frontal lobe lesions and amnesic patients. *Psychobiology, 17,* 3–11.

Joslyn, S., Loftus, E., McNoughton, A., & Powers, J. (2001). Memory for memory. *Memory & Cognition, 29,* 789–797.

Kalakoski, V., & Saarilouma, P. (2001). Taxi drivers' exceptional memory of street names. *Memory & Cognition, 29,* 634–638.

Karney, B. R., & Coombs, R. H. (2000). Memory bias in long-term close relationships: Consistency or improvement? *Personality and Social Psychology Bulletin, 26,* 959–970.

Kimball, D. R., Smith, T. A., & Muntean, W. J. (2012). Does delaying judgments of learning really improve the efficacy of study decisions? Not so much. *Journal of Experimental Psychology: Learning, Memory, and Cognition, 38*(4), 923–954.

Kolers, P. A., & Palef, S. R. (1976). Knowing not. *Memory & Cognition, 4,* 553–558.

Koriat, A. (1993). How do we know that we know? The accessibility model of the feeling of knowing. *Psychological Review, 100,* 609–639.

Koriat, A. (1997). Monitoring one's own knowledge during study: A cue-utilization approach to judgments of learning. *Journal of Experimental Psychology: General, 126,* 349–370.

Koriat, A. (2002). Comparing objective and subjective learning curves: Judgments of learning exhibit increased underconfidence with practice. *Journal of Experimental Psychology: General, 131,* 147–162.

Koriat, A., & Bjork, R. A. (2006). Illusions of competence during study can be remedied by manipulations that enhance learners' sensitivity to retrieval conditions at test. *Memory & Cognition, 34,* 959–972.

Koriat, A., & Levy-Sadot, R. (2001). The combined contributions of the cue-familiarity and accessibility heuristics to feelings of knowing. *Journal of Experimental Psychology: Learning, Memory, and Cognition, 27,* 34–53.

Koriat, A., Levy-Sadot, R., Edry, E., & de Marcas, S. (2003). What do we know about what we cannot remember? Accessing the semantic attributes of words that cannot be recalled. *Journal of Experimental Psychology: Learning, Memory, and Cognition, 29,* 1095–1105.

Kostic, B., & Cleary, A. M. (2009). Song recognition without identification: When people cannot "name that tune" but can recognize it as familiar. *Journal of Experimental Psychology: General, 138*(1), 146–159.

Kroneisen, M., & Makerud, S. E. (2017). The effects of item material on encoding strategies: Survival processing compared to the method of loci. *Quarterly Journal of Experimental Psychology, 70*(9), 1824–1836.

Leary, M. R. (1981). The distorted nature of hindsight. *Journal of Social Psychology, 115,* 25–29.

LePort, A. K. R., Stark, S. M., McGaugh, J. L., & Stark, C. E. (2017). A cognitive assessment of highly superior autobiographical memory. *Memory, 25*(2), 276–288.

Liu, Y., Su, Y., Xu, G., & Chan, R. C. K. (2007). Two dissociable aspects of feeling-of-knowing: Knowing that you know and knowing that you do not know. *Quarterly Journal of Experimental Psychology, 60,* 672–680.

Long, D. L., & Prat, C. S. (2002). Memory for Star Trek: The role of prior knowledge in recognition revisited.

Journal of Experimental Psychology: Learning, Memory, and Cognition, 28, 1073–1082.

Luna, K., Nogueira, M., & Albuquerque, P. B. (2019). Words in larger font are perceived as more important: Explaining the belief that font size affects memory. *Memory, 27*(4), 555–560.

Luria, A. R. (1968). *The Mind of a Mnemonist: A Little Book about a Vast Memory* (L. Solotaroff, Trans.). New York: Basic Books.

Mark, M. M., & Mellor, S. (1991). Effect of self-relevance of an event on hindsight bias: The foreseeability of a layoff. *Journal of Applied Psychology, 76*, 569–577.

Markant, D., DuBrow, S., Davachi, L., & Gureckis, T. M. (2014). Deconstructing the effect of self-directed study on episodic memory. *Memory & Cognition, 42*(8), 1211–1224.

Massen, C., Vaterrodt-Plünnecke, B., Krings, L., & Hilbig, B. E. (2009). Effects of instruction on learners' ability to generate an effective pathway in the method of loci. *Memory, 17*(7), 724–731.

McFarland, C., & Ross, M. (1987). The relation between current impressions and memories of self and dating partners. *Personality and Social Psychology Bulletin, 13*, 228–238.

McGuire, M. J., & Maki, R. H. (2001). When knowing more means less: The effects of fan on metamemory judgments. *Journal of Experimental Psychology: Learning, Memory, and Cognition, 27*, 1172–1179.

Meeter, M., Myers, C. E., & Gluck, M. A. (2005). Integrating incremental learning and episodic memory models of the hippocampal region. *Psychological Review, 112*, 560–585.

Metcalfe, J. (2002). Is study time allocated selectively to a region of proximal learning? *Journal of Experimental Psychology: General, 131*, 349–363.

Metcalfe, J. (2009). Metacognitive judgments and control of study. *Current Directions in Psychological Science, 18*, 159–163.

Metcalfe, J., & Finn, B. (2008a). Evidence that judgments of learning are causally related to study choice. *Psychonomic Bulletin & Review, 15*, 174–179.

Metcalfe, J., & Finn, B. (2008b). Familiarity and retrieval processes in delayed judgments of learning. *Journal of Experimental Psychology: Learning, Memory, and Cognition, 34*, 1084–1097.

Morris, P. E., Fritz, C. O., Jackson, L., Nichol, E., & Roberts, E. (2005). Strategies for learning proper names: Expanding retrieval practice, meaning and imagery. *Applied Cognitive Psychology, 19*(6), 779–798.

Morris, P. E., Jones, S., & Hampson, P. (1978). An imagery mnemonic for the learning of people's names. *British Journal of Psychology, 69*(3), 335–336.

Neath, I. (1998). *Human Memory: An introduction to research, data, and theory*. Belmont, CA: Thomson Brooks/Cole Publishing.

Neisser, U. (1982). Memory: What are the important questions? In U. Neisser & I. E. Hyman (Eds.), *Memory Observed: Remembering in Natural Contexts*. New York: Worth.

Nelson, T. O., & Dunlosky, J. (1991). When people's judgments of learning (JOLs) are extremely accurate at predicting subsequent recall: The "Delayed-JOL effect." *Psychological Science, 2*, 267–270.

Nelson, T. O., & Leonesio, R. J. (1988). Allocation of self-paced study time and the "labor-in vain effect." *Journal of Experimental Psychology: Learning, Memory, and Cognition, 14*, 676–686.

Nisbett, R. E., & Wilson, T. D. (1977). Telling more than we can know: Verbal reports on mental processes. *Psychological Review, 84*(3), 231.

Palombo, D. J., Alain, C., Söderlund, H., Khuu, W., & Levine, B. (2015). Severely deficient autobiographical memory (SDAM) in healthy adults: A new mnemonic syndrome. *Neuropsychologia, 72*, 105–118.

Palombo, D. J., Sheldon, S., & Levine, B. (2018). Individual differences in autobiographical memory. *Trends in Cognitive Sciences, 22*(7), 583–597.

Parker, E. S., Cahill, L., & McGaugh, J. L. (2006). A case of unusual autobiographical remembering. *Neurocase, 12*(1), 35–49.

Patihis, L. (2016). Individual differences and correlates of highly superior autobiographical memory. *Memory, 24*(7), 961–978.

Peynircioğlu, Z. F. (1990). A feeling-of-recognition without identification. *Journal of Memory and Language, 29*(4), 493–500.

Peynircioğlu, Z. F., & Tatz, J. R. (2019). Intensifying the intensity illusion in judgments of learning: Modality and cue combinations. *Memory & Cognition, 47*(3), 412–419.

Rajaram, S. (1993). Remembering and knowing: Two means of access to the personal past. *Memory & Cognition, 21*, 89–102.

Reder, L. M. (1987). Strategy selection in question answering. *Cognitive Psychology, 19*, 90–138.

Reder, L. M., & Ritter, F. E. (1992). What determines initial feeling of knowing? Familiarity with question terms, not with the answer. *Journal of Experimental Psychology: Learning, Memory, and Cognition, 18*(3), 435–451.

Rhodes, M. G., & Castel, A. D. (2008). Memory predictions are influenced by perceptual information: Evidence for metacognitive illusions. *Journal of experimental psychology: General, 137*(4), 615–625.

Rhodes, M. G., & Castel, A. D. (2009). Metacognitive illusions for auditory information: Effects on monitoring and control. *Psychonomic Bulletin & Review, 16*(3), 550–554.

Rhodes, M. G., & Tauber, S. K. (2011). The influence of delaying judgments of learning on metacognitive accuracy: A meta-analytic review. *Psychological Bulletin, 137*(1), 131.

Rubin, D. C., Schrauf, R. W., & Greenberg, D. L. (2003). Belief and recollection of autobiographical memories. *Memory & Cognition, 31*, 887–901.

Safer, M. A., Bonanno, G. A., & Field, N. P. (2001). "It was never that bad": Biased recall of grief and long-term adjustment to the death of a spouse. *Memory, 9*, 195–204.

Sanna, L. J., & Schwarz, N. (2004). Integrating temporal biases: The interplay of focal thoughts and accessibility experiences. *Psychological Science, 15*, 474–481.

Schreiber, T. A. (1998). Effects of target set size on feelings of knowing and cued recall: Implications for the cue effectiveness and partial-retrieval hypotheses. *Memory & Cognition, 26*, 553–571.

Schwartz, B. L. (1994). Sources of information in metamemory: Judgments of learning and feelings of knowing. *Psychonomic Bulletin & Review, 1*, 357–375.

Seel, S. V., Easton, A., McGregor, A., Buckley, M. G., & Eacott, M. J. (2019). Walking through doorways differentially affects recall and familiarity. *British Journal of Psychology, 110*(1), 173–184.

Soderstrom, N. C., & Bjork, R. A. (2014). Testing facilitates the regulation of subsequent study time. *Journal of Memory and Language, 73*, 99–115.

Son, L. K. (2004). Spacing one's study: Evidence for a metacognitive control strategy. *Journal of Experimental Psychology: Learning, Memory, and Cognition, 30*, 601–604.

Sprecher, S. (1999). "I love you more today than yesterday": Romantic partners' perceptions of change in love and related affect over time. *Journal of Personality and Social Psychology, 76*, 46–53.

Takahashi, M., Shimizu, H., Saito, S., & Tomoyori, H. (2006). One percent ability and ninety–nine percent perspiration: A study of a Japanese memorist. *Journal of Experimental Psychology: Learning, Memory, and Cognition, 32*, 1195–1200.

Thompson, C. P., Cowan, T. M. & Frieman, J. (1993). *Memory Search by a Memorist.* Hillsdale, NJ: Erlbaum.

Thompson, C. P., Cowan, T. M., Frieman, J., Mahadevan, R. S., & Vogl, R. J. (1991). Rajan: A study of a memorist. *Journal of Memory and Language, 30*, 702–724.

Thompson, R., Emmorey, K., & Gollan, T. H. (2005). "Tip of the fingers" experiences in deaf signers: Insights into the organization of a sign-based lexicon. *Psychological Science, 16*, 856–860.

Van Boekel, M., Varma, K., & Varma, S. (2017). A retrieval-based approach to eliminating hindsight bias. *Memory, 25*(3), 377–390.

Voss, J. L., Baym, C. L., & Paller, K. A. (2008). Accurate forced-choice recognition without awareness of memory retrieval. *Learning & Memory, 15*(6), 454–459.

Voss, J. L., & Paller, K. A. (2006). Fluent conceptual processing and explicit memory for faces are electrophysiologically distinct. *The Journal of Neuroscience, 26*(3), 926–933.

Wang, A. Y., & Thomas, M. H. (2000). Looking for long-term mnemonic effects on serial recall: The legacy of Simonides. *American Journal of Psychology, 113*(3), 331–340.

Wilding, J. M., & Valentine, E. R. (1997). *Superior Memory.* Hove, UK: Psychology Press.

Winkielman, P., & Schwarz, N. (2001). How pleasant was your childhood? Beliefs about memory shape inferences from experienced difficulty of recall. *Psychological Science, 12*, 176–179.

Wood, G. (1978). The knew-it-all-along effect. *Journal of Experimental Psychology: Human Perception and Performance, 4,* 345–353.

Xu, J., & Metcalfe, J. (2016). Studying in the region of proximal learning reduces mind wandering. *Memory & Cognition, 44*(5), 681–695.

Yates, F. A. (1966). *The Art of Memory.* Chicago, IL: The University of Chicago Press.

Young, K. D., Peynircioğlu, Z. F., & Hohman, T. J. (2009). Revelation effect in metamemory. *Psychonomic Bulletin & Review, 16,* 952–956.

CHAPTER 16

Memory in Infancy and Childhood

As we have seen repeatedly, memory is not stable and static. Every experience alters our memories, making things easier or harder to remember, distorting some things, and clarifying others. To further complicate this, people are in a constant state of development, moving from one age to another. These developmental changes have implications for how memory functions. Early on, some memory processes are poorly functioning or absent, whereas others are in a nearly adult form. This chapter examines memory through infancy and childhood. Throughout this overview, we can see how our memory and memory skills became more sophisticated and efficient.

Beginning with infancy, one of the first challenges is dealing with the fact that different methods are needed to test such young people, due to their lack of language. Following this, we explore aspects of memory that have been covered in earlier chapters to see how developed they are in infants and how they mature. Next, we cover the issue of infantile amnesia. After this, we move on to memory development in children. Again, we look at a number of different memory processes. Finally, we also look at the phenomenon of childhood amnesia.

INFANCY

The development of memory begins as soon as the nervous system can retain information. However, not all types of memory are available at the same time or for the same reasons. Here we consider the very early memories of infants. We first consider the challenges of testing preverbal humans to give you an idea of the barriers facing researchers. After this we look at changes in memory that occur during infancy (0–2 years of age). Finally, we cover the topic of infantile amnesia, or the inability to remember any events from when you were an infant.

Testing the Very Young

Testing infant memory is hard. A big challenge is that infants neither understand nor produce language, which is the medium of most studies of memory. Thus, researchers who study infant memory are faced with the problem of how to assess

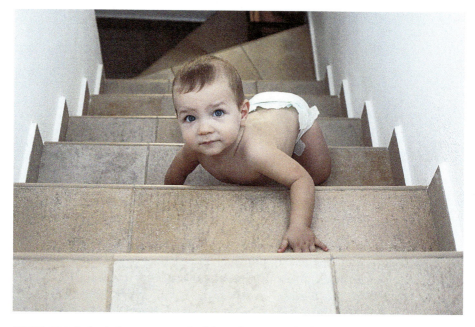

PHOTO 16.1 *Infants learn a great deal in a short period of time. The challenge for memory researchers is to figure out what infants do and do not know given that they lack the language skills of children and adults*

Source: Juan Aunion/Shutterstock.com

such nonverbal primates in a way that provides meaningful information. Several techniques have been created to do this (Hayne, 2004; Rovee-Collier & Cuevas, 2009). Each of these uses some motor activity that is already available to infants—that is, something that they do already. What the researcher does is assess how this behavior changes as a function of whether something is remembered. Here we look at four examples of methods that have been used to assess memory in infants.

One way to study infant memory is to use a gaze duration/direction or the **looking method** (Friedman, 1972). Infants spend a lot of time looking around the world in an effort to understand it. To assess infant gaze as a measure of memory, the infant may be placed in a caregiver's lap in the lab. To keep caregivers from unintentionally biasing the infant, they may be asked to listen to music over headphones. Moreover, any displays might be out their line of sight. This method is useful because infants spend more time looking at things that interest them, which are more likely to be new things. Things that are looked at less are recognized, and thus, are in memory. Increased looking times reflect more of an unconscious, implicit memory novelty preference than an explicit recognition of old items (Snyder et al., 2008).

Another way to determine what infants remember is to use the infants' natural sucking behavior. Babies love to suck on things. This is important because it helps the infant to eat, but they also suck on lots of other things that do not have any nutritional value, such as pacifiers. We can take advantage of **nonnutritive sucking** as a tool to study memory. Rate of sucking changes as a function of whether the infant encounters something old (in memory) or new. This is measured using high-tech pacifiers. When something is old, infants suck at a slower rate. However, when something new is introduced, they suck faster (Siqueland & DeLucia, 1969).

A third technique is a **conjugate reinforcement** paradigm (Rovee-Collier & Fagan, 1981). For this technique, infants lay on their backs in a crib. One end of a ribbon is tied around one of the baby's ankles, and the other end is attached to a mobile. Whenever the baby kicks, the mobile moves, which is a very cool thing for an infant. They can directly control something in the world. They soon pick up on the kicking–mobile movement relationship and spend a good deal of time kicking. Memory for this event can be tested by varying any number of things, such as the amount of time that has passed or the context that can serve as a cue. Essentially, if the infant remembers the situation, it kicks more often.

Finally, researchers have found that older infants can recall information using techniques such as **elicited imitation** (Bauer, 1996; 2002). In these studies, an experimenter does some task, such as assembling a simple toy, while the child watches. Then, after a delay, such as a month later, it is observed whether the infant does the task. This is evidence of recall because it requires the child to deliberately recall the steps needed. It has been found that some form of memory recall begins in infants as young as nine months and becomes stable by two years of age.

Stop and Review

To test infants, researchers have derived clever methods. This is needed because infants lack the ability to use language. Such methods include looking, nonnutritive sucking, conjugate reinforcement, and elicited imitation.

Memory and Infancy

Human memory is made up of many components that develop at different rates. This is guided by neurological changes, as well as the acquisition of abilities that increase memory, including the ability to crawl (around 9 months) and the acquisition of language (starting around 10 months) (Hayne & Simcock, 2009). Here, we look at different types of memory and how they progress during infancy.

Different types of memory development are associated with **neurological development** rates. For example, the thalamus and some medial temporal structures, which are important for more primitive types of memory, are nearly developed at birth, whereas the frontal lobes, which are important for controlling the flow of processing in memory are not completely functional until one year of age or older (Chugani et al., 1986). The prefrontal cortex and hippocampus continue to develop through infancy and into childhood (Bauer, 2007). There is a slow development of the dentate gyrus which receives information from other parts of the brain. Because the hippocampus is important to memory, if neural signals are not effectively getting into it, then declarative memories are not going to be as reliable. Thus, infant memory, to some degree, is influenced by the readiness of the nervous systems.

What about infant **sensory and short-term memories**? If you remember from Chapter 4, research shows that adults have a very large capacity in iconic memory, but are only able to move 4–6 items into short-term memory before iconic memory decays away. To test infants' iconic memory, Blaser and Kaldy (2010) used displays of multiple items (e.g., colored diamonds). The infants' task was to notice if any of these objects in the display had changed. Infants did this task as well as adults. Thus, they have iconic memories that can process 4–6 items before it decays away. Iconic memory seems to be well developed early on, even if the knowledge and skills for what to do with that information is not fully developed. Thus, infants can maintain information in the sensory registers to select things from the world.

While infants have reasonably well-developed sensory registers, their short-term memory is not at adult levels, although it matures over time. At six months, while infants might be surprised if an object is briefly occluded and then reappears, they are not if it is briefly occluded and changes shape, such as going from a red sphere to a red cube (Kibbe & Leslie, 2011). Thus, infants are holding in short-term memory information that there was something there but not exactly what. They have conceptual knowledge, such as whether an object was a doll or a ball, but do not remember perceptual qualities, such as its color (Kibbe & Leslie, 2019). As infants develop and acquire language, they start using names for objects to help maintain information in short-term memory (Mani & Plunkett, 2010). In addition, young infants (seven months old) show short-term memory serial position curves for pictures of adult faces, with primacy and recency effects. Moreover, the recency effect can be easily disrupted (Cornell & Bergstrom, 1983), suggesting that infants are prone to interference from other information. Overall, infants have some form of short-term memory that exhibits phenomena like adults, but their ability to control its contents needs to develop.

Infants have various forms of **nondeclarative memory**, such as the ability to learn new motor skills. They can associate the sights and sounds of their parents with care and comfort and acquire a large array of unconscious influences on behavior. Almost immediately, they develop skills to help them get along in the world (e.g., learning to eat). Thus, implicit memory is well on its way at an early age. As an illustration of early nondeclarative memory abilities, infants prefer familiar sounds they heard while in the womb, such as the sound of their mother's voice. Although nondeclarative memory is present at birth, if not before, it still must also go through a period of development (Rovee-Collier, 1997).

Complex forms of **episodic memory** are present even at very young ages. For instance, using the conjugate reinforcement paradigm, even three-month-old infants remember to kick five days later (Butler & Rovee-Collier, 1989). This is episodic memory because the kicking is context dependent. When the crib liner is the same during the second session as it was during the first, the kicking rate is higher as compared to when it is different. The crib liner is an episodic retrieval cue (see Chapter 7). The rudiments of episodic memory are present in infants, although the ability to form complex episodic memories and retain them requires development.

The ability to explicitly remember information for long periods of time increases in accuracy and duration as an infant matures (Hartshorn et al., 1998).

For example, using elicited imitation, Carver and Bauer (2001) found that nine-month-old infants can remember and reproduce previously viewed actions up to four weeks later. In contrast, 13-month-old infants can reproduce an action up to six months later. The pattern of retention durations is shown in Figure 16.1 (Bauer, 2007). This pattern of remembering is even evidenced in ERP recordings (Bauer et al., 2003). Other aspects of episodic memory also continue to develop. For example, around 24 months of age, prospective memory ability begins to emerge (Ślusarczyk et al., 2018).

Infant **semantic memory** is advanced enough to allow infants to abstract away from the original information (Mandler, 1988), although early schemas are grounded in perceptual experience (Mandler, 1992). Infants also create and use categories. As early as three or four months, they make basic level category distinctions, such as dogs and cats (Quinn et al., 1993) and subordinate category distinctions by six or seven months (Quinn & Tanaka, 2007). By at least nine months of age, infants can abstract new categories, such as those based on object shapes or colors, within a few minutes (Dewar & Xu, 2010). However, it is not until about 14 months of age that infants make distinctions based on superordinate categories, such as knowing that "drinking" and "sleeping" belong to the superordinate category *animals* and that "needs keys" and "giving a ride" belong to the superordinate

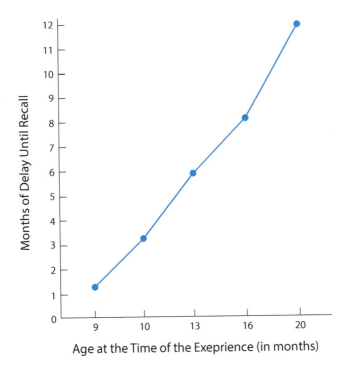

FIGURE 16.1 *Recall Intervals for Children 9 to 20 Months Old from a Number of Studies*

Source: adapted from Bauer, P. J. (2007). Recall in infancy. *Current Directions in Psychological Science, 16*, 142–146

category *vehicles* (Mandler & McDonough, 1996). Knowledge of finer level categories remains elusive until over two years old (Mandler et al., 1991). Thus, infants have the basic mechanisms for forming semantic memories, but do not yet have the kinds of knowledge needed to be as effective as adults.

Semantic memory also involves the identification of drawings and pictures. To do this, we must match a more abstract picture with a memory of a real object, which is not as simple as it sounds. To test this ability, Hochberg and Brooks (1962) raised their own child from birth to age 19 months in an environment in which objects in pictures were never named and where pictures were unavailable, to the point of not letting their child see picture books and removing labels from baby food jars. Despite this, at 19 months, their child was able to identify pictures and drawings with no problem. Thus, the ability to abstract information occurs without explicit practice or training.

Stop and Review

Memory development in infants reflects patterns of maturation. While some neural structures are well-developed early on, others are not. Some of the more developed memory systems in infants include the sensory registers, nondeclarative, and semantic memory abilities. However, other types of memory are undeveloped, including short-term memory and episodic memory (in terms of memory for specific events), although the rudimentary elements of these systems are in place.

Infantile Amnesia

What is the first thing that you remember? The very first thing. It is time to think about our memories from when we were infants. But wait. Where *are* they? This absence of early memories is **infantile amnesia**. Most adults, if they think about it, find that their earliest memory is not from infancy but from when they were between the ages of two and four (Mullen, 1994; Usher & Neisser, 1993).[1] These initial memories tend to have information about where the event took place and what happened, but few other details, such as who else was there, their thoughts at the time, the weather, their age, how long the event lasted, and what was worn, unless these are easily inferred or central to the memory (Wells et al., 2014). These very first memories tend to be earlier for women and people with higher levels of education (Kingo et al., 2013). They are often fragmented, such as a memory of standing in a room, whereas more episodic memories of whole events are regularly reported about a year later (Bruce et al., 2005). The phenomenon of infantile amnesia is surprising given that infancy is a time when we are actually learning a very large number of things.

As an example of infantile amnesia, my earliest memory is from when I was two and a half years old. My parents had just moved from Ohio to Wisconsin, and we were living in a trailer park until they could find a house. It was late December, and I remember ice creeping in underneath the door. Because my family was new

---

1 It is possible to have event memories from as early as 18 to 24 months, but not earlier (Howe et al., 2003), although most of these may be fictional (Akhtar et al., 2018). Also, note that because of the phenomenon of forward telescoping (see Chapter 12), initial memories may be earlier on average than reported (Wang & Peterson, 2016).

in town, some of my father's new coworkers wanted to help out. So, one of them came to the trailer one evening dressed as Santa Claus to give me a thrill. (He already had a Santa suit because he had discovered that when he wore it to a bar, someone always wanted to buy Santa a drink.) When he walked into the trailer, I was terrified. I remember crying and screaming and running into my bedroom to get away from this big, red, creepy-looking guy who had burst into my home and started ho-ho-hoing at me.

Occasionally, people report memories from earlier ages. However, we need to have a bit of skepticism before we accept these as real. The problem is that many of these "memories" were generated in response to seeing pictures, hearing stories told by older relatives, or other sources. Thus, they are not memories of the event itself, but are generated from mental images and mental models created at the time people heard those descriptions. Thus, while people are remembering an event from when they were very young, these may have been generated in the same way that false memories are (see Chapter 13). Keep in mind that people do not always report the same earliest memories. These are stable around 55–60% of the time (Ece et al., 2019; Kihlstrom & Harackiewicz, 1982).

TRY IT OUT

This project is for assessing memories from adults and plotting out infantile amnesia. First, put together a list of 30 nouns. These words will be used as cues for people to remember events.

You need at least 12 participants, but more is better. For each participant, read the words aloud. The task is to recall the first event from their childhood that the word suggests. They should write down a one- or two-sentence description of each memory. Be sure to tell them that they do not need to write down memories that they would not want other people to read about because they are too embarrassing or upsetting. Give people about a minute to write down a brief description of each event. After you have gone through your list of words, have your participants go through their events and write down how old they were at the time (alternatively, have them write down the date as close as they can get to it). This is the data of most interest. You will also need your participants' current age. If you get their birthdate, then you can be more precise.

After your participants have gone through and dated the events that they wrote down, collect their responses. Then, tabulate the age that the person reported being in terms of how many years old they were. This should give you a percentage of responses for each age (0, 1, 2, 3, etc.). Then plot the data as a function of age. What you should observe is that there are fewer and fewer memories as you plot younger and younger ages. Moreover, there should be hardly any memories for the age of two or younger. This is because of infantile amnesia.

What happens to memories before the age of two or so? Why do we have no conscious memories of this period of our lives? Nearly all the events are forgotten. There are several explanations for infantile amnesia. One of the first people to take note of infantile amnesia was Sigmund Freud (1899/1938). His explanation was rooted in his **psychodynamic view**. For Freud, many of our psychological problems involved sexual thoughts and desires. Infants are no exception. For Freud, when we are infants we go through a period of sexual thinking and wishing. Part of that involves a desire to be sexually intimate with our opposite-sexed parent. As we mature, we take on the rules and norms of our culture as part of the development of the superego. At this time, we learn that our incestual thoughts are taboo. To protect ourselves from this threatening and horrible knowledge about ourselves, our unconscious blocks from consciousness all memories from this time. This grand scale repression is so successful that people have no memory of when they were infants.

Freud's theory makes interesting reading, and it fits well into his broader theories. However, there are few people today who accept his view on infantile amnesia. Most contemporary explanations focus on other factors.

Modern Views

There are many ideas about what causes infantile amnesia, and there are likely multiple factors that contribute to it. There are several changes that move people from a state of not remembering much about their lives to the awareness that is autobiographical memory. The **multicomponent development theory** (Fivush & Nelson, 2004) embraces the idea that there are number of memory abilities or components that bring about this new type of memory, although it is still unclear whether infantile amnesia is brought about by poor memory storage or an inability to access whatever memories are there (Howe, 2019). Note that, unlike Freud's account, infantile amnesia is not really an amnesia—a catastrophic forgetting—but an inability to form long-lasting conscious, personal memories.

A **neurological account** is based on developmental changes in neural structures. Humans are born neurologically immature. The brain quadruples in size while developing to adulthood. The hippocampus, an important structure for creating new memories (see Chapter 2) is relatively underdeveloped at birth. It does not reach adult form until a child is a few years old (Nadel & Zola-Morgan, 1984). The dentate gyrus is particularly slow in developing, and there is a high rate of neurogenesis in this area, which may disrupt memories that are being stored (Josselyn & Frankland, 2012). The critical role of the hippocampus is to bind together information to create episodic and autobiographical memories, which lends support to the idea that it is involved in infantile amnesia. If an infant cannot create effective episodic and autobiographical memories because the neurological processes are just not fully there yet, then this would support the absence of memories from this time in our lives.

This role of the development of the hippocampus in infantile amnesia has also been tied to embodied processing (Glenberg & Hayes, 2016). This is rooted in the idea that the hippocampus is important for spatial processing, as evidenced by the presence of space cells, grid cells, and such. Thus, the offset of infantile amnesia may be a function of more spatial navigation by people around the age when infantile amnesia begins to lift, along with the increased use of navigation aspects of the hippocampus increasing at this time. The increased use of contextually based cells then improves long-term retention of episodic and autobiographical knowledge.

In addition to hippocampal development, infants have less developed frontal lobes. This part of the brain is important for binding contextual factors in memory, allowing for such things as source monitoring (see Chapter 13). This inability to link different aspects of experience leads to a reduced ability to form autobiographical memories (Newcombe et al., 2000). Finally, during infancy and early childhood, the ability to consolidate memories is underdeveloped, leaving people more prone to interference from later events (Bauer et al., 2007), thereby contributing to infantile amnesia. In general, the problem of infantile amnesia reflects a time when infants are acquiring but not retaining, complex and neurologically sophisticated episodic memories (see Chapter 12).

Another theory of infantile amnesia, the **schema organization view**, is that infants are trying to understand how the world works and are still developing their schemas (Chapter 9). Infantile amnesia is related to a development in the understanding of how adults think and talk about the world and the passage of time. For example, a child might remember what typically happens during a trip to McDonald's but not remember any of the details from a given trip. Young children with underdeveloped schemas may focus on inappropriate aspects of an event. As their schemas become more developed, they have difficulty retrieving the prior memories that were formed with old schemas. That said, it seems that young children can form episodic memories. The difficulty is that they are forgotten faster (Nelson & Gruendel, 1981).

An important thing to note about the time when infantile amnesia lifts is that this is also the time when **language development** is making big strides (Nelson, 1993). Infantile amnesia may reflect an inability to organize information into a coherent life narrative, which can then be used to help retrieval. Early on, infant memory has two roles: either as a generic schema-driven memory or as a repository for temporary episodic memories. With the advent of language, and the need to share experiences with others in our social context, autobiographical memory is developed. Thus, the chaotic jumble of memories that is infantile amnesia is displaced with the organization of the new autobiographical memory. This is supported by work showing that preverbal children do not translate nonverbal knowledge into verbal information after they learn how to talk about those events. The memories appear to stay nonverbal (Simcock & Hayne, 2002), which makes them harder to retrieve (Richardson & Hayne, 2007).

Finally, for the **emergent self view**, there are significant changes during infancy in how people understand themselves (Howe & Courage, 1993). Infantile amnesia is a function of our developing a sense of self as a unique and identifiable entity. Newborn infants lack a clear sense of self as a separate entity from the environment. The development of the self is divided into the acquisition of the "I" and the "me." The "I" is the subjective sense of self as a causal agent, whereas the "me" is the objective sense of self, such as your personal features. This latter sense emerges around 18 months and is well established by 24 months. Once this concept of self is established, autobiographical memory can be constructed around it. Again, the offset of infantile amnesia corresponds to the onset of autobiographical memory.

As noted earlier, the multicomponent development theory (Nelson & Fivush, 2004) is the idea that there are several memory abilities or components that emerge to bring about autobiographical memory. These components include not only the development of an adequate episodic memory system but also the development of language and narrative skills, an understanding of how adults think and talk about the world and the passage of time, as well as how people understand themselves. Thus, there are multiple causes that bring about an emergence from infantile amnesia.

These factors are influenced by the culture in which one grows up (Wang, 2003). Culture can influence the age at which people report their first memories. For example, children whose parents reminisce about the past, such as where the child went and what they saw, emerge out of infantile amnesia faster than children whose parents spend less time talking about events (Fivush & Nelson, 2004). These children also grow to be better at explaining things because they have a head start on understanding narrative structure and style. Thus, a critical influence is how parents talk with their children. Although what children report as their earliest memories changes as they grow older, even throughout their teens, these reports are more likely to remain stable when parents reminisce more with their children about events that happened (Reese & Robertson, 2019).

Finally, people in individualist cultures (e.g., Western and/or urban), come out of infantile amnesia six months to a year earlier than people in collectivist (e.g., Asian and/or rural) cultures (Göz et al., 2017; Wang, 2003). This may be because in collectivist cultures children interact differently with adults, with less of a focus on the self than in Western cultures.

Stop and Review

The inability of adults to remember most memories from when they were infants is infantile amnesia. This is in contrast to the furious pace that infants are acquiring new knowledge. Freud thought that this was a period of catastrophic forgetting, a genuine amnesia, in which we actively repress memories. Modern theories suggest that this is not a genuine amnesia, but an immature ability to form conscious, personal event memories. It is due to an immaturity of the nervous system, a lack of requisite semantic knowledge, such as schemas, a lack of language skills to organize and structure experiences, and an absence of a self-concept around which memories can be structured. These multiple causes converge, along with elements of culture, to help infants move from not being able to remember events for long, to being able to reliably retain memories.

CHILDHOOD

As people leave infancy and move into childhood, memory continues to develop. Here, childhood is the period from ages three to 17, although much of what we have to say applies to children under the age of 12. During this time, the nervous system continues to develop until people reach early adulthood. These changes, of course, influence memory. For example, the speed with which children execute memory processing increases exponentially until the mid to late teens (Kail, 1991). The nervous system is becoming more efficient.

Neurological and Short-Term/Working Memory Processes

As people progress through childhood, **neurological development** continues. For example, the dentate gyrus of the hippocampus continues its move towards adult form until the age of five. That said, hippocampal development continues into adulthood, and shifts emphasis from more memory pattern completion (emphasizing more generalized semantic memory processes) to more memory pattern separation (emphasizing more distinct episodic memories) (Keresztes et al., 2018). Moreover, there is a pruning of neural connections, with adults having fewer connections than children, although there is an overall increase in brain size (Bauer, 2009). Thus, the brain is becoming more fine-tuned and efficient at processing information and retaining it for longer.

Although the sensory registers are well developed (Engle et al., 1981), the ability to use **short-term/working memory** consistently improves. For instance, there is an increase in the rate and effectiveness of rehearsing information to keep it active. This increases the amount of information being rehearsed (Ornstein et al., 1975). In other words, memory span is getting larger. Short-term span improves from about two items for two-year-olds to about six items by the time a child is nine (Dempster, 1981). With a larger memory span, overall memory increases. Another factor that improves is the speed with which children articulate information. As a reminder, the word length effect is the finding that people remember fewer words as word articulation times increase. This is because longer words are more likely to decay in the phonological loop (see Chapter 5). As children age, they pronounce words faster. Thus, older children having larger memory span scores (Hulme et al., 1984). This relation between rehearsal speed and span is shown in Figure 16.2.

This increased articulation speed reflects a general increase in processing speed that occurs as children grow older (Kail, 1991). This increased speed influences both verbal and visual–spatial working memory (Kail, 1997), not just the maintenance of a list of words. Overall, working memory improves as children become better at processing knowledge.

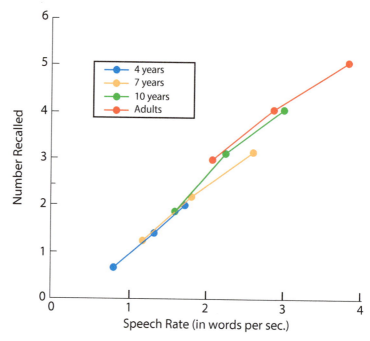

FIGURE 16.2 *Relation between Person's Speech Rate and Working Memory Span Scores Broken Down by Different Age Groups*

Source: adapted from Hulme, C., Thomson, N., Muir, C., & Lawrence, A. (1984). Speech rate and the development of short-term memory span. *Journal of Experimental Child Psychology, 38,* 241–253

STUDY IN DEPTH

As noted earlier, children generally score lower than adults on memory span tests. However, this can be influenced by a child's interests. A study by Lindberg (1980) directly compared two groups of 40 participants. One group was made up of college students at Marshall University (around the age of 20). The other was made up of third graders (around the age of nine).

Prior to testing, two lists of 30 items were created. One list had words from standard categorized word norms that are typically used in working memory span studies. The other list had items that the children had more familiarity with. These included the names of cartoon characters, children's books and film names, television show characters, as well as the names of teachers and rooms at their elementary school. Thus, college students were more likely to be familiar with the words on the first list, whereas the third graders were more likely to be familiar with those on the second list.

The lists were read at a slow rate of one word every three seconds. At the end of each list, people were to recall as many of the words as they could. They were to guess if they were unsure and not worry about spelling. After all, many third graders are not as good at spelling as college students. After they were done, their recall sheets were collected.

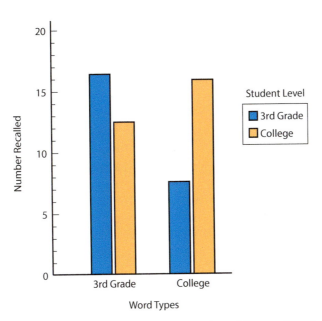

FIGURE 16.3 *Influence of Domain of Interest Words on Memory Span in Children and Adults*

Source: adapted from Lindberg, M. A. (1980). Is knowledge base development a necessary and sufficient condition for memory development? *Journal of Experimental Child Psychology, 30*, 401–410

What was found was that when children were given words pertaining to topics for which they had greater knowledge, such as the names of cartoon characters, memory spans improved to that of college students, but college students' memories were better for categorized lists of words, as shown in Figure 16.3. The ability to remember materials is at least partially a function of people's knowledge base. If items are drawn from children's knowledge bases, their performance is much better. This calls into question concerns about just how effective the working memory abilities of children may be, with children having better memories than they are sometimes given credit for.

Episodic Remembering and Forgetting

Like adults, children benefit from effective learning strategies. For example, even very young children benefit from some form of testing rather than simple restudy (Fazio & Marsh, 2019). More generally, in childhood there is an increase in information structure and organization, and this is reflected in **episodic memory** retrieval success (Bjorklund & Zeman, 1982). That is, how well children can learn new episodic information reflects an ability to structure and organize the materials. The better that they can organize it, the more they remember, and organization skills improve with age. For example, for memory for names of furniture found at home, younger children (around age ten) tend to organize memory based on furniture category (e.g., chairs, tables, etc.), whereas by age 16 children have switched over to organizing around spatial categories (e.g., living room, dining room, etc.) (Plumert, 1994). This second organization is more efficient and effective. Thus, children change their thinking to more sophisticated ways of structuring and organizing knowledge and experiences. This improves long-term retention.

Not only does increased age during childhood improve episodic memories for the past, but it also improves memory for the future. For example, there are age-related improvements in **prospective memory**. Children aged four to six are less effective at prospective memory, often forgetting to do something in the future. However, by the ages of 13 or 14, prospective memory is at adult levels. That said, there is the beginning of a decline through a person's twenties to forties (Maylor & Logie, 2010; Zimmermann & Meier, 2006). This contrasts with retrospective memory, which continues to improve throughout early adulthood.

Also developing during childhood is the ability to engage in mental time travel for **episodic future thinking**, which appears to emerge between three and four years of age, and shows a particularly large improvement from ages four to five (Atance 2008; Atance & O'Neill, 2005). In a way, this parallels young children's ability to retrieve memories for past events (Busby & Suddendorf, 2005). It should be noted that it is easier for children to imagine future events for other people than for themselves, suggesting that there are some delays in processing information about the self (Russell et al., 2010). While this ability does increase with age, as do other future-oriented abilities, such as delayed gratification and prospective memory, these developments do not seem to be strongly correlated with one another, suggesting that there are different underlying processes for each of them (Atance & Jackson, 2009).

The improvements observed during childhood are not only for the storage of information, but also for the retrieval of knowledge. This includes the management of **interference** from competing memory traces. Early on, during the preschool years, children are more prone to interference, particularly retroactive interference, which can result in more forgetting (Darby & Sloutsky, 2015a). That said, if there are long delays between related sets of information, such as 48 hours, then the retroactive interference effects can be attenuated because children have an opportunity to consolidate their knowledge (Darby & Sloutsky, 2015b). For older ages, such as around the age of 12, children show similar interference effects as adults (such as a fan effect), and they can better organize information to reduce that interference (Gómez-Ariza & Bajo, 2003). Moreover, inhibition appears to help children to the same degree as adults. Children show repeated practice and part-set cuing effects that are like adults (Zellner & Bäuml, 2005), as well as similar retrieval practice effects (Aslan & Bäuml, 2010). Finally, for directed forgetting, Harnishfeger and Pope (1996) tested six, eight, and ten-year-olds, along with college students and found that the ability to inhibit information increased with age, with ten-year-olds doing as well as the adults.

Semantic Memory

As children have more experience with the world, **semantic memory** becomes more complex. This does not mean that there is no complex semantic information at all in younger children. There can be if the child has taken the time and effort to learn it. Even at a particularly young age, a child can have a complex semantic network of a particular domain. For example, a portion of a four-and-a-half-year-old boy's knowledge of dinosaurs is shown in Figure 16.4 (Chi & Koeske, 1983). His semantic memory of dinosaurs is complex and well organized. Many of the armored dinosaurs are in a cluster and so are the large plant-eaters. When the boy recalled the names of dinosaurs, the ones he recalled most often were those with more semantic links.

For semantic memory, children also develop more complex schemas and scripts for commonly experienced aspects of the world. This is evident even around the age of three (Nelson & Gruendel, 1988). These schemas and scripts become more numerous and continue to develop as a child ages. Their scripts include more details and minor steps in whatever the process might be. The desire to develop and improve scripts and schemas in young children can be clearly seen in their need to cling to set routines where they can predict and understand what is happening.

For categorization, even young children show some proficiency. However, there are changes that do occur during development. For example, preschool children are likely to assume that members of the same basic level category have a similar internal structure (same kind of stuff inside) but do not do this for

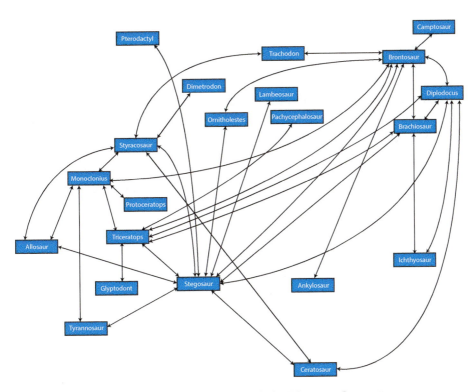

FIGURE 16.4 *A Boy's Semantic Memory Network for Dinosaur Concepts*

Source: adapted from Chi, M. T. H., & Koeske, R. D. (1983). Network representation of a child's dinosaur knowledge. *Developmental Psychology*, 19, 29–39

superordinate level categories until second grade (Gelman & O'Reilly, 1988). Another developmental shift is category use. While adults often view typical members as the best representative of a category (e.g., a prototype), younger children (around five years old) view more extreme examples as the best representative (Foster-Hanson & Rhodes, 2019). For example, the fastest cheetah would be more representative of the category "cheetah" than one that ran at an average speed for a cheetah. More adult ways of thinking about categories emerge as children age.

Another thing that changes with children's mental categories is how natural kind and artifact categories develop (Gelman, 1988). As a reminder, natural kind categories are for things in nature, such as plants and animals. Members of a natural kind category are often superficially similar. In comparison, artifact categories are items created by people for various uses and are defined by how we use them, not their appearance. For example, a screwdriver is more similar in appearance to a butter knife, but the knife is more likely to be classified with a fork. Categories are driven more by appearance for young, preschool children, which is a natural kind bias, but not by older children, who develop an alternative way to create categories that involves the memory processes needed for artifact categories.

Specialized Memory

The improvement in memory, as well as the emergence from childhood amnesia (see next section), is tied to the onset of a more coherent and elaborate life narrative as **autobiographical memory** skills continue to develop, particularly in adolescence (Habermas & Bluck, 2000; McLean, 2005). Autobiographical narrative memory structures memories of experienced events. It provides a sense of the meaning and flow of the events in people's lives as they move through adolescence. This is done, in part, by giving memory traces more temporal and causal coherence (such as developing a well-ordered narrative), as well as thematic organization. It also provides more links to join various elements of experience together, making it more likely that they will be remembered later. This autobiographical memory development is accompanied by increases in the ability to tell stories, as well as increases in general memory abilities (such as working memory) (Bauer & Larkina, 2019).

Autobiographically, children place a high priority on flashbulb memories, such as living through a hurricane (Fivush et al., 2004) or experiencing a tornado (Bauer et al., 2017), that are similarly detailed to those of adults. This is noteworthy given that autobiographical memories for non-traumatic experiences from around a similar time are less detailed than those of adults.

Given that there are developmental changes for a variety of memory systems as children grow older, how does this affect **memory and reality** judgments in children? An important aspect of this is source monitoring. In general, children are not as effective as adults at this, particularly for internal and external source monitoring, compared to reality monitoring (Lindsay & Johnson, 1991; Parker, 1995; Roberts & Blades, 2000). However, this does improve. Thus, young children have more difficulty accurately remembering where a given piece of knowledge was acquired.

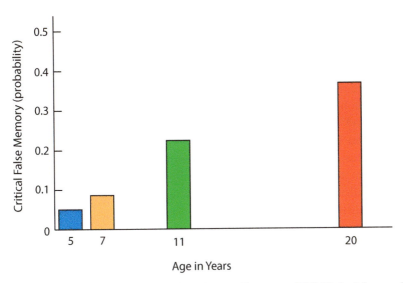

FIGURE 16.5 *Probability of Making a False Memory Error on a DRM False Memory Task*

Source: adapted from Brainerd, C. J. (2013). Developmental reversals in false memory: A new look at the reliability of children's evidence. *Current Directions in Psychological Science, 22*(5), 335–341

False memories generated using the DRM paradigm (see Chapter 13) change as children grow older. As seen in Figure 16.5, it starts out relatively small or absent in five-year-olds. Seven-year-old children show a small effect and 11-year-old children show a larger effect, but still smaller than adults (Brainerd, 2013). This is related to the fact that semantic memories, which are behind the generation of this false memory effect, are still developing. The more developed semantic memories are, the easier it is to draw inferences, and the more likely that gaps will be filled in and be confused as being real memories. The source of that knowledge is then lost, leading to a belief in the false memory.

The ability to distinguish what really happened, from what did not, plays into important **memory and the law** situations where children may be eyewitnesses who need to give testimony. As is detailed in Chapter 14, eyewitness memory is easily distorted when a witness has been exposed to misleading post-event information. Given this, how reliable are children's eyewitness accounts in the face of under-developed memory systems? The research is a bit mixed and complicated. Considering that, some simple points can be made (Ceci & Bruck, 1993). First, children can provide accurate eyewitness testimony. In the absence of external influences, a child's memory is like an adult's, provided that a child understands the event.[2]

Given that, it is also the case that children are more susceptible to misinformation than adults in some cases (Poole & Lindsay, 2001, but see Otgaar et al., 2016), even when they encounter a single instance of misinformation from an adult (Bruck & Ceci, 2004). This may occur because adults are often authority figures for children, making children less able to resist the misinformation. The children's reports do not

---

2 For a case study of seven- and nine-year-old children's eyewitness memories for their mother's murder, see McWilliams et al. (2013).

simply reflect greater compliance with what children may perceive as the demands or wishes of the adult asking the questions (Otgaar et al., 2012). This can be mitigated to some degree by repeated interviews, but only when their initial memories are fairly strong (Goodman & Quas, 2008).

In addition to issues of misleading post-event information, children may also have problems with lineup identification. In a meta-analysis of 91 studies, Fitzgerald and Price (2015) reported that children do more poorly with lineups. They are more likely to make false positives and are less likely to correctly identify a culprit. This may reflect development trends in the processing and storage of detail information in memory. Younger children (not yet seven), have difficulty storing detailed information about experienced events, whereas older children have an ability to store and retrieve such details (Strange & Hayne, 2013). That said, adolescents may do worse than younger children and adults when it comes to misidentifying bystanders as perpetrators (unconscious transference). This may be because they have lower inhibition control, make more inferential errors, and have more liberal decision-making criteria (Brackmann et al., 2019). These factors are obviously of importance to investigators trying to solve a crime.

Another important aspect of memory that is improving during childhood is **metamemory** (Bjorklund et al., 2009). For example, for a short-term memory serial position curve (see Chapter 4), to get the most out of the recency effect, we should recall the last items first before they are displaced out of short-term memory. We develop an implicit understanding of this, and adults often do recall items this way. However, young children lack this awareness and are less likely to start with the final items. This has a net effect of reducing the overall amount of knowledge retrieved. Samuel (1978) found that this recency effect strategy was used infrequently by first graders, but it was used progressively more often as people moved into the college years. Metamemory strategies also develop in terms of a general increased awareness of the need to rehearse information to maintain it. This sort of simple memory strategy begins to emerge in two-year-old children (DeLoache et al., 1985). For example, a toy might be hidden under an object, and children will continue to glance or point in that direction, suggesting an active attempt to maintain this information in memory.

Staying on the topic of metamemory, proneness to the hindsight bias decreases across childhood (Bernstein et al., 2011). This is shown in Figure 16.6. Preschoolers are less likely to realize that something they learned is not something that they knew all along. However, older children develop an awareness that there is a change in knowledge from not knowing something to knowing something. Young children's lack of awareness that they are storing new knowledge in memory may contribute to a lack of effort in trying to learn new things.

The ability to organize and structure information continues to mature during childhood (Paris & Lindaur, 1976). As a reminder, the more that information is structured, the better it is remembered later. An example of this is inferring that a spoon was used when reading the sentence "The truck driver stirred the coffee in his cup." If this inference is made, then the word "spoon" is an effective memory cue for this sentence. Older children are more likely to make implicit associations to help organize information and improve memory. This also assists in the emergence and development of autobiographical memory.

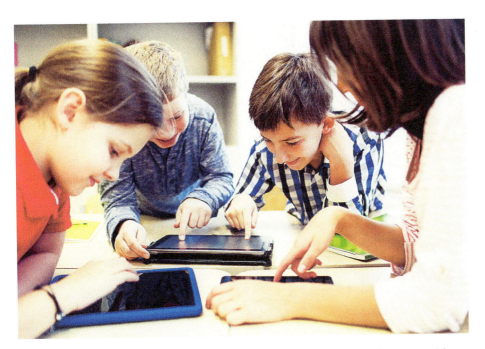

PHOTO 16.2 *Memory and learning skills continue to improve as children grow older. One of the greatest sources of this improvement is children's knowledge of how to control and use their memories*

Source: Syda Productions/Shutterstock.com

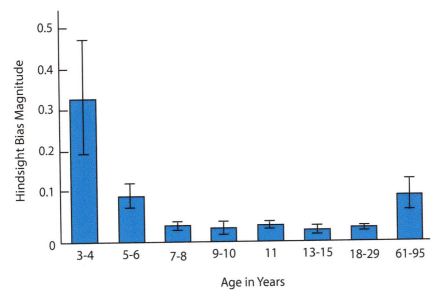

FIGURE 16.6 *Magnitude of the Hindsight Bias from Childhood to Old Age*

Source: adapted from Bernstein, D. M., Erdfelder, E., Meltzoff, A. N., Peria, W., & Loftus, G. R. (2011). Hindsight bias from 3 to 95 years of age. *Journal of Experimental Psychology: Learning, Memory, and Cognition, 37*(2), 378–391

Improve Your Memory

At this point there is not much you can do about your childhood memory. That part of your life has come and gone. However, there is some insight that can be gained from understanding why children forget things to develop ways to improve your own memory. As noted here, one of the biggest improvements is for children to gain an awareness of how their own memories work. As Chapter 15 detailed, our metamemory awareness is far from perfect. You, like most people, probably do not have the best insight into how your own memory works. You can improve how well you remember things by becoming more aware of when you may be over-estimating the likelihood of remembering something in the future. If you encourage yourself to use the principles that you have learned in this book, you will find that you will better learn and remember more things. You started along the trajectory of greater memory awareness and control as you matured as a child. Now, allow yourself to continue this process.

Stop and Review

Memory continues to develop in childhood. Short-term/working memory becomes more efficient, along with faster processing speed and better inhibition of irrelevant information. Episodic memories are more structured, allowing children to better process event knowledge, and they are less susceptible to interference. For semantic memory, children develop more elaborate and detailed categories, schemas, and scripts. These allow them to better organize and structure knowledge, and so remember more experiences. For autobiographical memory, life narratives become more complex and better structured. In terms of memory and reality, while children are better at monitoring source information, they become more susceptible to DRM false memories. Relatedly, although children can be effective eyewitnesses, they may be more prone to distortion from misleading information. Finally, as they grow, children become more aware of the limits and abilities of their own memories.

CHILDHOOD AMNESIA

As noted earlier, adults are unable to remember any events from when they are infants. This is infantile amnesia. After people emerge out of infantile amnesia, it is not the case that there is normal adult memory at that time. Instead, memory for experienced events is better, but it is still quite spotty. Thus, this is a period of **childhood amnesia** (Jack & Hayne, 2010). While infantile amnesia lasts up to around the age of three or so, childhood amnesia lasts up to around the age of seven or so. If you reflect on your own childhood, you are likely to find that your memories for events prior to the age of eight are quite spotty relative to your memories for other ages. This is worse than what would be expected based on normal forgetting curves.

Forgetting and Consolidation

So, why does childhood amnesia occur? One explanation is that children forget information faster than do adults (Bauer & Larkina, 2016). Figure 16.7 illustrates the rates of forgetting as people grow older. Thus, while children have more developed neurological structures, have reached a level of schema development and language processing to help them structure knowledge, and have acquired the ability to form episodic memories and embedded them in an autobiographical narrative, they still are not at adult levels in the ability to consolidate and retain event memories in a way that makes them available and accessible over long periods of time.

Life Narrative

As children reach the age of seven and beyond, the ability to consolidate memories improves. Thus, the rate at which information is forgotten improves as well (Bauer & Larkina, 2014). Part of this improvement may be related to the ability to form more complete narratives of experienced events. This makes the memories less episodic and more autobiographical (Bauer, 2015). By adolescence, the cultural life scripts children have for how a person's life should unfold are similar to those of adults (Tekcan et al., 2012). If younger children are encouraged to form narrative accounts of experienced events, then their memories for those events improve (Wang et al., 2015). Thus, the emergence from childhood amnesia is due to better memory consolidation and better autobiographical memory structures.

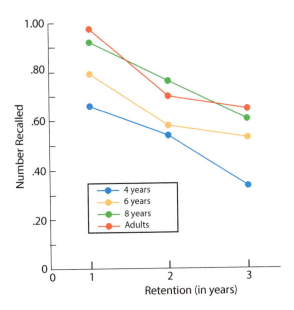

FIGURE 16.7 *Changes in the Rate of Forgetting over the Course of Development for Autobiographical Memories*

Source: adapted from Bauer, P. J., & Larkina, M. (2016). Predicting remembering and forgetting of autobiographical memories in children and adults: A 4-year prospective study. *Memory, 24*(10), 1345–1368

Stop and Review

While children have moved beyond infantile amnesia, their memories are still not up to adult levels. Up to the age of eight, episodic memories are spotty and fragmented. They are forgotten at a rate faster than one would expect. One reason for this is that children have not fully developed the ability to consolidate episodic memories. Also, around age eight there is an increase in the formation of the life narrative of autobiographical memory which helps provide structure to experiences, leading them to be better remembered.

PUTTING IT ALL TOGETHER

Infants and children go through a time of dramatic change in the ability to remember. When dealing with infants, the first challenge is to find a way to assess memory. Several methods have been developed, including the looking method, nonnutritive sucking, conjugate reinforcement, and elicited imitation. Neurologically, some neurological structures being well-developed at birth, whereas others are still in a relatively primitive state. The presence of some neurologically developed structures at birth is why some types of memory are ready to go, even if the content to fill them is not there yet. These include the sensory registers, nondeclarative memory, as well as some episodic and semantic memory abilities. The hippocampus is an important memory structure that continues to develop throughout childhood.

Some types of memories go through a great deal of change during childhood. Working memory capacity increases in the speed of processing as well as an increase in the cognitive control and metamemory skills needed to manipulate information. For episodic memory, there is development in the ability to effectively bind and maintain information. Finally, semantic memory acquires the content of world knowledge, which becomes more structured and organized all the time, boosting the retention of any memories that draw upon this knowledge.

The lag in memory abilities and content bring about periods of infantile and childhood amnesia. The emergence from these comes about with a continued improvement in the ability to consolidate declarative event memories in the cortex. There is also growth of appropriate semantic memories, the expansion of language abilities to structure and tag memories, and the emergence of a clear self-concept around which to structure autobiographical memory. More generally, infantile and childhood amnesia are the inverse of the onset and development of autobiographical memory. Autobiographical memory provides a means to organize and give meaning to your life. Overall, many elements come together to move infants and children from a state of inability to remember events, to the ability to do so regularly and reliably.

STUDY QUESTIONS

1. What are some of the various ways of testing infants' memories, and how do they work?
2. What memory systems are well developed in infancy, and which are still immature?
3. What is infantile amnesia? What are some major theoretical accounts for why it occurs and why does it go away?
4. What are some of the major changes in memory that are observed during childhood?
5. What important role does metamemory play in changes in memory during childhood?
6. What is childhood amnesia, and how does it relate to infantile amnesia?
7. As a child moves through adolescence, what role does autobiographical memory play in changes in memory?

KEY TERMS

- childhood amnesia
- conjugate reinforcement
- development
- elicited imitation
- emergent self view

- infantile amnesia
- language development
- looking method
- multicomponent development theory

- neurological account
- neurological development
- nonnutritive sucking
- psychodynamic view
- schema organization view

EXPLORE MORE

Here are some additional readings to explore that can provide you deeper insight into some of the ideas of how memory changes across infancy and childhood.

Atance, C. M. (2008). Future thinking in young children. *Current Directions in Psychological Science, 17*(4), 295–298.

Bauer, P. J. (2007). Recall in infancy. *Current Directions in Psychological Science, 16*, 142–146.

Ceci, S. J., & Bruck, M. (1993). Suggestibility of the child witness: A historical review and synthesis. *Psychological Bulletin, 113*, 403–439.

Jack, F., & Hayne, H. (2010). Childhood amnesia: Empirical evidence for a two-stage phenomenon. *Memory, 18*(8), 831–844.

Josselyn, S. A., & Frankland, P. W. (2012). Infantile amnesia: A neurogenic hypothesis. *Learning & Memory, 19*(9), 423–433.

REFERENCES

Akhtar, S., Justice, L. V., Morrison, C. M., & Conway, M. A. (2018). Fictional first memories. *Psychological Science, 29*(10), 1612–1619.

Aslan, A., & Bäuml, K-H. T. (2010). Retrieval-induced forgetting in young children. *Psychonomic Bulletin & Review, 17*(5), 704–709.

Atance, C. M. (2008). Future thinking in young children. *Current Directions in Psychological Science, 17*(4), 295–298.

Atance, C. M., & Jackson, L. K. (2009). The development and coherence of future-oriented behaviors during the preschool years. *Journal of experimental child psychology, 102*(4), 379–391.

Atance, C. M., & O'Neill, D. K. (2005). The emergence of episodic future thinking in humans. *Learning and Motivation, 36*(2), 126–144.

Bauer, P. J. (1996). What do infants recall of their lives? Memory for specific events by one-to two-year-olds. *American Psychologist, 51*, 29–41.

Bauer, P. J. (2002). Long-term recall memory: Behavioral and neuro-developmental changes in the first two years of life. *Current Directions in Psychological Science, 11*, 137–141.

Bauer, P. J. (2007). Recall in infancy: A neurodevelopmental account. *Current Directions in Psychological Science, 16*, 142–146.

Bauer, P. J. (2009). The cognitive neuroscience of the development of memory. In M. L. Courage & N. Cowan (Eds.) *The Development of Memory in Infancy and Childhood* (pp. 115–144). New York: Psychology Press.

Bauer, P. J. (2015). A complementary processes account of the development of childhood amnesia and a personal past. *Psychological Review, 122*(2), 204–231.

Bauer, P. J., Burch, M. M., Scholin, S. E., & Güler, O. E. (2007). Using cue words to investigate the distribution of autobiographical memories in childhood. *Psychological Science, 18*, 910–916.

Bauer, P. J., & Larkina, M. (2014). Childhood amnesia in the making: Different distributions of autobiographical memories in children and adults. *Journal of Experimental Psychology: General, 143*(2), 597–611.

Bauer, P. J., & Larkina, M. (2016). Predicting remembering and forgetting of autobiographical memories in children and adults: A 4-year prospective study. *Memory, 24*(10), 1345–1368.

Bauer, P. J., & Larkina, M. (2019). Predictors of age-related and individual variability in autobiographical memory in childhood. *Memory, 27*(1), 63–78.

Bauer, P. J., Stark, E. N., Ackil, J. K., Larkina, M., Merrill, N., & Fivush, R. (2017). The recollective qualities of adolescents' and adults' narratives about a long-ago tornado. *Memory, 25*(3), 412–424.

Bauer, P. J., Wiebe, S. A., Carver, L. J., Waters, J. M., & Nelson, C. A. (2003). Developments in long-term explicit memory late in the first year of life: Behavioral and electrophysiological indices. *Psychological Science, 14*, 629–635.

Bernstein, D. M., Erdfelder, E., Meltzoff, A. N., Peria, W., & Loftus, G. R. (2011). Hindsight bias from 3 to 95 years of age. *Journal of Experimental Psychology: Learning, Memory, and Cognition, 37*(2), 378–391.

Bjorklund, D. F., Dukes, C., & Brown, R. D. (2009). The development of memory strategies. In M. L. Courage & N. Cowan (Eds.) *The Development of Memory in Infancy and Childhood* (pp. 145–175). New York: Psychology Press.

Bjorklund, D. F., & Zeman, B. R. (1982). Children's organization and metamemory awareness in their recall of familiar information. *Child Development, 53*, 799–810.

Blaser, E., & Kaldy, Z. (2010). Infants get five stars on iconic memory tests: A partial-report test of 6-month-old infants' iconic memory capacity. *Psychological science, 21*(11), 1643–1645.

Brackmann, N., Sauerland, M., & Otgaar, H. (2019). Developmental trends in lineup performance: Adolescents are more prone to innocent bystander misidentifications than children and adults. *Memory & Cognition, 47*(3), 428–440.

Brainerd, C. J. (2013). Developmental reversals in false memory: A new look at the reliability of children's evidence. *Current Directions in Psychological Science, 22*(5), 335–341.

Bruce, D., Wilcox-O'Hearn, L. A., Robinson, J. A., Phillips-Grant, K., Francis, L., & Smith, M. C. (2005). Fragment memories mark the end of childhood amnesia. *Memory & Cognition, 33*, 567–576.

Bruck, M., & Ceci, S. (2004). Forensic developmental psychology: Unveiling four misconceptions. *Current Directions in Psychological Science, 13,* 229–232.

Busby, J., & Suddendorf, T. (2005). Recalling yesterday and predicting tomorrow. *Cognitive Development, 20*(3), 362–372.

Butler, J., & Rovee-Collier, C. (1989). Contextual gating of memory retrieval. *Developmental Psychobiology, 22,* 533–552.

Carver, L. J., & Bauer, P. J. (2001). The dawning of a past: The emergence of long-term explicit memory in infancy. *Journal of Experimental Psychology: General, 130,* 726–745.

Ceci, S. J., & Bruck, M. (1993). Suggestibility of the child witness: A historical review and synthesis. *Psychological Bulletin, 113,* 403–439.

Chi, M. T. H., & Koeske, R. D. (1983). Network representation of a child's dinosaur knowledge. *Developmental Psychology, 19,* 29–39.

Chugani, H. T., Phelps, M. E., & Mazziotta, J. C. (1986). Positron emission tomography study of human brain functional development. *Annals of Neurology, 22,* 487–497.

Cornell, E. H., & Bergstrom, L. I. (1983). Serial-position effects in infants' recognition memory. *Memory & Cognition, 11*(5), 494–499.

Darby, K. P., & Sloutsky, V. M. (2015a). The cost of learning: Interference effects in memory development. *Journal of Experimental Psychology: General, 144*(2), 410–431.

Darby, K. P., & Sloutsky, V. M. (2015b). When delays improve memory: Stabilizing memory in children may require time. *Psychological Science, 26*(12), 1937–1946.

DeLoache, J. S., Cassidy, D. J., & Brown, A. L. (1985). Precursors of mnemonic strategies in very young children's memory. *Child Development 56,* 125–137.

Dempster, F. N. (1981). Memory span: Sources of individual and developmental differences. *Psychological Bulletin, 89*(1), 63–100.

Dewar, K. M., & Xu, F. (2010). Induction, overhypothesis, and the origin of abstract knowledge: Evidence from 9-month-old infants. *Psychological Science.*

Eimas, P. D., & Quinn, P. C. (1994). Studies on the formation of perceptually based basic-level categories in young infants. *Child Development, 65,* 903–917.

Ece, B., Demiray, B., & Gülgöz, S. (2019). Consistency of adults' earliest memories across two years. *Memory, 27*(1), 28–37.

Engle, R. W., Fidler, D. S., & Reynolds, L. H. (1981). Does echoic memory develop? *Journal of Experimental Child Psychology, 32,* 459–473.

Fazio, L. K., & Marsh, E. J. (2019). Retrieval-based learning in children. *Current Directions in Psychological Science, 28*(2), 111–116.

Fitzgerald, R. J., & Price, H. L. (2015). Eyewitness identification across the life span: A meta-analysis of age differences. *Psychological Bulletin, 141*(6), 1228–1265.

Fivush, R., McDermott Sales, J., Goldberg, A., Bahrick, L., & Parker, J. (2004). Weathering the storm: Children's long-term recall of Hurricane Andrew. *Memory, 12*(1), 104–118.

Fivush, R., & Nelson, K. (2004). Culture and language in the emergence of autobiographical memory. *Psychological Science, 15,* 573–577.

Foster-Hanson, E., & Rhodes, M. (2019). Is the most representative skunk the average or the stinkiest? Developmental changes in representations of biological categories. *Cognitive Psychology, 110,* 1–15.

Freud, S. (1899/1938). Childhood and concealing memories. In A. A. Brill (Ed.), *The Basic Writings of Sigmund Freud.* New York: The Modern Library.

Friedman, S. (1972). Newborn visual attention to repeated exposure of redundant vs "novel" targets. *Perception & Psychophysics, 12,* 291–294.

Gelman, S. A. (1988). The development of induction within natural kind and artifact categories. *Cognitive Psychology, 20,* 65–95.

Gelman, S. A., & O'Reilly, A. W. (1988). Children's inductive inferences within superordinate categories: The role of language and category structure. *Child Development, 59,* 876–887.

Glenberg, A. M., & Hayes, J. (2016). Contribution of embodiment to solving the riddle of infantile amnesia. *Frontiers in Psychology, 7,* 10.

Gómez-Ariza, C. J., & Bajo, M. T. (2003). Interference and integration: The fan effect in children and adults. *Memory, 11,* 505–523.

Goodman, G. S., & Quas, J. A. (2008). Repeated interviews and children's memory: It's more than just how many. *Current Directions in Psychological Science, 17*, 386–390.

Göz, İ., Çeven, Z. İ., & Tekcan, A. İ. (2017). Urban–rural differences in children's earliest memories. *Memory, 25*(2), 214–219.

Habermas, T., & Bluck, S. (2000). Getting a life: The emergence of the life story in adolescence. *Psychological Bulletin, 126*(5), 748–769.

Harnishfeger, K. K., & Pope, R. S. (1996). Intending to forget: The development of cognitive inhibition in directed forgetting. *Journal of Experimental Child Psychology, 62*, 292–315.

Hartshorn, K., Rovee-Collier, C., Gerhardstein, P., Bhatt, R. S., Wondoloski, T. L., Klein, P., Gilch, J., Wurtzel, N., & Campos-de-Carvalho, M. (1998). The ontogeny of long-term memory over the first year-and-a-half of life. *Developmental Psychobiology, 32*, 69–89.

Hayne, H. (2004). Infant memory development: Implications for childhood amnesia. *Developmental Review, 24*(1), 33–73.

Hayne, H., & Simcock, G. (2009). Memory development in toddlers. In M. L. Courage & N. Cowan (Eds.) *The Development of Memory in Infancy and Childhood*, pp. 43–68. New York: Psychology Press.

Hochberg, J., & Brooks, V. (1962). Pictorial recognition as an unlearned ability: A study of one child's performance. *American Journal of Psychology, 75*, 624–628.

Howe, M. L. (2019). Unravelling the nature of early (autobiographical) memory. *Memory, 27*(1), 115–121.

Howe, M. L., & Courage, M. L. (1993). On resolving the enigma of infantile amnesia. *Psychological Bulletin, 113*, 305–326.

Howe, M. L., Courage, M. L., & Edison, S. C. (2003). When autobiographical memory begins. *Developmental Review, 23*(4), 471–494.

Hulme, C., Thomson, N., Muir, C., & Lawrence, A. (1984). Speech rate and the development of short-term memory span. *Journal of Experimental Child Psychology, 38*, 241–253.

Jack, F., & Hayne, H. (2010). Childhood amnesia: Empirical evidence for a two-stage phenomenon. *Memory, 18*(8), 831–844.

Josselyn, S. A., & Frankland, P. W. (2012). Infantile amnesia: A neurogenic hypothesis. *Learning & Memory, 19*(9), 423–433.

Kail, R. (1991). Processing time declines exponentially during childhood and adolescence. *Developmental Psychology, 27*, 259–266.

Kail, R. (1997). Processing time, imagery, and spatial memory. *Journal of Experimental Child Psychology, 64*, 67–78.

Keresztes, A., Ngo, C. T., Lindenberger, U., Werkle-Bergner, M., & Newcombe, N. S. (2018). Hippocampal maturation drives memory from generalization to specificity. *Trends in Cognitive Sciences, 22*(8), 676–686.

Kibbe, M. M., & Leslie, A. M. (2011). What do infants remember when they forget? Location and identity in 6-month-olds' memory for objects. *Psychological Science, 22*(12), 1500–1505.

Kibbe, M. M., & Leslie, A. M. (2019). Conceptually rich, perceptually sparse: Object representations in 6-month-old infants' working memory. *Psychological Science, 30*(3), 362–375.

Kihlstrom, J. F., & Harackiewicz, J. M. (1982). The earliest recollection: A new survey. *Journal of Personality, 50*, 134–148.

Kingo, O. S., Berntsen, D., & Krøjgaard, P. (2013). Adults' earliest memories as a function of age, gender, and education in a large stratified sample. *Psychology and Aging, 28*(3), 646–653.

Lindberg, M. A. (1980). Is knowledge base development a necessary and sufficient condition for memory development? *Journal of Experimental Child Psychology, 30*, 401–410.

Lindsay, D. S., & Johnson, M. K. (1991). Recognition memory and source monitoring. *Bulletin of the Psychonomic Society, 29*, 203–205.

Mandler, J. M. (1988). How to build a baby: On the development of an accessible representational system. *Cognitive Development, 3*, 113–136.

Mandler, J. M. (1992). How to build a baby: II. Conceptual primitives. *Psychological Review, 99*, 587–604.

Mandler, J. M., Bauer, P. J., & McDonough, L. (1991). Separating the sheep from the goats: Differentiating global categories. *Cognitive Psychology, 23*, 263–298.

Mandler, J. M., & McDonough, L. (1996). Drinking and driving don't mix: Inductive generalization in infancy. *Cognition, 59*, 307–335.

Mani, N., & Plunkett, K. (2010). In the infant's mind's ear: Evidence for implicit naming in 18-month-olds. *Psychological Science, 21*(7), 908–913.

Maylor, E. A., & Logie, R. H. (2010). A large-scale comparison of prospective and retrospective memory development from childhood to middle age. *Quarterly Journal of Experimental Psychology, 63*(3), 442–451.

McLean, K. C. (2005). Late adolescent identity development: Narrative meaning making and memory telling. *Developmental psychology, 41*(4), 683–691.

McWilliams, K., Narr, R., Goodman, G. S., Ruiz, S., & Mendoza, M. (2013). Children's memory for their mother's murder: Accuracy, suggestibility, and resistance to suggestion. *Memory, 21*(5), 591–598.

Mullen, M. K. (1994). Earliest recollections of childhood: A demographic analysis. *Cognition, 52*, 55–79.

Nadel, L., & Zola-Morgan, S. (1984). Infantile amnesia: A neurobiological perspective. In M. Moscovitch (Ed.), *Infant Memory*. New York: Plenum Press.

Nelson, K. (1993). The psychological and social origins of autobiographical memory. *Psychological Science, 4*, 7–14.

Nelson, K., & Fivush, R. (2004). The emergence of autobiographical memory: A social cultural developmental theory. *Psychological Review, 111*, 486–511.

Nelson, K., & Gruendel, J. M. (1981). Generalized event representations: Basic building blocks of cognitive development. In M. E. Lamb, A. L. Brown (Eds.). *Advances in Developmental Psychology* (pp. 131–158). Hillsdale, NJ: Erlbaum.

Nelson, K., & Gruendel, J. M. (1988). At morning it's lunchtime: A scriptal view of children's dialogues. In M. B. Franklin & S. S. Barten (Eds.), *Child Language: A Reader* (pp. 263–277). New York: Oxford University Press.

Newcombe, N. S., Drummy, A. B., Fox, N. A., Lie, E., & Ottinger-Alberts, W. (2000). Remembering early childhood: How much, how, and why (or why not). *Current Directions in Psychological Science, 9*, 55–58.

Ornstein, P. A., Naus, M. J., & Liberty, C. (1975). Rehearsal and organization processes in children's memory. *Child Development 46*, 818–830.

Otgaar, H., Howe, M. L., Brackmann, N., & Smeets, T. (2016). The malleability of developmental trends in neutral and negative memory illusions. *Journal of Experimental Psychology: General, 145*(1), 31–55.

Otgaar, H., Verschuere, B., Meijer, E. H., & van Oorsouw, K. (2012). The origin of children's implanted false memories: Memory traces or compliance? *Acta Psychologica, 139*(3), 397–403.

Paris, S. G., & Lindaur, B. K. (1976). The role of inference in children's comprehension and memory for sentences. *Cognitive Psychology, 8*, 217–227.

Parker, J. F. (1995). Age differences in source monitoring of performed and imagined actions on immediate and delayed tests. *Journal of Experimental Child Psychology, 60*, 84–101.

Plumert, J. M. (1994). Flexibility in children's use of spatial and categorical organizational strategies in recall. *Developmental Psychology, 30*, 738–747.

Poole, D. A., & Lindsay, D. S. (2001). Children's eyewitness reports after exposure to misinformation from parents. *Journal of Experimental Psychology: Applied, 7*, 27–50.

Quinn, P. C., Eimas, P. D., & Rosenkrantz, S. L. (1993). Evidence for representations of perceptually similar natural categories by 3-month-old and 4-month-old infants. *Perception, 22*, 463–475.

Quinn, P. C., & Tanaka, J. W. (2007). Early development of perceptual expertise: Within-basic-level categorization experience facilitates the formation of subordinate-level category representation in 6- to 7-month-old infants. *Memory & Cognition, 35*, 1422–1431.

Reese, E., & Robertson, S. J. (2019). Origins of adolescents' earliest memories. *Memory, 27*(1), 79–91.

Richardson, R., & Hayne, H. (2007). You can't take it with you: The translation of memory across development. *Current Directions in Psychological Science, 16*, 223–227.

Roberts, K. P., & Blades, M. (2000). Children's memory and source monitoring of real-life and televised events. *Journal of Applied Developmental Psychology, 20*, 575–596.

Rovee-Collier, C. (1997). Dissociations in infant memory: Rethinking the development of implicit and explicit memory. *Psychological Review, 104*, 467–498.

Rovee-Collier, C., & Cuevas, K. (2009). The development of infant memory. In M. L. Courage & N. Cowan (Eds.) *The Development of Memory in Infancy and*

Childhood (pp. 11–41). New York: Psychology Press.

Rovee-Collier, C., & Fagan, J. W. (1981). The retrieval of memory in early infancy. *Advances in Infancy Research, 1*, 225–254.

Russell, J., Alexis, D., & Clayton, N. (2010). Episodic future thinking in 3-to 5-year-old children: The ability to think of what will be needed from a different point of view. *Cognition, 114*(1), 56–71.

Samuel, A. G. (1978). Organizational vs. retrieval factors in the development of digit span. *Journal of Experimental Child Psychology, 26*, 308–319.

Simcock, G., & Hayne, H. (2002). Breaking the barrier? Children fail to translate their preverbal memories into language. *Psychological Science, 13*, 225–231.

Siqueland, E. R., & Delucua, C. A. (1969). Visual reinforcement of nonnutritive sucking in human infants. *Science, 165*(3898), 1144–1146.

Ślusarczyk, E., Niedźwieńska, A., & Białecka-Pikul, M. (2018). The first signs of prospective memory. *Memory, 26*(10), 1385–1395.

Snyder, K. A., Blank, M. P., & Marsolek, C. J. (2008). What form of memory underlies novelty preferences? *Psychonomic Bulletin & Review, 15*, 315–321.

Strange, D., & Hayne, H. (2013). The devil is in the detail: Children's recollection of details about their prior experiences. *Memory, 21*(4), 431–443.

Tekcan, A. İ., Kaya-Kızılöz, B., & Odaman, H. (2012). Life scripts across age groups: A comparison of adolescents, young adults, and older adults. *Memory, 20*(8), 836–847.

Usher, J. N. A., & Neisser, U. (1993). Childhood amnesia and the beginnings of memory for four early life events. *Journal of Experimental Psychology: General, 122*, 155–165.

Wang, Q. (2003). Infantile amnesia reconsidered: A cross-cultural analysis. *Memory, 11*, 65–80.

Wang, Q., Bui, V. K., & Song, Q. (2015). Narrative organisation at encoding facilitated children's long-term episodic memory. *Memory, 23*(4), 602–611.

Wang, Q., & Peterson, C. (2016). The fate of childhood memories: Children postdated their earliest memories as they grew older. *Frontiers in Psychology, 6*: 2038.

Wells, C., Morrison, C. M., & Conway, M. A. (2014). Adult recollections of childhood memories: What details can be recalled? *Quarterly Journal of Experimental Psychology, 67*(7), 1249–1261.

Zellner, M., & Bäuml, K-H. (2005). Intact retrieval inhibition in children's episodic recall. *Memory & Cognition, 33*, 396–404.

Zimmermann, T. D., & Meier, B. (2006). The rise and decline of prospective memory performance across the lifespan. *Quarterly Journal of Experimental Psychology, 12*, 2040–2046.

CHAPTER 17

Memory and Aging

As outlined in Chapter 16, the development of memory in infants and children takes time, but it gets better. This is obvious even to the most casual observer. There is also a strong expectation of memory change at the other end of life as we progress into old age. The stereotype is that old people are more forgetful, and there is some truth to this. However, natural aging does not negatively affect all types of memory. There are some things that stay the same or even improve.

We start this chapter by covering issues involved with testing older adults and the neurological changes that occur during the natural aging process. After this we look at some things that decline and change as people grow older. Because the news is not all bad, we also look at memory processes that stay the same or improve with age. A more general change in cognition as we grow older is how we process emotions and emotional information. Finally, although they are not caused by aging, but are so strongly correlated with advanced age, we consider various dementias and how they influence memory.

TESTING OLDER ADULTS AND NEUROLOGICAL CHANGE

When assessing the influence of the natural aging process on memory in older adults, some basic issues need to be considered. Two primary ones are how older adults are tested and changes that occur in the nervous system. We consider each of these in turn.

Testing Older Adults

When studying memory in older adults, one issue that must be resolved is how changes in memory are assessed? There are two general ways to do this. One is to do a **cross-sectional study**, in which a group of older adults is compared with a group of younger adults, typically college students. In these cases, the younger adults are treated as the control group, against which the older adults are compared. This is the type of study that is done most often. This is because these studies can be done relatively easily and quickly. Because younger and older adults differ in systematic ways, the results can be enlightening.

However, there are some issues with cross-sectional studies. An issue that is more of a concern for older adults than younger adults is the variability among people. There is typically more variability in performance for older adults than for younger adults (Williams et al., 2005). As an example, the change in the amount of response time variability across the life span is shown in Figure 17.1. Note that while older adults are more variable than younger adults overall, there are some older adults who are less variable than even most younger adults.

Part of this variability reflects the range of ages of the people involved. The younger adults are often college students, typically from 18 to 22 years old. This is not a large age range. However, for older adults, the age range is often broader, involving people anywhere from their early sixties to their nineties. Thus, there is a span of many decades. People at these different ages are not all the same, and this increased variability makes it harder to detect changes. Some studies split the older adults into two groups, often called the young-old and the old-old. For example, the young-old might be people from 60–75 and the old-old would be people age 76 and up.

Apart from the wider range of ages, there is increased variability even if older adults are limited to a narrow age range. Compared to older adults, younger adults are more homogeneous. By the time people reach older adulthood, they have had a broader range of experiences, are feeling the impact of multiple decades worth of life choices, and any innate differences have had more time to manifest themselves. Thus, older adults are more likely to show larger differences among one another, and this increased variability complicates studies of aging and memory.

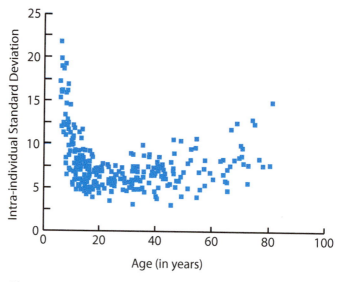

FIGURE 17.1 *Changes in the Amount of Intra-Individual Variability (How Variable a Given Person's Responses Are) for Response Times across the Life Span*

Source: Williams, B. R., Hultsch, D. F., Strauss, E. H., Hunter, M. A., & Tannock, R. (2005). Inconsistency in reaction time across the life span. *Neuropsychology, 19*(1), 88–96

Finally, the life experiences of people from different age cohorts are different, including the education and social contexts that people have experienced. Researchers need to be mindful that any age differences could be due to different experiences, and not age. Again, given the wide range of ages in groups of older adults, there is more variety of experience for those people than with younger adults.

Another way of assessing age-related changes in memory is do a **longitudinal study** in which the same people are tested at multiple points in time. One advantage is that it avoids many of the problems with cross-sectional studies. Because the same people are tested repeatedly, any differences in memory are more likely to be due to age-related changes. This is because people serve as their own controls. Even with the greater variability among older adults, because you know where each person is starting off at the beginning of the study, researchers can better target age-related memory changes.

There are some insightful longitudinal studies of age-related memory change; for example, the Betula study of memory, health, and aging done in Sweden (Nilsson et al., 2004). This study, begun in 1988, involves testing a large set of people every five years. At the beginning of the study participants ranged in age from 35 to 80 years of age. The wide range of ages allows researchers to do both cross-sectional and longitudinal comparisons. One finding was that age-related declines in declarative memory may be over-exaggerated in cross-sectional studies. A comparable longitudinal analysis showed smaller changes (Rönnlund et al., 2005).

Another illustration of the utility of longitudinal studies is a study by Salthouse (2016). In this study, people across a range of ages were tested twice, 2–3 years apart. As seen in Figure17.2, while younger adults improve over the two testing

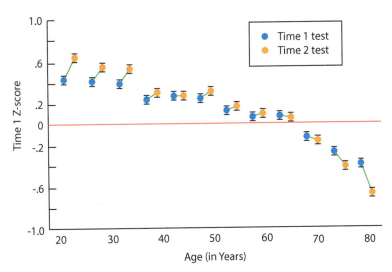

FIGURE 17.2 *Changes in the Memory Performance across Many Different Ages Using Longitudinal Testing*

Source: adapted from Salthouse, T. A. (2016). Continuity of cognitive change across adulthood. *Psychonomic Bulletin & Review, 23*(3), 932–939

sessions, this benefit goes away as people age, and declines are actually observed for older adults.

Given their advantages, why are longitudinal studies not done exclusively? Well, there are some difficulties. First, they take a lot of time, money, and effort. Second, it takes a long time to get the data. Memory research is a scientific endeavor, and our understanding is constantly changing. If you have a decades long study, it could be that issues that were thought to be important turn out not to be, or are better measured a different way, and new ways of understanding memory emerge. By the later study decades, the data collected from the early years might not be as informative or as insightful as a cross-sectional study. Third, there is an issue of people dropping out of the study over time. The reasons for dropping out are important if those people who did worse do not return to the study. This makes the effects of aging look better than they are. A final concern is that the same people are getting the same or similar tasks multiple times. Any experience they have with a task changes how they do later, even if it is years down the road.

Neurological Changes

Age-related neurological change is a universal phenomenon seen across cultures (Park et al., 1999). A basic change that occurs is in the rate or speed of neural firing, which is slower for older adults. Consequently, older adults take longer to engage in any cognitive process than do younger adults. This is one reason why your following distance behind cars will likely become larger as you grow older. At some level you are aware that your reflexes are not as fast as they used to be, and you implicitly give yourself more time to stop. Thinking more abstractly, the more complex a mental task is, the more noticeable the slowdown. Thus, memory processes that take more time overall are even slower for older adults.

Age-related changes in neural processing have led to **speed theories** of memory and aging. These changes can affect memory in many ways. For example, during processing, it is more likely that forgetting will occur for some of the information in the stream of thought, and performance declines (Salthouse, 1996), leading to problems.

In addition to neural speed, other parts of the brain are changing. The frontal lobes undergo the greatest change (Albert & Kaplan, 1980) and are less effective in older adults (Rypma et al., 2001). This reduces the ability to control the flow of information. The dorsolateral prefrontal lobe (on the top and sides in the front) is more affected than is the ventromedial prefrontal lobe (on the bottom and middle) (MacPherson et al., 2002). The dorsolateral prefrontal lobe is more responsible for the central executive of working memory, controlling the flow of thought. This results in a decline in executive memory functions, which can have several negative effects. For example, this can lead to difficulties retrieving long-term memories (e.g., Craik et al., 2018). In contrast to this part of the frontal lobe, the ventromedial prefrontal lobe is more involved in emotional and social tasks, such as regulating one's feelings.

The age-related decline in the frontal lobes leads to a decline in the ability to inhibit irrelevant information (Hasher & Zacks, 1989), as captured by **inhibition**

theory. When older adults try to remember things, related but irrelevant information is activated, thereby clogging the stream of thought. In a sense, one reason that older adults have trouble with memory is not that they are remembering too little, but that they are remembering too much. That said, there are multiple inhibition mechanisms, and aging influences these to different degrees (Rey-Mermet et al., 2018).

With aging, there are also changes in the temporal lobes. Related to this are changes with the hippocampus, which shows declines in the ability to engage in LTP (Jessberger & Gage, 2008). As a reminder, LTP is critical for the formation of new long-term memories. Thus, older adults show global problems with learning and retrieving memories.

One way for older adults' brains to compensate for these declines is to decrease cerebral lateralization (Colcombe et al., 2005) in which one hemisphere of the brain (left or right) becomes more dominant or does more of the processing than the other. Lateralization occurs initially because a group of nearby cells can make the necessary computations faster than groups that are spread out and need to pass information along the corpus callosum. In older adults, there is less lateralization (Reuter-Lorenz & Cappell, 2008). This may be because older adults need a larger array of cells to do the same job that a more localized portion would handle in younger adults.

Stop and Review

Aging brings about changes in memory. Most research involves cross-sectional studies in which younger adults, often college students, are compared with older adults. Alternatively, longitudinal studies can be done in which a set of people are assessed repeatedly over time. A primary neurological change with aging is a slower rate of neural firing. More globally, there are declines in portions of the frontal and temporal lobes, which influence the effectiveness of memory. There is also some degradation of hippocampal functions, such as LTP, which makes the acquisition of some types of knowledge harder. Finally, there is decrease in the lateralization as older adults engage in more whole-brain processing.

SOME THINGS CHANGE

In line with the stereotype, there are several age-related declines in memory. This section covers these changes. We start by discussing changes in core memory abilities, such as short-term/working memory, episodic memory, and semantic memory. We then discuss changes in more specialized topic areas.

Core Memory

First, older adults have reduced **short-term/working memory** capacities (Craik & Byrd, 1982). Thus, they are less able to coordinate information, especially when working memory demands are large. One example of this change is seen during text comprehension. In a study by Light and Capps (1986), people heard brief three- to five-sentence stories in which the final sentence contained a pronoun that referred back to a story character. What was manipulated was the distance between the character and the pronoun by varying the number of sentences between them. The greater the distance, the more performance declined, especially for older adults. Data showing this disruption is given in Table 17.1. Because older adults have less memory capacity, they have more difficulty holding on to a name and are more likely to forget it. As a result, when the pronoun is heard, they have a harder time determining to whom it referred.

Not only is working memory capacity affected, but so is the ability to engage in other working memory processes. For example, mental rotation is slower in older than younger adults (e.g., Gaylord & Marsh, 1975). This is due not only to decreased processing speed of mental rotation itself, but also to the time needed to initiate this process. For example, an EEG study by Zhao et al. (2019) found that electrophysiological markers of the onset of mental rotation were delayed by about 150 milliseconds in older adults relative to younger adults.

A noticeable age-related change in **episodic memory** is a decline in the ability to recall and recognize information (Zacks et al., 2000). These age-related memory differences are larger for recall than recognition (Rhodes et al., 2019), but are definitely present for both (Fraundorf et al., 2019). Part of the difficulty is with binding information together to store complex episodic memories. This could even lead to the binding of irrelevant information into a memory trace (Campbell et al., 2010). Thus, certain characteristics of an experience, such as context and features, may not be stored as effectively. As a result, older adults show smaller von Restorff effects (Bireta et al., 2008; but see Gallo et al., 2007), smaller bizarre imagery effects (Nicolas & Worthen, 2009), smaller encoding specificity effects (Duchek, 1984), and smaller adaptive memory effects (Stillman et al., 2014).

For **prospective memory**, there are some declines with old age (Einstein & McDaniel, 1990; Maylor, 1993), depending on the type of prospective memory. Older adults show declines for both time-based and event-based prospective memory, but more so for time-based prospective memory (Einstein et al., 1995; see Henry et al., 2004, for a meta-analysis).

TABLE 17.1 *Effects of Aging on the Percentages of Accurate Resolutions of Anaphors*

	Young	Old
Number of intervening sentences		
Zero	65.1	64.1
One	61.8	58.3
Number of intervening sentences		
Zero	64.9	63.4
Two	61.3	54.7

Source: adapted from Light, L. L., & Capps, J. L. (1986). Comprehension of pronouns in young and older adults. *Developmental Psychology, 22*, 580–585

Prospective memory, remembering to do something in the future, can show age-related declines. One illustration of this is a study by Einstein and McDaniel (1990). They recruited 24 students at Furman University who ranged in age from 17 to 24 years old. Another 24 were alumni of Furman who agreed to participate and ranged in age from 65 to 75. These were community dwelling older adults who drove themselves to the study.

For the study, people were seated at a computer. The primary task was a short-term memory test in which people were to learn lists of words and report them back. Each list was four to nine words long for the younger adults, and three to eight words long for the older adults. There were 42 trials. Each list was drawn from a set of 26 one- and two-syllable words. Thus, the words were repeated during the study. On each trial, people saw a "Prepare for Trial" signal for a second and a half. Then, they saw a list of words shown at a rate of one word every three-quarters of a second. At the end of a list, people were given a "recall" signal in which they were to verbally report all the words that they could remember, in the order that they saw them. People were given three minutes during these recall periods. Three practice trials were given to familiarize people with the task.

The secondary task was the prospective memory task. People were told to press a key on the keyboard whenever they heard the word "rake". As such, this is event-based prospective memory. This critical word appeared on three trials. The dependent measure was the rate at which people remembered to press the key in response to seeing this word.

What was found was that older adults remembered to do the prospective memory task less often than the younger adults. On average, younger adults did it 77% of the time, whereas the older adults did it 58% of the time. Thus, the older adults had some prospective memory difficulty.

That said, it should be noted that older adults tend to do better in naturalistic settings (such as remembering appointments) (Bailey et al., 2010). This may reflect better time management and the use of strategies that compensate for other declines in prospective memory. For example, time-based prospective memory in older adults is better when they lay out a plan (e.g., taking medication) ahead of time rather than just rehearsing information (Chasteen et al., 2001) or if the prospective task occurs with some regularity (Rose et al., 2010).

Older adults spend more time thinking proactively than younger adults do (Gardner & Ascoli, 2015). The difficulty older adults have with prospective memory may reflect difficulties self-initiating a memory process as needed (Craik, 1986). Older adults are less able to monitor themselves, and so, are more likely to not start something, such as a prospective memory task (Albiński et al., 2012), perhaps because of declines in frontal lobe processing (e.g., Lamichhane et al., 2018).

For episodic future thinking, older adults appear to think less specifically about future events than younger adults (e.g., Williams et al., 1996). Their future thoughts tend to be more general, with fewer details. This may be a result of older adults focusing more on emotionally positive aspects of events and avoiding thinking about negative aspects (Jumentier et al., 2018).

In terms of **forgetting**, older adults also have trouble regulating the retrieval of information from long-term memory. For example, they are more susceptible to associative interference and show larger fan effects than do younger adults (Gerard et al., 1991). They also show smaller retrieval practice effects (Aslan & Bäuml, 2012). Both are consistent with the idea that older adults have difficulty suppressing related and irrelevant information (Healey et al., 2013). Thus, as older adults try to remember something, they experience more interference from related memories, thereby making retrieval slower and less accurate.

In terms of directed forgetting, older adults do less well than younger adults (Andrés et al., 2004; Zacks et al., 1996; for a meta-analysis see Titz & Verhaeghen, 2010). This is more likely to happen using the item method and selective directed forgetting, than the list method (Zellner & Bäuml, 2006). This decline in directed forgetting has been attributed to declines in inhibitory processes (but see Sahakyan et al., 2008). For example, if asked to recall items that they were previously told to forget, older adults recall more to-be-forgotten items than younger adults because this information was not sufficiently inhibited.

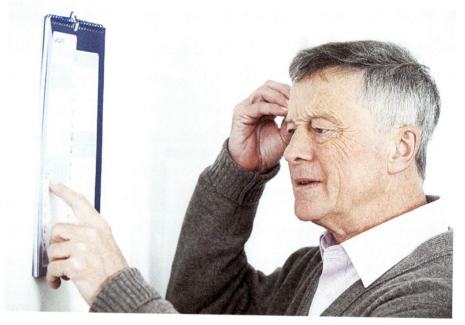

PHOTO 17.1 *Some aspects of memory, such as semantic memory and higher order memories, are preserved, or even improve, with age*

Source: Syda Productions/Shutterstock.com

Specialized Topic Areas

For spatial memories, older adults do worse on some tasks than others. For example, they appear to have difficulty with the spatial direction to other locations (Richmond et al., 2018). Overall, older adults may find it harder to create mental maps and retrieve information from them (Iaria et al., 2009).

For **autobiographical memory**, older adults' memories are dominated more by salient landmark events, self-relevant information, and emotionally positive events (Dijkstra & Kaup, 2005). They also become more generic, with fewer details, for both retrospective memories and future thoughts (Addis et al., 2008). However, this is truer for deliberate autobiographical memories than for spontaneous ones (Schlagman et al., 2009), although spontaneous memories are more emotionally positive, overall. Older adults also focus more on the semantic than the episodic aspects of autobiographical memory, and these memories are experienced more from an observer than a field perspective and are more likely to be classified as "known" rather than "recollected."

In terms of **memory and reality**, older adults show several declines. First, they are less effective at source monitoring and are more likely to make reality monitoring errors, confusing perceived and imagined events, perhaps because of declines in memory for perceptual and contextual information (Hashtroudi et al., 1990). They are also more likely to make destination errors and forget to whom they have told something in the past (causing them to tell the same story multiple times) (Gopie et al., 2010). Older adults are also more likely to have source monitoring errors for perceptually similar sources (e.g., two women) (Ferguson et al., 1992). Older adults decreased ability to integrate different types of source information leads to an increased likelihood of exhibiting cryptomnesia (McCabe et al., 2007) and false fame effects (Dywan & Jacoby, 1990). This can also be seen in ERPs recorded during source monitoring, with younger adults' ERP waves showing greater discrimination than older adults' (Dywan et al., 1998).

As noted later, older adults place more emphasis on semantic memories, such as categories and schemas. Therefore, they are more likely to report general knowledge-based false memories, such as the DRM false memory effect (see Chapter 12) (Norman & Schacter, 1997). This increase in false memory reports can be attributed to declines in the ability to monitor reality, as well as changes in inhibitory processing (Askey & Playfoot, 2018). Both of these changes reflect declines in overall frontal lobe functioning (Butler et al., 2004; but see Chan & McDermott, 2007).

Older adults are more likely to create false event memories (Gallo & Roediger, 2003) which may involve script-consistent information that was not actually encountered (LaVoie & Malmstrom, 1998). They are also more likely to misidentify positive attributes as corresponding to the choices they selected (Mather & Johnson, 2000). Some of the increase in false memories is due to older adults being less able to use conscious-based recollections and relying more on familiarity (Jacoby & Rhodes, 2006). That said, age-related changes in source monitoring do not always occur. When two sources are defined based on value characteristics, such as being told that John always tells the truth and Mary always tells lies, older and younger adults do equally well at identifying the source of a memory (Rahhal et al., 2002).

For issues related to **memory and the law**, older adults are just as likely as younger adults to have memory influenced by misleading post-event suggestions. However, older adults are more confident in these memory errors (Dodson & Krueger, 2006). They are also more likely to have trouble picking perpetrators out of a lineup, with confidence unaffected (Colloff et al., 2017). Again, these misinformation errors may be caused by source monitoring problems. For example, older adults are more likely to pick a person from a police lineup even if that person was not the perpetrator but had only been seen in a series of mugshots (Memon et al., 2002).

There are several age-related changes in **metamemory**. Older adults are less accurate in their judgments of learning (JOLs) than younger adults (Bieman-Copland & Charness, 1994), which may be due to declines in conscious recollection processes (Daniels et al., 2009). Thus, older adults are less able to assess whether they have learned something. However, older adults do effectively use relative accuracy and their use of JOLs to guide their study time (Dunlosky & Hertzog, 2000; Miles, & Stine-Morrow, 2004). They adjust their JOLs based on the nature of the information being learned, such as whether it is difficult or easy.

Another difficulty that older adults have with metamemory is for feeling of knowing (FOK) judgments. Their FOK ratings are poorer than younger adults', although primarily for episodic, rather than semantic, knowledge (Souchey et al., 2000), and they may experience more problems with a tip-of-the-tongue state (White & Abrams, 2002). Relatedly, older adults are more confident in their recognition errors, which rely more on levels of familiarity than explicit recollection. This could be due to declines in medial temporal lobe activity and their increased reliance on overall cortical activity (Chua et al., 2009). Overall, older adults have declines in conscious recollective experiences but not with more unconscious familiarity-based memory (Prull et al., 2006).

Finally, older adults are more likely to show larger hindsight bias effects compared to younger adults (Bernstein et al. 2011; Groß & Bayen, 2015). This may be due to an increased reliance on memory for newer, correct knowledge over memory for an original knowledge state (Groß & Pachur, 2019), possibly due to a decline in the ability to inhibit related and irrelevant information (Coolin et al., 2016). Specifically, after we learn something, to remember what it was like prior to learning, we need to inhibit the newer knowledge, which can intrude on thinking, causing misremembering of mental states prior to learning. Thus, this is an example of how inhibitory processing declines disrupt metamemory.

Overall, older adults have some troubles with memory. Moreover, they may have some insight into this change. For example, according to the Seattle Longitudinal Study, if complaints of forgetting increase over time, there is also a trend for performance on memory tasks to get worse (Hülür et al., 2018).

However, all aspects of memory do not inevitably get worse with age. In the next section we highlight some things that stay the same or even improve. Before that, it is important to understand that your attitude has a strong influence on how memory performs. If you *think* that memory gets worse with age, then performance will be worse (Hess et al., 2003; see Lamont et al., 2015 for a meta-analysis). This can occur

TABLE 17.2 *Effects of Age-Positive and Age-Negative Words on Memory: Difference in Pre- and Postexposure Conditions*

	Older Adults		Younger Adults	
	Negative	*Positive*	*Negative*	*Positive*
Immediate recall	−1.77	0.98	−0.36	−0.10
Learned recall	−0.46	0.49	0.43	0.07
Delayed recall	−1.11	0.20	0.33	−0.07
Photo recall	0.14	1.50	0.77	0.24
Auditory recall	−0.64	−0.20	−0.47	−0.60

Source: generated from data reported in Levy, B. (1996). Improving memory in old age through implicit self-stereotyping. *Journal of Personality and Social Psychology, 71*, 1092–107.

at a subconscious level. In a study by Levy (1996), older adults were given a series of memory tests. Prior to this they were subliminally exposed to a number of age-positive words, such as "wisdom," "sage," or "guidance," or age-negative words, such as "senile," "dementia," and "decrepit." Although the older adults were not aware that they had seen the words, their performance was affected. Data from this study are shown in Table 17.2. Older adults did worse following age-negative words, but better following age-positive words. There was no such influence for the younger adults. Thus, the implicit age-related stereotypes that are activated can impact how well memory works.

When goals are set for people to improve memory, both younger and older adults respond well, and this is sometimes greater for the older adults (West et al., 2003), although not always (Chasteen et al., 2005). Older adults may be more prone to discounting their abilities and may be making their situation worse with self-handicapping thoughts. If we emphasize people's ages prior to doing a memory task, such as filling out a questionnaire asking people to rate various positive and negative adjectives describing older adults, this can set up a *stereotype threat* situation. This activates negative age-related ideas from the culture. This then leads older adults to do worse on memory tasks than they would otherwise (Bouazzaoui et al., 2016).

Stop and Review

A common idea is that memory gets worse as we grow older. There is a decline in short-term/working memory capacity, with older adults less able to keep as much information active. There are also declines in episodic memory, which older adults find harder to form. Older adults also have trouble with prospective memory, although these effects are larger in the laboratory than in everyday life. In terms of forgetting, older adults are less able to regulate interference at retrieval, possibly due to a decline in inhibitory processes. Relatedly, older adults are not as efficient at some types of directed forgetting. For autobiographical memory, older adults report fewer details and tend to focus on positive events. For memory and reality, older adults are more prone to false memories and are more confident in their memory errors. Finally, older adults are less aware of their own memory contents and processes than are younger adults. Many of these age-related deficits are worsened by negative social stereotypes about aging and memory.

SOME THINGS STAY THE SAME

While aging is associated with declines in memory, there are some aspects that remain constant and even improve. This follows on ideas outlined by Hess (2005) that note that traditional views of memory and aging may overemphasize age-related declines, miss areas of stability or improvement, not take into account adaptive developmental changes, and ignore that there is a greater degree of variability between people when older adults are considered.

Core Memory

There are several aspects of memory that are not negatively affected by the aging process. **Nondeclarative memories** show some stability with age, perhaps because they are neurologically more robust. For example, other than an overall change in processing speed, there is little in the way of age-related changes in priming (Fleishman et al., 2004). Similarly, procedural skills, such as golf putting, as shown in Figure 17.3, are learned similarly at nondeclarative memory level by younger

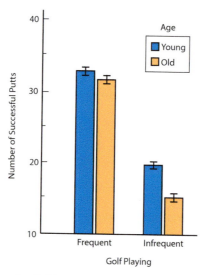

FIGURE 17.3 *Data for Golf Putting Success Showing that Older Adults Who Maintain Their Skill (Frequent Golfers) Show No Skill Deficit Compared to Younger Adults*

Source: generated from data reported in Chauvel, G., Maquestiaux, F., Hartley, A. A., Joubert, S., Didierjean, A., & Masters, R. S. (2012). Age effects shrink when motor learning is predominantly supported by nondeclarative, automatic memory processes: Evidence from golf putting. *Quarterly Journal of Experimental Psychology, 65*(1), 25–38

and older adults (Chauvel et al., 2012). Thus, motor skills that are acquired earlier in life can remain largely intact into old age.

As noted in the previous section, there is no doubt that **episodic memory** declines with age. However, this decline has limits. Some aspects of episodic memory stay at a high level and may even improve. The distinction between what is and is not remembered is a distinction between quantitative and qualitative aspects of memory (Small et al., 1999). There is a near uniform quantitative decline in episodic memory, with older adults remembering less. However, qualitative aspects of memory are preserved. That is, the way information is remembered stays the same. Older adults show as much information structuring during remembering as do younger adults and may even show an increase (Kahana & Wingfield, 2000). Moreover, older adults benefit as much as younger adults do by engaging in distributed rather than massed practice (Balota et al., 1989; Maclean et al., 2017).

Younger and older adults use mental models similarly in memory (Radvansky et al., 1990). Thus, older adults have preserved abilities to update their understanding (Radvansky & Dijkstra, 2007). For example, they are as likely to forget information after walking through a doorway as younger adults (Radvansky et al., 2015). This more fundamental type of knowledge (as compared to words) may remain robust during development. This can be seen in Figure 17.4. While younger adults outperform older adults at the surface form and textbase levels, they do not at the mental model level (Radvansky et al., 2001). This preserved memory is seen in everyday tasks, such as remembering news events (Frieske & Park, 1999). Compared to younger adults, older adults better remember the content of news stories and the sources of those

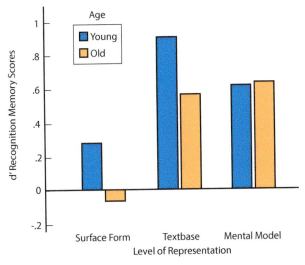

FIGURE 17.4 *Poorer Recognition Memory for Older Adults, Relative to Younger Adults, at the Surface Form and Textbase Levels, but Preserved Recognition Memory for Older Adults at the Event Model Level*

Source: generated from data reported in Radvansky, G. A., Zwaan, R. A., Curiel, J. M., & Copeland, D. E. (2001). Situation models and aging. *Psychology and Aging, 16*(1), 145–160

stories. Relatedly, older adults show similar flashbulb memory effects as younger adults (Kvavilashvili et al., 2010). Thus, higher level comprehension and memory is preserved in older adults.

Although older adults show some declines in inhibitory processes during memory retrieval, they do not show declines in the suppression of irrelevant concepts in the repeated practice paradigm (Aslan et al., 2007). This suggests that not all types of inhibitory processes are compromised in old age. Similarly, the greater dependency older adults have on the organization of information in memory may lead them to be more susceptible to things such as part-set cuing (Marsh et al., 2004). This organizational dependency is also revealed in the finding that, like younger adults, older adults are similarly likely to forget information when recalling in groups, in which one's retrieval plan is disrupted (Henkel & Rajaram, 2011).

One of the biggest areas of stability and improvement for older adults is with **semantic memory** (Rönnlund et al., 2005). Over a lifespan, people are exposed to a broad range of information, and this knowledge continues to accumulate. Older adults often outperform younger adults on measures of semantic knowledge, such as vocabulary tests. This is not related to educational factors, such as the older adults getting a "better" education. Moreover, the structure of semantic memory is largely unchanged, as evidenced by the finding that semantic priming effects remain stable (Balota & Duchek, 1988), including both automatic (Howard et al., 1981), more consciously controlled priming (Burke et al., 1987), and mediated priming (Bennett & McEvoy, 1999). Older adults can reliably draw on a broader range of real-world knowledge than younger adults.

Because of the preservation and expansion of semantic memory for older adults, as episodic memory declines, there is a greater reliance on information in semantic memory, such as schemas and scripts (Light & Anderson, 1983; Umanath & Marsh, 2014). Thus, older adults focus on more important (relative to less important) information (Castel et al., 2007). Older adults rely on their schemas so much that they may have more trouble suppressing them when they are irrelevant (Arbuckle et al., 1994).

Not only do older adults update their episodic memories as effectively as younger adults do, they are better able to forget and modify their semantic understandings when they get something wrong. For example, they are less likely to be misled by information that is inconsistent with their world knowledge (Umanath & Marsh, 2012). They are also better able to correct semantic misunderstanding when they get new information (Metcalfe et al., 2015) and retain these corrections longer than younger adults (Sitzman et al., 2020), thereby showing superior age-related memory.

As noted earlier, the information that is more readily forgotten, and most likely to suffer because of aging, is memory for details. Keeping in mind fuzzy trace theories, memory is composed of detailed, specific memories and more general, gist-related memories. As the aging process proceeds, episodic memory declines, but semantic memory improves. As a result, older adults' memories are more likely to be influenced by general information, rather than memory for details (Koutstaal,

2006), which is not observed when older adults do not have prior knowledge (Koutstaal et al., 2003).

This differential emphasis on semantic and episodic memory is also seen with social judgments. Older adults are more likely to make predictions of other people's future behavior based on a general, schematic understanding, rather than specific episodic information about the person (Hess et al., 1998). However, not all social judgments are biased toward schematic information. If people are asked to rate how likable a person is, younger and older adults use schematic and specific information similarly (Hess & Bolstad, 1998). Thus, while older adults are more dependent on their semantic knowledge, they can disregard it when needed.

The stability and reliance on semantic knowledge can lead it to be activated and used, even though we do not want it to be, as is the case with social stereotypes. Older adults are in a position in which their semantic knowledge is intact, but their ability to suppress unwanted information is compromised. As a consequence, older adults are more likely to activate stereotypes and be influenced by them, even when they are trying to be egalitarian (Radvansky et al., 2009; Stewart et al., 2009). Thus, older adults may, at times, be prejudiced against their will. That said, it is also possible for older adults to deactivate stereotypes if they are discounted in some way (such as explicitly noting that a baby sitter was male) (Radvansky et al., 2009).

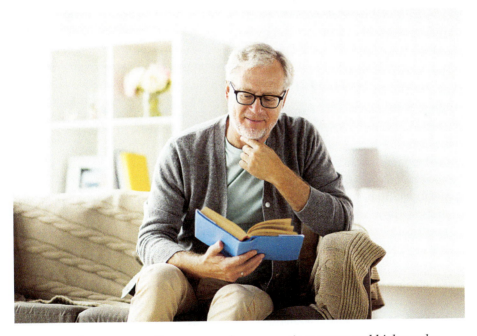

PHOTO 17.2 *Some aspects of memory, such as semantic memory and higher order memories, are preserved, or even improve, with age*

Source: Syda Productions/Shutterstock.com

Specialized Topic Areas

There are age-related changes in **metamemory**. Not only do older adults have generally superior semantic memories, they also have a greater awareness of this expanded knowledge base (Kavé & Halamish, 2015). When learning new things, they appear to rely on the region of proximal learning as much as do younger adults (Price & Murray, 2012). On another topic, Bayen et al. (2006) found no major effect of aging on the hindsight bias (see Figure 17.4). Hindsight judgments are similar in younger and older adults.

Aging and Emotion

Overall, older adults showed an enhanced ability to regulate their emotions (Urry & Gross, 2010). They also more often show mood congruency effects in memory (Knight et al., 2002). Although older adults are less efficient than younger adults at source monitoring and some prospective memory tasks, these age differences disappear if the information is emotional (May et al., 2005). A similar age-invariant finding is observed for emotional information in working memory, particularly for positive materials (Mikels et al., 2005). It should be noted that this emotion influence is only observed if people think about the emotional aspects of an event at the time. It does not occur automatically (Emery & Hess, 2008).

With old age there is a tendency to emphasize positive over negative information, which is known as the **positivity effect** (Reed & Carstensen, 2012; but see Murphy &

Improve Your Memory

Some parts of memory remain stable or improve with age. Is there anything that you can do to make it more likely that you will be one of those people who show less of a mental decline? In short, the answer is, to some degree, "yes." Hertzog et al. (2008) outlined a number of steps that you can take to address age-related changes in memory and keep any deficits to a minimum. They cover the intellectual, social, and physical activities you can engage in to aid memory. In short, the more that you stay active in several complex intellectual, social, and physical activities, the more successfully you will age, and the smaller your deficits will be. So, be active in a wide variety of things throughout your life, and you will have fewer problems as you grow older.

On top of this, the broader your knowledge base is when you enter old age, the more that you will have to work with. So, to put yourself in the best position, expose yourself to many different experiences. Read a wide variety of books, watch lots of different kinds of shows and movies, go out to plays and concerts, go visit different places, and so on. People who are intellectually active throughout their lives (college professors, for example) can show smaller or no memory deficits in some areas (Shimamura et al., 1995).

Isaacowitz, 2008). This reflects a greater interest in close interpersonal relationships and a desire to control emotions as we age. As a consequence, older adults show poorer memory for negative information than do younger adults (Charles et al., 2003; but see Grühn et al., 2005). Even after negative public events (e.g., a bombing), older adults memories grow less negative with time more so than do younger adults' memories (Ford et al., 2018). This is consistent with fMRI work which shows that while there are preserved connections between the dorsolateral prefrontal cortex (BAs 9 & 46) and the amygdala, preserving emotional control, the connections from the amygdala and the hippocampus are weakened, suggesting a decline in emotional influences on memory (St. Jacques et al., 2009).

Stop and Review

There are areas where memories remain intact or improve with old age. Nondeclarative memories remain largely intact, so long as skills are practiced. For episodic memory, there are declines in the quantity of what is remembered, but the quality of those memories improves. Older adults also update their memories as efficiently as younger adults. Perhaps the biggest area in which memory is preserved or improves with aging is semantic memory. Older adults have better vocabularies, schemas, and scripts than younger adults. This may lead them to depend more on their semantic knowledge to compensate for deficits they experience in episodic memory. Finally, older adults have more emotional control than younger adults and put a greater premium on positive experiences.

DEMENTIA

Dementia is a condition in which there are serious impairments in many aspects of thinking, only one of which is memory, but without an impairment of consciousness. People often think of dementias as illnesses of the elderly. However, dementia is not caused by natural aging. It is true that while many older adults will acquire some form of dementia (11% over the age of 65, and 32% over the age of 85), many younger people contract these diseases as well (Brandt & Rich, 1995). However, because dementia often emerges with advanced age, it is covered in this chapter. The memory problems that occur with dementia include a decline in the ability to learn new information and a loss of prior memories. Because of widespread brain degradation, this memory loss can even extend to well-ingrained memories. In this section we consider several more prominent dementias. These include Alzheimer's disease, Parkinson's disease, Huntington's disease, and the dementia associated with multiple sclerosis.

Alzheimer's Disease

Alzheimer's disease was first described by Alois Alzheimer in 1907. It is one of the most rapidly expanding health concerns that we have. As the population ages, more people will succumb to its effects. This disease occurs only in certain people because of specific neurological conditions. It is not a natural consequence of growing old. While far too many older adults will contract Alzheimer's, most will not.

Alzheimer's disease is a cortical dementia marked by severe degradation in brain structure and function. With Alzheimer's disease, the mind and memory deteriorate. Three primary changes occur (Hodges, 2000). The first is a loss in the number of neurons and neural connections, primarily focused in the frontal and temporal lobes, which are critical for memory, with the sensory and motor areas being better preserved. Second, there are **neurofibrillary tangles** that occur within neurons and impede their ability to effectively transmit a signal. They grow over time, eventually pushing other neural structures, such as the nucleus, mitochondria, and ribosomes, to one side, and disrupting their function and filling up the interior of the axons and dendrites. Finally, a third change is the presence of **amyloid plaques** which are growths of old neural tissue with a core of amyloid proteins that occupy the regions around neurons and are surrounded by microglia. These plaques are about 70 microns in diameter, much larger than the neurons, which are often 10 to 30 microns in diameter. Their presence makes it difficult for neurons to function because they degenerate axons.

In addition, with Alzheimer's disease there are also changes in the cholinergic system (Bartus et al., 1982), particularly the manufacturing of the neurotransmitter acetylcholine (ACh), which is critical to learning and memory. The decrease can be mediated somewhat by people taking an ever-increasing list of medications that have been found to affect the symptoms of this disease.

No one knows for sure exactly what causes Alzheimer's. However, several preconditions are known that indicate the likelihood of contracting the disease (Small, 1998). There is a strong genetic component. If a relative has Alzheimer's, there is a 25 to 50% probability that a person will develop it as well. If not, then the probability is only 10%. In identical twins, if one twin contracts the condition, there is a 40 to 50% chance that the other will as well, and a 10 to 50% chance for fraternal twins. There is a higher rate of occurrence of the disease in people with Down's syndrome, also suggesting a genetic component.

There are also external, environmental influences. For example, people who have suffered head traumas or long periods of depression are more likely to succumb. There are some protective factors. People who have been exposed to estrogen or antioxidants may be less likely to get the disease. Similarly, people who experience body inflammations, such as arthritis, are less likely to contract Alzheimer's. There may also be some DNA combinations that are more resistant to this condition. Thus, there are many factors that impact whether a person will one day have to live with Alzheimer's disease.

People with Alzheimer's disease suffer from working memory problems. These tend not to be problems maintaining information but with controlling the flow of thought in the central executive. They have normal working memory spans for verbal and spatial information. However, they do not show normal recency effects for larger sets of information. In terms of central executive problems, they have trouble managing memories under dual-task conditions where a person needs to keep track of two things at once. As such, they can become more easily confused and overwhelmed.

Alzheimer's disease has a profound effect on episodic memories, although there is a temporal gradient, with newer memories being more likely to be compromised than older memories (e.g., Sadek et al., 2004). This temporal gradient of memory loss can be extensive, reaching back several decades. As the disease progresses, there are losses of earlier and earlier memories that can result in changes and losses in a person's identity (Addis & Tippett, 2004). The temporal gradient of memory loss suggests that a factor in this condition is in encoding. It is even difficult for Alzheimer's patients to form new flashbulb memories (Budson & Gold, 2009). Neurological work using fMRI scanning has shown that the prefrontal lobes of Alzheimer's patients are not functioning as well as normal people's (Corkin, 1998). The rate with which they forget episodic information, once it has been encoded, is the same as for people without the disease (White & Ruske, 2002). Thus, the episodic memory problems can be viewed as a form of anterograde amnesia (see Chapter 10). Retrieval, while difficult, is less of a problem, at least in the earlier stages of the disease. This deficit is more profound with recall than with recognition.

Although semantic memory is initially more resistant, it does eventually succumb. Alzheimer's patients may lose the ability to recall the names of objects and may substitute similar words—for example, using "tiger" or "animal" for "lion." Thus, there is a degree of noise and error in semantic memory. This can also be seen in how semantic memories are lost. Memory of how something is used to interact with other objects—that is, its functional relations—is lost sooner than knowledge about its parts and properties, with knowledge about categorical relations being the most resistant to loss (Johnson & Hermann, 1995). Also, with regard to semantic memory, these people have trouble processing new semantic categories (Nosofsky et al., 2012). Patients with Alzheimer's disease are more likely to have trouble remembering public information as compared to autobiographical information (Greene & Hodges, 1996). Here is a case where stable, semantic information is more vulnerable than episodic information.

Although many memory systems are affected by Alzheimer's disease, some systems are less affected than others. For example, implicit memory processes are more intact. This also spills over into related metamemory processes. Using the remember–know distinction, Alzheimer's disease patients show declines in memory for information that is marked as "remember" but not when it is marked as "know" (Barba, 1997). Also, Alzheimer's patients have trouble making accurate source monitoring decisions (Mammarella & Fairfield, 2006). That said, some implicit memory processes are disrupted. For example, Alzheimer's patients often show impaired semantic priming.

Parkinson's Disease

The diseases we look at next—Parkinson's, Huntington's, and multiple sclerosis—are subcortical dementias. This contrasts with Alzheimer's disease, which is a cortical dementia. It should be noted that not everyone who contracts these other diseases becomes clearly demented. These subcortical dementias are often associated with movement difficulties, as well as with more minor problems in memory and thinking.

With **Parkinson's disease**, there is damage to or loss of neurons in the basal ganglia and the substantia nigra. This is accompanied by a disruption in dopamine processing. This damage produces problems in coordinating movements, such as tremors, "pill rolling" (rubbing fingers together as if rolling a pill), problems in facial expression, and difficulty in walking. Parkinson's disease usually begins around the age of 50. In addition to the movement problems, there are cognitive and emotional deficits, including problems with memory (Brandt & Rich, 1995; Pirozzolo et al., 1982). There may be working memory problems, such as with updating spatial information in the visuo-spatial sketchpad. For example, when people with Parkinson's travel through a new space with twists and turns, they may become more disoriented (Montgomery et al., 1993). In addition, they may experience problems identifying locations of previously seen pictures on a simple display grid (Pillon et al., 1997). They do not keep track of spatial contextual information like normal people would.

In addition, people with Parkinson's may have central executive and episodic buffer troubles (Altgassen et al., 2007; Brown & Marsden, 1988). In fact, the visuo-spatial deficits may actually be a result of more central executive and episodic buffer problems (Altgassen et al., 2007). They have some difficulty controlling their stream of thought and how they use memories. For example, they have difficulty changing strategies and will continue doing things the way they have always done them before (Canavan et al., 1989). They also having difficulty evaluating the importance of events in a semantic schema or script, although they can order scripted information quite well (Zalla et al., 2000).

With Parkinson's disease, like with Alzheimer's disease, the loss of episodic memories follows a temporal gradient, with older memories being more preserved than newer ones. However, the extent of the temporal gradient is far more subtle and is not as noticeable. Finally, while the forgetting of event content is less compromised in Parkinson's disease than in Alzheimer's disease, the opposite is true for event date memories. People with Parkinson's disease may have difficulty locating events in time (Sagar et al., 1988) or putting information in a correct sequence, such as a telephone number. Part of the problem may be with trouble in coordinating retrieval strategies and not encoding or consolidating (Godbout & Doyon, 2000). Specifically, when recalling the components of a common script, such as going to the doctor, Parkinson's disease patients are more likely to leave out minor components, retrieve script components in the incorrect order, and have more irrelevant intrusions.

Huntington's Disease

Huntington's disease is characterized by uncontrolled muscle spasms, resulting in jerky movements. It is caused by damage to the basal ganglia and the caudate nucleus. It often strikes around the age of 40, and the victim generally dies by the age of 60. In addition, there are problems in memory (Brandt & Rich, 1995). Huntington's patients have problems with the central executive of working memory, resulting in a reduced memory span and difficulties in dual-task situations (Hodges, 2000). However, the rate of forgetting in episodic memory may be preserved along with recognition memory. Importantly, there is no temporal gradient to forgetting, but it is more uniform across time (Sadek et al., 2004). This suggests that the problem is with the retrieval rather with than the encoding and storage of memories.

With Huntington's disease, there may be problems with free recall, but not recognition, consistent with the idea that patients are having trouble planning how to retrieve information. In general, the memory deficits are milder and like those observed with Parkinson's. However, they are more likely to have trouble with nonverbal information, such as memory for faces, spatial layouts, or visual images. In the earlier stages of Huntington's disease, patients may be aware of the memory problems they are experiencing, but as the disease progresses, this awareness slips away (de Langavant et al., 2013). Finally, these people may have trouble with procedural memory, even though this memory system is often preserved in people with neurologically related memory losses.

Multiple Sclerosis

Multiple sclerosis (MS) involves a demyelinization of various neurons. Although MS is generally associated with muscle control problems, it can also affect memory. There appears to be some atrophy of cells in area CA1 of the hippocampus, which is important for creating declarative memories, as well as damage to portions of the frontal lobe, which is important for controlling the processing of information in memory (Benedict et al., 2002; Sicotte et al., 2008). One of the larger areas of impact is short-term memory. There are problems in both creating and retrieving memories (Pelosi et al., 1997), and MS patients appear to have awareness of their memory deficits (Randolph et al., 2001). There is also a decline in the speed with which short-term memory is scanned, but not working memory capacity per se (Janculjak et al., 2002). Again, there is a greater disturbance of explicit over implicit memory. Finally, MS patients may have trouble with the retrieval of autobiographical memories (Ernst et al., 2015).

Stop and Review

Memory can be devastatingly altered by dementia. Alzheimer's disease, the most common form of dementia, results in memory being systematically destroyed as drastic changes are made in the cortex. Other conditions, such as Parkinson's disease, Huntington's disease, and multiple sclerosis, are subcortical diseases that can each have a memory loss component to them. How each condition affects memory depends on the brain structures that are damaged. For example, while Alzheimer's and Parkinson's diseases have memory losses that exhibit a temporal gradient, suggesting a problem in consolidation, Huntington's disease has a flat loss gradient, suggesting a problem in memory retrieval.

PUTTING IT ALL TOGETHER

Aging involves memory gains and losses. How well people do as they age is revealed by cross-sectional and longitudinal studies. As you age, many of your nondeclarative skills hang around, and may even improve, with practice. The expansion of world knowledge in semantic memory will help you better organize your experiences that are kept in memory. This is a source of wisdom that comes with aging. When processing event information, as an older adult you will be better able comprehend, draw inferences, and remember your experiences at higher, abstract levels of thinking. Finally, as an older adult you will be better able to regulate your emotions. Part of this involves placing a greater emphasis on emotionally positive information and experiences, which is known as the positivity effect.

The gains you make as you progress through life can compensate for the losses. For example, your neurons will not fire as rapidly as they do now. There also will be changes in your frontal lobes, which are involved in the control of thought and action. This may explain problems with the control of memory that you experience as you age, with short-term/working memory shrinkage, and with prospective memory and directed forgetting. This also drives some of the loss in inhibitory control, which can lead to problems dealing with retrieval interference, such as fan effects. Cortical changes are involved with source memory problems. In addition, there are changes in the temporal lobes and the hippocampus, which are important for making new memories. Thus, it will be less likely that you will retain the details of events in episodic memory. This can lead you to be more dependent on your semantic memories, as well as relying more on feelings of familiarity rather than conscious recollection.

The biggest changes in memory that can occur are if you are unfortunate enough to contract some form of dementia. This is most likely to be Alzheimer's disease, a cortical dementia in which there is a decline in the number of neural connections, the presence of neurofibrillary tangles within neurons, and amyloid plaques outside of and around neurons. As this disease progresses, memory and thinking are compromised. You may also be afflicted with a subcortical dementia, such as Parkinson's disease, Huntington's disease, and multiple sclerosis.

STUDY QUESTIONS

1. What are some of the advantages and disadvantages of studying aging and memory using cross-sectional studies?
2. What are some of the advantages and disadvantages of studying aging and memory using longitudinal studies?
3. What are some major neurological changes that occur with old age that can affect memory?
4. What are the dominant theories of age-related changes in memory? In what ways do they overlap? In what ways are they different?
5. How are short-term/working memory abilities affected by the natural aging process? What are the implications of these changes?

6. What aspects of episodic memory become worse as a person ages? Think about this in terms of both retrospective and prospective memory abilities.

7. What changes in long-term memory occur that cause older adults to be more likely to forget information? How effective are older adults at deliberately forgetting things?

8. How does aging affect autobiographical memories in older adults?

9. How are issues related to memory and reality influenced by aging, and what implications does this have for legal settings?

10. What problems do older adults experience with regard to metamemory processing?

11. What role do social attitudes and stereotypes play in age-related problems with memory?

12. What influence does the natural aging process have on nondeclarative memories?

13. What aspects of episodic memory remain intact into old age?

14. Why does semantic memory improve for older adults, and how does this increase in semantic memory influence other kinds of memory processes?

15. How are higher-level processing and memory affected by old age?

16. What are the changes in emotional processing that occur with aging? What are the impacts of these changes on aging and memory?

17. What can you do to help preserve your memory ability when you move into old age?

18. What are the characteristics of Alzheimer's disease? What parts of the brain are affected? How is memory affected?

19. What are some of the subcortical dementias? What parts of the brain are affected? How is memory affected?

KEY TERMS

- Alzheimer's disease
- amyloid plaques
- cross-sectional study
- dementia
- Huntington's disease
- inhibition theory
- longitudinal study
- multiple sclerosis (MS)
- neurofibrillary tangles
- Parkinson's disease
- positivity effect
- speed theories

EXPLORE MORE

Here are some additional readings for you to further explore issues related to memory and aging.

Chasteen, A. L., Bhattacharyya, S., Horhota, M., Tam, R., & Hasher, L. (2005). How feelings of stereotype threat influence older adults' memory performance. *Experimental Aging Research, 31*(3), 235–260.

Einstein, G. O. (2004). *Memory Fitness: A Guide for Successful Aging*. New Haven, CT: Yale University Press.

Logie, R. H., & Maylor, E. A. (2009). An internet study of prospective memory across adulthood. *Psychology and Aging, 24*, 767–774.

Naveh-Benjamin, M., & Ohta, N. (2012). *Memory and Aging: Current Issues and Future Directions*. Philadelphia, PA: Psychology Press.

Radvansky, G. A. & Dijkstra, K. (2007) Aging and situation model processing. *Psychonomic Bulletin & Review, 14*, 1027–1042.

REFERENCES

Addis, D. R., & Tippett, L. J. (2004). Memory of myself: Autobiographical memory and identity in Alzheimer's disease. *Memory, 12*, 56–74.

Addis, D. R., Wong, A. T., & Schacter, D. L. (2008). Age-related changes in the episodic simulation of future events. *Psychological Science, 19*(1), 33–41.

Albert, M. S., & Kaplan, E. (1980). Organic implications of neuropsychological deficits in the elderly. In L. W. Poon, J. L. Fozard, L. S. Cermak, D. Arenberg, & L. W. Thompson (Eds.), *New Directions in Memory and Aging* (pp. 403–432). Hillsdale, NJ: Erlbaum.

Albiński, R., Sedek, G., & Kliegel, M. (2012). Differences in target monitoring in a prospective memory task. *Journal of Cognitive Psychology, 24*(8), 916–928.

Altgassen, M., Phillips, L., Kopp, U., & Kliegel, M. (2007). Role of working memory components in planning performance of individuals with Parkinson's disease. *Neuropsychologia, 45*(10), 2393–2397.

Andrés, P., Van der Linden, M., & Parmentier, F. B. R. (2004). Directed forgetting in working memory: Age-related differences. *Memory, 12*, 248–256.

Arbuckle, T. Y., Cooney, R., Milne, J., & Melchior, A. (1994). Memory for spatial layouts in relation to age and schema typicality. *Psychology and Aging, 9*, 467–480.

Askey, C., & Playfoot, D. (2018). Examining theories of cognitive ageing using the false memory paradigm. *Quarterly Journal of Experimental Psychology, 71*(4), 931–939.

Aslan, A., & Bäuml, K.-H. T. (2012). Retrieval-induced forgetting in old and very old age. *Psychology and Aging, 27*(4), 1027–1032.

Aslan, A., Bäuml, K. H., & Pastötter, B. (2007). No inhibitory deficit in older adults' episodic memory. *Psychological Science, 18*(1), 72–78.

Bailey, P. E., Henry, J. D., Rendell, P. G., Phillips, L. H., & Kliegel, M. (2010). Dismantling the "age–prospective memory paradox": The classic laboratory paradigm simulated in a naturalistic setting. *Quarterly Journal of Experimental Psychology, 63*(4), 646–652.

Balota, D. A, & Duchek, J. M. (1988). Age-related differences in lexical access, spreading activation, and simple pronunciation. *Psychology and Aging, 3*, 84–93.

Balota, D. A., Duchek, J. M., & Paullin, R. (1989). Age-related differences in the impact of spacing, lag, and retention interval. *Psychology and Aging, 4*(1), 3–9.

Barba, G. D. (1997). Recognition memory and recollective experience in Alzheimer's disease. *Memory, 5*, 657–672.

Bartus, R. T., Dean, R. L., Beer, B., & Lippa, A. S. (1982). The cholinergic hypothesis of geriatric memory dysfunction. *Science, 217*, 408–417.

Bayen, U. J., Erdfelder, E., Bearden, J. N., & Lozito, J. P. (2006). Interplay of memory and judgment processes in effects of aging on hindsight bias. *Journal of Experimental Psychology: Learning, memory, and Cognition, 32*, 1003–1018.

Benedict, R. H. B., Bakshi, R., Simon, J. H., Priore, R., Miller, C., & Munschauer, F. (2002). Frontal cortex atrophy predicts cognitive impairment in multiple sclerosis. *Journal of Neuropsychiatry and Clinical Neurosciences, 14*(1), 44–51.

Bennett, D. J., & McEvoy, C. L. (1999). Mediated priming in younger and older adults. *Experimental Aging Research, 25*, 141–159.

Bernstein, D. M., Erdfelder, E., Meltzoff, A. N., Peria, W., & Loftus, G. R. (2011). Hindsight bias from 3 to 95 years of age. *Journal of Experimental*

Psychology: Learning, Memory, and Cognition, 37(2), 378–391.

Bieman-Copland, S., & Charness, N. (1994). Memory knowledge and memory monitoring in adulthood. *Psychology and Aging, 9*, 287–302.

Bireta, T. J., Surprenant, A. M., & Neath, I. (2008). Age-related differences in the von Restorff isolation effect. *Quarterly Journal of Experimental Psychology, 61*, 345–352.

Bouazzaoui, B., Follenfant, A., Ric, F., Fay, S., Croizet, J. C., Atzeni, T., & Taconnat, L. (2016). Ageing-related stereotypes in memory: When the beliefs come true. *Memory, 24*(5), 659–668.

Brandt, J., & Rich, J. B. (1995). Memory disorders in the dementias. In A. D. Baddeley, B. A. Wilson, & F. N. Watts (Eds.), *Handbook of Memory Disorders* (pp. 243–270): Chichester, UK: Wiley.

Brown, R. G., & Marsden, C. D. (1988). Internal versus external cues and the control of attention in Parkinson's disease. *Brain, 111*, 323–345.

Budson, A. E., & Gold, C. A. (2009). Flashbulb, personal, and event memories in clinical populations. In O. Luminet & A. Curci (Eds.), *Flashbulb Memories: New Issues and New Perspectives* (pp. 141–162). New York: Psychology Press.

Burke, D. M., White, H., & Diaz, D. L. (1987). Semantic priming in young and older adults: Evidence for age constancy in automatic and attentional processes. *Journal of Experimental Psychology: Human Perception and Performance, 13*, 79–88.

Butler, K. M., McDaniel, M. A., Dornberg, C. C., Price, A. L., & Roediger, H. L. (2004). Age differences in veridical and false recall are not inevitable: The role of frontal lobe function. *Psychonomic Bulletin & Review, 11*, 921–925.

Campbell, K. L., Hasher, L., & Thomas, R. C. (2010). Hyper-binding: A unique age effect. *Psychological Science, 21*(3), 399–405.

Canavan, A. G. M., Passingham, R. E., Marsden, C. D., Quinn, N., Wyke, M., & Polkey, C. E. (1989). The performance on learning tasks of patients in the early stages of Parkinson's disease. *Neuropsychologia, 27*, 141–156.

Castel, A. D., Farb, N. A. S., & Craik, F. I. M. (2007). Memory for general and specific value information in younger and older adults: Measuring the limits of strategic control. *Memory & Cognition, 35*, 689–700.

Chan, J. C. K., & McDermott, K. B. (2007). The effects of frontal lobe functioning and age on veridical and false recall. *Psychonomic Bulletin & Review, 14*, 606–611.

Charles, S. T., Mather, M., & Carstensen, L. L. (2003). Aging and emotional memory: The forgettable nature of negative images for older adults. *Journal of Experimental Psychology: General, 132*, 310–324.

Chasteen, A. L., Bhattacharyya, S., Horhota, M., Tam, R., & Hasher, L. (2005). How feelings of stereotype threat influence older adults' memory performance. *Experimental Aging Research, 31*(3), 235–260.

Chasteen, A. L., Park, D. C., & Schwarz, N. (2001). Implementation intentions and facilitation of prospective memory. *Psychological Science, 12*, 457–461.

Chauvel, G., Maquestiaux, F., Hartley, A. A., Joubert, S., Didierjean, A., & Masters, R. S. W. (2012). Age effects shrink when motor learning is predominantly supported by nondeclarative, automatic memory processes: Evidence from golf putting. *Quarterly Journal of Experimental Psychology, 65*(1), 25–38.

Chua, E. F., Schacter, D. L., & Sperling, R. A. (2009). Neural basis for recognition confidence in younger and older adults. *Psychology and Aging, 24*, 139–153.

Colcombe, S. J., Kramer, A. F., Erickson, K. I., & Scalf, P. (2005). The implications of cortical recruitment and brain morphology for individual differences in inhibitory function in aging humans. *Psychology and Aging, 20*, 363–375.

Colloff, M. F., Wade, K. A., Wixted, J. T., & Maylor, E. A. (2017). A signal-detection analysis of eyewitness identification across the adult lifespan. *Psychology and Aging, 32*(3), 243–258.

Corkin, S. (1998). Functional MRI for studying episodic memory in aging and Alzheimer's disease. *Geriatrics, 53*, S13–S15.

Craik, F. I. M. (1986). A functional account of age differences in memory. In F. Lix & H. Hagendorf (Eds.), *Human Memory and Cognitive Capabilities, Mechanisms, and Performances* (pp. 409–422). Amsterdam: Elsevier.

Craik, F. I. M., & Byrd, M. (1982). Aging and cognitive deficits: The role of attentional resources. In F. I. M. Craik & S. Trehub (Eds.), *Aging and Cognitive Processes* (pp. 191–211). New York: Plenum Press.

Craik, F. I. M., Eftekhari, E., Bialystok, E., & Anderson, N. D. (2018). Individual differences in executive functions and retrieval efficacy in older adults. *Psychology and Aging, 33*(8), 1105–1114.

Daniels, K. A., Toth, J. P., & Hertzog, C. (2009). Aging and recollection in the accuracy of judgments of learning. *Psychology and Aging, 24,* 494–500.

de Langavant, L. C., , Fénelon, G., Benisty, S., Boissé, M. F., Jacquemot, C., & Bachoud-Lévi, A. C. (2013). Awareness of memory deficits in early stage Huntington's disease. *PloS One, 8*(4), e61676.

Dijkstra, K., & Kaup, B. (2005). Mechanisms of autobiographical memory retrieval in younger and older adults. *Memory & Cognition, 33,* 811–820.

Dodson, C. S., & Krueger, L. E. (2006). I misremember it well: Why older adults are unreliable eyewitnesses. *Psychonomic Bulletin & Review, 13,* 770–775.

Duchek, J. M. (1984). Encoding and retrieval differences between young and old: The impact of attentional capacity usage. *Developmental Psychology, 20*(6), 1173–1180.

Dunlosky, J. & Hertzog, C. (2000). Updating knowledge about encoding strategies: A componential analysis of learning about strategy effectiveness from task experience. *Psychology and Aging, 15,* 462–474.

Dywan, J., & Jacoby, L. L. (1990). Effects of aging on source monitoring: Differences in susceptibility to false fame. *Psychology and Aging, 5,* 379–387.

Dywan, J., Segalowitz, S. J., & Webster, L. (1998). Source monitoring: ERP evidence for greater reactivity to nontarget information in older adults. *Brain and Cognition, 36,* 390–430.

Einstein, G. O., & McDaniel, M. A. (1990). Normal aging and prospective memory. *Journal of Experimental Psychology: Learning, Memory, and Cognition, 16,* 717–726.

Einstein, G. O., McDaniel, M. A., Richardson, S. L., Guynn, M. J., & Cunfer, A. R. (1995). Aging and prospective memory: Examining influences of self-initiated retrieval processes. *Journal of Experimental Psychology: Learning, Memory, and Cognition, 21,* 996–1007.

Emery, L., & Hess, T. M. (2008). Viewing instructions impact emotional memory differently in older and younger adults. *Psychology and Aging, 23,* 2–12.

Ernst, A., Noblet, V., Denkova, E., Blanc, F., de Seze, J., Gounot, D., & Manning, L. (2015). Functional cerebral changes in multiple sclerosis patients during an autobiographical memory test. *Memory, 23*(8), 1123–1139.

Ferguson, S. A., Hashtroudi, S., & Johnson, M. K. (1992). Age differences in using source-related cues. *Psychology and Aging, 7,* 443–452.

Fleischman, D. A., Wilson, R. S., Gabrieli, J. D. E., Bienias, J. L., & Bennett, D. A. (2004). A longitudinal study of implicit and explicit memory in old persons. *Psychology and Aging, 19,* 617–625.

Ford, J. H., DiBiase, H. D., Ryu, E., & Kensinger, E. A. (2018). It gets better with time: Enhancement of age-related positivity effect in the six months following a highly negative public event. *Psychology and Aging, 33*(3), 419–424.

Fraundorf, S. H., Hourihan, K. L., Peters, R. A., & Benjamin, A. S. (2019). Aging and recognition memory: A meta-analysis. *Psychological bulletin, 145*(4), 339–371.

Frieske, D. A., & Park, D. C. (1999). Memory for news in young and old adults. *Psychology and Aging, 14,* 90–98.

Gallo, D. A., Cotel, S. C., Moore, C. D., & Schacter, D. L. (2007). Aging can spare recollection–based retrieval monitoring: The importance of event distinctiveness. *Psychology and Aging, 22,* 209–213.

Gallo, D. A., & Roediger, H. L. (2003). The effects of associations and aging on illusory recollection. *Memory & Cognition, 31,* 1036–1044.

Gardner, R. S., & Ascoli, G. A. (2015). The natural frequency of human prospective memory increases with age. *Psychology and Aging, 30*(2), 209–219.

Gaylord, S. A. & Marsh, G. R. (1975). Age differences in the speed of a spatial cognitive process. *Journal of Gerontology, 30*(6), 674–678.

Gerard, L., Zacks, R. T., Hasher, L., & Radvansky, G. A. (1991). Age deficits in retrieval: The fan effect. *Journal of Gerontology, 46*(4), P131–P136.

Godbout, L., & Doyon, J. (2000). Defective representation of knowledge in Parkinson's disease: Evidence from a script-production task. *Brain and Cognition, 44,* 490–510.

Gopie, N., Craik, F. I. M., & Hasher, L. (2010). Destination memory impairment in older people. *Psychology and Aging, 25*(4), 922–928.

Greene, J. D. W., & Hodges, J. R. (1996). The fractionation of remote memory: Evidence from a longitudinal study of dementia of Alzheimer type. *Brain, 119,* 129–142.

Groß, J., & Bayen, U. J. (2015). Adult age differences in hindsight bias: The role of recall ability. *Psychology and Aging, 30*(2), 253–258.

Groß, J., & Pachur, T. (2019). Age differences in hindsight bias: A meta-analysis. *Psychology and Aging, 34*(2), 294–319.

Grühn, D., Smith, J., & Baltes, P. B. (2005). No aging bias favoring memory for positive material: Evidence from a heterogeneity–homogeneity list paradigm using emotionally toned words. *Psychology and Aging, 20,* 579–588.

Hasher, L., & Zacks, R. T. (1989). Working memory, comprehension, and aging: A review and a new view. *Psychology of Learning and Motivation, 22,* 193–225.

Hashtroudi, S., Johnson, M. K., & Chrosniak, L. D. (1990). Aging and qualitative characteristics of memories for perceived and imagined complex events. *Psychology and Aging, 5,* 119–126.

Healey, M. K., Hasher, L., & Campbell, K. L. (2013). The role of suppression in resolving interference: Evidence for an age-related deficit. *Psychology and Aging, 28*(3), 721–728.

Henkel, L. A., & Rajaram, S. (2011). Collaborative remembering in older adults: Age-invariant outcomes in the context of episodic recall deficits. *Psychology and Aging, 26*(3), 532–545.

Henry, J. D., MacLeod, M. S., Philips, L. H., & Crawford, J. R. (2004). A meta-analytic review of prospective memory and aging. *Psychology and Aging, 19,* 27–39.

Hertzog, C., Kramer, A. F., Wilson, R. S., & Lindenberger, U. (2008). Enrichment effects on adult cognitive development: Can the functional capacity of older adults be preserved and enhanced? *Psychological Science, in the Public Interest, 9,* 1–65.

Hess, T. M. (2005). Memory and aging in context. *Psychological Bulletin, 131,* 383–406.

Hess, T. M., Auman, C., Colcombe, S. J., & Rahhal, T. A. (2003). The impact of stereotype threat on age differences in memory performance. *The Journals of Gerontology Series B: Psychological Sciences and Social Sciences, 58*(1), P3–P11.

Hess, T. M. & Bolstad, C. A. (1998). Category-based versus attribute-based processing in different-aged

adults. *Aging, Neuropsychology, and Cognition, 5,* 27–42.

Hess, T. M., Follett, K. J., & McGee, K. A. (1998). Aging and impression formation: The impact of processing skills and goals. *Journal of Gerontology: Psychological Sciences, 53B,* P175–P187.

Hodges, J. R. (2000). Memory in the dementias. In E. Tulving & F. I. M. Craik (Eds.) *The Oxford Handbook of Memory* (pp. 441–459). Oxford: Oxford University Press.

Howard, D. V., McAndrews, M. P., & Lasaga, M. I. (1981). Semantic priming of lexical decisions in young and old adults. *Journal of Gerontology, 36,* 707–714.

Hülür, G., Willis, S. L., Hertzog, C., Schaie, K. W., & Gerstorf, D. (2018). Is subjective memory specific for memory performance or general across cognitive domains? Findings from the Seattle Longitudinal Study. *Psychology and Aging, 33*(3), 448–460.

Iaria, G., Palermo, L., Committeri, G., & Barton, J. J. S. (2009). Age differences in the formation and use of cognitive maps. *Behavioural Brain Research, 196*(2), 187–191.

Jacoby, L. L., & Rhodes, M. G. (2006). False remembering in the aged. *Current Directions in Psychological Science, 15,* 49–53.

Janculjak, D., Mubrin, Z., Brinar, V., & Spilich, G. (2002). Changes of attention and memory in a group of patients with multiple sclerosis. *Clinical Neurology and Neurosurgery, 104,* 221–227.

Jessberger, S., & Gage, F. H. (2008). Stem-cell-associated structural and functional plasticity in the aging hippocampus. *Psychology and Aging, 23,* 684–691.

Johnson, M. K., & Hermann, A. M. (1995). Semantic relations and Alzheimer's disease: An early and disproportionate deficit in functional knowledge. *Journal of the International Neuropsychological Society, 1,* 568–574.

Jumentier, S., Barsics, C., & Van der Linden, M. (2018). Reduced specificity and enhanced subjective experience of future thinking in ageing: The influence of avoidance and emotion-regulation strategies. *Memory, 26*(1), 59–73.

Kahana, M. J., & Wingfield, A. (2000). A functional relation between learning and organization in free recall. *Psychonomic Bulletin & Review, 7,* 516–521.

Kavé, G., & Halamish, V. (2015). Doubly blessed: Older adults know more vocabulary and know better what they know. *Psychology and Aging, 30*(1), 68–73.

Knight, B. G., Maines, M. L., & Robinson, G. S. (2002). The effects of sad mood on memory in older adults: A test of the mood congruence effect. *Psychology and Aging, 17*, 653–661.

Koutstaal, W. (2006). Flexible remembering. *Psychonomic Bulletin & Review, 13*, 84–91.

Koutstaal, W., Reddy, C., Jackson, E. M., Prince, S., Cendan, D. L., & Schacter, D. L. (2003). False recognition of abstract versus common objects in older and younger adults: Testing the semantic categorization account. *Journal of Experimental Psychology: Learning, Memory, and Cognition, 29*, 499–510.

Kvavilashvili, L., Mirani, J., Schlagman, S., Erskine, J. A. K., & Kornbrot, D. E. (2010). Effects of age on phenomenology and consistency of flashbulb memories of September 11 and a staged control event. *Psychology and Aging, 25*(2), 391–404.

Lamichhane, B., McDaniel, M. A., Waldum, E. R., & Braver, T. S. (2018). Age-related changes in neural mechanisms of prospective memory. *Cognitive, Affective, & Behavioral Neuroscience, 18*(5), 982–999.

Lamont, R. A., Swift, H. J., & Abrams, D. (2015). A review and meta-analysis of age-based stereotype threat: Negative stereotypes, not facts, do the damage. *Psychology and Aging, 30*(1), 180–193.

LaVoie, D. J., & Malmstrom, T. (1998). False recognition effects in younger and older adults' memory for text passages. *Journals of Gerontology: Psychological Sciences, 53B*, P255–P262.

Levy, B. (1996). Improving memory in old age through implicit self-stereotyping. *Journal of Personality and Social Psychology, 71*, 1092–107.

Light, L. L., & Anderson, P. A. (1983). Memory for scripts in young and older adults. *Memory & Cognition, 11*, 435–444.

Light, L. L., & Capps, J. L. (1986). Comprehension of pronouns in young and older adults. *Developmental Psychology, 22*, 580–585.

Maclean, A. C., Bell, M. C., & Simone, P. M. (2017). Interference effects, age, and the spacing benefit. *American Journal of Psychology, 130*(3), 295–302.

MacPherson, S. E., Phillips, L. H., & Della Sala, S. (2002). Age, executive functioning, and social decision making: A dorsolateral prefrontal theory of cognitive aging. *Psychology and Aging, 17*, 598–609.

Mammarella, N., & Fairfield, B. (2006). The role of encoding in reality monitoring: A running memory test with Alzheimer's type dementia. *Quarterly Journal of Experimental Psychology, 59*, 1701–1708.

Marsh, E. J., Dolan, P. O., Balota, D. A., & Roediger, H. L. (2004). Part-set cuing effects in younger and older adults. *Psychology and Aging, 19*, 134–144.

Mather, M., & Johnson, M. K. (2000). Choice-supportive source monitoring: Do our decisions seem better to us as we age? *Psychology and Aging, 15*, 596–606.

May, C. P., Rahhal, T., Berry, E. M., & Leighton, E. A. (2005). Aging, source memory, and emotion. *Psychology and Aging, 20*, 571–578.

Maylor, E. A. (1993). Aging and forgetting in prospective and retrospective memory tasks. *Psychology and Aging, 8*, 420–428.

McCabe, D. P., Smith, A. D., & Parks, C. M. (2007). Inadvertent plagiarism in young and older adults: The role of working memory capacity in reducing memory errors. *Memory & Cognition, 35*, 231–241.

Memon, A., Hope, L., Bartlett, J., & Bull, R. (2002). Eyewitness recognition errors: The effects of mugshot viewing and choosing in young and old adults. *Memory & Cognition, 30*(8), 1219–1227.

Metcalfe, J., Casal-Roscum, L., Radin, A., & Friedman, D. (2015). On teaching old dogs new tricks. *Psychological Science, 26*(12), 1833–1842.

Mikels, J. A., Larkin, G. R., Reuter-Lorenz, P. A., & Carstensen, L. L. (2005). Divergent trajectories in the aging mind: Changes in working memory for affective versus visual information with age. *Psychology and Aging, 20*, 542–553.

Miles, J. R., & Stine-Morrow, E. A. L. (2004). Adult age differences in self-regulated learning from reading sentences. *Psychology and Aging, 19*, 626–636.

Montgomery, P., Siverstein, P., Wichmann, R., Fleischaker, K., & Andberg, M. (1993). Spatial updating in Parkinson's disease. *Brain and Cognition, 23*, 113–126.

Murphy, N. A., & Isaacowitz, D. M. (2008). Preferences for emotional information in older and younger adults: A meta-analysis of memory and attention tasks. *Psychology and Aging, 23*, 263–286.

Nicolas, S., & Worthen, J. B. (2009). Adult age differences in memory for distinctive information: Evidence from the bizarreness effect. *Quarterly Journal of Experimental Psychology, 62*, 1983–1990.

Nilsson, L. G., Adolfsson, R., Bäckman, L., de Frias, C. M., Molander, B., & Nyberg, L. (2004). Betula: A prospective cohort study on memory, health and aging. *Aging Neuropsychology and Cognition, 11*(2–3), 134–148.

Norman, K. A., & Schacter, D. L. (1997). False recognition in younger and older adults: Exploring the characteristics of illusory memories. *Memory & Cognition, 25*, 838–848.

Nosofsky, R. M., Denton, S. E., Zaki, S. R., Murphy-Knudsen, A. F., & Unverzagt, F. W. (2012). Studies of implicit prototype extraction in patients with mild cognitive impairment and early Alzheimer's disease. *Journal of Experimental Psychology: Learning, Memory, and Cognition, 38*(4), 860–880.

Park, D. C., Nisbett, R., & Heeden, T. (1999). Aging, culture, and cognition. *Journals of Gerontology: Psychological Sciences, 54B*, P75–P84.

Pelosi, L., Geesken, J. M., Holly, M., Hayward, M., & Blumhardt, L. D. (1997). Working memory impairment in early multiple sclerosis: Evidence from an event-related potential study of patients with clinically isolated myelopathy. *Brain, 120*, 2039–2058.

Pillon, B., Ertle, S., Deweer, B., Bonnet, A.-M. Vidailhet, M., & Dubois, B. (1997). Memory for spatial location in "de novo" parkinsonian patients. *Neuropschologia, 35*, 221–228.

Pirozzolo, F. J., Hansch, E. C., Mortimer, J. A., Webster, D. D., & Kuskowski, M. A. (1982). Dementia in Parkinson's disease: A neuropsychological analysis. *Brain and Cognition, 1*, 71–83.

Price, J., & Murray, R. G. (2012). The region of proximal learning heuristic and adult age differences in self-regulated learning. *Psychology and Aging, 27*(4), 1120–1129.

Prull, M. W., Dawes, L. L. C., McLeish M., A., Rosenberg, H. F., & Light, L. L. (2006). Recollection and familiarity in recognition memory: Adult age differences and neuropsychological test correlates. *Psychology and Aging, 21*, 107–118.

Radvansky, G. A. & Dijkstra, K. (2007) Aging and situation model processing. *Psychonomic Bulletin & Review, 14*, 1027–1042.

Radvansky, G. A., Gerard, L. D., Zacks, R. T., & Hasher, L. (1990). Younger and older adults' use of mental models as representations for text materials. *Psychology and Aging, 5*, 209–214.

Radvansky, G. A., Lynchard, N. N. A., & von Hippel, W. (2009). Aging and stereotype deactivation. *Aging, Neuropsychology and Cognition, 16*, 22–32.

Radvansky, G. A., Pettijohn, K. A., & Kim, J. (2015). Walking through doorways causes forgetting: Younger and older adults. *Psychology and Aging, 30*(2), 259–265.

Radvansky, G. A., Zwaan, R. A., Curiel, J. M., & Copeland, D. E. (2001). Situation models and aging. *Psychology and Aging, 16*, 145–160.

Rahhal, T. A., May, C. P., & Hasher, L. (2002). Truth and character: Sources that older adults can remember. *Psychological Science, 13*, 101–105.

Randolph, J. J., Arnett, P. A., & Higginson, C. I. (2001). Metamemory and tested cognitive functioning in multiple sclerosis. *Clinical Neuropsychologist, 15*, 357–368.

Reed, A. E., & Carstensen, L. L. (2012). The theory behind the age-related positivity effect. *Frontiers in Psychology, 3*: 339.

Reuter-Lorenz, P. A., & Cappell, K. A. (2008). Neurocognitive aging and the compensation hypothesis. *Current Directions in Psychological Science, 17*, 177–182.

Rey-Mermet, A., Gade, M., & Oberauer, K. (2018). Should we stop thinking about inhibition? Searching for individual and age differences in inhibition ability. *Journal of Experimental Psychology: Learning, Memory, and Cognition, 44*(4), 501–526.

Rhodes, S., Greene, N. R., & Naveh-Benjamin, M. (2019). Age-related differences in recall and recognition: A meta-analysis. *Psychonomic Bulletin & Review, 26*(5), 1529–1547.

Richmond, L. L., Sargent, J. Q., Flores, S., & Zacks, J. M. (2018). Age differences in spatial memory for mediated environments. *Psychology and Aging, 33*(6), 892–903.

Rönnlund, M., Nyberg, L., Bäckman, L., & Nilsson, L-G. (2005). Stability, growth, and decline in adult life span development of declarative memory: Cross-sectional and longitudinal data from a population-based study. *Psychology and aging, 20*(1), 3–18.

Rose, N. S., Rendell, P. G., McDaniel, M. A., Aberle, I., & Kliegel, M. (2010). Age and individual differences in prospective memory during a "Virtual Week": The roles of working memory, vigilance, task regularity, and cue focality. *Psychology and Aging, 25*(3), 595–605.

Rypma, B., Prabhakaran, V., Desmond, J. E., & Gabriei, D. E. (2001). Age differences in prefrontal cortical activity in working memory. *Psychology and Aging, 16,* 371–384.

Sadek, J. R., Johnson, S. A., White, D. A., Salmon, D. P., Taylor, K. I., DeLaPena, J. H., Paulsen, J. S., Heaton, R. K., & Grant, I. (2004). Retrograde amnesia in dementia: Comparison of HIV-associated dementia, Alzheimer's disease, and Huntington's disease. *Neuropsychology, 18,* 692–699.

Sagar, H. J., Cohen, N. J., Sullivan, E. V., Corkin, S., & Growdon, J. H. (1988). Remote memory function in Alzheimer's disease and Parkinson's disease. *Brain, 111,* 185–206.

Sahakyan, L., Delaney, P. F., & Goodmon, L. B. (2008). Oh, honey, I already forgot that: Strategic control of directed forgetting in older and younger adults. *Psychology and Aging, 23,* 621–633.

Salthouse, T. A. (1996). The processing-speed theory of adult age differences in cognition. *Psychological Review, 103*(3), 403–428.

Salthouse, T. A. (2016). Continuity of cognitive change across adulthood. *Psychonomic Bulletin & Review, 23*(3), 932–939.

Schlagman, S., Kliegel, M., Schulz, J., & Kvavilashvili, L. (2009). Differential effects of age on involuntary and voluntary autobiographical memory. *Psychology and Aging, 24,* 397–411.

Shimamura, A. P., Berry, J. M., Mangels, J. A., Rusting, C. L., & Jurica, P. J. (1995). Memory and cognitive abilities in university professors: Evidence for successful aging. *Psychological Science, 6*(5), 271–277.

Sicotte, N. L., Kern, K. C., Giesser, B. S., Arshanapalli, A., Schultz, A., Montag, M., Wang, H., & Bookheimer, S. Y. (2008). Regional hippocampal atrophy in multiple sclerosis. *Brain, 131*(4), 1134–1141.

Sitzman, D. M., Tauber, S. K., & Witherby, A. E. (2020). How do older adults maintain corrections in knowledge across a lengthy delay? *Psychology and Aging, 35*(1), 112–123.

Small, B. J., Dixon, R. A., Hultsch, D. F., & Hertzog, C. (1999). Longitudinal changes in quantitative and qualitative indicators of word and story recall in young-old and old-old adults. *Journal of Gerontology: Psychological Sciences, 54B,* P107–P115.

Small, G. W. (1998). The pathogenesis of Alzheimer's disease. *Journal of Clinical Psychiatry, 59,* 7–14.

Souchey, C., Isingrini, M., & Espagnet, L. (2000). Aging, episodic memory feeling-of-knowing, and frontal functioning. *Neuropsychology, 14,* 299–309.

Stewart, B. D., von Hippel, W., & Radvansky, G. A. (2009). Age, race, and implicit prejudice: Using process dissociation to separate the underlying components. *Psychological Science, 20,* 164–168.

Stillman, C. M., Coane, J. H., Profaci, C. P., Howard Jr, J. H., & Howard, D. V. (2014). The effects of healthy aging on the mnemonic benefit of survival processing. *Memory & Cognition, 42*(2), 175–185.

St. Jacques, P. L., Dolcos, F., & Cabeza, R. (2009). Effects of aging on functional connectivity of the amygdala for subsequent memory of negative pictures. *Psychological Science, 20,* 74–84.

Titz, C., & Verhaeghen, P. (2010). Aging and directed forgetting in episodic memory: A meta–analysis. *Psychology and Aging, 25*(2), 405–411.

Umanath, S., & Marsh, E. J. (2012). Aging and the memorial consequences of catching contradictions with prior knowledge. *Psychology and Aging, 27*(4), 1033–1038.

Umanath, S., & Marsh, E. J. (2014). Understanding how prior knowledge influences memory in older adults. *Perspectives on Psychological Science, 9*(4), 408–426.

Urry, H. L., & Gross, J. J. (2010). Emotion regulation in older age. *Current Directions in Psychological Science, 19*(6), 352–357.

West, R. L., Thorn, R. M., & Bagwell, D. K. (2003). Memory performance and beliefs as a function of goal setting and aging. *Psychology and Aging, 18,* 111–125.

White, K. G., & Ruske, A. C. (2002). Memory deficits in Alzheimer's disease: The encoding hypothesis and cholinergic function. *Psychonomic Bulletin & Review, 9,* 426–437.

White, K. K., & Abrams, L. (2002). Does priming specific syllables during tip-of-the-tongue states facilitate word retrieval in older adults? *Psychology and Aging, 17*, 226–235.

Williams, B. R., Hultsch, D. F., Strauss, E. H., Hunter, M. A., & Tannock, R. (2005). Inconsistency in reaction time across the life span. *Neuropsychology, 19*(1), 88–96.

Williams, J. M. G., Ellis, N. C., Tyers, C., Healy, H., Rose, G., & Macleod, A. K. (1996). The specificity of autobiographical memory and imageability of the future. *Memory & Cognition, 24*(1), 116–125.

Zacks, R. T., Hasher, L., & Li, K. Z. H. (2000). Human memory. In F. I. M. Craik and T. A. Salthouse (Eds.), *Handbook of Aging and Cognition* (2nd ed.). Mahwah, NJ: Erlbaum.

Zacks, R. T., Radvansky, G. A., & Hasher, L. (1996). Studies of directed forgetting in older adults. *Journal of Experimental Psychology: Learning, Memory, and Cognition, 22*, 143–156.

Zalla, T., Sirigu, A., Pillon, B., Dubois, B., Agid, Y., & Grafman, J. (2000). How patients with Parkinson's disease retrieve and manage cognitive event knowledge. *Cortex, 36*, 163–179.

Zellner, M., & Bäuml, K-H. (2006). Inhibitory deficits in older adults: List-method directed forgetting revisited. *Journal of Experimental Psychology: Learning, Memory, and Cognition, 32*, 290–300.

Zhao, B., Della Sala, S., & Gherri, E. (2019). Age-associated delay in mental rotation. *Psychology and Aging, 34*(4), 502–511.

CHAPTER 18

Formal Models of Memory

Verbal descriptions of memory are nice. They give us a feel for how it operates, but they can be vague. Worse, alone they may not distinguish among the different theories of memory. A more precise language is needed to capture the subtle flavors and nuances of memory, and that language is mathematics. By casting ideas in a mathematical language, thereby creating a **formal model**, we can look at finer qualities of memory that are not possible with verbal descriptions. This mathematical expression is often done using computer models. A formal model of memory forces us to be explicit about how things work. Our assumptions are laid bare. For verbal descriptions it is easy to fudge things and make assumptions without realizing it. Moreover, formal models allow for more accurate predictions. If psychology is to continue to succeed as a science, there should be a reasonable level of predictability to be able to predict what will happen on average. An example of a reasonable prediction is knowing that people remember more if they spread studying out over several short sessions rather than a single long one.

Formal models provide a degree of precision and accuracy that is not possible with verbal descriptions. Formal models play the important role of pointing out theoretical errors and allowing a range of researchers to test various aspects of a theory (Farrell & Lewandowsky, 2010). Hintzman (1990) stated the following:

> The common strategy of trying to reason backward from behavior to underlying process (analysis) has drawbacks that become painfully apparent to those who work with simulation models (synthesis). To have one's hunches about how a simple combination of processes will behave repeatedly dashed by one's own computer program is a humbling experience that no experimental psychologist should miss.
>
> (p. 111)

This chapter covers several formal models of memory. First, we look at two simple models of recognition and recall, and how a formal comparison of these has led to interesting and unexpected insights. Next, we cover four classes of theories: (1) network models of memory that emphasize associative structure; (2) global matching models that assume that memory is accessed as a whole, and that structure emerges from this process; (3) parallel distributed models that use the nervous system as their inspiration; and (4) dual process models that assume there are two fundamentally different types of memory processes.

Before turning to the models themselves, you should be aware that they rely heavily on quantitative descriptions. However, this chapter has relatively few formulas. The intent is to provide you with a general overview of how these models characterize memory while neither assuming a degree of mathematical sophistication nor the ability to apply that knowledge.

SIMPLE MODELS OF MEMORY

We first examine two relatively simple models of memory and then move on to more developed ideas. The first theory is the threshold model of recognition, followed by the generate–recognize model of recall.

Threshold Model

The first simple model of memory, the **threshold model** (Murdock, 1974), is the idea that there is a threshold of activation that a memory trace must exceed for it to be identified as "old" (or recognized). Moreover, according to some versions, such as the two-high-threshold model (Snodgrass & Corwin, 1988), there may also be some threshold below which information is clearly identified as "new." Memories that fall between these two thresholds are ambiguous, and so people may make a guess as to what response to make. This is shown in Figure 18.1.

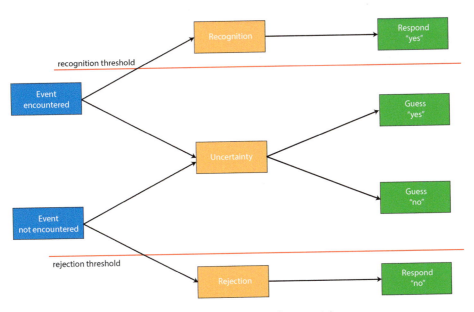

FIGURE 18.1 *Illustration of the Threshold Model of Recognition*

These thresholds are subjective levels that people use (consciously or unconsciously) to evaluate whether items are old. Now, not all memories that people consider old have been encountered before. Some are new, but for some reason, people recognize them as old. These incorrect responses are essentially guesses. Thus, we must account for how much guessing is going on to better evaluate memory. For example, if people answer "yes" to all of the old items on a test, but never say "yes" to a new item, then we can conclude that memory is very good. However, if people answer "yes" to all of the old items, but also always answer "yes" to all the new items, this is a much less impressive feat. As you can see, we need to correct for guessing.

To **correct for guessing** the threshold model uses the probability of correctly recognizing, as well as the probability of incorrectly identifying something as old (a guess). Here p is the probability of correct recognition, and g is the probability of guessing correctly. The "|" sign stands for "given that." Given this, the probability of giving a correct "yes" response can be written as:

$$P (\text{"yes"} \mid \text{old item}) = p + (1 - p)g$$

Using this formula and logic, the terms can be rearranged to gain an estimate of the likelihood that people are recognizing rather than guessing.

$$p = \frac{P(\text{"yes"} \mid \text{old item}) - P(\text{"yes"} \mid \text{new item})}{1 - P(\text{"yes"} \mid \text{new item})}$$

There are other versions of the threshold model (e.g., Starns & Ma, 2018). One example of a different version is whether the retrieval process used during recognition is discrete or continuous. For a discrete process model, the assumption is that features are retrieved from memory in an all-or-none manner. The two-high threshold model is a discrete process model.

In comparison, for continuous process models, the assumption is that information is retrieved along a continuum, such as memory strength. Examples of continuous process models are theories based on **signal detection theory** (see Chapter 3). As a reminder, when a memory of an old item exceeds the threshold, we correctly recognize it. This is a **hit**. When an old item's activation level fails to reach the threshold, it is rejected. This is a **miss**. When a new item is rejected because the memory does not exceed the threshold (because it is new), this is a **correct rejection**. Finally, if a new item has a representation in memory that exceeds the threshold, we inappropriately identify it as old. This is a **false alarm**. Signal detection approaches also play a role in the global matching models discussed later in the chapter.

While most formal models of memory assume that retrieval involves continuous processes, there is some evidence that both types of processes may be used but under different circumstances (McAdoo et al., 2018).

Memory researchers, as with other disciplines, borrow tools from other sciences to help them solve problems. One example of this is signal detection theory. There are also models of memory that use mathematical principles of quantum probability theory (Trueblood & Hemmer, 2017) from the field of particle physics. Thus, there are many ways to capture what memory is doing, and the inspiration for these may sometimes come from surprising sources.

Generate–Recognize Model

Another simple model is the **generate–recognize model** of recall (Bahrick, 1970; Kintsch, 1970). This model assumes that recall, particularly free recall, is a two-stage process. Recall is not just recognition with a higher threshold. Instead, recall involves a search of memory, whereas recognition simply involves people indicating whether items are familiar. Still, it would be nice if the retrieval involved in recall were not completely different from recognition. The generate–recognize model tries to accomplish both of these aims.

The first stage of the model is a generate component, which is unique to recall. During this phase people take the available retrieval cues to generate a set of memory traces whose contents can be reported. This is done by activating information in memory that is associated with the cues, followed by the information that is associated with that, and so on. For example, if you remember that some of the items on your grocery list were in the dairy section, this will help activate your memory for butter, which may then remind you that you also need to get some bread. This information is cross-referenced to generate a set of possible responses. In the second stage, people apply the standard recognition processes to the information that was generated in the first stage. For example, you may retrieve bread as something to buy at the grocery store but then realize that this is not something that you need to get on this trip.

The generate–recognition model, although relatively simple, makes clear predictions about how retrieval operates, and this relatively simple model of memory continues to be used to explain memory (e.g., category cued recall, Hunt et al., 2016). One prediction is that recall is harder than recognition because there are more steps involved. Another is that recall is more influenced by associations between concepts in memory. Finally, this model also predicts that everything that affects recognition also affects recall because recognition is a subprocess of recall.

Recognition Failure

As described in Chapter 3, recall and recognition are common ways to assess memory. The generate–recognition model is an explanation of how recall and recognition may be related to one another. This section provides a quantitative comparison of this relationship. In some ways recall and recognition are similar—for example, they are both direct memory measures—but there are differences, such as the degree to which they are influenced by the organization of information during learning. Suppose people learn lists of words that are either grouped by categories (organized) or are presented randomly (unorganized). In general, the organized list is better recalled than the unorganized list. However, recognition is less affected (Kintsch, 1968).

However, there is a problem. In some studies, there are a few items that are recalled but not recognized. This is called **recognition failure**, and it is a problem for generate–recognize models. If the processes that operate during recognition also operate during recall, then anything that is recalled should be recognized. However, recognition failure regularly occurs. This consistency is shown in Figure 18.2. If everything that could be recognized was also recalled, then the data points should fall along the diagonal (with some random error), but this does not occur. Instead, there is a systematic deviation, with points falling above the diagonal, indicating recognition failure. A formal description of this is the **Tulving–Wiseman function** (Tulving & Wiseman, 1975). Here, Rn stands for recognition, and Rc stands for recall. (As a refresher, p stands for "probability that," and "|" stands for "given that.")

$$p(\text{Rn} \mid \text{Rc}) = p(\text{Rn}) + .5\,[p(\text{Rn}) - p(\text{Rn})^2]$$

The explanation for this function is that recall and recognition use different types of retrieval cues (Flexser & Tulving, 1975). Recall uses cues to prompt retrieval, whereas recognition uses the item itself. For example, whenever I need to make copies on my departmental copier, the machine asks for the last four digits of my phone number. Sometimes I find this hard to remember without first recalling the first three digits. I have my phone number stored in such a way that retrieving

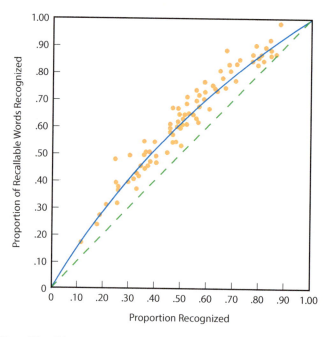

FIGURE 18.2 *Data Plot Illustrating Recognition Failure and the Tulving-Wiseman Function*

Source: Flexser, A. J., & Tulving, E. (1975). Retrieval independence in recognition and recall. *Psychological Review, 85*, 153–171

the last four digits is highly associated with the context of the first three. If I saw only the last four digits, it would not surprise me if I did not recognize it as part of my phone number. This differentially based retrieval that uses different memory cues, with some independence between recall and recognition, is at odds with the generate–recognize model and is brought to light only with a formal analysis of the data.

To address this issue with the generate–recognize model, there has been an appeal to the idea that recall and recognition have some overlapping processes. Jacoby and Hollingshead's (1990) modification was a generate–*sometimes* recognize model. Here, the recognition step is sometimes skipped if the generate process is rapid. When information is generated so easily, no recognition is needed. Thus, recognition failure could occur because this step is sometimes skipped, causing something to be recalled without being recognized.

STUDY IN DEPTH

Guynn et al. (2014) did a study that supports the generate–recognize model assuming that information that is generated is only *sometimes* recognized (Jacoby & Hollingshead, 1990). This was done using 72 students from the University of New Mexico. They investigated this issue by varying how people encoded information. We focus only on part of this rather complex study.

At learning, people encoded items by emphasizing either item-specific or relational information (see Chapter 7). For *item-specific* processing, people either read a series of words or did an anagram task of unscrambling the first two letters of words (e.g., "utrtle"). The anagram task places a greater emphasis on item-specific processing because people focus mental effort on individual words, and less on how the words may be related to one another. In comparison, for *relational* processing, people either simply wrote words down or sorted them into experimenter-provided categories (e.g., four-footed animals). Category sorting places emphasizes relational processing because items are related to the categories. After learning, all participants had a 3-minute distractor task of solving math problems.

To assess the generate–recognize model, they gave one of two memory tasks. One was a category production task. People were given category names (e.g., four-footed animals) and were told to generate as many members of that category as possible. This emphasizes the process of generation over recognition because people need to generate items from memory. There is no need for recognition because there is no need to compare what is generated with what was encountered before. Any influence of the prior learning is largely implicit. The second task was category-cued recall. People were given category names and were to use them to help remember any of the items that were encountered previously. This involves both generating information from memory, as well as a recognition process to assess whether the generated items were encountered before.

The pattern of performance, shown in Figure 18.3, is that item-specific processing (anagram solution) had a minor impact on the category generation, but had a greater impact on cued recall. Thus, item-specific encoding influenced recognition, but not generation. In comparison, relational learning (category sorting) influenced the generation

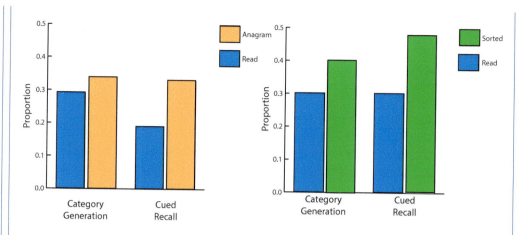

FIGURE 18.3 *Partial Plot of Data of Guynn, McDaniel, Strosser, Ramirez, Castleberry, and Arnett's (2014) Data Exploring the Viability of Modified Generate-Recognition Model of Recall*

Source: created from data reported in Guynn, M. J., McDaniel, M. A., Strosser, G. L., Ramirez, J. M., Castleberry, E. H., & Arnett, K. H. (2014). Relational and item-specific influences on generate–recognize processes in recall. *Memory & Cognition, 42*(2), 198–211

component because performance was different in both the generation and cued recall tasks. Moreover, while there was a difference between categorized and uncategorized items, there was no difference when the anagram task was done, suggesting that the generation component was unaffected by category sorting. Thus, generation and recognition processes could be separately affected and both are involved during recall.

Stop and Review

Simple models capture basic aspects of memory. For the threshold model, memories are retrieved when activation exceeds a threshold, similar to signal detection models. The generate–recognize model of recall incorporates all the essential characteristics of recognition into the retrieval process. As appealing as the generate–recognize model is for its simplicity, the recognition failure effect suggests caution. That said, a generate–sometimes–recognition model may overcome this.

NETWORK THEORIES

In Chapter 1 we saw that the work of Aristotle had a profound influence on memory theories through his ideas about associations. The influence of associations on memory is seen with priming, encoding specificity, and the structure of semantic memory. Some formal models have taken ideas of associative structure and used them as the fundamental basis for their theories of memory. A clear way to see this is with network models. Here, memory is captured by having large numbers of smaller units, often called **nodes**, joined together in a tangled web of associations by an even larger number of **links**.

Semantic Networks

The first major **network theory** of memory was by Collins and Quillian (1969; 1972) to capture semantic memory in the service of a computer program that would be able to use human language in a natural way (a goal that, while getting closer, is still far off). In **Collins and Quillian's network model**, the nodes were simple concepts, like *bird* or *canary*, and the links were of several types. Figure 18.4 shows a portion of a network, with property associations and categorical associations. For property associations, some concepts are properties of other concepts that they are associated with. For example, *feathers* is a property of *bird*, *yellow* is a property of *canary*, and so on. Other associations were superordinate category relations—for example, "A canary is a bird." In semantic networks, information is generally stored in one location in the network using a cognitive economy. That is, rather than expending effort endlessly replicating concepts, individual concepts can be instantiated in the network only a few times or even just once.

When people access a concept in memory, like *canary*, a search process begins with activation moving along all the links associated with that concept. This is **spreading activation**. A way to think about spreading activation is as electricity flowing through the wires of a circuit. Through spreading activation, if the concept *feathers* was also accessed, the links associated with it would be searched. When two search paths meet to create an intersection, people can verify that the concepts are associated and stored in memory. If the two searches do not form an intersection, because they are not connected in memory, then the information is not something that is known. For example, if you were asked whether a canary has feathers, the nodes for *canary* and *feathers* would be activated, and the activation would spread along the links associated with these nodes. These spreads of activation would meet,

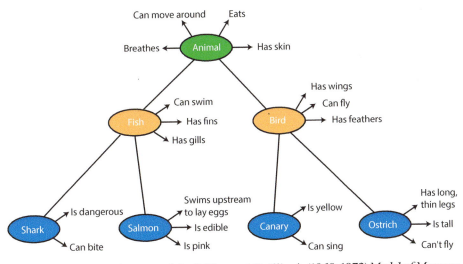

FIGURE 18.4 *Portion of a Network in Collins and Quillian's (1969, 1972) Model of Memory*

Source: adapted from Collins, A. M., & Quillian, M. R. (1969). Retrieval time from semantic memory. *Journal of Verbal Learning and Verbal Behavior, 8,* 240–247

and you could verify that the fact is known. However, if you were asked whether a canary has gills, the nodes for *canary* and *gills* would be activated, and the activation would spread along the links associated with these nodes. However, these spreads of activation would not meet, and you could verify that this is something not known.

A prediction of this model is that the speed with which information is retrieved is a function of the distance between two nodes in a network. For example, people should be faster to verify that "A canary is yellow" than "A canary has feathers." Although initial studies supported this idea (Collins & Quillian, 1969), subsequent work revealed problems. For example, if nodes are far from one another, it should take longer to verify those facts. However, some facts are verified more quickly than should be possible according to these models (Rips et al., 1973). For example, people verify that "A pig is an animal" faster than "A pig is a mammal," even though the opposite is predicted.

While Collins and Quillian's network was hierarchical, this was replaced with the idea that memory is structured in terms of degree of relatedness (Ashcraft, 1976; Collins & Loftus, 1975). Figure 18.5 illustrates this kind of memory network.

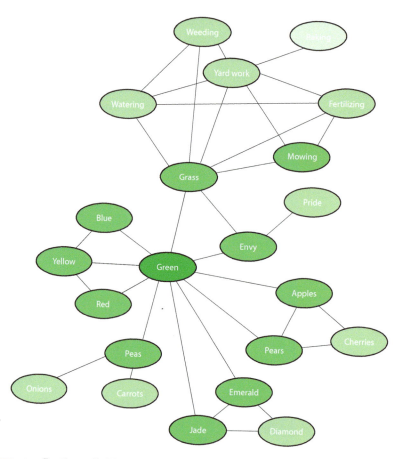

FIGURE 18.5 *Portion of a Network in Collins and Loftus's (1975) Model of Memory*

Source: adapted from Collins, A. M., & Loftus, E. F. (1975). A spreading activation theory of semantic processing. *Psychological Review, 82,* 407–428

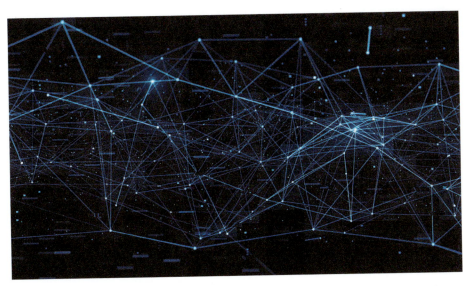

PHOTO 18.1 *For many people, it is easy to think of memory as being a network of inter-related and inter-connected ideas*

Source: arleksey/Shutterstock.com

For example, *green* is closely associated with colors because there are more links to other colors. However, *green* is less associated with *raking* because, in this network, there are not many links between the *green* and the *raking* nodes. Also, the relative strength of associations is captured by the length of the links connecting the concepts, with shorter links standing for stronger associations. For example, while *emerald* is associated with both *green* and *diamond*, it is more closely associated with *diamond* than *green*, because the association is stronger. The approach of trying to understand how semantic networks are structured continues to influence lines of research (Morais et al., 2013).

Network models provide straight-forward accounts of **priming**. As a reminder, when people encounter information, this not only activates those concepts but makes related concepts more available as well. For a network model, priming occurs because a concept is activated, and this activation spreads along the links to related concepts. Therefore, it is easier to shift your thinking to related ideas (because they are already primed) rather than do something completely different.

An attractive idea behind network theories of memory is that everything is defined in terms of everything else, much like a dictionary. However, this is also a major problem (Johnson-Laird et al., 1984), as there is no clear way to ground knowledge in the world, an issue that theories of embodied or grounded cognition seek to address.

ACT

Another network model of memory is the **ACT** (Adaptive Control of Thought) model (Anderson, 1990). Of all the models discussed here, this is the most comprehensive. For ACT, knowledge is stored in a **propositional network**. A proposition is a

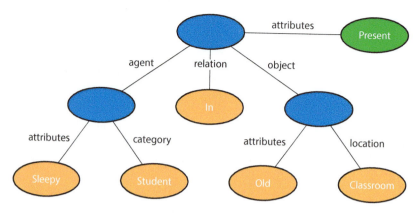

FIGURE 18.6 *ACT Model Propositional Network for the Sentence "The Sleepy Student Is in the Old Classroom"*

simple idea unit. In the memory network, a proposition is two nodes and a link. Information is retrieved through a process of spreading activation, as with other network models. An example of a propositional network for the sentence "The sleepy student is in the old classroom" is given in Figure 18.6. This sentence is made up of several propositions that are organized by the network.

One property of ACT is the distinction between type nodes and token nodes. **Type nodes** are general concepts, like those seen in the semantic networks. For example, a *bird* type node stands for birds in general. In addition, **token nodes** correspond to specific instances. For example, a *bird* token node would stand for a specific bird, such as "that robin over there."

The ACT model also has the idea that there is a limited amount of activation available. Not all associations with a concept in memory are searched equally well, simultaneously, and to a high degree. Instead, activation is a limited resource. The more associations with a concept, the more finely divided the activation becomes, and retrieval time is slowed down accordingly. This is ACT's explanation for the fan effect (see Chapter 8). The more facts people learn about a concept, the more associations that are linked to it. When they need to verify any one of those facts, the number of associations with that concept divides up the activation, and retrieval along any one of those pathways is slowed (Anderson, 1974).

Another characteristic of ACT is the distinction between production and declarative memory. The network of propositions is the declarative memory part of the model. The other part is **production memories**, which are the mental steps people go through to get from one state of knowing to another. Productions manipulate information and are executed when appropriate conditions in working memory match the relevance of the production. They are basically, "if ... then" statements in long-term memory. If a condition is present, then the information is manipulated in a specified way. For example, when you learned addition in your elementary school math class, you developed production memories for how to manipulate the number information as it was encountered in problems you were given.

TRY IT OUT

The aim of this Try It Out is for you to observe the fan effect, as predicted by the ACT model. For this task you first need a set of sentences for participants to memorize. The important thing when creating your list is to make the sentences relatively simple and for there to be two identifiable concepts in each sentence with which other sentences can potentially share associations. For example, you may have your participants memorize sentences about people in locations of the form "The *person* is in the *location*" such as "The banker is in the museum." For each sentence, there should be one to three associations with each concept. For example, there could be one to three locations that each person is in, and one to three people in each location. In Anderson's (1974) original experiment, he had 28 such study sentences. After you create your study sentences, you also want to create a set of foil sentences for the recognition test. These incorrect sentences should be recombinations of concepts from studied sentences. For example, if people memorized "The banker is in the museum" and "The architect is in the hotel," then the unstudied sentences could be "The banker is in the hotel" and "The architect is in the museum."

For this study you need at least 16 participants. At the beginning, have your participants memorize the sentences. Do this by presenting the sentences one at a time in a random order. Fix the amount of time people can see each sentence, such as seven seconds. After people go through the entire list, have them try to answer questions about the two types of concepts, such as "Where is the *person*?" and "Who is in the *location*?" If there is more than one answer for a question, then the person should have to recall all of them. If they get an answer wrong, tell them the correct answer. After going through all the test questions, have people go back and study again. Repeat this study–test procedure until a participant can answer all the test questions. At that point, they will have memorized the facts and are now ready for the recognition test.

For the recognition test, use the entire sets of studied and foil sentences. These should be presented one at a time. The task is to indicate whether each sentence was studied or not. Because people memorized the sentences, accuracy is going to be very high. You need to collect response times. Try to use a computer to do this. To get better data, repeat the number of times each studied and foil sentence is presented. Perhaps eight times each.

Average the response times for each fan level (number of associations) for the two concepts in the study sentences. What you should observe is that as the number of associations increases, there is an increase in response time. This illustrates the prediction of the ACT model that a greater number of associative links "fanning" off of a concept node divides the amount of spreading activation. The more finely this activation is divided, the longer it takes to build up and retrieve any one idea and the slower the response time.

Productions are initially slow and cumbersome to execute. However, they become more automatic and unconscious with practice. For example, when you solve a math problem—such as "574 × 63 = ?"—you invoke mental procedures to arrive at the correct answer. The more practice you have, the stronger the productions become, and the easier it is to solve the problems. At some point, your ability to solve such math problems is nearly automatic.

Production memories interact with the declarative memory through working memory. For ACT, working memory is that part of the declarative network that is currently active along with the productions that are operating on it. The addition of a production memory makes ACT a powerful tool. It allows for explanations of memory based not only on how information is structured but how people manipulate it and the consequences this has for long-term memory.

Latent Semantic Analysis (LSA)

The idea of relating concepts to one another, the essence of most network models of memory, has been incorporated into other theories, even if they are not strictly network models. One of these is **Latent Semantic Analysis**, or **LSA** (Landauer & Dumais, 1997). In LSA, many texts (nearly a million) are fed into the program. From that input, a high-dimensional space (over 300 dimensions) is created to evaluate the co-occurrences of words in the language. Meaning is determined by assessing which words occur in similar contexts. Thus, if two words are perfect synonyms of each other, they would occur in the same contexts, although they would rarely ever occur together (that would be redundant). Thus, values derived from LSA can be indices of how similar two concepts are in memory (Kintsch, 2014).

Knowledge is represented in LSA as the relations among concepts in the high-dimensional semantic space. In this way, the model "acquires" a large set of knowledge in a way that mimics human performance, without a programmer directly hardcoding the relations among concepts. This is the latent part of latent semantic analysis. These relations fall out of the high-dimensional structure. This model has been successfully applied to several tasks including grading essay exams (Steinhart, 2001), metaphor comprehension (Kintsch & Bowles, 2002), and problem solving (Quesada et al., 2001).

Stop and Review

Network theories of memory have been very influential. Semantic network models provided clear, testable predictions that were initially verified in studies with people. However, subsequent work discredited the hierarchical structure idea. Network models continue to develop. The concept of spreading activation pervades a lot of thinking about memory retrieval, especially in accounts of priming. The ACT model has a propositional network for storing information in long-term memory, along with a production memory for altering the contents of memory. Finally, LSA uses co-occurrences in a sophisticated way to automatically derive contextualized meanings.

GLOBAL MATCHING MODELS

For network models, knowledge is stored in a complex, highly organized, and highly integrated structure. Portions of the network become activated to meet the demands of the current task. In comparison, for **global matching models**, memories are accessed through processes that consider the entire set of traces available. Relation between different memories occurs at retrieval. That is, structure in memory emerges out of the process of retrieval rather than being a part of long-term storage, as with network models.

In these models information is either stored as separate memory records, in what are called **multiple trace models**, or as patterns of information imposed on a common framework, in what are called **distributed storage models**. In global matching theories, multiple memory traces are activated in parallel. What is retrieved is a function of (1) the familiarity of the memory probe, (2) the degree of overlap between the probe and the memory traces, and (3) the amount of activation of the memory traces related to the probe (Clark & Gronlund, 1996).

In general, global matching models have evolved out of signal detection theories of retrieval (see Chapter 3). The availability of memory traces is a function of their familiarity (discrimination), and successful retrieval involves activation reaching a given threshold (bias). Two multiple trace models, SAM and MINERVA 2, are considered here. We also examine two distributed storage models, TODAM and CHARM.

Search of Associative Memory (SAM)

One multiple trace model is the **Search of Associative Memory**, or **SAM** (Gillund & Shiffrin, 1984; Raaijmakers & Shiffrin, 1980; 1981), which arose out of the development of Atkinson and Shiffrin's modal model of memory (Malmberg et al., 2019). For SAM, memories are stored in traces that contain content, associative, and contextual information. Remembering occurs when a cue (something in the world or a thought) overlaps with features in a trace, causing it to become active and potentially be retrieved. Memory retrieval is probabilistic—that is, the probability that a given trace is remembered is a function of its relation to the memory probe and its strength relative to other traces. The greater the strength, the higher the probability of retrieval.

For example, if you are asked if you recently saw a blue bandana, all your memories involving "blue" and "bandana" would be activated. A memory of an actual blue bandana would match more than other memories with those features, and so would be most likely to be retrieved. Still, there is a probability, albeit small, that you might first retrieve a memory of a red bandana, before rejecting it, searching memory again, and retrieving the memory of the blue bandana.

The **recall** process for SAM is shown in Figure 18.7. Initially, people are given a recall cue, such as a question. To organize the information that needs to be recalled, even if it is a modestly complex set, people create a retrieval plan to keep track of the information. This retrieval plan generates a series of probe cues to access

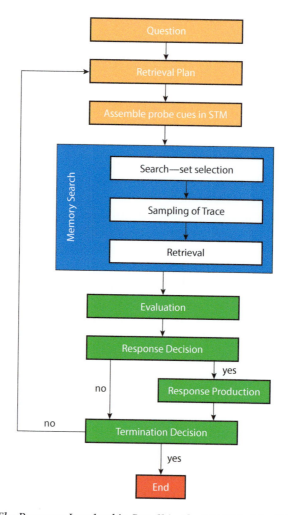

FIGURE 18.7 *The Processes Involved in Recall in the SAM Model of Memory*

Source: Raaijmakers, J. G. W., & Shiffrin, R. M. (1981). Search of associative memory. *Psychological Review,* *88*, 93–134

memory traces using a global matching process. During the memory search, the SAM model first restricts itself to a subset of traces that are more likely to be relevant. It then searches through them, starting with the stronger ones and moving to the weaker ones. This search process, which focuses on memory traces more resonant with the retrieval cues, closely resembles spatial foraging behavior in animals (Hills et al., 2012). In other words, a patch of memory is searched until the likelihood of retrieving a new memory trace is low, then the search moves on to another patch.

These memory traces are recovered into short-term memory, where they are evaluated and either reported (output) or not (similar to a generate–recognize model). Then people either continue to search memory for more information or quit. The decision of when to stop searching is guided by the probability of more retrieval attempts being successful (Dougherty et al., 2014). Thus, information is retrieved

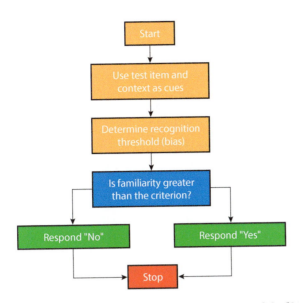

FIGURE 18.8 *Processes Involved in Recognition in the SAM Model of Memory*

Source: Gillund, G., & Shiffrin, R. M. (1984). A retrieval model for both recognition and recall. *Psychological Review, 91,* 1–67

through a sampling process that is influenced, but not completely determined, by how much memory traces are related to a retrieval cue. Traces that more closely match a cue are more likely to be retrieved and evaluated. If they are relevant, they are reported; otherwise, they are not.

In comparison, for **recognition**, whether an item is recognized is a function of the sum of all the traces related to a probe, as shown in Figure 18.8. Information in both the recognition probe and its context are used to sample memory. This makes contact with all of those traces that share those features with the probe and the context. Context information helps narrow down the set of traces, thereby making retrieval more accurate. If the familiarity value that is returned from this sampling process is above threshold, then people accept the information as old (it is recognized). Otherwise, it is classified as new (it is not recognized). Thus, something may be recognized because people have many weak memories, not just a single strong memory.

Thus, recognition extracts memories one at a time, starting with those that resonate most strongly with the retrieval cue. This includes both information in the cue itself, as well as the surrounding context. If this process produces a response that is strong enough, then people recognize the information as old. Otherwise, it is rejected as new.

MINERVA 2

Another multiple trace model is **MINERVA 2** (Hintzman, 1986) (MINERVA 1 did not last very long). This theory assumes that memory traces are strings of features. Each feature, either content or context information, is represented by a value indicating its presence or absence. For MINERVA 2, what is retrieved is not a single memory trace (as in SAM). Instead, what is returned is a new trace called an **echo**, which is a weighted composite of all the traces that were activated. We examine two characteristics of the echo in detail: echo intensity and echo content.

Echo intensity is the activation strength of the echo that is returned by retrieval. This is a function of the intensity of the traces that were tapped by retrieval (see Figure 18.9). This is analogous to the familiarity value returned in SAM. The greater the overlap between the cue and the echo, the greater the activation. Thus, if a memory probe activates memory traces with a high degree of overlap, then echo intensity is greater. For example, you have many memories of people speaking your name. Thus, if your name were a memory probe, the echo would have a high level of intensity because of the high degree of overlap. In contrast, you are likely to have very few to no memory traces about St. Ignatius High School football during the early 1980s. Although this information makes contact with some memories—such as those about football, high school, and history of the 1980s—there is likely little overlap with this memory probe as a whole, and the echo intensity is weak, thereby indicating that this information is not known. Echo intensity is also useful in determining event frequency (e.g., how often have you been to the grocery store in the past two weeks?). More high-intensity echoes reflect frequent occurrences, whereas low-intensity echoes reflect rare events (Hintzman, 1988).

The other aspect of an echo is **echo content** which is the weighted average of the contents of all the memory traces activated by a probe. Those memory traces with a greater overlap carry more weight and have a greater influence over echo content. Thus, what is returned during retrieval is a composite or blending of many traces. Thus, MINERVA 2 produces effects in memory such as the influence

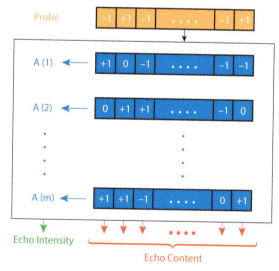

FIGURE 18.9 *Echo Intensity and Content in MINERVA 2*

Source: Hintzman, D. L. (1986). "Schema abstraction" in a multiple-trace memory model. *Psychological Review, 93,* 411–428

of schemas (Hintzman, 1986), without having to actually create and store schemas. This is because features of specific events get averaged out, and what is left are general abstract components. For example, if you are given the concept "grocery store," this activates all memories about grocery stores that you have in long-term memory. What you remember is a weighted average of all those grocery store experiences, with the individual contexts averaged out.

When people try to remember a single event, the precision of the memory cue is important. The more closely a memory trace corresponds to the cue, the larger a role it plays in the structure of the echo. But there is always some contribution of other overlapping traces, even if that contribution is weak. In this way, memory retrieval is always a distorting process. What is remembered is always a composite of several memories. To compound this distortion further, the echo that is returned is then stored as a new memory trace. Thus, MINERVA 2 captures the idea that memory is constantly changing because of experience, and even by the act of remembering.

Although the MINERVA 2 retrieval process is constantly distorting, this same process also helps it narrow in on a trace. By using the echo that was returned to help focus the memory search, thereby activating a smaller and smaller set of memory traces, people have more accurate retrieval compared to getting only the first returned, most averaged, memory trace. This process is shown in Figure 18.10.

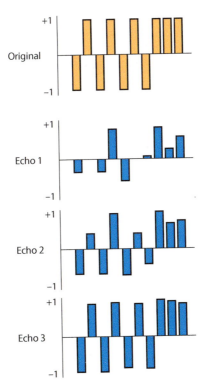

FIGURE 18.10 *Echo Improvement in MINERVA 2*

Source: Hintzman, D. L. (1986). "Schema abstraction" in a multiple-trace memory model. *Psychological Review, 93*, 411–428

Initially, the composition of the echo only remotely resembles what is being searched for. However, over time, by using the echoes that were generated as part of the memory search process, the correspondence gets better and better.

Further Work

Work continues on models of memory. For example, **REM**, for **Retrieving Effectively from Memory** (Shiffrin & Steyvers, 1997), combines properties of SAM and MINERVA 2, as well as other sources, to provide a wider-ranging, more effective account of memory. Like SAM, REM assumes that information is stored in multiple memory traces and that memory is searched in a trace-by-trace, probabilistic fashion. Moreover, information is represented as a vector of features, like MINERVA 2. In addition, unlike other models, REM assumes that there is a probability of an error in the information stored in a memory trace. Work on the REM model has further inspired work on another model, **SARKAE**, for **Storing And Retrieving Knowledge And Events**, that pushes these ideas further as a model of memory that can account for both specific knowledge of individual events or experiences and more general knowledge that transcends the idiosyncrasies of singular experiences (Nelson & Shiffrin, 2013).

A feature that all these models have in common is that they are exclusively activation models. That is, memory retrieval occurs only using the activation of memory traces. When a memory trace is no longer being actively processed, its activation decays to some baseline level. However, as you have read in other chapters, memory retrieval also involves the active inhibition of strong but inappropriate memory traces. The introduction of inhibitory processes in these sorts of models is rare, but it has been done, as with the **Hydrogen model** (Radvansky & Tamplin, 2013).

TODAM and CHARM

Formal models like SAM and MINERVA 2 are multiple trace models that store each experience separately in memory. Any blending of information occurs during retrieval. Now we consider two global matching models that involve distributed storage. This is sensible if one thinks about how the brain stores information. It is not a system where each experience is stored at a separate place in the cortex. Instead, many different memories are imposed on the same neural structure, and the information is distributed throughout this structure.

Two of these models are **TODAM**, for **Theory of Distributed Associative Memory** (Murdock, 1982a; 1982b; 1993), and **CHARM** for **Composite Holographic Associative Retrieval Model** (Eich, 1982; 1985). These models developed out of a verbal learning tradition to account for memory for item and associative information, as well as serial order information, with an emphasis on memory for paired associates.

These models assume that information is represented as vectors of features, with a different memory trace for each item. What is important is that associative

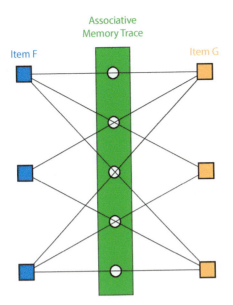

FIGURE 18.11 *Process of Convolution in Models like TODAM and CHARM*

Source: Eich, J. M. (1982). A composite holographic associative recall model. *Psychological Review, 89,* 627–661

information is stored as a convolution of the two item memory vectors. So, what is a convolution? A convolution process is illustrated in Figure 18.11. Each item vector is combined with every element of the vector of another memory trace to create the composite vector trace. Thus, information from both items is distributed across a shared set of memory elements. This is an efficient way of encoding information about items and associations, using relatively few resources. Because of the regular structure of these convoluted vectors, the original traces can be extracted using a correlation process. The properties of the convoluted vector are correlated with the values of a memory probe, allowing for the extraction of the previous information.

One metaphor that has been used to describe these models is that of ripples on a pond (Murdock, 1982a). Different objects, such as a textbook, a computer, or a roommate, make different types of waves when thrown in the water. If several objects are thrown in the pond, all the waves are superimposed on the same surface. With enough sophistication, one could examine the wave patterns to determine what objects were thrown in and where.

Stop and Review

Global matching models do not make strong assumptions about how information is organized. Instead, organization is a result of the retrieval process. The SAM model is based on a probabilistic access of traces as a function of the match with the retrieval cue. Other models, such as MINERVA 2, account for how memory is changed by the act of remembering. More recent models include REM and SARKAE which combine elements from different models. Other global matching models, such as

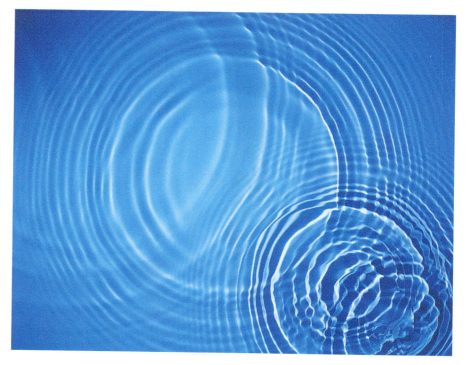

PHOTO 18.2 *Distributed storage global matching models of memory such as TODAM and CHARM assume that memories are laid out on the same structure, much like ripples overlay one another on water*

Source: luckypic/Shutterstock.com

CHARM and TODAM, explore how multiple traces can be superimposed on a limited representational structure, as would be expected with the neurons of the brain.

PARALLEL DISTRIBUTED PROCESSING (PDP) MODELS

An important idea in TODAM and CHARM is that memory traces are overlaid on shared collections of units. The brain is only so big, and the same neurons contribute to representing multiple memories. This idea has been elaborated on a grand scale for **parallel distributed processing**, or **PDP**, models (McClelland & Rumelhart, 1986; Rumelhart & McClelland, 1986).

PDP models store information in a single structure, with multiple memories superimposed on one another in a common representational framework. This is done as a network of nodes and links like a semantic network. However, rather than a node being connected to those concepts that are associated with it, in a PDP model each node is massively interconnected with a very large number of other nodes. In many cases, memories are distributed across several shared components. In these models, individual nodes do not represent concepts. Instead, in a PDP model, it is the pattern of activation that produces the representation, learning, and memory.

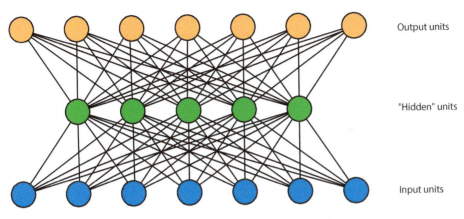

Output units

"Hidden" units

Input units

FIGURE 18.12 *Sample Parallel Distributed Processing Network*

The most prevalent types of PDP models are what are called **connectionist models** or **neural networks**. These theories use the structure of the nervous system as their inspiration. The brain is, in a real sense, a distributed representation. Information is not stored in individual neurons. Instead, it is captured by the pattern of neural firing over large sets of neurons. Thus, any given neuron participates in the representation of many different memories, along with what other neurons are doing. Connectionist models are not only found in psychology, but also in computer science, biology, and so on, because this is such a powerful means of representing and processing information. In computer science, this approach has been worked up to a high degree in what are known as *deep networks*.

A simple connectionist network is shown in Figure 18.12. First, as you can see, there are the nodes and links. The model is a collection of "units" interconnected to other units (and potentially to themselves as well). The units in these models could correspond to neurons, and the links to axonal connections with other neurons. These nodes are massively interconnected with each other, forming layers of nodes, like the layers of cells in the brain. Information is represented as a pattern of activation in the nodes of the network. These patterns are established by shifting the weights of the connections among the various nodes. Thus, learning is a shift in connection strengths, to allow new patterns to emerge.

Units are divided into "layers," consistent with the fact that brain cells are often grouped into layers along paths of information processing. A simple connectionist model contains three layers: an input layer, an output layer, and a "hidden" layer, whose presence allows for great flexibility in adjusting to experience. In deep networks, there are a very large number of hidden layers.

Learning

Information is represented in these models in the "strength" of the connections between the units. These strengths are called connection *weights*. Some connections are excitatory and some are inhibitory. This is like changing the strength of connections between neurons. A model is operating well when the pattern of activity at the output stages bears a stable and consistent relationship to the pattern at the input stage.

The shifting of connection weights during learning is a gradual process. Every experience alters the connections in some way. Some become stronger, whereas the others become weaker or not affected at all. Over time, differences in the representation of different types of knowledge can emerge. Figure 18.13 shows shifts in the activation levels of several output nodes in a network that has been trained on several concepts. The more training there has been, the more differentiated the representations. Notice that concepts that have similar meanings are represented by similar patterns of activation. Thus, a connectionist model can capture memory characteristics such as semantic similarity.

The ability of PDP networks to alter themselves rather fluidly is one of their biggest assets. It is also one of their biggest deficits. Specially, if a model is trained on a particular set of items, it will learn those readily. However, if the model is then trained up on a new set of items, without continued training on the old items, it will exhibit **catastrophic forgetting**. That is, the new pattern of weights will over-write

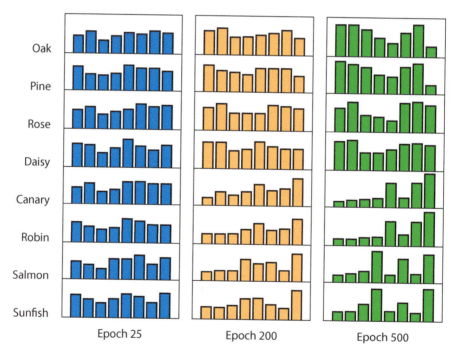

FIGURE 18.13 *Representational Improvement across Various Epochs (Training Cycles) in a Parallel Distributed Processing Model. The Height of the Bars Corresponds to the Activation Level of a Set of Output Nodes for Each of the Concepts*

Source: McClelland, J. L., McNaughton, B. L., & O'Reilly, R. C. (1995). Why there are complementary learning systems in the hippocampus and neocortex: Insights from the successes and failures of connectionist models of learning and memory. *Psychological Review, 102*(3), 419–457

and destroy the old ones, causing the network to lose its prior knowledge (McCloskey & Cohen, 1989). While this has been used to explain some of the limits on working memory capacity (Endress & Szabó, 2020), this process is in contrast to human forgetting in long-term memory that shows much more gradual rates of forgetting. Thus, PDP models need to allow for the long-term retention of knowledge along with flexible encoding of new information. This may be done by having both slow and fast networks that work in tandem.

Retrieval

After a memory is established in a PDP network, at some point it may be necessary to retrieve it. Norman et al. (2007) reported a PDP model that simulated the retrieval inhibition observed in a retrieval practice paradigm (see Chapter 8). This is a complex model in which there are separate networks for hippocampal (episodic) and cortical (semantic) memory systems with (direct or indirect) recurrent connections among network elements for learning and which uses oscillating patterns of activity (akin to the cortical synchronization of theta waves). Using this model, Norman et al. simulated the pattern of results found with humans.

Stop and Review

PDP models are advanced and complex models. The way they process information is inspired by the organization and processing of neurons in the brain. Information is encoded in a complex of massively interconnected units by changing the pattern of weights between them. In PDP models, there is a great deal of flexibility because any given unit does not stand for anything. Information is represented and processed in a distributed fashion across the entire network. While this is a promising way to model memory, PDP models cannot depend exclusively on distributed representation but often need a symbolic or "localist" representation to be meaningful (Bowers, 2017).

Dual Process Theories

One characteristic of the models we have covered so far is that retrieval is a single process, possibly involving some version of a signal detection theory. However, other theories take the view that retrieval involves **dual processes**. One is a **familiarity** process that uses a signal detection-like process in which information is identified as old (remembered) when it exceeds a threshold (like most formal models of memory). The other is a **recollection** process that involves the conscious retrieval of components that are associated with the to-be-retrieved information (Mandler, 2008; Yonelinas, 2002). During recognition, familiarity may use continuous processes (values of memory strength), whereas recollection may use discrete processes (an experience is recollected or not) (Yonelinas, 1994). Both typically work together, but we sometimes find ourselves in situations where one process produces one result and the other produces another (but see Donaldson 1996; Rotello & McMillan, 2006). For example, suppose you meet someone who seems familiar, but you cannot remember his or her name or how you know him or her. This is remembering with familiarity but not recollection.

Atkinson and Juola

One of the earliest dual process models was Atkinson and Juola's (1973; 1974) model. For this view, people first try a fast familiarity process to see if information is recognized. If this initial process fails, then a more deliberate and effortful search is made of long-term memory. This more effortful search produces a richer set of knowledge that is associated with recollection. Thus, in this model, recollection is conditional on familiarity failure.

More Recent Views

Subsequent dual process theories assume that recollection and familiarity operate concurrently (Mandler, 1980). Because familiarity uses less information, it often finishes before recollection. Moreover, familiarity is more unconscious and automatic, whereas recollection is more conscious and effortful (Jacoby, 1991). Familiarity provides more quantitative information about the strength of the memory trace(s). In comparison, recollection provides more qualitative features associated with the information (e.g., who? what? where? when? why?) (Yonelinas, 2002). It has also been the suggested that there may be three processes available for memory retrieval, namely familiarity, recollection, and reconstruction (Brainerd et al., 2009).

Improve Your Memory

The primary purpose of constructing formal models of memory is to allow memory researchers to better predict how memory will do under various conditions. This is because our intuitions and mental reasoning can often be wrong. The same is true for your own assessment of how your memory works and when it will and will not be effective. Additionally, formal models give an idea about what you can do to improve your memory. Specifically, when you are trying to learn some new information for a class, your job, or some other aspect of your life, try to keep track of your time and how much you are learning. Tally how much you can remember later. Then, over time, plot your performance and look to see how you have done. Having a more solid base on which to understand your own performance, rather than relying exclusively on your intuition, should help you more effectively budget your time so that you come out ahead when it is time to demonstrate or use the knowledge.

One Process or Two?

One of the rules of thumb in science is, when all else is equal, accept the simplest solution. This principle is **Occam's razor**. The idea is to trim out all the irrelevant stuff. If this is the case, then why have a dual process theory of memory if a single process model will do just fine? One reason is that recollection and familiarity seem to involve double dissociation. That is, there are things that affect one process more than the other, and vice versa. For example, recollection is more influenced than familiarity by (1) different levels of processing, (2) generation effects, and (3) full versus divided attention during learning or retrieval. In contrast, familiarity is more affected than recollection by (1) changes in modality (e.g., first hearing something (auditory) and then later reading it (visual)), (2) perceptual priming, (3) changing response bias (i.e., being more liberal or conservative), (4) familiarity information being forgotten more rapidly (Yonelinas, 2002), and (5) the influence of novelty (Kishiyama & Yonelinas, 2003).

Moreover, familiarity and recollection involve different neurological structures. Familiarity depends more on the temporal cortex surrounding the hippocampus and on the operation of the cortex as a whole. Thus, brain damage typically has a smaller effect on familiarity than on recollection. In contrast, recollection depends more on the hippocampus and the frontal lobes. The influence of the hippocampus is seen in amnesics with hippocampal damage. The influence of the frontal lobes on recollection is also seen in older adults who have age-related changes in frontal lobe functioning. Similar results are observed in people with sustained frontal lobe damage (Yonelinas, 2002). Given this, a theory that includes both processes is needed.

Stop and Review

It is possible that memory retrieval involves dual processes, as suggested by Atkinson and Juola. This typically involves a simpler, automatic, familiarity-based process and a more complex, deliberative, conscious recollection-based process. Evidence for dual process theories comes from work showing double dissociations.

PUTTING IT ALL TOGETHER

To best understand memory, we should be able to make reasonable predictions about how it works under different conditions. This is best done using formal models of memory. Some models assume that memory retrieval involves a single process. This includes the threshold model, which is a simple model of memory. It also includes semantic network models that describe the structure of memory using associative relations among concepts and the spread of activation among them. Latent Semantic Analysis is another example, which, in this case, uses large amounts of input data with a large number of dimensions. Single process models also include multiple trace models (SAM and MINERVA 2), distributed storage models (TODAM and CHARM) that assume that memories are activated in a global matching process. Finally, there are PDP models that use the structure of the nervous system for inspiration. Other models involve a complex of multiple processes, as with the generate–recognize model, the ACT model with its propositional network and production memory, and dual process models of memory that assume that there are at least two memory processes operating during retrieval: a familiarity component and a recollection component. Whatever the approach that is taken, the overarching goal is to bring a greater degree of understanding and predictability to our understanding of what goes right and wrong with human memory.

STUDY QUESTIONS

1. What are two simple models of recognition and recall? What evidence is there to suggest that such basic ideas may be in error?
2. How is signal detection theory related to threshold models of memory?
3. What were some of the first network models of memory, and how did they structure information?
4. By what processes are memories retrieved from or activated in a network model of memory?
5. In what ways is LSA like and different from more traditional network models of memory?
6. What are the primary characteristics of global matching models of memory?
7. What are some of the ways that information is thought to be stored and retrieved in global matching models?
8. What is the difference between multiple trace and distributed representation models of global matching models of memory?
9. What are some of the major features of PDP models of memory?
10. What are the two types of processes that are operating in dual process models? What evidence supports this idea?

KEY TERMS

- ACT
- catastrophic forgetting
- CHARM
- Collins and Quillian's network model
- connectionist models
- correct for guessing
- correct rejection
- distributed storage models
- dual processes
- echo
- echo content
- echo intensity
- false alarm
- familiarity
- formal model
- generate–recognize model
- global matching models
- hit
- Hydrogen model
- links
- LSA
- MINERVA 2
- miss
- multiple trace models
- network theory
- neural networks
- nodes
- Occam's razor
- PDP

- priming
- production memories
- propositional network
- recall
- recognition failure
- recollection

- REM
- SAM
- SARKAE
- signal detection theory
- spreading activation
- threshold model

- TODAM
- token nodes
- Tulving–Wiseman function
- type nodes

EXPLORE MORE

Here are some additional readings to allow you to explore issues more deeply concerning formal models of memory.

Anderson, J. R. (1990). *The Adaptive Character of Thought*. New York: Psychology Press.

Hintzman, D. L. (1986). "Schema abstraction" in a multiple-trace memory model. *Psychological Review*, *93*, 411–428.

Kanerva, P. (1988). *Sparse Distributed Memory*. Cambridge, MA: MIT press.

Mandler, G. (2008). Familiarity breeds attempts: A critical review of dual-process theories of recognition. *Perspectives on Psychological Science*, *3*, 390–399.

McClelland, J. L., & Rumelhart, D. E. (1986). *Parallel Distributed Processing, Vol. 2: Psychological and Biological Models*. Cambridge, MA: MIT press.

Raaijmakers, J. G. W., & Shiffrin, R. M. (1980). SAM: A theory of probabilistic search of associative memory. *The Psychology of Learning and Motivation*, *14*, 207–262.

Rumelhart, D. E., & McClelland, J. L. (1986). *Parallel Distributed Processing, Vol. 1: Foundations*. Cambridge, MA: MIT press.

Yonelinas, A. P. (2002). The nature of recollection and familiarity: A review of 30 years of research. *Journal of Memory and Language*, *46*, 441–517.

REFERENCES

Anderson, J. R. (1974). Retrieval of propositional information from long-term memory. *Cognitive Psychology*, *6*, 451–474.

Anderson, J. R. (1990). *The Adaptive Character of Thought*. New York: Psychology Press.

Ashcraft, M. H. (1976). Priming and property dominance effects in semantic memory. *Memory & Cognition*, *4*, 490–500.

Atkinson, R. C., & Juola, J. F. (1973). Factors influencing speed and accuracy of word recognition. *Attention and Performance*, *6*, 583–612.

Atkinson, R. C., & Juola, J. F. (1974). Search and decision processes in recognition memory. In D. H. Krantz, R. C. Atkinson, R. D. Luce, & P. Suppes (Eds.), *Contemporary Developments in Mathematical Psychology* (pp. 243–293). San Francisco, CA: Freeman.

Bahrick, H. P. (1970). Two-phase model for prompted recall. *Psychological Review*, *77*, 215–222.

Bowers, J. S. (2017). Parallel distributed processing theory in the age of deep networks. *Trends in Cognitive Sciences*, *21*(12), 950–961.

Brainerd, C. J., Reyna, V. F., & Howe, M. L. (2009). Trichotomous processes in early memory development, aging, and neurocognitive impairment: A unified theory. *Psychological Review*, *116*, 783–832.

Clark, S. E., & Gronlund, S. D. (1996). Global matching models of recognition memory: How the models match the data. *Psychonomic Bulletin & Review, 3,* 37–60.

Collins, A. M., & Loftus, E. F. (1975). A spreading–activation theory of semantic processing. *Psychological Review, 82,* 407–428.

Collins, A. M., & Quillian, M. R. (1969). Retrieval time from semantic memory. *Journal of Verbal Learning and Verbal Behavior, 8,* 240–247.

Collins, A. M., & Quillian, M. R. (1972). How to make a language user. In E. Tulving & W. Donaldson (Eds.), *Organization and Memory* (pp. 309–351). New York: Academic Press.

Donaldson, W. (1996). The role of decision processes in remembering and knowing. *Memory & Cognition, 24,* 523–533.

Dougherty, M. R., Harbison, J. I., & Davelaar, E. J. (2014). Optional stopping and the termination of memory retrieval. *Current Directions in Psychological Science, 23*(5), 332–337.

Eich, J. M. (1982). A composite holographic associative recall model. *Psychological Review, 89,* 627–661.

Eich, J. M. (1985). Levels of processing, encoding specificity, elaboration, and CHARM. *Psychological Review, 92,* 1–38.

Endress, A. D., & Szabó, S. (2020). Sequential presentation protects working memory from catastrophic interference. *Cognitive Science, 44*(5), e12828.

Farrell, S., & Lewandowsky, S. (2010). Computational models as aids to better reasoning in psychology. *Current Directions in Psychological Science, 19*(5), 329–335.

Flexser, A. J., & Tulving, E. (1975). Retrieval independence in recognition and recall. *Psychological Review, 85,* 153–171.

Gillund, G., & Shiffrin, R. M. (1984). A retrieval model for both recognition and recall. *Psychological Review, 91,* 1–67.

Guynn, M. J., McDaniel, M. A., Strosser, G. L., Ramirez, J. M., Castleberry, E. H., & Arnett, K. H. (2014). Relational and item-specific influences on generate-recognize processes in recall. *Memory & Cognition, 42*(2), 198–211.

Hills, T. T., Jones, M. N., & Todd, P. M. (2012). Optimal foraging in semantic memory. *Psychological Review, 119*(2), 431–440.

Hintzman, D. L. (1986). "Schema abstraction" in a multiple-trace memory model. *Psychological Review, 93,* 411–428.

Hintzman, D. L. (1988). Judgments of frequency and recognition memory in a multiple-trace memory model. *Psychological Review, 95,* 528–551.

Hintzman, D. L. (1990). Human learning and memory: Connections and dissociations. *Annual Review of Psychology, 41,* 109–139.

Hunt, R. R., Smith, R. E., & Toth, J. P. (2016). Category cued recall evokes a generate–recognize retrieval process. *Journal of Experimental Psychology: Learning, Memory, and Cognition, 42*(3), 339–350.

Jacoby, L. L. (1991). A process dissociation framework: Separating automatic from intentional uses of memory. *Journal of Memory and Language, 30*(5), 513–541.

Jacoby, L. L., & Hollingshead, A. (1990). Toward a generate/recognize model of performance on direct and indirect tests of memory. *Journal of Memory and Language, 29,* 433–454.

Johnson-Laird, P. N., Hermann, D. J., & Chaffin, R. (1984). Only connections: A critique of semantic networks. *Psychological Bulletin, 96,* 292–315.

Kintsch, W. (1968). Recognition and free recall of organized lists. *Journal of Experimental Psychology, 78,* 481–487.

Kintsch, W. (1970). Models for free recall and recognition. In D. A. Norman (Ed.), *Models of Human Memory* (pp. 331–373). New York: Academic Press.

Kintsch, W. (2014). Similarity as a function of semantic distance and amount of knowledge. *Psychological Review, 121*(3), 559–561.

Kintsch, W., & Bowles, A. R. (2002). Metaphor comprehension: What makes a metaphor difficult to understand? *Metaphor and Symbol, 17,* 249–262.

Kishiyama, M. M., & Yonelinas, A. P. (2003). Novelty effects on recollection and familiarity in recognition memory. *Memory & Cognition, 31,* 1045–1051.

Landauer, T. K., & Dumais, S. T. (1997). A solution to Plato's problem: The latent semantic analysis theory of acquisition, induction, and representation of knowledge. *Psychological Review, 104,* 211–240.

Malmberg, K. J., Raaijmakers, J. G., & Shiffrin, R. M. (2019). 50 years of research sparked by Atkinson and Shiffrin (1968). *Memory & Cognition, 47*(4), 561–574.

Mandler, G. (1980). Recognizing: The judgment of previous occurrence. *Psychological Review, 87,* 252–271.

Mandler, G. (2008). Familiarity breeds attempts: A critical review of dual-process theories of recognition. *Perspectives on Psychological Science, 3,* 390–399.

McAdoo, R. M., Key, K. N., & Gronlund, S. D. (2018). Stimulus effects and the mediation of recognition memory. *Journal of Experimental Psychology: Learning, Memory, and Cognition, 44*(11), 1814–1823.

McClelland, J. L., McNaughton, B. L., & O'Reilly, R. C. (1995). Why there are complementary learning systems in the hippocampus and neocortex: Insights from the successes and failures of connectionist models of learning and memory. *Psychological Review, 102*(3), 419–457.

McClelland, J. L., Rumelhart, D. E., & PDP Research Group. (1986). *Parallel Distributed Processing, Vol. 2: Psychological and Biological Models.* Cambridge, MA: MIT press.

McCloskey, M., & Cohen, N. J. (1989). Catastrophic interference in connectionist networks: The sequential learning problem. *The Psychology of Learning and Motivation, 24,* 109–165.

Morais, A. S., Olsson, H., & Schooler, L. J. (2013). Mapping the structure of semantic memory. *Cognitive Science, 37*(1), 125–145.

Murdock, B. B. (1974). *Human Memory: Theory and Data.* Potomac, MD: Erlbaum.

Murdock, B. B. (1982a). A theory for the storage and retrieval of item and associative information. *Psychological Review, 89,* 609–626.

Murdock, B. B. (1982b). A distributed memory model for serial–order information. *Psychological Review, 90,* 316–338.

Murdock, B. B. (1993). TODAM2: A model for the storage and retrieval of item, associative, and serial-order information. *Psychological Review, 100,* 183–203.

Nelson, A. B., & Shiffrin, R. M. (2013). The co-evolution of knowledge and event memory. *Psychological Review, 120*(2), 356–394.

Norman, K. A., Newman, E. L., & Detre, G. (2007). A neural network model of retrieval-induced forgetting. *Psychological Review, 114,* 887–953.

Quesada, J.F, Kintsch, W., & Gomez, E. (2001) A computational theory of complex problem solving using the vector space model (part I): Latent semantic analysis, through the path of thousands of ants. In Cañas (Ed.) *Cognitive Research with Microworlds,* 117–131.

Raaijmakers, J. G. W., & Shiffrin, R. M. (1980). SAM: A theory of probabilistic search of associative memory. *The Psychology of Learning and Motivation, 14,* 207–262.

Raaijmakers, J. G. W., & Shiffrin, R. M. (1981). Search of associative memory. *Psychological Review, 88,* 93–134.

Radvansky, G. A., & Tamplin, A. K. (2013). Suppression in retrieval practice, part-set cueing, and negative priming memory: The Hydrogen model. *Quarterly Journal of Experimental Psychology, 66*(7), 1368–1398.

Rips, L. J., Shoben, E. J., & Smith, E. E. (1973). Semantic distance and the verification of semantic relations. *Journal of Verbal Learning and Verbal Behavior, 12*(1), 1–20.

Rotello, C. M., & McMillan, N. A. (2006). Remember–know models as decision strategies in two experimental paradigms. *Journal of Memory and Language, 55,* 479–494.

Rumelhart, D. E., & McClelland, J. L. (1986). *Parallel Distributed Processing, Vol. 1: Foundations.* Cambridge, MA: MIT press.

Shiffrin, R. M., & Steyvers, M. (1997). A model for recognition memory: REM—retrieving effectively from memory. *Psychonomic Bulletin & Review, 4,* 145–166.

Snodgrass, J. G., & Corwin, J. (1988). Pragmatics of measuring recognition memory: Applications to dementia and amnesia. *Journal of Experimental Psychology: General, 117*(1), 34–50.

Starns, J. J., & Ma, Q. (2018). Guessing versus misremembering in recognition: A comparison of continuous, two-high-threshold, and low-threshold models. *Journal of Experimental Psychology: Learning, Memory, and Cognition, 44*(4), 527–539.

Steinhart, D. (2001). Summary Street: An intelligent tutoring system for improving student writing through the use of Latent Semantic Analysis. Unpublished doctoral dissertation, Institute of Cognitive Science, University of Colorado, Boulder.

Trueblood, J. S., & Hemmer, P. (2017). The generalized quantum episodic memory model. *Cognitive Science, 41*(8), 2089–2125.

Tulving, E., & Wiseman, S. (1975). Relation between recognition and recognition failure of recallable words. *Bulletin of the Psychonomic Society, 6,* 79–82.

Yonelinas, A. P. (1994). Receiver-operating characteristics in recognition memory: Evidence for a dual-process model. *Journal of Experimental Psychology: Learning, Memory, and Cognition, 20*(6), 1341–1354.

Yonelinas, A. P. (2002). The nature of recollection and familiarity: A review of 30 years of research. *Journal of Memory and Language, 46,* 441–517.

Memory Methods

This appendix provides you with methods that can be used to calculate various indices of memory that you might not have encountered elsewhere in your coursework. The qualities of these methods are discussed in Chapter 3, as well as other places throughout the book.

This appendix is divided into three sections. The first describes a signal detection analysis method using measures of discrimination and bias. The second is a measure of clustering that can be applied to recall data. The third is the process dissociation procedure to provide estimates of implicit and explicit memory.

SIGNAL DETECTION ANALYSIS

As noted in Chapter 3, signal detection analyses correct for guessing and separate the influences of discrimination and bias in people's responses. Signal detection analyses are typically applied to yes–no recognition data—that is, when people are presented with individual items and are asked to indicate whether each item is old or new. A popular measure of signal detection is d' (Tanner & Swets, 1954), which takes into account both the hit rate (H) and the false alarm rate (FA), which are both conveyed as proportions (i.e., 0 to 1). Using Z-scores, it is defined as:

$$d' = Z(H) - Z(FA)$$
$$\beta = \text{Exp}\,((Z(FA^2) - Z(H^2)) / 2)$$

An alternative to β to calculate the bias, or criterion, level is C, which is:

$$C = ((Z(H) + Z(FA))) / 2$$

Measures of discrimination and bias can be derived with a spreadsheet program (Sorkin, 1999) using:

$$d' = \text{NORMSINV}(H) - \text{NORMSINV}(FA)$$
$$\beta = \text{NORMDIST}(z_c,\ d',\ 1,\ 0)/\text{NORMDIST}(z_c,\ 0,\ 1,\ 0)$$

where

$z_c = NORMSINV(1 - FA)$

Finally, the way to calculate the alternative bias measure C, is:

$C = - (NORMSINV(H) + NORMSINV(FA)) / 2$

An alternative nonparametric measure of discrimination is A' (following Donaldson, 1992, and Snodgrass & Corwin, 1988; see also Pollack, 1970). Here is the equation for calculating A' when the number of hits is greater than or equal to the number of false alarms:

$A' = .5 + [(H - FA) * (1 + H - FA)] / [4H * (1 - FA)]$

However, when the number of hits is less than the number of false alarms, the following formula should be used:

$A' = .5 - [(FA - H) * (1 + FA - H)] / [4FA * (1 - H)]$

B''_D (Donaldson, 1992) is a measure of bias, like β, but based on the same principles as A'. Here is how to calculate B''_D:

$B''_D = [(1 - H) * (1 - FA) - HFA]/[(1 - H) * (1 - FA) + HFA]$

Here, an A' of .5 corresponds to chance discrimination (i.e., no discrimination). That is, when A' values are around .5, it is unlikely that people are reliably recognizing old information and rejecting new information. An A' value of 1 corresponds to perfect discrimination. That is, perfectly detecting old information in memory and rejecting new information. A' values of less than .5 indicate below chance identification. This may mean that people are using memory in a consistent and reliable way but not in the way you are hypothesizing. If A' is negative, then you have calculated it wrong.

For bias, positive B''_D values correspond to conservative responses. That is, people are being careful about what they are willing to identify as recognized. In contrast, negative B''_D values correspond to liberal responses. That is, people are willing to say that any given item has been encountered before and is remembered. B''_D values of zero correspond to no bias. B''_D values greater than 1 or less than −1 indicate that you've done something wrong in your calculations.

CLUSTERING

Another thing you may want to know is how information is structured or organized in memory. One way to do this is test if people have structured information in a way that you think they will. For example, if you know that experts tend to organize information in a certain way, you can assess the degree to which a person's own organization in memory matches the expert. This would tell you something about the level of expertise.

One measure of organization is the Adjusted Ratio of Clustering (*ARC*) score (Roenker et al., 1971). *ARC* scores are applied to recall test data. Essentially, people recall a set of information that was learned earlier. Then, using a preconceived idea about how information could be organized in memory, you assess the degree to which the organization approaches that ideal, taking chance into account. The formula for calculating an *ARC* score is:

$$ARC = (R - E(R)) \, / \, (maxR - E(R))$$

Here, *R* stands for the number of observed categorical repetitions—that is, how many times during a person's recall two items from the same predetermined category were recalled together—for example, recalling two animal names one after the other. *E(R)* is the number of categorical repetitions that would be expected by chance given the categories being tested for and how much the person actually recalled. In a sense, this is the amount of error that might be expected. The formula for calculating *E(R)* is:

$$E(R) = \frac{\Sigma_i n^2}{N} - 1$$

Here, *n* is the number of items recalled from a given category *i*, and *N* is the number of items recalled by a person. Finally, *maxR* is the maximum number of repetitions possible if clustering perfectly conformed to expectations, again given the categories being tested and the amount of information recalled. The formula for calculating *maxR* is:

$$maxR = N - k$$

Again, *N* is the number of items recalled by a person, and *k* is the number of categories present in a person's recall. This calculation will result in a number something like a ratio, although not quite. Perfect clustering results in an *ARC* score of 1, whereas chance clustering results in a score of 0. Variations in the degree of clustering result in values between these two. It is possible to get negative *ARC* scores. This indicates clustering below chance. If this value is a relatively large negative number, it might suggest that people have mentally organized information in a way other than the categories that you defined.

A related measure is the *ARC'* score (Pellegrino, 1971) which uses sequential order across multiple recall attempts, rather than categorical groupings. Here is a simplified version for pairs of repetitions (rather than triples or larger units). The formula is like the *ARC* score. The formula for *ARC'* is:

$$ARC' = O(ITR) - E(ITR) \, / \, max(ITR) - E(ITR)$$

Here *ITR* refers to intertrial repetitions. *O(ITR)* are the number of observed repetitions, which is found by counting the number of times an item follows another. For example, if people were to recall the months of the year, this would count as 1 if July followed June on trial *t* and *t+1*. The formula for *E(ITR)*, the number of times a repetition would occur across trials by chance, is:

$$E(ITR) = (N-1)!(M-3+R) / N!$$

Here *M* is the number of items recalled on trial *t*, *N* is the number recalled on trial *t+1*, and *R* is the number of items pairs that are recalled on trial *t*, but one or both of these items are not recalled on trial *t + 1*. The explanation point is a mathematical symbol of a factorial function. Finally, the formula for *max(ITR)*, the maximum number of intertrial repetitions that could occur, is:

$$max(ITR) = M - 3$$

PROCESS DISSOCIATION

The process dissociation procedure (Jacoby, 1991) is a way to separate out the influence of conscious and unconscious memory. Although this method is imperfect, it does a reasonable job. Essentially, you compare performance in two conditions. In one, both conscious and unconscious processes work in the same way. This is the *inclusion condition*. In the second, these processes would work in opposition to one another. This is the *exclusion condition*. By looking at the difference in performance in these two conditions, you can derive estimates of how each is being affected by the manipulation of interest.

In the inclusion condition, people do some task that would involve implicit and explicit memory working together—for example, asking a person to report words, such as animal names, that had been seen earlier on a list of animal names. This can be done using either conscious or unconscious influences. In the inclusion condition people can do the task using both explicit and implicit memory to produce words that were on the previous list. This is expressed as:

$$I = R + F - RF$$

Here, *I* stands for the inclusion condition, *R* stands for recollection, the explicit, conscious process—and *F* stands for familiarity—the implicit, unconscious process. Thus, the rate of remembering old items on the inclusion condition reflects the rate of explicitly recollecting items, plus the rate of remembering items based on implicit familiarity, minus the portion where the two overlap (e.g., if you recall something consciously, the additional unconscious familiarity does not give you an additional benefit).

In contrast, in the exclusion condition, people are asked to do something that puts implicit and explicit memory in opposition. For example, people might see a list of animal names at the initial part of the study. Then, they would be asked to report a list of animals if they did not use any from the list heard earlier. Thus, words from the previous list that are reported are almost certainly due to unconscious memory because if people consciously remembered them, they should not report them. This is expressed as:

$$E = F(1 - R)$$

Here, E stands for the exclusion condition. Thus, the rate of remembering old items is the rate at which the implicit memory processes retrieve information, minus those that are rejected because they are also consciously remembered. By separating out performance in the exclusion and inclusion conditions, we are left with the contribution of explicit memory. This is expressed as:

$$R = I - E$$

What is due to implicit memory can also be estimated. The estimate for familiarity is:

$$F = i / (1 - I + E)$$

REFERENCES

Donaldson, W. (1992). Measuring recognition memory. *Journal of Experimental Psychology: General, 121,* 275–277.

Jacoby, L. L. (1991). A process dissociation framework: Separating automatic from intentional uses of memory. *Journal of Memory and Language, 30*(5), 513–541.

Pellegrino, J. W. (1971). A general measure of organization in free recall for variable unit size and internal sequential consistency. *Behavior Research Methods & Instrumentation, 3*(5), 241–246.

Pollack, I. (1970). A nonparametric procedure for evaluation of true and false positives. *Behavior Research Methods & Instrumentation, 2*(4), 155–156.

Roenker, D. L., Thompson, C. P., & Brown, S. C. (1971). Comparison of measures for the estimation of clustering in free recall. *Psychological Bulletin, 76*(1), 45–48.

Snodgrass, J. G., & Corwin, J. (1988). Pragmatics of measuring recognition memory: applications to dementia and amnesia. *Journal of Experimental Psychology: General, 117*(1), 34–50.

Sorkin, R. D. (1999). Spreadsheet signal detection. *Behavior Research Methods, Instruments, & Computers, 31*(1), 46–54.

Tanner, W. P., & Swets, J. A. (1954). A decision-making theory of visual detection. *Psychological Review, 61*(6), 401–409.

AUTHOR INDEX

SUBJECT INDEX